CW01461098

QUICK BED-SIDE PRESCRIBER

A HOME GUIDE

QUICK BED-SIDE PRESCRIBER

WITH NOTES ON

CLINICAL RELATIONSHIP OF REMEDIES AND HOMOEOPATHY IN SURGERY

By

J. N. SHINGHAL
F.R.H.S. (Cal.)

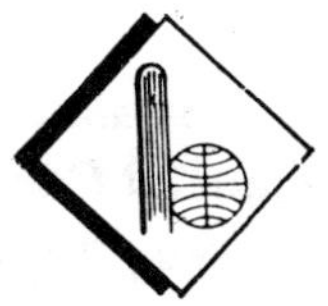

B. JAIN PUBLISHERS PVT. LTD.
DELHI

Note

Any information given in this book is not intended to be taken as a replacement for medical advice. Any person with a condition requiring medical attention should consult a qualified practitioner or therapist.

First Edition : 1970
Second Edition : 1973
Third Edition : 1976
Fourth Edition : 1978
Reprint Edition : 1979, Feb. 1980, Dec. 1980, 1981, 1982, 1983
Fifth Edition : Nov. 1983
Sixth Edition : Dec. 1984, 1987, 1988, 1990, 1991, 1992, 1993, 1994, 1996, 1998, 2000, 2001, 2002, 2003

Published by :
Kuldeep Jain
For
B. Jain Publishers (P.) Ltd.
1921, Street No. 10, Chuna Mandi,
Paharganj, New Delhi 110 055 (INDIA)
Phones: 3670430; 3670572; 3683200; 3683300
FAX 011-3610471 & 3683400
Email: bjain@vsnl.com
Website: www.bjainindia.com

Printed in India by:
Unisons Techno Financial Consultants (P) Ltd.
522, FIE, Patpar Ganj, Delhi - 110 092

Price: Rs. 220. 00

ISBN: 81-7021-192-1
BOOK CODE: B-2492

THE AUTHOR

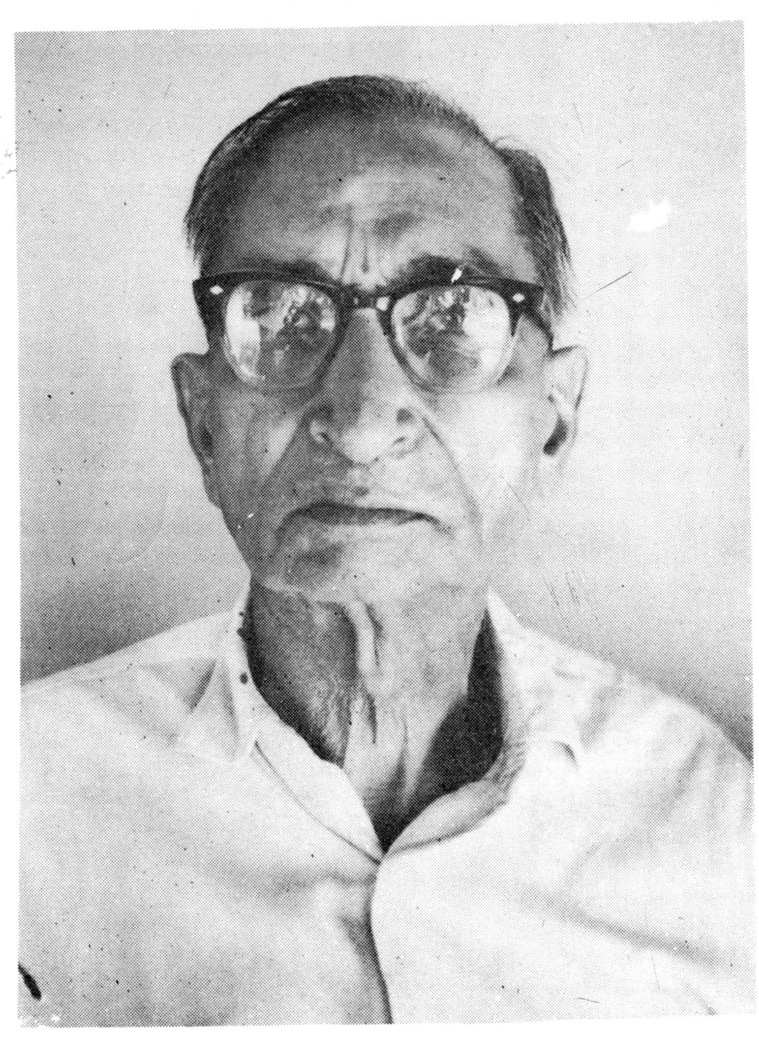

AUTHOR'S WIFE

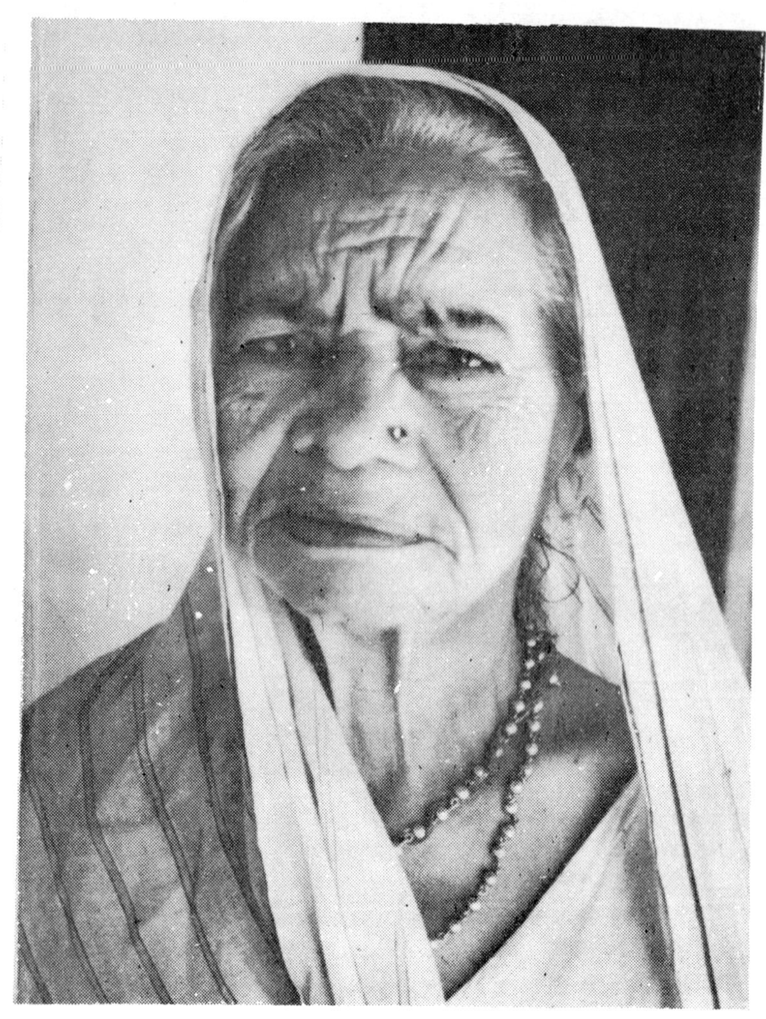

Smt. Sharbati Devi

CONTENTS

PREFACE TO THE FIFTH EDITION

Since this 'Prescriber' is not unfamiliar to most of Homoeopaths, so it needs no lengthy preface.

The Jain Publishing Co., Delhi approached me in 1979 with a request that hundreds of orders for supplying the book both from Indian and Foreign Homoeopaths were pending with them, so either I might revise the book or allow them to reprint the existing edition as printing of the revised edition will take a long time.

I was busy then in writing the second book "Graphic Picture of Selected Remedies" and could not afford to revise the Book.

Lest the reputation of publisher—who is one of the biggest Publishers of Mecical Books—should suffer for not supplying the book in time, so I acceded to their second alternative request for reprinting of the existing edition of the book. Thus the book has already seen the light of the day tenth times.

Incidently the book has carved out for itself truly a good name in the chorus of warm unsolicited tributes that it has been receiving month after month from Homoeopaths of many parts of the country as well as from foreign countries, is an indication.

This edition appears with some additional features and new materials to make it more useful and serviceable.

I have tried to elaborate and make more illuminating some of the existing alphabetical headings with added cross references in order to help the busy practitioner to find out the right medicines without much ado.

Again I have included treatments for some more diseases which did not find place in previous editions. This was necessitated by my own need as patients suffering from such diseases came to me for consultation or sent letters to me for their treatment both from India and foreign countries.

The time of puberty is very critical and delicate in a girl's life and several derangements occur in her life in certain cases. I have massed them together under one head "Derangements at Puberty."

Pains in certain parts of the body are sometime so terrific that the sufferer wants instant reliefs. The physician is equally anxious to give him or her instant relief without delay. The Preventives need early administration of a drug to save the patient to fall a prey to an epidemic illness or other ailments. I have grouped together such Pains, Prophylactics and Preventives under a separate chapter V.

I have included some more *'Nosodes'* which are more helpful and efficacious these days in the treatment of certain maladies. I have included some more drugs for external applications in some diseases.

I have again taken advantage of experiences of some more eminent and famous physicians in the science of healing and am greatly indebted to them. Their names along with the books authored by them appear in the Bibliography and in certain cases their names have been mentioned below the headings and in certain cases deliberately not mentioned.

I need not repeat what I have mentioned clearly in previous editions that I claim no originality and my sole aim is to benefit the patients by utilising experiences of other authors and not for any pecuniary gain. I have given only salient and most significant symptoms of certain diseases most succinctly and suggested treatment only to a few efficacious medicines otherwise the book might become bulky like certain Materia Medica thus jeopardise its name as a Quick Bed-Side Prescriber.

If this revised edition continues to serve the same purpose of relieving the sufferings, distresses of even a few ailing patients then I shall consider myself fully rewarded.

The greatest Healer is Lord (Shri Rama) and while ending this preface I earnestly pray to Him for curing or even minimising the sufferings of such patients who utilise this book for their troubles.

199, Din Dayal Upadhya Marg **J.N. Shingal**
New Delhi—110002

EXCERPTS FROM THE FOURTH EDITION

The third edition of Quick Bed-Side Presciber is almost finished and the book is going to the Press for the fourth time.

It is gratifying to learn from different quarters both from India and from Foreign countries that the book is serving the main purpose of helping in relieving and mitigating the distress and sufferings of ailing humanity which was the sole object for which it was written.

I must thank the Professionals as well as Lay Practitioners who have patronised it.

I have recasted the Chapter II 'Homoeopathy in Paediatrics'.

I have also added a useful Appendix III indicating the remedies predominently aggravated by heat and cold.

I pray to Shri Rama (God) that this book may continue to prove helpful and useful to those for whom it is intended.

1st. January, 1978 **J.N. Shinghal**
96, Press Road,
New Delhi-110002

EXCERPTS FROM THE THIRD EDITION

The first edition of the Prescriber was printed at Bareilly at the instance of my late son, Shri C.N. Shinghal, District Agricultural Officer, Bareilly.

This book received such a popular appreciation and approbation and its demand was so great that the first edition was finished within a short period beyond my expectations.

The new publisher, Dr. Prem Nath Jain of Jain Publishing Co., New Delhi approached me for revising the Prescriber.

By this time the saddest tragedy of my life occurred in the young tragic death of my said son, Shri C.N. Shinghal causing such a festering wound which is hardly ever to heal up. It was a stunning blow on my head which has unnerved me and from which it is scarcely possible to recover. "Let Thy will be done".

Under the above unfortunate circumstances I refused point-blankly the publishers that I was unable to revise the second edition.

Since they had to meet the public demand so for second edition they got a reprinted copy of the first edition and so obviously it is an exact replica of the first edition.

Now it is a turn for the third edition within such a spell of short period.

But for incessant demands for this Prescriber and the persistent exhortations and wishes of my friends and well-wishers revised and enlarged edition of this Prescriber would never have seen the light of the day.

I have since then further been benefited by clinical experiences of the other talented and eminent physicians whose names together with names of their respective books are now mentioned in the Bibliography.

I have taken the liberty of including their pointers in this edition. For clarity of comprehension and for facility of understanding I have, in most of the cases, reproduced the very words and language as used by these authors. I owe a deep gratitude to all these eminent and learned physicians for making use of their mature experiences.

I absolutely lay no claim to my own originality for Homoeopathy is a vast ocean of science and I am merely an humble explorer standing on its banks gathering pearls from whatever source I can lay my hands upon.

I am not unaware of limitations of a treatise like this Prescriber. Within a short compass it can not, nor it is intended to be a guide in all cases.

This Prescriber will furnish the ready reference to the busy Practitioner and will provide him with therapeutic pointers to select the correct remedies and that too quickly and without much ado.

When a Practitioner's comprehension seems to be shrouded due to the complicated nature of a case or for absence of both objective and subjective symptoms, this Prescriber will particularly come to his rescue by hitting upon the right medicine. This Prescriber may prove a labour saving device and a ready and easy reckoner in such cases ; more so in emergent cases.

A comprehensive chart about the relationship of medicines has been added. It will prevent the pitfalls of prescribing incompatible and antidotal medicines along with or after the principal drug. This chart will also prove very handy in prescribing drugs for second prescriptions to effectuate a perfect cure.

On the occasion of Hahnemann's Birthday Celebrations on **11**th April, 1971, held at Y.M.C.A. Hall, Chowringhee, Calcutta, a Fellowship was conferred on me at the hands of Honourable Mr. Justice A.N. Sen, Judge of Calcutta High Court, in recognition of the merit of this Prescriber.

My son, Dr. R.N. Shinghal, M.S., Assistant Professor of Surgery, Maulana Azad, Medical College and Surgeon, Irwin Hospital, New Delhi has helped me considerably in correcting the proofs of the book.

I expect from the possessors of the Prescriber and the patients who are cured with its aid, the good wishes and prayers for *shanti*, of my soul.

24th March, 1976
96, Press Road,
New Delhi-110002

J.N. Shinghal
F.R.H.S. (Cal.), R.M.P.

EXCERPTS FROM 'AN APOLOGY'

(First Edition)

A word of apology and not a preface to this book "QUICK BED-SIDE PRESCRIBER" is required here for my transgressing the vast science of Homoeopathy, which, actually, is the preserve of the giants in this science.

Ever since my school days I felt interested in the science of medicine. My late father Nyaya Ratna and Dharma Raj, Munshi Mithan Lal—a Tazimi Sardar, Judicial and Finance Minister and Member of State Council, Alwar State—of fragrant memories—had a big library of medical books both on Ayurvedic and Unani systems of medicines. Whenever I got time I read large number of them.

There were some original works on Unani system in Persian and since I was a student of Persian language, I read them in the original. There were other books also on such subjects as Allopathy, Hydropathy, Naturopathy, Chromopathy and on Dietetics and I left nothing of them unread. My father encouraged me in this direction. He engaged a qualified physician and ran a sort of charitable dispensary, in which work, I assisted him also.

Thus I inherited from him a bias in favour of medical science.

During the course of my official duties, in the year 1938, I was posted to Agra and lived under the same roof as of Dr. S.C. Sircar, the well-known Homoeopath of Agra. I attended his clinics also and I saw several wonderful cures under Homoeopathic treatment.

After this my official duties brought me on deputation to Delhi Municipality in 1948. The President of Delhi Municipal Committee was Dr. Yudhvir Singh, who was a famous Homoeopath. I attended his clinics in New Delhi for some time, whenever my duties permitted me.

Thereafter, fortunately for me, I chanced to meet Dr. B.C. Guha, M.D., L.R.C.P. & S. (Edin.), the well-known and reputed Homoeopath of Delhi. I requested him to help me and guide me in the study of Homoeopathy. To my agreeable surprise, he unhesitatingly agreed and assured me that he will make me a first class Homoeopath. He then prescribed for me a graded course of Homoeopathic Books and advised me to proceed step by step.

I again made a bold request to him to allow me to attend his clinics. He readily and willingly consented to my attending his clinics.

Inspite of my pre-occupation then with my official duties, I always managed to snatch some time to attend his clinics. I did this for a number of years, though, per-force, with unavoidable breaks.

I had thus the benefit of the experience of Dr. Guha taking up cases, repertorising them and prescribing the remedies in my presence for a number of years.

Most of these prescription have been tried and tested in the free dispensary run by me known as "SHARBATI HOMOEOPATHIC POOR DISPENSARY" after the name of my wife.

Armadale, Simla East
July 18, 1959

J.N. Shinghal,
Homoeopath

EXCERPTS FROM "ADDENDA"

(First Edition)

The foregoing notes were completed in 1959. But since then much water has flown in Ganga. With a view to brevity my original idea was to confine this Prescriber to everyday common ailments or to those cases which came to my knowledge during the course of my practice. But I had to revise my idea for I had still to explore several standard works in cases of complicated and chronic diseases coming for treatment before me. I, therefore thought of making this Prescriber more or less self contained so that a busy practitioner may not have, in its presence, to have to look to other books and delay in finding a cure.

Various diseases and their different remedies according to symptoms, which did not find place in the previous notes have been included. The alphabetical order instead of pathological classification has been maintained. Red-line symptoms at different phases of diseases have been given to do away with the confusion which a new practitioner often comes across. I have, however, left out certain diseases, which in actual practice, are known to be incurable and also these requiring surgical intervention. In such cases I have mentioned palliatives only.

I have taken liberty to take advantage of clinical experience of wizards of Homoeopathy and have, in a number of cases, unhesitatingly quoted their experience *in extenso* in their own words and in certain cases added their name also. I acknowledge humbly all such authorities and sources, though some names may have been omitted or overlooked unacknowledged inadvertently and in other cases deliberately not mentioned. I lay no claim to originality.

However, I have kept in view the requirements of "QUICK BED-SIDE PRESCRIBER" as the name of this treatise implies, so that the Practitioner may have the greatest ease, facility and confidence in selecting quickly the correct remedy. This compilation fulfils, to a large extent, my life-long ambition and mission to serve the suffering humanity without any pecuniary gains.

21st August, 1970 **J.N. Shinghal**

32, Lake Square
New Delhi-110002

FOREWORD

(About First Edition)

It is with pleasure that I read the book "QUICK BED-SIDE PRESCRIBER" compiled by Mr. J.N. Shinghal. Mr. Shinghal is an ardent student of Homoeopathy and has taken great pains in collecting the material for the book. The main question is whether there was need for such a reference book for whom it will be helpful. In my opinion, this type of Homoeopathic Quick Prescriber will be of immense help to the beginner, whereas for the veteran it can also offer suitable hints many a time, especially at the bed-side. Naturally, a book of this nature can not do perfect justice to the principal method of selection in Homoeopathy, *i.e.* selection by repertorisation. The main difference between this type of reference book and a good repertory is that former suggests one or two important remedies for a group of symptoms, the latter suggests a number of possible remedies of different degrees of efficacy for a single prominent symptom. But a book like this will, from practical point of view, be very helpful in selecting the proper remedy quickly, specially when attending patients outside the office and in most cases the selection will be right. But before one takes to this type of a reference book one must possess a thorough knowledge of the Homoeopathic Materia Medica. The book is surely not meant for those who have no adequate knowledge of the individual Homoeopathic drug stock. We should be thankful to Mr. Shinghal for having undertaken to compile a book of this nature which is likely to be of immense benefit to all types of Homoeopaths.

I wish him every success in this endeavour and also wish that it reaches the hands of many Homoeopaths in India and abroad for their own benefit.

Sd/- **B.C. Guha**

M.D. (Berlin), L.R.C.P. & S. (Edin.)

Consultant Physician in Homoeopathy.

12th May, 1969

90/17, Connaught Circus,

New Delhi-110001.

Testimonies of Two Supreme Court Judges, Govt. of India about Quick Bed-Side Presciber

S. K. Dass, I.C.S.
Retd. Judge of Supreme Court

Phone : 681945
A/59, Kailash Colony,
New Delhi-110048
Dated 13-7-1980

I have had occasion to see and consult Dr. J.N. Shinghal's 'Quick Bed-Side Prescriber'.

I am not a homoeopath, and am not in a position to express any expert opinion. I must, however, say that the book which is meant for both medical practitioners and laymen, is a very useful publication—its arrangement, its brief but pointed reference to characteristic yet significant symptoms of various ailments and the relevant Homoeopathic remedy are extremely useful.

I understand that it is not professionally correct to indicate the strength and dosage of a particular remedial medicine in a book like this, because dosage and strength will depend on the patients' condition and state of the disease, yet I feel that some indication of the usual dosage and strength may improve the usefulness of the book.

I have no doubt that the book will serve the purpose for which it has been written.

Sd/-
S. K. Dass

Hon'ble Justice A.N. Sen
Judge Supreme Court of India

Dear Shri Shinghal,

I have received your letter. I have had occasion to go through the book 'Quick Bed-Side Prescriber' written by you.

I have found the book to be very useful. This book will be of great help to the members of every household.

I am not surprised that this book has already run into a few editions because of the heavy demand.

I am happy to learn that you have written another book called "Graphic Pictures of Selected Remedies". I shall be happy to receive a copy of the same.

Sd/-

April 20, 1983 **A. N. Sen**
New Delhi.

REVIEW

(About the First Edition of the Book)

Bed-Side prescribing has always been a problem for the practitioner of Homoeopathy, specially lay Homoeopaths. Even the veteran amongst Homoeopaths many a times requires the aid of some "Prescriber" or Repertory, may be Clarke's *Prescriber* or Boenninghausen's *Pocket Book* or Boericke's *Materia Medica*.

The present book is a successful effort of an earnest and honest Homoeopath and Bed-Side Prescriber will certainly love to have a copy always with him.

Shri J.N. Shinghal, whom I had the privilege of knowing since my days in the Agra College, where he was two years senior to me, was an honest and efficient officer of U.P. Government and after his retirement he studied Homoeopathy with earnestness and perseverence. His association with Dr. Guha, the great Homoeopath of New Delhi, proved a boon for him and the reader will find that the "QUICK BED-SIDE PRESCRIBER" does not lack in practical pointers, so important sometimes for correct prescription.

The alphabetical arrangement has made this small Prescriber more valuable for even lay prescriber. Shri Shinghal has taken great pains in compiling the small book. It is more diffcult to compile a smaller volume than a bigger one. Here one has to be brief without sacrificing the fairness and importance of the symptoms

OPINION

Dr. Sushila Nayar, M.D. an eminent nationalist, a close co-worker and Personal Physician of Mahatma Gandhi and ex-Union Minister of Health says about first edition of "Quick Bed-Side Prescriber" as below :

I have known Shri Shinghal as an honest and dedicated civil servant for many years. He was a responsible officer in the Rehabilitation Department of Delhi State when I was the Minister Incharge from 1952 to 1955 and I had many occasions to see Shri Shinghal's humanism, but it was a surprise to me when he asked me to write a preface for a medical book that he had written, I do it with great pleasure.

I am much impressed by the fact that Shri Shinghal has put in a great deal of study and diligence to learn Homoeopathy as an extra curricular activity so to say. He may not be an institutionally qualified Homoeopath but those who know this science well, vouch-safe for the depth of his knowledge and experience and the "Bed-side Prescriber" proves this if any further proof was necessary. He had gone for the healing art merely as a labour of love and has no pecuniary interest in it.

In India medical facilities are still woefully inadequate inspite of a tremendous increase in the out-put of doctor since independence. Moreover modern medicine is very expensive for the majority of our people and they find it much more convenient to turn to Homoeopathy and other forms of treatment. I have myself seen some very difficult skin conditions respond to Homoeopathic treatment in a miraculous manner. I am sure the "Bed-Side Prescriber" will serve a very real need for all Practitioners of Homoeopathy and I do hope it will help them serve humanity better which is the sole objective with which Shri Shinghal has written this book.

11-9-1971
New Delhi.

Sd/-
Sushila Nayar

Quick Bed-Side Prescriber

A

Abdomen—See "Chapter V for details."

Abdomen—cavity opened with burning pain—If the abdomen cavity has been opened and the wall of the abdomen takes unhealthy look and there are stinging burning pains then *Staphysagaria* is the remedy. (*Staph*). See "Stretches".

Abdomen—colic disorders—Acute ; caused by incompatible food. After eating, sour taste in the mouth. Pressure in the stomach for one or two hours after eating. Tightness about the waist. Bloating of the stomach with stony weight in the stomach. Frequent and ineffectual desire to pass stool, passes only a small quantity at each attempt but passing even a small quantity relieves him. Colic. (*Nux-v.*). See "Digestion" and "Dyspepsia" under different heads.

Abdomen—dropsy of abdomen—Abdomen very much distended The stomch in dropsical conditions becomes very irritable. It seems as if nothing passes through it. He finally becomes paralysed in the bowels. The kidneys are not acting. (*Apoc*). See "Dropsy" under its different headings.

Abdomen—emptiness and weakness—A sense of emptiness and weakness in abdomen after stool which may be normal and this is relieved by either passing flatus or eructations. (*Ambra*).

Abdomen—enlarged, children delayed dentition—Enlarged specially of children, body emaciated with large head ; difficult and delayed dentition. Sweating on head while asleep ; vomiting and diarrhoea. Everything smells sour. (*Calc*). See "Head of children large."

Abdomen—pendulous after confinement—(1) Pendulous abdomen after confinement. (*Podo*). See "Pregnancy" under different heads and "Confinement—abdomen pendulous."

(2) For large abdomen—(*Sepia* ; *Coloc*.). See "Part 2 of Labour prophylactic" for difficult labour.

Abdomen—lump—The lump near liver region. The following may be tried according to symptoms :—

(*i*) *Conium* 200.

(*ii*) Feeling the lump in the pit of stomach—*Kali-c*. to be taken on empty stomach—first thing in the morning.

(*iii*) Watery excresceness, spongy tumours. *Thuja* 1000.

(*iv*) A powerful remedy for stony glands. *Calc-f.*

(*v*) *Thuja* 30 after it, give *Graph* 1 M. every 6th day.

(*vi*) *Tuberculinum* 1 M. as an intercurrent medicine. 3 weeks after it, given *Graph* 1 M. See "Tumour-in abdomen."

Abdomen—operation to prevent sepsis—See "Chapter V for details."

Abdomen—pains—after decayed food—Causing the patient to turn and twist in all directions. Liver and spleen enlarged. Pain in the abdomen is usually a burning pain which is relieved by warm application. Digestive troubles after decayed food, or animal matter, or alcoholic drinks and chewing tobacco. But should have (*i*) burning pain, (*ii*) restlessness and (*iii*) thirst for little quantity of water. (*Ars*). See "Swelling of abdomen."

(*b*) For pain in stomach, give *Belladonna* 200 mixed in water every 5 minutes until pain stops. See "Pain-abdominal burning" and "Pain in thighs".

(*c*) (*i*) If the patient feels pains on empty stomach. (*Anac*-30, four times daily.), (*ii*) If the pains occur after eating. (*Abies-n*., 30 four times daily).

(*d*) *Mag phos*. may be given for most of the pain particularly pain in the abdomen ; it will be very helpful as Antispasmodic.

Abdomen—distended wind—Abdomen distended with wind after eating (*Kali-c*). See "Flatulence" under its different heads and "Wind trouble".

Abortion—habitual—Habitual abortion, at the third month or later ; unusual bleeding during pregnancy or at a later stage, *i.e.* fifth or seventh months. (*Sep.*) For "Threatened abortion" compare (*Puls*). See also 'Miscarriage" under its different headings.

Abortion—every second or third month—(*a*) Habitual abortion, pain in small of back and genitals. Discharge of dark blood. (*Sabin*). The flow is bright red and clotted.

(*b*) *Helonias* prevents abortions which occur as a result of slightest over-exertion or irritating emotions.

Abortion, prophylactic for abortion—See "Chapter V for details".

Abortion tendency to miscarriage due to different causes—In women who habitually miscarry at a certain period of pregnancy *Viburnum opulus* should be given from sometime before.

(*i*) When arising from an accident—*Arn* 3, 1 hour.

(*ii*) When due to emotional disturbance—*Cham.*, 1 hour.

(*iii*) When due to syphilis in mother or child, give *Leuticum* (*Syphilinum*) 30, globules twice a week throughout pregnancy.

(iv) When previous children have been rickety-*Sil. 6, 8* hourly throughout pregnancy with necessary intermissions.

(*v*) When due to parental Tuberculosis (*Bacill-30,* once a month.)

(*vi*) When due to disease of placenta. (*Phos.*)

(*vii*) Vaginismus with emaciation and constipation. Muscular fibres of uterus do not develop proportionately as the foetus increases in uterus and this causes abortion. (*Plumb-e.*)

(*viii*) When the attack is caused by violent efforts such as lifting a weight or by a strain of the side or false step. Pain worse later part of night and during rest. Must change position for relief. (*Rhus-t.*). But if the effect is followed by profuse flooding of bright red blood and slight pain. (*Cinamonum*).

(ix) Haemorrhages : Continuous.—*Ip.*, *Sabin* , *Arn.* and *Cinnamon* ; for intermittent :—*Puls.*, with bright red colour blood : *Ip, Arn.* darkened :—*Sabin, Cham.* and *Secale.*, Convulsions :—*Ip, Hyos, Cham., Plat-met.*, blows on the abdomen : *Arn., Strains* : *Rhus, Cinnamon.* The dose should be 10 globules in half a tumbler full of boiled water, of which solution a dessert spoonful may be administered every two hours or oftener according to condition.

(x) When there is tendency to-abortion specially with a gonorrhoeal history give *Thuja* in mother tincture.

(c) Treatment of consequences :—For weakness of back, weakness of legs and weaknesss of eyes :—*Kalic-c.* ; for retained placenta :—*Sep.* ; for expulsion of foetus :—*Coffea.*, *Puls.*, or *Secale* : when kindeys do not secrete sufficient urine. (*Stram.*) See "Miscarriage" under its different heads.

(*d*) Threatened abortions, specially in habitual abortions. (*Helon.*)

(*i*) Pains fly across the abdomen form side to side ; doubling the patient up—a powerful restrainer of abortion (*Cimic.*). This will suit cases with habitual disposition.

(*ii*) *Secale cornutum* will be useful for abortion in the later months while *Sabina* for abortion specially about the third month. (*See., Sabin*).

(*iii*) *Caulopyhllum* is very useful remedy in false labour pains and also as a preventive for abortion. There is severe pain in the back and sides of abdomen ; scanty flow and uterine contractions. (*Caul.*). See "Miscarriage and its tendency."

Abortion-producing—*Goss.* to be given in M.T. in drop doses.

Abortion-threatened—(*a*) Threatened, flow ceases and then returns with increased force ; pains spasmodic (*Puls.*)

(*b*) Pain beginning in the back and going around to loins and to uterus, ending in cramps. This is the most remarkable indication. Dr. Nash has checked an impending abortion, and in one case even after a slight flow of blood was present (*Vib-o.*)

For abortion, see (*Sepia*). Compare for habitual abortion (*Caul*) See Miscarriage threatened", and . (5) of Pregnancy—its affection. and "Miscarriage habitual".

Abrasion—Slightest abrasion or scratch of the skin suppurates. *Petroleum* (compare *Hepar sulph.*).

Abscess of various types and recurring including cold abscess—(1) Painful and trobbing without much swelling with or without redness. (*Bell., or Apis.*)

(2) Great pain killer in boils—*Hep.,* every half an hour.

(3) Small boils in crops—(*Arn.*)

(4) Abscess near rectum (*Calc-s, grain IV, 3 hrs.*).

(5) Fistulous opening (*Fla-ac., 6 drops, 6 hrs.* (Clarke.)

(6) When hardness, heat and swelling are felt, give *Bell.* and *Merc-v.* alternately every 3 hours For long-continued abscess or when there are several-*Sang.* twice a day and *Ars.* night and morning. (Dr. Laurie.)

(7) *Tarent-c.* is for the exceeding painful and inflamed abscess; the neighbouring glands are swollen and painful.

(8) Terrible burning. Inflammation of connective tissue in which there exists a purulent focus. (*Anthrac.*).

(9) Continued tendency to relapse. Give *Sulf.* and *Sil.* alternately.

(10) Abscess about the parotid (gland situated near ear) axillary (near armpit) gland. The pus is bloody and pain is intense. Also useful in suppurative condition of eyes. (*Rhus-t.*)

(11) Suppurative conditions specially where symptoms of blood poisoning are present. Dr. Dewey says that *Echinacea* has achieved merited reputation to cure such cases and there is no question as to its efficacy.

(12) According to Dr. W.E. Leonard *Pyrogen* is a valuable remedy in recurring abscess conditions. It will clear up the system and prevent recurrence.

(13) For syphilitic and tubercular abscess. (*Kali-iodatum*).

(14) If an abscess forms and fails to point and surroundings present a purplish hue. (*Lach.*)

(15) Abscess—multiple. (*Vespa.*)

(16) Abscess—cold. (*Carb-ac.*) See "Boils", "Lumber abscess" and "Sore-cold".

Abscess-in armpit—Full of pus and swelling. (*Hep-s. 6,* four times a day.)

Abscess-formation—will abort.—Pus formation. *Merc-sol.* will abort the action if given in the beginning. Foul mouth and profuse perspiration guiding symptoms. To be followed by *Hep.* which will dry the wound. To be tried in all abscess formation. (*Merc-sol.*).

Abscess-inflamed—Boils ; inflammation tending to suppurate or refusing to heal ; inflammation of bone ; soft tissues and glands : pus offensive (*Silicea*).

Abscess—around the knee joint necrosed—4 or 5 abscesses in and around the knee joint. The ulceration attacked tibia, which was half eaten of and the necrosed bone protruded through the surface was cured with *Calc. hypophorica* first trituration. See "Caries." See "Inflammation tendency to pus."

Abscess-mastoid—Dr. Arschangouni claims *Capsicum* to be the best remedy for this trouble, while Dr. Dewey recommends *Nitric acid*. See "Mastoid abscess."

A

Abscess-pus formed—Where pus has formed *Hepar* hastens bursting of abscess and the cure. Where suppuration seems inevitable, it may open the abscess. Painful to be touched. (*Hep.*)

When suppuration continues indefinitely, then *Silica* will bring healthy action and promote granulation and after it *Fl-ac*. See "Boils" under its different heads and "Pus formation."

Abscess-severe pain—In any abscess where there is a great burning and stinging pain. Danger of gangrene. (*Tarentula-c.*).

Absent-mindedness—(1) The patient is absent-minded. He is very forgetful. Buys things in market and leaves them behind. He omits letters or words when writing (*Lac-c*).

(2) Even things spoken about a moment ago are forgotten. Constant loss of memory (*Ailanthus glandulosa.*)

(3) In the case of old people where age has taken the keenness out of all mental faculties (*Bar-c*).

(4) Cannot remember even the simplest words or facts (*Ambra.*).

See also "Forgetfulness", "Memory loss" and "Mind feeble and confused."

Abusiveness—(1) Wants to curse and swear (*Anac.*)

(2) Wants to abuse without being offended (*Hyos.*)

If this does not help, then (*Lyss.*)

Mental shock during—

Accidents—Mental shock during—*Arnica* will put them in proper frame of mind. See "Shock in injury."

Acidic craving for—Craving for acids and refreshing things (*Verat*).

Acidity—excessive—Excess of acidity, yellow, creamy coating at the back part of roof of the mouth ; sour eructations and vomiting (*Natrum Phos.*) See "Craving under its different heads."

Acidity with wind (also heart burn)—*Sul ac.* with gastralgia and eructations of wind *Arg-n.* 4 hourly. See "Flatulence" "Wind trouble" and "Hyper-acidity."

(1) Burning in upper part of abdomen goes even up to throat ; sometimes vomiting, much flatulence. (*Caps. 30*, four times daily.)

(2) Sour rising after meals. Heaviness in the stomach. Much offensive flatus. There is flatulence in stomach or upper part of abdomen. (*Carb-v.*)

(3) Heart-burn ; sour eructations ; sets teeth on edge. Chronic acidity. Nausea with chilliness. (*Sul-ac.*)

(4) Intensely acrid eructations. Acidity worse at night on lying down. Acrid vomiting. (*Rob.*)

(5) An excellent anti-acid powder particularly in peptic ulcer :–

Calc-c. 1x.
Carb-v. 2x.
Taka diastase 1 oz.
Sac lac 8 oz.

Mix together. Take 1/4 teaspoonful in a little water before each meal. (Dr. W.K. Bond). See "Dyspepsia also Acid dyspepsia."

Acne (pimples on the face and also on different parts of body)—(1) Pimples on the face at the age of puberty, *Asterias rubens* is the head remedy. If it fails, then try *Kali-b.*, and *Radium bromide* 30.

(2) *Ars-i.*, and *Sul-i*, may be tried in inveterate cases and also *Hydrc.*

(3) Pimples which suppurate with white pus need *Hep. Sulphur* is an intercurrent remedy when well selected medicines fail to respond. (Rai Bahadur Bishamber Das).

(*b*) (1) Thickly set clusters of pustules on face, with much itching : *Kali-b.* ; red pimply eruptions on face and forehead :— *Led.* ; pimples on face in syphilitic subjects : *Nit-ac.* ; pimples on face, nose and lips, red papulous eruptions on cheeks and around chin. *Bor.* (Dr. Bhanja).

(2) Pimples of the size of pea in different parts of body, the slightest scratch or injury inclines to ulceration. (*Hep.*) night and morning.

(3) Obstinate cases with tendency to pustulation are curable with *Ant-t.*

(4) Dr.Clarke says, "I know of no remedy of such universal usefulness in simple acne as *Kali-br. 30* while Dr. Cushing recommends *Ars-b. 4x* as very efficacious. See "face acne" and "pimples".

(5) Acne (black pores) "*Aur., Dros*".

(6) Acne Rosacea (coppery—red eruption on the face) *Aur. mur.*

(7) Patient suffering from the worst possible outbreak of acne ; worried and extremely constipation. (*Nat-mur.*).

(8) For women who have scanty menses. (*Sanguinaria*).

(9) Small red pimples on face with gastric derangements and white coated tongue. (*Antim Crudum*).

(10) Acne specially on the wings of the nose. (*Thuja*).

Acne, at puberty.—Of anaemic girls at puberty—(*Calc-p*). See ' Pimples".

Acne-due to different causes—If acne is of arthritic nature then urea. If vaccinical acne then *Thuja, Sabina*. *Silicea*, and *Maland.* ; if acne from masturbation then *Bellis perennis* ; if it is due to phthisis then Bacill. and if Pustullar and scarring then *Vaccinum* and *Variolinum*.

Acrid fluids (discharges from eyes, nose, etc.)—The acrid nature of all fluids that excoriate the surface they touch viz. saliva, nasal discharge eye-discharge, stool and menstrual discharge. (*Am-c*). See "Saliva producing rawness and constant spitting".

Acridity—Acridity (irritation) is the key-note of the kind of action characteristic of *Arum-t.*

Acute condition if within 24 hours—Think of *Acon.* always in all acute conditions within 24 hours of its onset. *Acon.* is followed well by *Sulph.*

Acute gastritis—*Ant-c.*, is a very useful remedy. It is most useful remedy if the disease is caused by overloading the stomach ; nausea persists · tough contents vomitted. See also "Gastric trouble" and "Dyspepsia" under different heads.

Adenoid growths, breathing with open mouth—

(*a*) In thin children, large pale tonsils (*Calc-p.*)

(*b*) (1) In children with consumptive family history begin with *Bacillinum* 200 once a fortnight. R. B. Bishamber Das recommends that in each case, the treatment should begin by administering, this fortnightly. He suggests *Mercurius iodatus flavus* as another excellent remedy for treatment of adenoids. (2) *Hydrastis* is perfectly homoeopathic to the totality of symptoms produced by adenoid morbid growth. (3) For enlarged tonsils and adenoid-*Agraphis*. See "Tonsils and adenoids".

(*c*) Dr. Lambrechts of Antwerp puts lint saturated with this medicine 1 part to 6 parts of glycerine for about 15 minutes in each nostril with great success (*Hydrastis.*)

(*d*) Dr. Clarke of London regarded *Agraphis nutans* as a leading remedy for adenoids and breathing with open mouth to avoid surgery. See "Nose adenoids", "Mouth open in sleep".

(*e*) (*i*) *Bar-c.*, is a useful remedy specially in children who have recurring attacks of acute tonsillitis. (*Bar-c.* 30 four times a day. After sometimes, go on increasing potency up to C.M.).

(*ii*) Adenoids are greatly benefited and often times permanently cured by a weekly dose of *Tuber.*

(*f*) *Bromine 3x* is an excellent remedy for sequelae of surgical removal of Tonsils and adenoids. (Dr. Sukarkar).

(*g*) *Teucri scords* is a useful remedy for adenoids.

(*h*) Dr. Kent cured such cases cent percent by giving *Tuberculinum* alone.

Adenoid-external treatment—Cotton tampon well saturated in *Hydrastis* mother tincture 10 gms. and pure **glycerine** in 60 gms. if put into the nose at bed time will give a great relief and obtain atrophy of the adenoid vegetation. See "Tonsils adenoids".

Adipsia (absence of thirst)—

(1) Complete obsence of thirst ; loathing sour thing—(*Ferrum-ac*).

(2) Constant loss of thirst—(*Ledum*).

(3) Neither thirst nor appetite, the thought of food is disgusting—(*Sarsaparilla*).

See "Thirsts under different heads".

Administration—of medicine—One or two drops of liquid may be given in a spoonful of water for a dose. Three to five pills or 2 to 5 grains of powder may be given dry on the tongue or dissolved in spoonful of water.

Instead of the above method, a solution may be prepared by mixing about 10 drops of the liquid with 4 ounces of water (boiled and cooled water preferred) 10 grains of powder with the same quantity of water of this solution, a tablespoonful may be given to adults for a dose, a teaspoonful to children. The solution must be well-stirred or shaken after mixing the medicine and also before administration. In acute cases potency 30 doses may be repeated.

In acute cases ; fevers, neuralgia etc., doses may be given every hour or oftener. In chronic cases 1 to 4 doses may be given. The medicines are best administered on the empty stomach—at least half an hour before or an hour after meals. For children 2 drops or 2 pilules for a dose and for infants half a drop or half pilule for a dose. See "Dose" also.

Those who are accustomed to take coffee and tea or to smoke should not take medicine immediately before or after but should have an interval of half an hour. (Guide to Health by Father Muller). *Nux-vom.* should be administered at night time while *Sulf* should be given in the morning.

Affections—after suppressions of skin troubles—Affection originating from suppression of itches or chronic skin troubles like eczema. (*Causticum*).

Afraid of being alone—*Sepia*. Compare *Phos.* See also "Fear" under its different heads.

After pains—Dr. Farrington says that *Caulophyllum* and *Xanthoxylum* are particularly useful for severe after-pains, while Dr. Herring recommends *Cuprum* for most distressing after-pains, particularly in women who have borne many children. See "Pregnancy—its affections" under its different heads.

Ague (malaria or intermittent fever) with diarrhoea and vomiting—*China* is specific for true ague. Give every half an hour during the chill. *Ip.* when there is much nausea and vomiting. *Ph-a.* two or more doses if the sweating be profuse.

(1) Of the remedies most useful to reduce high temperature, *Bell.* tops the list ; then comes *Gels.*, *Verat-v.*

(2) Dr. Allen says that for a high temperature (103°-105°) with little or no remission, the patient is literally being consumed with fever, *Sulph.* is the remedy.

(3) For long lasting heat with bone pains, nausea and vomiting, *Eup-per.* is good.

(4) Severe long lasting heat with great thirst calls for *Nux-v.* and *Sec.*

(5) For high fever of phthisis *Bapt.* is excellent.

(6) Tendency to copious diarrhoea and vomiting, prostration, faintness, coldness and sweating—*Verat.* See "Malaria" and "Fever" under their different heads.

(7) Continuous fever with weakness. System depleted. Tongue thickly furred ; yellow, shiny coating. Bitter taste. No appetite. (*Chin-a*. 200 two hourly before fever).

(8) Bilious vomiting during fever. Thirst in the morning before rigour. Pain in the bones. Perspiration following upon the onset of hot stage (*Caps*. 6).

(9) Headache. Pain in all joints. Thirst precedes or accompanies rigor. (*Cimex*. 30).

Aggravation—Some complaints are aggravated under certain conditions :

(1) All complaints on motion—*Bry*.

(2) After the least food or drink—*Staphysargia*.

(3) By mental exertion—*Nat. carb*.

(4) Of chronic asthma in damp weather—*Nat-s*.

(5) Of diarrhoea from warm to cold weather, damp or dry—*Dulc*.

Air-raid—anxiety and fear—Use *Arg-n*., *Arn*. and *Ign*., according to symptoms.

Air-sickness—Those not habituated to such travelling feel a sort of revolt in stomach by downward motion and sudden dip upsets most people. Give 3 or 4 doses of *Borax* before flight. It should be of 30 potency. May also be given on the appearance of signs of uneasiness. The other medicines which will help are *Nux-v*. or *Petr*. and they may also be taken before the flight.

Air-traveller fatigue—For people who have to travel a great deal specially by air and over great distances, *Arnica* will prevent mental and physical fatigue and exhaustion. See "Fatigue'.

Albumin-in urine in dropsy and typhoid—(1) *Apis mellifica*, also when present during pregnancy.

(2) Urine scanty with albumen and dropsical swelling of the whole body (*Hell*.). See "Urine in dropsy".

(3) *Albumin* in urine during or after typhoid (*Ph-a*). See 'Urine albuminous and other casts".

(4) For lessening the amount of albumin in urine give *Tr. Carsphyllus 3x*, five drops in water thrice daily.

Albuminuria (inflammation of kidney)—(1) Pale, profuse urine with albumin casts and great reduction of urine, nausea and pain in stomach. (*Aur-c.*) 10 drops before meals and at bed time.

(2) High grade of kidney inflammation, urine scanty, bloody or highly albuminous—*Canth.* (freshly prepared).

(3) For albuminuria of pregnancy—*Helon.*

(4) Urine scanty, suppressed, high-coloured, loaded with casts. burning and patient apathetic—*Apis.* Compare *Kalmia*. See "Kidney affections" and "Urine albuminous and other casts".

Allergy—Allergy is a condition of unusual or exaggerated specific susceptibility to a substance which is harmless to the majority of persons given in like amounts and under similar condition, *e.g.* fish, berries, egg white, and various foods producing symptoms such as urticaria, nausea, vomiting, pains, purging, migraines, asthmatic attacks and many other symptoms of various natures. Drugs and medicines that would be borne by the majority, would produce allergic symptoms and even toxic manifestation in those specifically sensitive.

Some of the remedies are given below for most common allergies.

(*i*) Susceptibility to parsley (a kind of plant containing volatile oil) can be cured by *Petroselinum* 30, says Dr. James W. Ward.

(*ii*) Asthma due to susceptibility to the protein substance in eggs cured by repeated doses of *Egg White*.

(*iii*) For hay fever. (*Ambrosia artemesiaea in potency*).

(*iv*) Allergy for wheat which causes eczema. (*Psor.*)

(*v*) Allergy to straw berries which produce urtcaria ; somtimes there is difficulty in breathing as if a weight were on the chest. (*Fragaria vesca*).

(*vi*) Allergy to sugar or cane sugar. (*Saccharum off.*).

(*vii*) Allergy to milk which causes urticaria. (*Urtica-urens*).

(*viii*) Allergy to eggs, starches, milk, honey, ragwood, pollens onions, wheat, animal food. (*Natrum-m.*).

(*ix*) Allergy to eggs. (*Ferrum met*).

(*x*) Sensitive to hair dyes which produce eczema. Allergy to feathers and chocolates. Cured hay fever in a patient using pillow feathers. Allergy to cooked animal food. (*Sulf.*).

(*xi*) For all allergic diseases, having elective affinities for the skin, mucous membranes and other parts and organs particularly for lungs. (*Argentum Nitrite*).

(*xii*) *Tuberculinum* and *Sulf* are the head remedies for removing allergy against, milk, milk products, eggs, sardines, cooked animal food etc. *Tuberculinum* should be given first in 200 dilution. If no improvement is achieved with 2 doses given every week, try *Sulf* 200 a dose every week. If this potency does not respond it may be increased to 1 M, a dose or two need only be given every fortnight.

Allergy-skin—(a) Any true treatment for skin allergies whether it be urticaria, allergic dermatitis or anglo-neuratic oedemas must therefore aim at raising the individual's resistance against known or unknown allergents.

When the skin allergy is worse from heat *Apis.* is thought of and when worse from cold *Arsenic alb.* is administered. When the allergy results after consumption of alcoholic beverages *Choloratum* is used, when damp weather is the cause *Dulcamara* is made use of. Besides this, *Urtica urens* 6, *Nat. phos 6x*, and *Nat Sulph 6x* are also commonly used.

(*b*) Allergic reactions to antibiotics (*Sulf.*).

(*c*) If after eating there is oedema or puffness of the cellular tissue in all parts of body attended with redness, burning stinging and skin develops urticarious inflammation with red and white areola, then give *Apis Mel.* 200.

(*d*) Allergy to smell of flower causing asthma. (*Ailan-g.*)

Allergic catarrh—Cold in nose, throat or larynx. Morning coryza with violent sneezing. A watery discharge drips from the nose constantly burning like fire and excoriates the upper lips and the wings of the nose until there are rawness and redness. Pain in the head and forehead. The patient gets such coryza every year in August (*All-c*). See "Catarrh" and "Coryza" under their different heads and "Nose watering causing rawness".

Alcoholism—(1) For anti-doting bad effects of liquor such as gastric trouble, restlessness, giddiness, (*Nux-v*).

(2) Drunkard without energy, without strength of will, unable to refuse wine, vomits after the least excess in drinks (*Petr*).

(3) Craving for wine, patient pale, shrivelled and cold, cannot tolerate the slightest amount of food (*Sul-ac.*). See "Drunkenness".

Alopecia—(1) Itching of the head and falling off of the hair ; the new hair break off (*Acid-Fluor.*).

(2) The hairs come out in lumps, leaving bare patches ; eye lashes also fall out. (*Aloes.*).

(3) Baldness, specially of crown in young people ; scalp sensitive to touch. (*Baryta carb.*).

(4) Hair falls out when combing, specially during confinement and lactation ; enormous dandruff. (*Cantharis.*).

(5) Premature Baldness. (*Silicea.*).

(6) Hair falls out in single spot and white hair grows there (*Vinca minor*). See "Baldness" and "Hair-grey".

A

Alopecia-areata—Bald patch on head about the size of a paisa with wens on scalp. First give *Bacill 30* ; later on *Tuberculinum C* and ultimately *Thuja 30*.

Alternation of heat and cold feeling—The patient feels hot once and soon after feels chilly and again hot and so on (*Merc-s*).

Amenorrhoea-absence of menstruation in fat girls—

(1) Especially young plethoric girls. (*Acon.*).

(2) Dr. Jahr recommends *Platina* which acts promptly.

(3) *Cocculus* is useful when condition is accompanied with cramps and leucorrhoea.

(4) For too short, too scanty and insufficient (*Puls*). In anaemic girls *Ferrm met*. It helps raising the hemoglobin content in the blood. See "Menstruation" under its different heads.

Amenorrhoea—absence of menses in dropsy—In dropsical conditions, the menses and uterus fail to perform their function, and amenorrhoea comes on with dropsical conditions. A low state of weakness and nervous excitement sets in (*Apoc.*).

Amputation neuritis—(1) *Allium cepa.* is a wonderful remedy for traumatic neuritis often met with the stump after amputation or serious injury. The pains are almost unbearable (*All-c*) See also "Stumps neuritis" and "Injury-stump".

(2) When there are tearing, stitching pains worse in bed at night after amputation of foot. (*Am-m.*)

(3) Precludes any after suffering from amputation. (*Hyper.* internally and if possible then locally as well).

This *Hyper.* supersedes the use of morphia after operation. See "Neuritis in stump" and "Post operative complication."

Anaemia—general weakness—(*a*) Emaciated in cheek and around the neck. General weakness. Nervous prostration or irritability. Whether the anaemia is caused by loss of fluids, menstrual irregularity, loss of semen, grief or other mental diseases. Emaciation notwithstanding the patient eats. General paleness, shortness of breath, palpitation, loss of weight and throbbing headache (*Nat-m.*). See "Weakness-anaemia with mental prostration".

(*b*) For anaemia and under nourished conditions specially in splenic anaemia give 10 drops doses of *Rubia tinctorum*. See "Chlorosis anaemia".

Anaemia in infants—(*a*) Thin and puny with tendency to rickets (*Sil.*, *8* hourly). See "Rickets" and "Emaciation with sweating in head in children."

(*ii*) Pernicious progressive (*Pic-a.*).

(*iii*) With profuse and exhausting sweat during sleep—(*China*).

(*iv*) From exhausting diseases or haemorrhages—(*Chin.*, 4 hourly).

(*v*) Anaemia after fevers when patient is pale with puffiness of extremity (*Ferr-met.*) *Ferr-ac* is specific for anaemia to be given in M. or C.M.

(*vi*) Anaemia of infants and aged.—For puny, weak limbed children and those who grow too fast. (*Iridium*). It is also useful for the aged persons exhausted by disease.

Anaemia—face bloated—Patient is pale and anaemic in look. Oedema and bloating of the face. The bloating is all around the eyes or all over the face (*Phos.*).

(*b*) In *Kali carb* the upper lids bloat. In *Apis.* lower lids bloat.

Anaemia-pernicious—(1) Excessive debility and prostration. Extreme anxiety. Considerable oedema ; marked desire for acids ; rapid emaciation ; anaemia may be due to malaria or toxic influence. *Ars.* takes first rank in cases of pernicious anaemia. It is one of the most valuable remedies in the treatment of chlorosis. form of anaemia most common in young women characterised by a marked reduction of hemoglobin in the blood, but with a slight diminution in number of red cells) and anaemia.

(2) Pernicious anaemia. Weakness and trembling. Tongue dry in centre, constitution broken down by venereal diseases. Great sensitiveness of skin of right half of body. (*Crotal.*)

(3) Anaemia from gastro-intenstinal troubles : Sedentary habits, high living and debauchery. (*Nux-v.*)

(4) Anaemia in young girls at puberty. Menses too early, short, scanty, pale followed by exhaustion. Abnormal craving for indigestible substances. (*Alumn*)

(5) *China* for pernicious anaemia with profuse and exhausting sweat during sleep.

(6) Hysterical headache, sallowness, brown stains on face, bruised pain in limbs, constipation, coldness of hands and feet, swelling of feet and ankles. (*Sep.* a dose night and morning.)

(7) Debility of nerves from seminal loss, excessive grief perspiration or leucorrhoea. (*Ph-a.*)

(8) Pernicious-anaemia responds well to *Arsenic-alb.* where there is extreme weakness and anxiety.

(9) Anaemia after malaria-where the patient eats well but is still emaciated, constipated and dipressed (*Nat-mur*)

Anaemia-with thread worms—Patient passes thread worms. Appetite by spells. Frontal headache. Abdominal pains. Vertigo. Averse to milk. Craves meat and sweet, (*Sulf*) See "Worms" and "Emaciation" under different heads.

Anaemia—secondary—Resulting from loss of fluids as in lactation or haemorrhages or from excessive menstrual flow or excessive diarrhoea. (*Cinchona*).

Anaesthesia—specially chloroform—Antidote-*Phos.* See "Chloroform" under its different heads.

Anasarca—There is great distention and vomiting in people with anasarca. He drinks and vomits. He vomits his food also. He has a sense of pressure in the episgastrium region below the two ribs and in the chest. Abdomen has also share of dropsy in the whole picture of dropsy. Aggravated by cold (*Apoc.*) ; compare *Apis*, , which is hot. See "Dropsy" under its different headings.

Aneurism (dilation of artery)—(1) Violent, long lasting palpitation of the heart by lying on left side : short breathing when ascending, great weakness. (*Baryta carb.*).

(2) The following two remedies may be given complementary to ensure complete recovery.

(*i*) *Carbo animalis.*

(*ii*) *Lycopodium.*

Anger-complaints from—(*a*) Colic or other complaints as a consequence of anger (*Coloc.*)

(*b*) Another excellent remedy for bad effects is (*Staphy*).

(1) Trembling when he cannot give vengeance to his anger. Tries his best to quarrel with somebody to revile him (*Aurum-foliatum*).

(2) *Aurum metallicum* ; *Nux-v.* for anger from least contradiction.

(3) Anger in children which may result in diarrhoea, cough or convulsions ; quarrelsome children. Give in C.M. dilution—one dose every fortnight-*Cham.* See "Sensitiveness—offended on trifling." and "Rage fits of".

(4) Anger with violence followed by repentance (*Crocus sativa*).

Anger of children—Child fretful and restless. Child cries without any cause and child wants this or that thing but throws them away whenever offered. The child is quiet when carried about. Child peevish. *Cham.* is an excellent remedy for irritability and other symptoms of infants and children. (*Cham.*) The other remedies that may have similar anger in children but not always consoled by their being carried about are *Aconite, Bryonia, Coloc*, *Lyc.*, and *Nux-v.* See "Crying of child".

Angina pectoris—palpitation and pain—Nervous spasmodic palpitation, constricting pains around heart. (*Mag-p.*)

(*i*) Severe pains when the heart's action suddenly ceases and the patient becomes unconscious, pulse weak and feeble, impending suffocation *Cimic. Act-rac* and also *Cactus grandiflorus* for insufficiency and rapid action.

(*ii*) Sudden and terrible pain on the left side of the chest radiating over the heart and the left arm. *Crataegus* is the head remedy for all heart troubles. It is a heart tonic.

(*iii*) In acute attacks when the heart's action is rapid and tumultuous, oppressed breathing, face flushed, palpitation. Such conditions are readily cured by *Aml-n.* May be inhaled also 3 drops on cotton. See "Emphysema".

(*iv*) Pain in the heart with rheumatic symptoms—*Act-rac.*

(*v*) If there is organic disease and weakening of the heart muscle *Ars-i*, *3x.* gr. night and morning immediately after food.

(*vi*) *Cuprum aceticum* is of great value in curing angina pectoris.

(*vii*) Violent precordial pain extending to the axilla and down the arm and forearm to fingers, with numbness of extremity. Pulse feeble and rapid. Sinking sensation at the cramping pain from chest to abdomen. It works like Nitro glycerine (*Lactrodectus Mactons*). See "Pain in right arm".

(*viii*) Dr. Leo Bonnin recommends that small doses of Nitro-glycerine (*Glonoine*) in homoeopathic dilutions often woks wonders since it is best able to quickly open the vessels thus allowing blood to flow again to the heart.

(*ix*) Anguishing substernal pain which radiates to neck and arms, irregular pulse, tendency to syncope, palpitation and sharp stitches in heart, pulse weak and irregular or full and bounding with aggravation from the least motion (*Spigelia*) Dr. Dewey. See "Heart".

(*x*)' Functional irregularties of the heart from a reflex nerve disturbance. Numbness of left arm, hearts' action ceases suddenly and impending suffocation. terine disorders combines with rheumatism and heart trouble (*Actea racemosa*).

(*xi*) When the pain shoots to the *apex.* and down, the particularly left arm palpitation, breathlessness and low blood-pressure. *Cactus-g.* is successful remedy.

(*xii*) The patient robust firm and sturdy with breathing difficulty, becoming worse with exertion and pain produced by motion. (*Bryonia.*)

(*xiii*) Excruciating pain and agony .caused by spasm or contractions of the coronary artery which supply the heart muscles. (*Ergot*).

Angina pectoris—stitches—Stitches in cardiac region. Worse by motion. (*Bry*). See "Heart—angina pectoris".

Ankle ulcer.—Ulcer around ankles and lower legs. (*Psor*).

Ankles swollen—(*a*) *Apis.*, 4 hrs.

(*b*) When there is a chronic sprain of the ankles with oedema. (*Stront* c). See "Sprained joints sore and ankles".

Ankles weakness—Weakness of ankles. They turn easily specially in children who are late in learning to walk. (*Nat.m.*, or *Sil.*)

(2) For pale children. (*Cal-c.*)

(3) Thin and rickety children. (*Sil.*)

(4) Almost in all cases. (*Calc-p.*)

Annoyance—(*i*) Least disturbance causes annoyance. **(*Cocc.*)** See "Peevish".

(*ii*) Caused by noise or light. (*Ars.*).

(*iii*) Trifling matters cause annoyance. (*Con.*).

(*iv*) If annoyance is followed by cold, chill, vomiting or diarrhoea. (*Bryo, Vèrat a.* or *Nux. v.*).

(*v*) When food or drink taken immediately after being vexed produces bitter taste, headache, or cough or vomiting then *Cham*.

(*vi*) Never smile on face. Terrible storm of temper. Violent rage. (*Tuber.*).

Antibiotic— *Pyrogen* is a broad spectrum antibiotic and acts like Mystins and Pencillin in allopathy. In allopathy fevers, especially puerperal, *Pyrogen* has demonstrated its great value as a homoeopathic dynamic antiseptic. For all discharges, which are horribly offensive such as menstrual, lochial, diarrhoea, vomit, sweat and breath and for great pain and violent burning in abscesses, it should be used. It should also be used for septicaemia following abortion. It can also be used when there is insufficient reaction or insufficient improvement. Give a few doses of *Pyrogen 200* once a week. It should not be repeated too frequently. See "Fever septic."

Antidote—To alcohol : *Agar.*

To chloroform. *Phosphorus* is the natural antidote to chloroform. It will stop chloroform vomiting. See "Chloroform antidote."

Lead poisoning and caustic. *Colocynthis* is the best antidote for lead poisoning and caustic.

Mercury. To Mercury and its over use—*Aur-m.*

Antidote to Opium and Morphine habit.—5 drops of *Ip.* tincture for every grain of opium and morphine.

Quinine. *Ipecacuanha* remedies many of the bad effects of quinine in malaria.

Stimulants, like wine, coffee, tea and other drugs *Nux-v.*

Stretches—Of all stretches. *Staphy.*

Aspirin.—*Mag-Phos* or *Antipyr*.

Coaltar drugs and fumes of gases—*Carbo-v.*

Infected vaccination wound.—*Malandrinum.*

Pencillin—*Asphodestra 3x.*

Radium burns—*Cadmium iod.* along with *Phosphorus.*

Antibiotics—*Sulf.*

Aluminium poisoning—*Cadmium Oxide.*

Antidote to Insulin—*Insulin.*

Antiseptic Homoeopathic—*Calendula* is a homoeopathic Dettol. A solution of *Calendula mother tincture* one part with six parts of hot water applied hot is the best application for open wounds, cuts etc. It reduces pain considerably and promotes healing. Kent says that external injuries are healed beautifully by Calendula. One teaspoonful of *Calendula if* one and a half ounce of hot water applied hot. See "Wound incised clear out."

Anti-psoric—*Sulphur* creates reaction in the body and then the indicated medicine acts. See "Blocks".

Anti psoric : *Am-c* See "Blocks".

Charcoal fumes poisoning : *Ammon carb.*

Anti sycotic—*Thuja* paves the way for right medicine to cure. Sometimes sycotic constitution acts as a block to the action of the indicated remedies and *Thuja* is supreme to remove the sycotic block. See "Blocks".

Anti syphilitic—*Mercury* See "Blocks".

Anti-tetanus serum of Homoeopathy—Give *Hypericum 6* and *Ledum 200* alternately four hourly for two days.

Anus-abscess—Painful abscess about the anus in case of fistula. (*Calc-s.*) See "Condylomata."

Anus-cutting of piles—Anal sphincter for treatment of piles (*Staphy.*).

Anus fissure—(*a*) Sharp, cutting pain during and after stool with constipation *Nit-ac.* 6 hr. (*b*) Fissure burning like fire, stool forced with great effort. Knife like pains. (*Ratanhia.*). See "Fissure" and "Rectum aches".

Anus Pain—See "Chapter V for details".

Anus itching—(1) Itching and burning in anus preventing sleep which may be very great driving patient to desperation. He is compelled to bore with the finger into the anus ; so violent is the itching that the patient cannot let it alone. Cold application relieves the itching whereas ointments may increase the burning. (*Aloe.*) Compare *Ratanhia.*

(2) Violent itching and crawling in anus and rectum. (*Ignatia*).

(3) For itching and redness of children (*Sulph*). See "Itching Anus".

Anus-oozing—Moisture oozing from Anus. (*Antim-crud.*). Compare *Sepia.*

Anxiety—Anxiety is an emotion from which anyone may suffer to a greater or lesser extent. *Argentum Nitricum* taken before examination, speaking or public appearances affects a calming influence almost immediately. See "Fear of Examination". (Dr. M.G. Blackie).

Apoplexy—Populary known as 'stroke' or 'fit'. Haemorrhage in the brain tissue marked by sudden unconsciousness, partial or complete thrombosis of cerebral vessles—(1) Apoplexy occurring suddenly without warning with palpitation. Cold moist skin and convulsion of facial muscles. (*Laur.*)

(2) Involuntary stool and urine, twitching of muscles, inability to swallow ; falls down suddenly with a scream ; red face. (*Hyos*).

(3) Motor paralysis and paralysed part becomes thinner ; speech imperfect and stammering ; paralysis of the tongue. (*Cupr-met.*).

(4) Coma with dusky face and stertorus breathing, lies unconscious, laboured pulse, snoring, eyes half opened, redness

and bloatedness. *Opium* is a head remedy and most important in bad cases, should be given in 30th dilutions 3 times a day. If *Opium* fails then try *Apis mellifica* for complete stupor.

(5) If apoplexy is due to weakness of brain, *Formica* strengthens the brain and stops recurrence.

(6) Dr. E.G. Jones uses *Ferrum Phosphoricum* in the 3x trituration in hot water and states that it will usually restore the patient to consciousness in a short-time and control the haemorrhage.

(7) Complete stupor—*Apis mellifica*.

(8) Redness of face ; restlessness ; when due to chill or fright. (*Acon*).

(9) Dr. W.H. Butler believes that *Arnica* 30 is a sheet-anchor for dissolving blood clots most favourably in a number of cases.

(10) Threatened apoplexy or cerebral congestion when there is numbness, vertigo, headache and flushed face. (*Lithium carbonicum*).

(11) Apoplexy of old or tendency thereto. (*Baryta carb*).

(12) Pain in back of head. Bursting feeling, complete insensibility ; no mental grasp of anything. Eyes half closed. Paralysis of brain. *Delirium*. (*Opi*).

(13) Violent confusion of head with red face while exercising. Headache which comes up from the nape of the neck and spreads over the head (*Strontiana carbonica*).

(14) Frequent abstraction of mind, giddiness with congestion. Pain deep in the brain especially left side. Stiffness of joints. Face pale and puffy. (*Lach*).

(15) Great redness of the face with congestion in head. Full and rapid pules, pupils dilated. Give in 6th dilution and repeat every 15 minutes during attack. (*Bell*).

(16) For complete stupor apoplexy give *Apis* when *Opium* fail.

Appendicitis, also septic—Great tenderness to pressure on one spot ; fearful pain in ileo-caecal region. Deathly sensation in stomach pit. *Iris tenax* is the specific remedy for appendicitis. Compare *Echi., Bell., Lach.*

(1) Start treatment well with *Iris tenax* which is specific and is to be given as routine prescription. Give *Sulphur* as intercurrent remedy to complete the cure.

(2) When the pain is constant, the patient never free from pain, bowels filled with gas, with griping, better by bending backward. Give *Dioscorea* in hot water, 5 drops of its M.T. will relief pain and give ease to the patient.

(3) High degree of pain which may be cutting, twisting, or cramping. (*Coloc.*)

(4) When acute attack is over, in order to stop recurrence of attacks, give *Lyco.*, in high dilutions of 1000 fortnightly or monthly.

(5) Pain, fever, headache-*Bell.* one-hourly.

(6) Tense pain region, worse from touch or motion and vomiting (*Plumb.*)

(7) Patients who become exceedingly nervous from abdominal pain. (*Ignatia*)

(8) *Lyco.* and *Lach.* may be given advantageously on the onset of appendicitis.

(9) When the acute attack of appendicitis has subsided then in order to prevent its recurrance give *Psor.*

(10) *Cadmium iod* prevents necrosis in appendicitis while *Plumb-iodat* is very useful in appendicitis with peritonitis.

(11) For aggravation of pain on tossing in bed. (*Bryo-C.M.*).

(12) *Echinacea* is claimed to have acted brilliantly in septic appendicitis ; the tincture 1x and 3x are the strengths used. No indications except septic condition ; tiredness is characteristic.

Appendicitis-preventive against recurring attack and necrosis—See "Chapter V for details."

Appetiser—*Cinchona Rubra* and *Gention mother tincture* in combination, 10 drops to be taken before meals is an in appetiser. (*Dr. Ellis Barker*). See " No. (3) of Tonic."

Appetite of child scattered—(*a*) Cina appetite is very sporadic (scattered). At one time there is keen appetite and at another time there is total absence. Child can always be hungry and wants to eat something. Wants things and throws them away in anger when offered (*Cina*).

(*b*) Very hungry but cannot eat enough to satisfy. (*Lac-c*).

(*c*) Increased hunger in rickety children (Ol-j).

Appetite absence—(*i*) If the patient has no appetite and has good deal of thirst with chilliness and reluctance to uncover he requires *Apocynum cannabinum* in dropsy. (*Apoc.*).

(*ii*) Loss of appetite, emaciation, anaemia and burning thirst with copius pale urine (*Acet-ac*).

(*iii*) Bitter taste, tongue coated yellow at back. Main cause indigestion. (*Nux-v*).

(*iv*) Simple loss of appetite or after acute illness. Give mother tincture half an hour before meals (*Gent. 1.*).

(*v*) Complete loss of appetite for food, drinking, without disgust or bad taste for these things (*Ignatia*). See "Loss of appetite."

(*vi*) Complete loss—complete loss of appetite (*Thuj*). See "Hunger" under its different head.

(*vii*) Give *Iodum 3x* in a half tumbler of boiled water about half an hour before meals for absence of appetite. See "Hunger lost".

Appetite increased or ravenous—(1) Ravenous hunger and much thirst. Anxiety and worried if he does not eat. Loss of flesh yet hungry and eating well. The patient wants to eat all the time and feels comfortable while the stomach is full or being filled, relieved by eating with progressive emaciation. Foul ulceration and salivation. Liver and spleen sore and enlarged. Removes worms.*Iodum* (to be used in tincture form). Compare *Calc carb.* and *Ferrum met.*

(2) Canine hunger before epileptic attack. (*Hyoscyamus.*)

(3) Awakened by canine hunger *Acid phos.* See "Hunger canine".

Arteriosclerosis—(1) The hardening of arterial walls.—When large blood-vessels and aorta are involved with severe headache, worse at night and when lying down. (*Baryta mur*.).

(2) Congestion in the chest and head, strong palpitation ; *Hypertrophy* of the heart. (*Aurum-mur.*).

(3) Senile arteriosclerosis, fatty degeneration, failing compensation. (*Strophanthus*).

(4) Give *Carduus marianus* 5 drops of the trincture T.D.S. which will give marked benefit to the patient.

Arthritis-inflammation of a gouty hyper-sensitivation with rheumatic constitution—Adults and aged persons with arthritic or rheumatic constitution but the sensation of pain is far in excess of pain. Alongwith this-hyper-sensitivation, the patient must be peevish and snappish which is the peculiar mental condition of *Cham.* There is numbness with pain ; violent pains are usually at night and compel the patient to leave the bed and walk about (*Cham* in *200 dilution*).

(*i*) Swelling of terminal finger joints with pain ; swelling of knees—(*Colch.*) This is a good remedy for gout.

(*ii*) Pain in wrists and ankles with fever. Diminishes the amount of urates. (*Trimethyl*).

(*iii*) Pain in soles of feet and heels—(*Tartaric acid.*).

(*iv*) Tonic spasms of the toe of right foot, very painful (*Cupr-acet.*). (*b*) Swelling of great toe. (*Eupatorium perfoliatum*).

(*v*) Rheumatism of right shoulder blade or joint, wrist, ankle or knee-joint. (*Stic.*).

(*vi*) Rheumatism particularly of elbow and knee joints with great swelling, redness and high fever. (*Sal-ac.*).

(*vii*) For gout accompanied with diabetes. (*Phaseol.*).

(*viii*) Sharp pains in fingers, thumb, knees, toes and in step. (*Elat.*) See "Rheumatism" under its different headings and also "Gout. including arthritis deformans".

(*ix*) Arthritis deformans : *Picric acid.*

(*x*) In rheumatoid arthritis according to Dr. Blackie *Senguinaria* for a shoulder joint. *Ruta* or *Pulsatilla*, particularly for the knee, *Rhus tox* for lumbago, jaw or any place where there is relief from continuous movement., *Calcarea.*, *Hyp.*, *Phos.* for hands and wrist., *Natrum Phosph* for elbow, *Cadmium* salts for upper back and many other.

Arthritis-due to gonorrhoea—The limbs feel as though paralysed. There are drawing pains in the bones and then there is tingling of parts. The skin is dirty, covered with spots here and there and the perspiration is most profuse and offensive. (*Thuj.*) See "Gonorrhoea arthritis."

Arthritis-pain—See "Chapter V for details."

Arthritis-prevention of deformities—See "Chapter V for details."

Ascites-dropsy of abdomen—Abdomen very much distended The stomach in dropsical conditions becomes very irritable. It seems as if nothing passes through it. He finally becomes paralysed in the bowels. The kidneys are not acting. Dropsy from disease of liver. (*Apoc.*)

(*i*) Disorders of the heart and lungs in dropsy of renal origin. Puffiness of the face with oedema about the eye-lids, transparent skin, thirst and vomiting. Albumin in the urine (*Ars.*, 2 hourly.).

(*ii*) Acute dropsical swellings with suppression of urine. (*Scil.*, 2 hourly.).

(*iii*) Dropsy from organic disease of the heart-*Ars-i.* *3x.* *Gr III* after meals.

(*iv*) Dropsy from congestion of kidney, dull aching pain in renal region, dark, smoky, urine, urine scanty, diarrhoea. (*Ter*).

(*v*) Dropsy with enlargement of liver and spleen. Diarrhoea with pain in lower part of back. A prompt diuretic when the urine is suppressed (*Liatris spicata mother tincture in 10 drops doses*).

(*vi*) Dropsy from organic disease of the heart, small frequent irregular pulse, nausea, vomiting, diarrhoea, burning in stomach, scanty, dark albuminous urine. Suppressed, dilated heart. Swelling of the feet, continuous sleepness, cold sweat, dropsical swelling of genitals. (*Dig. 30*). See "Dropsy" under its different headings.

(*vii*) For ascites due to cirrhosis of liver. (*Crot-t.*)

(*viii*) Swelling of legs with acute pains during movement.

Swelling of the face. General dropsical conditions. The intolerence of smell of food or cooking of food is the ranking symptom. (*Colch.*). See "Dropsy liver, kidney or heart."

Asiatic cholera—Usual rice water stool, vomiting and purging ; stool profuse, gushing and prostrating. Rapid sinking of forces : cold sweat and cold breath ; face hippocratic ; whole body icy cold. (*Verat.*). Compare *Camph.* and *Cupr-met.* See also "Cholera" under its different heads and "Collape-cold sweats in cholera, measles eruptive fever".

Assimilation-defective in children inspite of nourishment—Children who sweat on head easily ; emaciated and badly nourished children. Child may be hungry, wanting food too often but not gaining weight due to bad assimilation. Large head, big belly, thin limbs, emaciated face ; cannot walk or learning to walk late. Constipated. Does not grow according to age. Face looks old and creased as in monkey, (*Sil.*). Compare *Calc-c.* See "Weakness in rickety children." "Children's debilitating diseases".

Asphyxia-due to charcoal fumes—*Bovista.*

Asphyxia Neonatorum (inability of newborn to respire)—*Ant-t.* first one globule dry on the tongue. If it fails then *Opium* in the same manner. *Laurocerasus* is useful when there is gasping without breathing, blueness of face and twitching of face muscles. See "Sub-head 12 of Pregnancy disorder of".

Asthenopia (Weakness of ocular muscles or visual power due to errors of refraction or over-use.) :

(1) Asthenopia due to muscular defects and errors of accommodation. Coloured Light produces dizziness. (*Art-v.*).

(2) *Onosmodium* is very useful remedy in eye strain with dull heavy sore aching eyes. No inflammatory trouble but patient is troubled with headaches and weakness.

Dr. A.B Nortan finds this remedy gives prompt relief to many annoying symptoms.

(3) *Ruta* is also a most valuable remedy for affections of eyes from over work where every tissue of eyes is irritable. Eyes burn, feel hot like balls of fire.

(4) Similarly *Euphrasia* is one of the best remedies in eye affections ; it has inflammation of lids, which appear red and ulcerated with profuse excoriating discharge ; photophobia : pustules near the corner of cornea. Reading or writing brings pain in eyes ; it is specially useful in granular ophthalmia. *Ruta* and *Euphrasia* are very old remedies for eyes affections. The great English poet Milton has composed a verse for their usefulness.

"Purge with Euphrasy and Rue.
The visual nerve, for he had much to see."

(5) *Asthenopia* from irritated conjunctiva, granular lids, loss of power of internal rectus (straight muscle of the eye). (*Alumina*).

Asthma-children—(*a*) Specially in children : dry, hacking, cough in afternoon with pain in pit of stomach ; worse cold drinks. (*Thuja*).

(*b*) A child who in trying to ease the breathing lies flat on back and arms stretched out while sleep. (*Psorinum*).

Asthma-chronic—Worst in dry cold air. Better in damp air. (*Hep.*)

Asthma-attack—(*i*) To be given alternately during attack. It will act as a palliative and will ease the breathing and the cough. (*Acon. IX and Ip. IX*).

(*ii*) Attack occurring early morning frequently induced by disorders of stomach. There is also flatulence. Relieved by lying on back or by changing sides or sitting up. (*Nux-v.3,* 15 minutes).

(*iii*) Convulsive breathing, nausea or vomiting, cold sweat on the face. (*Verat-v.* 3, 15 minutes).

(*iv*) Attack comes on in night after midnight. Irritable and full of fears, compels the patient to sit which affords him relief. Sensitive to every atmospheric change, intolerance of cold weather. Expectoration must be swallowed. Wheezing (*Kali-c.,* not to be repeated too often).

(*v*) *Dysponoea* with thick and purulent mucus, with or without bronchitis. An excellent remedy for asthma. Acts best in stout and corpulent patient. (*Blatta orientalis.* Lowest potency during attack, high after it is over).

(*vi*) Grasping at throat with sense of choking, sticky mucus and saliva. Dry cough dependent on cardiac lesions. Cannot lie down, intense sneezing which relieves breathing (*Naja.*). Compare *Adrenalin.*

(*vii*) Asthma aggravated by emotions, by cares and repeated griefs. (*Ignatia*). Dr. Clarke suggests that in most cases a course of *Bacillinum-30—200* once a week will be of marked advantage while Rai Bahadur Bisambar Das recommends :

1. *Tuberculinum* ; 2 *Thuja* ; 3. *Nat-s* ; 4. *Med.*, and 5. *Syph.*—to be given intercurrently in potency not below 200 or 1M or C.M. in addition to indicated medicines. No other medicine to be given 2 or 3 days before and after their use.' If desired results achieved, then further drugging to be avoided.

Asthma-pain—See "Chapter V for details."

Asthma—of old persons—(*a*) Asthma on attempting coition. Asthma of old persons and children in feeble condition. (*Ambra.*) See "Cough of old people."

(*b*) Expectoration :—Expectoration brick shade. May be given half hourly during the attack. (*Bry.*)

(*c*) With nausea :—Of old people with chronic asthmatic cough. Nausea to be present. While breathing a feeling of suffocation from accumulation of mucus. (*Ip*) (*d*) Hysterical—These patients some times get hystericla asthma ; all sorts of disturbance in breathing. Asthmatic attacks at least once a day, all her life, brought on by every bodily exertion, coition, especially by every satisfying meal. Worst at night. (*Asaf*)

(*e*) With perspiration—Of old people where the patient appears as if dying and patient feels hot and perspires and wants fanning during attack. Useful in desperate cases. (*Carb-v.*)

(*f*) In midnight—of old people—Worse after **12** in night ; springs out of bed, unable to lie down for fear of suffocation. Must sit up to breathe. Respiration is wheezing. The air passages seem constricted. (*Ars.*) It is safest medicine for asthma and when given during attack it will have magic effect. (*Ars.*)

(*g*) (1) An old patient suffering from asthma for last 20 years. Worse when he wakes up in the morning also worse at night. Aggravation in summer. Has allergic cold. Feels comfortable when lying flat with hands raised above head during attack. (*Bacillinum 1M & 10M, at intervals.* Ultimately *Psorinum* in increasing potency). See "No. (1) of Asthma-general".

(2) An old patient suffering from bronchial asthma of a long standing, constipation and frequent urination. Attacks worse every monsoon with cough and cold with profuse expectoration. Irritable. Better when alone. Vaccinated and inoculated. (*Natrum-sulph.*) in increasing potencies up to 50 M. In between *Bacillinum 200* and 1M ultimately one dose of *Thuja 10M.* for vaccination and inoculation.). See "Eczema general No. (1)."

(3) A patient was suffering from bronchial asthma since a very long time. Attacks worse at night between 3 and 4 a.m. Constipated and hot patient. Cold drinks and ice-cream make

him worse. Better in open air in monsoon. Suffered from various skin troubles. Family history of asthma. Developed attacks when weather became warm. Vaccinated. (*Sulf* in increasing potencies from 200 onwards up to 50M ; later on *Carb-v.30 and Ant c. 30*. Lastly *Caust* from 200 in increasing onwards potencies). (*Dr. Wadia.*)

(4) A young lad suffering from bronchial asthma. Having constant cough and cold. During attack vomiting any food and drink. Attacks come prior to any examination or keeping an appointment. Worse lying flat, better being propped up or leaning forward on a pillow. Vaccinated. Likes cold weather. Very sensitive and intelligent. Fond of salts, prefers to be alone and all times nervous. Family history of asthma (After attack give *Gels. 30* Then *Arg-n. 200*. Lastly *Nat-m.* in increasing potencies for completing cure) (*Dr Wadia.*)

(5) Hurried and difficult breathing as if every breath would be his last breath. (*Apis* 30.) (*Dr. Bhanja.*)

(6) Attacks during rain and damp weather mostly at 4 and 5 a.m. ; must hold chest when coughing. Cough with thick, ropy greenish expectoration. According to Dr. Leonard "Looseness of bowels at each attack" is a guiding symptom for *Nat-s.*

(7) Asthma continually recurring with some gouty tendency. (*Stram.* 30)

(8) For paroxysms of nervous asthma ; it gives relief at once. (*Cuprum.*)

(9) *Lobelia-inflata* gives relief in acute asthma if administered from 2nd to 6th dilution.

(10) Asthma as a result of anger. (*Cham.*)

(11) Asthma worse in dry cold weather and better in damp weather (*Hep.*). For patients extremely sensitive to damp weather. (*Nat-s.*)

(12) Asthma with difficult exhalation at marked coughing and aggravation at night. Cough so violent, seems as if each

spell would be termination. (*Meph.* to be given from 1x to 3x dilutions in repeated doses.)

(13) In asthma there is this difference which is very valuable. *Hepar-Sulph.* is worse in dry cold weather and better in damp weather. *Natrum Sulph.* exactly opposite of this. Extremely sensitive to damp. There is no remedy that has amelioration so strongly in damp weather. (*Dr. Nash*).

(14) If *Mer. biniod* in 3x or 2x is given at bed time then it will abort an attack of asthma and will prevent the expected attack developing during night.

(15) Cardiac asthma. Losses breath on any exertion. During spasm or asthma 10 drops of *Sumbul* in hot water will give relief and in continued small doses will cure. See "Cardiac Asthma and Dyspnoea."

(16) An efficacious remedy for wheezing and oppression in bronchitic patients. Asthma with profuse tenacious expectoration which relieves. Cannot breathe when lying down. (5 drops doses of *Tr. Grindelia.*)

(17) Worse from day-light to sun-set. Brighter in the evenings. Only improved by lying on face ; worse by wet, damp weather and thunder storms. When other remedies fail to act give *Medorrhinum* as an intercurrent remedy. Also useful when alternate or co-existence of asthma with rheumatism.

(18) If the patient finds relief in breathing by lying on face on knee elbow position. (*Medorrhinum*).

Asthma-palliative during attack—*Aconite IX* and *Ipec. IX* be given alternately during the attack. It will act as a palliative and will ease the breathing and the cough.

Astigmatism (myopic)—It is a disease of the eye for structural error or malformation, congenital or accidental of the lens, in which the rays of light from a point do not converge to a point on the retina. Hyperaesthesia rays of retina, great sensibility of retina. Pain, extending back into head ; lachrymation ; and impaired vision. *Myopic astigma.*

Useful in restoring power to the weakness of ciliary muscle. (*Lilium tig.*) See "Eyes" under different head.

Atomic radiation—In this age of nuclear technology *Phosphorus* is specific for the bad effects of atomic radiation. (*Phos.*)

Atrophy of nipples and breast—short nipples or development slow—(*a*) Nipple short, flat, atrophied so that instead of projecting depression exists. According to Dr. Jahr *Sarsaparilla* is the best medicine for this difficulty 1 or 2 drops of liquid in water every 4 or 6 hours. See "Muscular atrophy No. 5 under muscles."

(*b*) If the mammae develop themselves too slowly at the age of puberty (*Nux-m.*, *Conium* dose as above). See "Nipple-atrophy."

Automatic motion of one arm and leg—There are automatic movements of one leg or arm while the other appears paralysed. (*Helleborus*).

Aversion to milk and to other things—The patient says "Oh, I cannot drink milk, if I take milk it gives me diarrhoea." Who would think of anything but *Nat-c.*, for such a case. (*Aeth-c.*). See :"Diarrhoea milk upsets."

(*i*) Aversion to amusement. (*Ig.*)

(*ii*) To family members, to business or profession. (*Sep.*)

(*iii*) To doing anything mental or physical. . (*Cad.*) See "Milk not digested with diarrhoea."

Axilla (armpits) different complaints—(*a*) Itching eruption in axilla. Eruption with inflamed glands—*Elaps corallinus* (*Corel snake*) 30, 4 hourly.

(*b*) Pain in right extending down arm. Pustules and Eczema, (*Jug-c.*)

(*c*) Irritation, eruption, abscess in arm. Itching and eruption of small red pustules. (*Jug-r.*, 4 hourly.)

(*d*) Perspiration excessive. (*Kali-c.* 4 hourly.)

(*e*) Perspiration offensive. (*Nit-ac.*, 4 hourly.)

(*f*) Perspiration like garlic. (*Lyc.*, 4 hourly.)

(*g*) Inflamed glands. (*Bar-c.*, 4 hourly.) (*Clarke*). See "Perspiration offensive of body" and "Sweat offensive foot."

(*h*) Tumour of axilla. (*Tell.*)

Azoospermism—Absence or diseased condition of spermatoza in the semen :

(1) Absence of spermatoza in impotency due to sexual neuresthenia. Chronic prostatic discharge. (*Damiana*)

(2) Absence of spermatoza accompanied with impotency ; insufficient erections or absence of erections. Want of energy in coition. Emissions provoked by presence of women. (*Conium mac.*).

B

Back-ache—(1) The patient is to have the back-ache in bed and must sit up to turn over as turning or twisting the body aggravates when standing. The pain is mostly located in the lumbar-region and is often in connection with haemorrhoids. (*Nux-v.*).

(2) (*a*) Violent pain in sacro-lumbar region. Slightest effort to move may cause sweat and attempt to vomit. Sensation of heavy weight at coccyx, dragging downward, (*Ant-t.*). (*b*) Excruciating back-ache. Aching in legs. (*Variolinum*). See also "Lumbago back-ache or pain in loins."

(3) Severe backache, even touching it caused pain; the pain extending to head. (*Tellurium*)

Back-aching due to different causes :

(1) From over-exertion (*Arn.,*) 3 hourly.

(2) In pregnant women with sense of weakness in the back. (*Kali-c*).

(3) With scanty urine. (*Ter.*)

(4) With oxalates in urine. (*Ox-ac.*), 4 hourly.

(5) With piles—(*Aesc.*), 6 hourly.

(6) Back-ache in small-pox. (*Verat-v.*), 6 hourly. See "Small-pox backache."

(7) Pain in lumbar and sacral region down thighs and hips, spine sensitive, stiffness in neck and back. Rheumatic pains in muscles of back-neck. (*Cimicifuga racemosa*). See "Lumbago-backache or pains in loins."

Back-ache—burning sensation—Burning sensation of heat in the back. In any acute or chronic condition where this peculiar symptom is present, *Phosphorus* is likely to help in the whole case and not in the burning alone. (*Phos.*). See "Burning sensation."

Back-ache low down; scarcely able to rise or walk—(1) Specially low down in the back, through the sacrum and the hips; constant dull back-ache ; walking is almost impossible ; scarcely able to rise or walk after sitting. Ache centres in its action in the lower back and pelvic region and ever prominent is its characteristic. (*Aesc.*). See "Pelvis—lower back."

(2) *Cimicifuga* is useful for the violent aching when pain is due to some uterine complaints. See "Pains in pelvis".

Back-old hurt—Painfulness of the back on rising from a seat which is the result of old hurt is often cured by *Rhus-t*, followed if necessary by *Calc-c*.

(3) *Gnaphalium* will cure chronic back-ache which is worse from continued motion, better resting specially on back. The more chronic back ache, the better indicated is this remedy (*Gnaph.*)

Back pain-in the back during menstruation—Delayed first menstruation. Menses usually late and scanty in flow. Flow sometimes stops and flows again Nausea ; diarrhoea during or after menses. Tearful. (*Puls*). Compare *Act-rac*. See also "Menstrual flow with pain in back".

Back-ache, patient prone to backache—Pain anywhere and also in back, patient worst after bath, relief from warm application. Stiff in getting up in the morning. Restless and must move about although it may be painful at first.(*Rhust-tox.*) in high potency gives quick and lasting relief.

Back-ache stiff spine—Stiffness of the whole spine ; tightness in the muscles of the back. Violent; shooting, burning pains, Crawling, creeping fromication worse by stooping. (*Agar*). See also "Spine-stiffness."

Back-ache due to wetting or over-lifting—Affections of the muscles of back and even the spinal membrane, sprain, or by exposure, by sleeping on damp ground, or in bed with damp sheets or getting wet in rains while perspiring or too much bathing in lake or river or over-lifting particularly from stretching high up to these things. There may or may not be cold or fever in such circumstances. (*Rhust-t*). *Dulc.* is also a great remedy for back troubles from taking cold. See "Lumbago stiffness."

Back-ache violent and sudden kink—(1) Violent aching down the back. (*Act-rac.*).

(2) *Secale cornutum* has sudden catch or kink in the back. (*Sec.*).

Back-ache pains—See "Chapter V for details."

Backward children—who do not develop properly and look idiotic—(1) Head and belly big. Feeble and slow ; slow to understand and slow to execute. Profuse perspiration of head and forehead, skin pale. Acidity in stomach. (*Calc-c.*)

(2) Lack of intelligence. Mental confusion. Slow to understand and slow to move. Inattentive and unsteady. Fears everybody, strangers more. Swollen tonsils and swollen abdomen. Dwarfish, does not grow and develop (*Bar-c.*)

(3) Extremely violent and nervous, angry ; crying ; howling ; beating, biting ; wishes to run away. Easily frightened and starts up, out of its sleep with wild looks. Cannot remain alone Fears darkness, wants light. (*Stram.*)

R.B. Bishamber Das recommends that the treatment of above type of children should start with *Tuberculinum 200* which should be given at interval of one month each as an intercurrent remedy with above remedies. Similarly *Syphilinum 200* should be given as intercurrent remedy along with *Bar-c.* and *Stram.* at an interval of one month. Not more than two remedies should be given in each course of three to four months.

Tuberculinum and *Syphilinum* which should be given at intervals of one month each along with the other two remedies which are also to be used in two hundred dilution to be given alternately. Higher dilution than 200 should be used when no improvement is seen or when improvement is stopped. See also "Children late in learning to talk and walking" and "Idiocy" and "walking-delayed in children" under its different heads.

Baldness—Great falling out of hair. Premature baldness and grey hair. Complete Bald without eyebrows and eyelashes. Patients loved sweet things and suffered from indigestion. *(Lyco.)*.

(1) Falling of hair in pregnancy. Losing hair after chronic head-ache. *(Nat-m.* and *Sepia.)*

(2) Baldness due to syphilis. The hair will fall and not grow. *(Ustilago maydis.* Also *Fluoric-acid)*

(3) Falling of hair from head, also from eye-brows, lashes and genitals. *(Ph-ac.)*. Compare *Petrol.*

(4). Falling of hair due to dry white scaly dandruff. *(Thuja.)*

(5) Falling off with dryness. (*Kali-c.*)

(6) Senile whitening of hair. Start treatment with *Thyroidin* in 30 dilution.

(7) For grey hair *Lyc.* 30 and *Phos-acid* 30 may be tried one after the other. If no result is achieved within three months, the remedies may be given alternately in 1000 dilution every fortnight.

(8) To grow hair rapidly and to become dark. (*Wiesbaden* 200).

(9) Bald spots on the sides of head. The head sweats easily. The most important remedy is *Graph.*

(10) Falling off hair from general debility. (*Ph-a.*)

(11) Bald spots on the head. which are dry and scaly. Dandruff, roots of hair get grey and hair comes out in bunches. *(Phos.)*

(12) Falling off the hair with great itching of the scalp. *(Vinca minor.)*

(13) Falling off hair in child birth or in severe illness, *(Carbo-v.)*. See also "Hair" under its different heads and also "Falling out of hair."

(14) Much itching of scalp, scalp and roots of hair very sensitive to touch; great falling of hair. *(Sep.)*

(15) Baldness. Losing of hair from crown. *(Bar-c.)*. See "Alopecia."

(16) *Rosmarinus* has a long standing reputation as a remedy for Baldness, headache and flogging mental powers.

Barber's itch—*Rhus-t.* is an excellent, remedy and should be tried first. *Lach.* when there are cracks with oozing and reappearance after sticky discharge with itching like eczema suppression. *(Graph.)*

(1) Internally Dr. Baehr is said to have got best results from *Graphites*. Dr. Jahr applauds highly *Mezereum* and *Calc-c.* He reports some brilliant results with *Calc-c., Nit-ac.* and *Aur-m.* and are also highly recommended by Dr. Baehr. Compare *Sulph iodatum.*

(2) Herpes with burning, much itching. Vesicles of bluish colour. Worse in open air. *(Ran-b.)*. See also "Itch" under its different heads.

Bathing-dread—Dread of bathing, children hate to be washed or bathed. *(Sulf.)* See "Dread".

Beard—*(a) Anatherum* for falling off hair of beard.

(*b*) For falling off hair from beard another excellent medicine is *Sphingurus*. See "Hair" under its different heads.

Bed-sores :—

(1) Centre covered with dry bloody crust. (*Arg-n.*)

(2) Bed-sores in hips and sacral region. (*Arn-m.*)

(3) In Typhoid. (*Bapt.*)

(4) Of dark blue colour provided the characteristic dark blue colour is present. (*Lach.*). Paint all kinds of bed-sores with *Calendula* thrice daily.

(5) *Hypericum oil* and ointment are particularly useful in applying to bed-sores.

B. coli-infection—(1) *Thuja* is specific. 1M dilution every week later on once a month.

(2) *Tincture Berberis vul* M.T. 10 drops may be given in a cup of warm water after every three hours.

(3) According to Dr. Ghosh *B. coli* in 20th or 30th potency may be given. He recommends *Methylene blue* in 6th potency.

Birth-mark :—

(1) Treatment to be started with *Thuja*. The mother tincture of the same to be applied externally morning and evening.

(2) *Radium-brom.* to be given once a week along with *Thuja*. On that day, *Thuja* should not be given.

(3) *Vaocininum 200* dilution to be used as an intercurrent remedy once a fortnight. No other medicine to be given that day. See "Freckles spots brown and yellow saddle on face" "Naerus "

Bee-stings—An excellent remedy for bee-stings. Outer application in mother tincture cures and gives instantaneous relief. *Urtica urens, also Led p.* See also "Bites" and "stings".

Biliousness—(1) For jaundice, biliousness and other liver troubles. (5 drops of M. T. of *Chelidonium T. D. S.*) See "Jaundice."

(2) Bilious attacks. (*Berberis aquifolium. IX.* Tincture.).

Bilious-attack—Attack with vomiting of bile or acid, violent headache, diarrhoea. (*Iris-v.*).

(3) Complete suppression of bile, white stools and yellow skin. (*Chin.* 2 hrly.)

(4) After over-indulgence in alcohol or over-eating, constipation, sedentary persons. (*Nux-v.*, 1/2 hourly.)

(5) After fat or rich food. (*Puls.* 1/2 hourly.)

(6) Persons who suffer from acidity, sinking at pit of stomach in forenoon, constipation and piles. (*Sulph.*)

(7) Abdominal flatulence, constipation and scanty urine, (*Lyc.*) See "Flatulence-lower region."

(8) Persons of costive habit, subject to one sided headache. (*Kali-c.*). See also "Vomiting" under its different heads.

Bilious-diarrhoea—*Chamomilla* is the best remedy. It has green, slimy stool like chopped eggs. *Cham.* should be followed by *Merc-s.* and *Sulf.* See "Diarrhoea with colic."

Bilious-fever—(1) For febrile heat. *Acon., Bry., Chin., Nux-v.*

(2) For headache. *Bry.* and *Nux-v.*

(3) For good deal of vomiting *Ant-t., Ars., Ip.*

(4) For constipation with torpid stool. *Ars-a., Bry, Nux-v., Verat-a.*

(5) For diarrhoea *Ars-a.,Merc-s., Puls.* aud *Cham.* See "Fever" under its different heads.

Bilious-temperament—*Podo.* is specially adapted to persons of bilious temperament. It affects chiefly the duodenum, small intestines, liver and rectum.

Bilious-colic-pain—See "Chapter V for details."

Biliary colic-colic from the passage of gall-stones :

(1) For severe Pains *Coloc.*

(2) Cutting pains, changing locations and radiating and there is much flatulence. Some physicians think *Dioscorea* to be specific for gall-stones.

(3) Colic from gall-stone, followed by jaundice, pains come on spasmodically and are confined to a small spot. *Berb.*

(4) *Verat.,* is often very excellent to relieve the sufferings. See also "Gall-stone colic."

Birth control—(*a*) Three doses of *Nat-m. 200X* taken by women on the first, second and third day after cessation of the monthly course produces such reactions that fertilisation during the month becomes unlikely. Three doses must be repeated after every menses till conception is not desired.

(*b*) If *Puls. 200* is taken 4 days continuously before the regular date of menstruation, it will be sufficient to prevent conception.

(*c*) According to Dr. P. Banerjee the following medicines prevent pregnancy : (*i*) *Testis* 3X, 3 grains twice daily for seven days may be given from the day of cessation of menstruation each month. In many a case it prevents pregnancy. This medicine is a kind of nosode.

(*ii*) *Cyclamen M.T.*, 5 drops or *Xanthoxy M.T.*, 5 drops for 7 to 10 consecutive days from the day after cessation of menstruation. They also act in preventing conception. See "Oral contraceptive".

Bites—also teeth bites from chewing—(1) Bad effects from stings and bites have been cured by *Acet-ac. (Acet-ac.)*

(2) An excellent remedy for bee stings. (*Urt-u.*)

(3) Specific for dog bites. (*Lach.*). See "Dog bite wound"

(4) Serpent bites or other venomous insects. (*Ced.*) See "Snake bite."

(5) An antidote to snake poisoning. Its use renders the body immune to the influence of snake poison. (*Golondrina*) See "Serpent bite."

(6) The strong tincture of *Arnica* applied to a wasp sting prevents pain and swelling within 2 hours. See also "Insect-bites."

(7) Teeth bites inside of cheek from chewing. (*Caust.*). See "Teeth aches".

(8) For scorpion bites give *Ledum p. 200* internally and apply its Tincture locally.

Bites-animals—Rats, dogs, scorpion and cats. (*Ledum.*) Dog and cat bites to be painted externally with *Calendula M.T.* See "Stings" "Rat-bite" and "Snake bite".

Bites-prevention of complications—Rat bites, dog bites, cat bites, etc., are made safe by use of *Ledum* from its subsequent complication of tetanus or any other form of septic condition.

Ledum will prevent not only the subsequent inflammatory complication but will also prevent the shooting pains that naturally come when nerves are involved in the injury. There will be no trouble subsequently if *Led.* can be given at once. See "Cat bites—prevention of complications."

Bites-prevention of injuries, effects from bites of rabid animal, snake poison and rabies—See "Chapter V for details".

Bladder-with involuntary urine—(1) Burning and cutting, or sticking pain in urethra especially of the female urethra during and after urinating, *Berb.*, mother tincture. 2 drops 1/2 hour-4 hours.

(2) Involuntary passage of urine in sleep, *Senega 6* hrly. during day or during night. *Bell.* 6 hrly. See "wetting bladder".

(3) Burning in region of kidneys, bladder and ureter, strangury (painful urination). *Terebinthina* 1/2 hrly. (*b*) For attacks of pain in bladder, give *Kali-c.*, every half hourly and for stone give *Cantharis*. See also "Cystitis-inflammation of bladder" and "Stone in bladder."

(4) For pains in the bladder, ureters of kidneys dependent upon the passage of gravel, uric acid etc. give *Hydrange. arb 200 or 10 m* in Q Form. It will relieve the pain and work as sedative.

Bladder-irritation frequent urination—Frequent and troublesome calls to urinate and attended by inflammation may arise from the state of digestive organs. *Nux-v.* will usually be of service ; when occasioned by disorder of liver, *Merc* ; by nervous excitability or irritation. *Bell.* or *Cham.* and if an accompaniment of hysteria. *Ig.* ; for pain in bladder. (*Stry.*).

Bladder polyuria (excessive frequent secretion of urine) along weight—Urine about every half an hour; night and day; the urine high coloured and scalding. Burning during and sometimes after passing urine. Reduction of weight and loss of sleep. Continuous teasing and dribbling drop by drop, smarting and burning night and day disappears under *Arg-n. 30*. See also "Urine frequent and painful", "Cystitis inflammation of bladder" and "Under" urine its different heads.

Bladder-weakness of bladder with micturition—Micturition impeded. One is obliged to wait a while before the urine passes. Never able to finish the urinating (*Hepar*). See also "Micturition painful and uncontrollable".

Bladder-weakness of bladder after labour—Paralytic weakness of the bladder after a woman has gone through strenuous labour causing retention of urine afterwards is miraculously removed by *Causticum*. See "Cystitis-inflammation of bladder", "Labour retention of urine".

Bleeding-of any kind—See "Haemorrhage of any kind".

Bleeding-bright—Must be of bright red colour and from any out-let of body. (*Ferr-P.*). See also "Haemorrhages" under their different heads.

Bleeding-copious—Copious bleeding from the nose and other orifices mostly in the morning. (*Ambra.*). See "Nose bleeding in morning".

Bleeding-dark—Blood must be dark. Ulcers bleed. (*Lach.*).

Bleeding-dark does not easily coagulate—The blood from any orifice, nose, uterus, bladder, bowel etc. does not easily coagulate and is dark in colour. (*Am-c.*).

Bleeding-during pregnancy—Unusual bleeding during pregnancy or at later stage *i.e.,* 5th or 7th month. Habitual abortion at the 3rd month or later. (*Sep.*). See also "Pregnancy", "Haemorrhage—during pregnancy if abortion apprehended" and "Pregnancy bleeding".

Bleeding-from lungs—Coughing bloody sputum or bleeding from lungs. (*Acalypha Indica* 6th potency every half an hour during attack). See "Pneumonia with blood discharge."

Bleeding-from mucous membranes—From mucous membranes, *e.g.* nose, stomach, rectum and ulcer. (*Acet-ac*).

Bleeding-from navel—From navel of infants. (*Abrot.*). See also "Navel bleeding".

Bleeding-from rectum—Persistant bleeding, haemorrhage from anus, the blood being watery. (*Sanguisuga.*).

Bleeding-tendency from extracted teeth or any organ—*Phos.* patient has a bleeding tendency. Even slight wounds bleed a good deal. Extracted teeth bleed red blood for hours. The patient may bleed from every orifice of the body or from any internal organ. Bleedings from nose while blowing. (*Phos.*). See "Haemorrhage from any orifice".

Bleeding-from vein—For violent projectile bleeding after cutting of any vein apply *Tinc Ferr-Phos., 9 X.*, to that part and bandage it.

Blepharitis-inflammation of the edges of eyelids—(1) Loss of eyelashes. *Blepharitis marginals.* (*Petroleum.*) (2) Eruptions on lids which become red with margin covered with scales or crust. For keratitis (inflammation of the cornea), photophobia and blepharitis, give *Chrysarobinum* 30 dilution internally. Externally four grains of this medicine with one ounce Vaseline to be applied. (3) In acute cases when the suppuration is about to set in or has already taken place. The lids are inflamed with throbbing pain. (*Hepar sulph.*). See "No. (*b*) of eyelid drooping".

Blindness due to lightning—*Phosphorus* is specific for cure of such blindness. (*Phos 30* or *200*).

Blindness-sudden also night blindness :

(1) *Lycopodium* is the head remedy.

(2) During pregnancy. Night and day blindness in women during pregnancy. (*Ran-b.*).

(3) When the cause is not known. (*Hell*).

(4) When due to paralysis of opitic nerve. (*Bov.*)

(5) Night blindness with or without glaucoma or myopia. (*Phys.*).

(6) Sudden blindness. (*Acon*). See "Night blindness".

(7) In hysteria. (*Ferr-met.*)

(8) After lightning stroke. (*Phos.*)

(9) From grief or blindness due to haemorrhage in the eye, (*Gels.*). See "Nervous blindness", "Night blindness" and "Sudden appearance of symptoms and blindness".

Blinking of the eyes—(1) The patient fears darkness and of being left alone ; blinking eye-lid with nervous debility (*Lyc.*).

(2) Constant blinking of eye-lid. (*Euphr.*)

(3) Blinking of eye-lids during and after reading. (*Crocus*; *Calc-c.*).

Blisters-in feet about nails—Blisters in feet due to walking, ulcers in heels. Painful affections of fingers about nails (*All-c.*). See "Heels painful".

Blister-in mouth during fever or menses—Pearl like blisters in the mouth or near its corner during fever or menses. (*Nat-m.*). When *Nat-m.* fails, then try *Ignatia*. See "Fever blister."

Blisters-in mouth extremely painful—White blisters on side, close to root, painfully sore. Tip of tongue very painful. (*Thuja.*). Crusty in typhoid fever. (*Phos-ac.*) See also "Mouth blisters near corner."

Bloating-dropsy—In dropsy the face has a look of anguish, bloated, puffed and swollen. It is also bloated, under the eye. (*Apoc.*). See also "Dropsy" under its different heads.

Bloating lids-upper and lower—See "Number 29 of eyes".

Bloating-stomach—Bloating of stomach with a stony weight in the stomach. (*Nux-v.*). Patient is never happy after a good meal. (*Nux-v.*) See "Flatulent dyspepsia" and "Distension".
Blocks—Cure of a chronic trouble usually fails on two grounds :—(*i*) Either by wrong selection of a remedy which is very common or (*ii*) by "Blocks."

The road to cure is often blocked by some toxic effects of a disease-virus which has perhaps taken a place long ago and is still acting in the body. Until these blocks are removed, the remedy will not act.

Rarely the right remedy doses act as a block remover but often one has to use a different block remover which is allied to the original toxin. This shows the importance of taking the history of a case with special reference to its antecedents. Unless previous history is known properly in proper sequence, the sequence of disease cannot be ascertained and hence the block created by them cannot be removed. Usually the block is removed by "Nosode" connected with the original disease. Hence *Diphtherinum* will usually remove the sequence of diphtheria or will remove the block in another disease which takes place subsequent to diphtheria infection. The same may happen in respect of typhoid, cholera, mumps, measles, small-pox, etc., etc. The difficulty is, it is not always possible to have a *Nosode* connected with the original-disease. *Nux-vom*. removes blocks of those who have been drugged by mixtures, bitters, herbs and so-called vegetable pills under allopathic treatment.

There are, of course, some homoeopathic medicines which are supposed to be block removers, e.g. *Thuja*. for vaccination. *Sulphur* for psoric conditions etc. But usually the real block removers are *Nosodes* derived from the original toxins. See also "Creating reaction" and "Nosodes."

Blood dysentery—Blood dysentery, tenesmus not relieved by passing of stool. Stool hot, bloody, slimy (muddy), offensive with cutting pains and shreds of mucous membrane. But there must be tenesmus or urging of the bladder and rectum at the same time and urine passing in drops with much pain along with the stool, *i.e.*, the tenesmus of rectum must extend to the bladder area with symptoms of bladder also in order that *Merc-c*. may act or vice-versa, *i.e.* alongwith the symptoms of bladder the constant urging for urination, there should be urging to stool. *Merc-c*. has more intense symptoms which appear suddenly and vehemently. (Compare *Nux-v*. which must have absolute relief for some time after stool.). (*Merc-c*). See "Dysentery blood with urging for urination."

Blood-poisoning—*Ammonium carb.* has a state analogous to blood poisoning. Such as in erysipelas and in malignant form of Scarlet fever with prostration, great dyspnoea so that it seems as if the heart were giving out. (*Am-c.*). See "Septicaemia-blood poisoning for relieving fever."

Blood poisoning-in infective fever e.g. measles, diphtheria or small-pox—The blood is going rapidly to decomposition with black oozing from the mouth. Foul odour comes from the mouth and the nose. The child is going into a state of stupor, continued dreamy state while awake. The child is rapidly going into a comatose condition as a result of malig nant infection. Bloody discharge from nose or mouth. General prostration *e.g.* diphtheria, measles, small-pox, etc. (*Ailanthus glandulosa*). See "Measles not coming out properly."

Blood pressure high and low—(*a*) *Adrenaline* arrests the rise in high blood pressure and stimulates the heart. *Bar-m.* acts wonderfully in high blood pressure of old people. *Cactus* may be given when blood pressure is low, vertigo and palpitations when lying on side. Think of *Glonine* when there is oppression in the region of heart, vertigo, black spots before eyes and feels difficulty in going up-stairs.

(*b*) *Lach.* is the head remedy for high blood pressure. It should be tried first and will be of help in majority of cases. It is to be given in high potency, say, of 1 M. (*Lach.*).

(*c*) *Aurum-met.* is to be given when pressure is due to suppressed anger or resentment or due to over-sensitiveness followed by roaring in head, violent headache or vertigo. *Tuberculinum* is to be thought of as an intercurrent remedy in persons who are wasting in health. (R.B. Bishambar Das).

(*d*) *Ferrum phos. 3X, Kali-m. 3X* and *Calc. phos. 3X.* Put all 3 in 4 oz of fairly hot water in bottle. One teaspoonful every 1/2 hr. at lesser intervals according to severity of case. See "High blood pressure or hypertension" and "Low blood pressure."

(*e*) *Cannabis indica* highly emotional, talkative and excitable. No conception of time, space and place.

(*f*) *Baryta mur.* for old age, with high difference of systolic and diastolic pressure alongwith arteriosclerosis.

(*g*) *Bryonia,* high blood pressure accompanied with vertigo and splliting headache.

(*h*) *Adrenaline chloride* will lower the blood pressure and is useful as a palliative.

(*i*) When there are no clear symptom to indicate any remedy then Dr. W. Lang suggests alternate daily one dose of each medicine of *Cratagus, Glonoine* and *Passiflora.* It will keep the patient comfortable and prevent further deterioration in his general condition Dr. Stuwart agrees with this.

Blood purifier—(1)*Gunp.* is a great antipsoric remedy and is a great blood purifier. It helps to clear up many skin troubles. Should be given for a long time in 3X potency.

(2) *Echinacea* is another blood purifier. It is useful in every blood disease such as pimples, boils and small-pox.

It should be given in mother tincture 5 to 10 drops per dose.

Blood-spitting (Haemoptysis)—(1) Dr. Jousset says that we could positively rely upon *Ip.* and *Mill.* if given alternately.

(2) Drs. Holocombe and Thomas have used *Acal. I,* successfully in haemorrhage from lungs. Dr. Clofton says that in haemoptysis from pulmonary tuberculosis there is no other remedy equal to it in value.

(3) *Phos* is a favourite remedy for pulmonary haemorrhage but the dose must not be given too high. Low attenuation is recommended. See "Haemoptysis."

Blood-urine (Haematuria)—(1) Dr. Jahr advises to give *Cannabis indica* if no other remedy is specially indicated. If this does not afford relief then *Canth.* may be given. (2) *Millefolium* has shown great excellence as a specific remedy in bloody urine with painfulness of kidneys. (*Mill.*). See also "Haematuria."

Blotches-purple—Purple blotches on back of hands, palmer surface stiff. *Primula-obconica.*

Blushing—Sanguine temperament. Blushing and flushing easily, exited from slightest opposition. (*Ferrum met.*)

Boils—(1) When the boils are very large and recur in a person subject to them. Boil does not mature but remains blue. (*Lyco.*). (2) Small boils in ear. (*Pic-a.*). (3) Boil near anus, with fistula. (*Berb.*). (4) If repeated painful boils appear which resist ordinary treatment then *Echi. M.T.* 5 to 8 drops may be given thrice daily. (5) If at the commencement of dangerous and poisonous boils *Hyper. 200* is given internally then it cuts short its course. See "Abscess."

Boils-associated with internal disease—Whenever treating a severe form of disease, and an eruption comes to the surface, like a carbuncle or erysipelas and does not give relief to the patient then there is danger. Such malignant boils, carbuncles, appearing in a patient with some external trouble, *Am-c.* is the remedy very often in such condition. (*Am-c.*). See "Suppressed skin trouble."

Boils-in axilla—*Carbo-animalis 200* be given on alternate days. It is said to be infallible in such trouble. See "Axilla Complaints."

Boils-in crops—(1) Coming in crops in various parts of body or a single boil is succeeded by another as soon as first boil is healed. (*Sulf.*). (2) Tendency to small painful boils one after another in small boils in crops. (*Arn-m.*). See "(3) of Abscess." (3) *Berberis* prevents the recurrence of boils. (*Dewey*).

(4) If small boils appear in crops then give *Bryo.* in repeated doses while *Sulf.* may be given as an intercurrent remedy.

(5) *Luet.* is associated with succession of abscesses.

(6) Crops of boils on nape, nose face and mattery spots-Acne ; all over shoulder, glands of neck swollen. (*Thuja occ. 30* infrequently administered.)

B

Boils-carbuncles—(1) (*a*) Carbuncles with diabetes. Pus discharge from several openings with a very foul odour. Give *Carbolic acid* in 200 dilution. (*b*) In carbuncles *Anthracinum* is an excellent remedy when burning with high fever. To be given every fortnight in 1000 potency. One dose will cure or greatly improve the condition. (*c*) Carbuncles with burning as if coals were put on affected parts. *Ars-a*, is indicated when *Anthracinum* fails. (*d*) Carbuncles, burning and stinging pains. Gangrene. *Tarentula cubensis* is specific for carbuncles and septic boils. (2) It is also useful for exceedingly painful and inflamed abscess when neighbouring glands are painful and swollen. (*Tarent-c.*). See "Carbuncles" under its different heads and "Gangrene."

Boils-chronic, bed sore and carbuncles—Malignant chronic ulcers, bed sore, carbuncle provided the dark blue colour is present. (*Lach.*). See also "Carbuncles" under its different heads "Bed sores."

Boils-children—Specially of children surrounded with little bluish red area and also for eczema of children. (*Sep.*).

Boils-discharge from—*Hepar. sulph.* or *Calc. sulph.* can be excellent remedies in making the boils discharge and clear quickly.

Boil-habit and recurring—Those who have recurring boils, *Ech.* is an excellent remedy to break this habit.

Boils-nose—Crops of boils in nose, intensely painful, successively appear in nose, green fetid pus. (*Tuberculinum 200.*)

Boils painful covered by scab—See "Sore painful covered by scab."

Boils-pus aborted—*Hep.* in high potency will check formation to be followed by *Merc-s.* See also "Pus" under its different heads.

Boils-throbbing, swelling, painful—Great redness, throbbing and swelling, painfulness. *Bell.* is often the first remedy. (*Bell.*).

Tarentula cubens 30 is almost specific for boils and carbuncles. See "Gum-boil throbbing."

Bones-an abnormal growth and swelling—(1) An abnormal out-growth of bones. (*Merc-c.* or *Rhus-t.*). (2) Out-growth and swelling of bones in general. (*Kali-i.*). See "Caries of bones soft" and "Nosodes". (3) Enlargement of bone with or without cause. *Calc-f.* may be given in alternation with *Calc-p.* See "Bones-enlargement."

Bones-ache—(1) Great aching in the bones as if they would break. *Ammonium carbonicum.* (2) Bone pains general and severe. Pains in arms and wrists and back. Pains in limbs and muscles in influenza. (*Eupatorium perfoliatum*). See "Pain".

Bones-curvature and carious—(1) For curvature of bones, ricket and diseases of hip joint. (*Silicea.*). (2) For curvature of bones of spine and caries of vertebra and ricket with sour sweat. (*Calc-c.*). (*Dewey*). See also "Curvature of bones."

Bones-enlargement—Enlargement of bones with or without caries. (*Calc-f.*). See "Bones-an abnormal growth."

Bones-fracture and its non-union—(1) For union of bone. For formation of bones or conversion of tissues into bone. (*Calc.*). (2) For bones broken by injury or in fracture whether the fracture of bones is simple or compound use *Symphytum* in 1 M. potency. (3) *Ruta-graveolens* for non-union resulting from defective callus. See "Fracture" under its different heads. "Union of bones" and "Injury fracture."

Bone-inflammation—(1) Inflammation of bone due to injury. (*Ruta.*)

(2) Inflammation of bone due to fracture. (*Symphytum.*)

(3) For big bony over-growth anywhere in the body

marked ; action upon the jaw or elsewhere in the body, Nodosities, Necrosis. (*Hekla lawa.*) See "Bones-an abnormal growth" and "Swelling under different heads."

Bones-injuries and hardened spots over nodules—In bone injuries ; Deficient callus ; Formation of deposits in the fibrous membrane infesting the surface of bones. Hardened spots over nodules or growths left after bruises. Pain in the long bones. (*Ruta.*)

Bones-pains due to injury or fracture—(1) Pains in bones, pains in the periosteum as in syphilis mostly aggravated in the night. Old syphilitical bone pain in the head, very distressing. (*Asaf.*). (2) Pain in long bone whether due to injury, fracture or rheumatism. (*Ruta.*). See "Fracture pains" and "Pains in shin bones."

Bones-rickets with diarrhoea and debility—(1) *Calc-c.* is very highly spoken of both by Dr. Jahr. and Baehr when given in higher attenuation resulting in curative effects promptly. According to Dr. Farrington *Calc-p.* is excellent to prevent rickets. (2) The head comparatively large, offensive sweat, face pale, bone poorly developed. Drs. Jahr, Jousset, Dewey and Hughes applaud *Silicea* highly when *Calc-c.* fails. (3) *Phos-acid* is useful for diarrhoea in rickets according to Dr. Jousset while Dr. Dewey says that it is useful in extreme debility found in rickets. See "Ricket."

Bones-swelling of fingers and knees—Swelling of terminal finger joints with pain. Swelling of knees and other joints with irritability. (*Colch.*) See "Gout" under its different heads.

Boring into the nose in acute diseases with discharge and swelling—Tingling sensation in the mucous membrane of the mouth and nose. Children when they are suffering from acute disease they scratch and pinch their lips and bore into the nose even when they are bleeding from scratching. This has been a guiding symptom in acute diseases like typhoid, scarlet fever, and other type of continued low fever conditions with delirium, excitement and maniacal manifestations, the tingling and itching sensation must be so intense that the pain of bleeding is not felt. Acrid discharge from nose. Along with this excoriating discharge, the glands of the neck and even the parotid (situated near the ear) may be inflamed and are sore. (*Arum-t.*). See also "Finger boring-during sleep" and "Nose-children scratching in acute diseases".

Brain-concussion—*Arnica* 3 drops half hourly, *Kali-phos. 30,* 2 hours, See "Concussion of brain or spine".

Brain-congestion—Like *Bell.*, *Gels.* has congestion of brain but neither the fever nor congestion is so intense as in *Bel.* (*Gels.*). See also "Congestion of brain."

Brain-fag—(1) *Phos. acid* 2 drops 6 hourly. (2) Loss of memory (Funk) before an examination (*Anacardium*). See "Examination fear", "Examination nervousness" and Memory" under different heads.

Brain-inflammation—See "Inflammation of brain".

Brain-tumour—*Sulphur C.M.* 1 dose at first and then *Tuberculi. C.M.* 1 dose after 15 days ; other medicines i.e. *Conium mac. 200, Cal. iod. 200, Iodium 200, Cal. fluor. 200, Merc. iod.* arrest and absorb bony brain tumour of the scalp etc. See "Tumours in different heads."

Brain-pain—See "Chapter V for details."

Brain-undeveloped though body fully developed—Lack of development of the mind and brain while the body is fully developed. Such people are simple tongued and behave like children. Fear, simplicity, and innocence. Play with dolls and say foolish things. Childishness in girls of 18 to 25 years of age. Late incoming to womanhood. Backward mentally and physically, are dwarfish, do not grow and develop. Bashful. Aversion to strangers. (*Baryta-carb.*) It is slow in action, bears repetition.

Brain-tumour—See "Tumour in brain".

Breasts-congestion with flow of milk after weaning—(1) *Puls.* most useful followed by *Calc-c.* (2) For constant flow of milk. *Bell.*, *Calc-c.*, *Bry.* are the best remedies, See "Weaning-engorgement of breast", "Milk ceasing" and "Mastitis".

Breast-enlargement in a boy at the time of puberty—*Conium 1000* 1 dose once a fortnight and watch the progress for a fortnight before repeating the dose.

Breasts-pain in menses with abscess—(1) Pain in the breasts at menstrual period. Breasts hot and painful. Abscess of the mammae. (*Bry.*). (2) Breasts sore and inflamed. *Bell.* and *Bry.* most useful. See "Tumours-fatty". (3) Pain between two breasts. (*Raph.*).

Breast-not developing according to age—Females whose breast do not attend full growth and maturity according to age may be given *Lecithin 6X* 3 grains. and *Calc. phos. 12X* 4 tablets alternately 4 times a day.

Breast-tumours—Benign, mammary tumour, menses too early, too profuse, long lasting. Dysmenorrhoea. (*Tuberculinum 200* compare *Merc-iod.*).

Breathlessness—Shortness of breath going upstairs. Disinclination to walk. (*Calc.*). See "Dyspnoea" and "Choking."

Breathlessness-cardiac—See "Emphysema",

Breathing-oppressed must sit up—Breathing is much oppressed. Must sit up to breathe as the patient cannot lie down to breathe. The air passages seem constricted. (*Ars-a.*). During attack, give *Tr. Cactus* 200 in drops in water, follow it with *Tr. Ars.* 200, 4 drops in water every 5 minutes or earlier. See also "Dyspnoea", "Respiration", "Cough oppressed breathing with prostration."

Breathing-stertorous noisy and snoring with prostration—Rattling sound produced when the larynx and air passages are obstructed by mucus. (*Op.* 6th potency.). See "Catarrh of nose blocks" and "Mouth open in sleep".

B

Bowels-intussusception-slipping of one part of intestine into another—(1) Sudden pain with screaming, great restlessness, abdomen distended, passing blood and mucus through the rectum. Give *Aconite* in ·30 dilution every 15 minutes. Acts better in higher dilution of 1000.

(2) With colic and fetid vomiting. (*Plumbum*). (3) With violent colic and convulsion. (*Opium*). (4) Rushes about, better by bending double and pressing abdomen, great anguish, (*Verat-a.*). See "Hernia' under its different heads.

Bowels-pain—Pains in the bowels which cause frequent micturition. (*Terebinthina*).

Bright's disease (inflammation of kidney) with face puffed—(1) In the digestive complaints of Bright's disease with nausea, vomiting, drowsiness, difficult breathing, *Apoc.*, will be found of frequent use. (*Apoc.*). (2) Lachrymation from eyes. Whole face puffed up. Sickly and tired. Cannot endure any covering, almost thirstless ; urine scanty but very offensive and smelling strongly (*Nit-ac.*). (3) Uraemia with unconsciousness : pupils dilated and insensible to light ; convulsions, strong urinous odour from the body. Give *Hellebours* in 30 dilution every two hours. (4) Violent nephritis with scanty dark albuminous urine containing casts. *Kali-chlor.*—most effective of all homoeopathic remedies in Bright's disease. (5) In early stages of congestion of kidneys. Urine bloody with pains along the ureters and in the back (*Terebinth.*). (6) Albumin in urine which becomes black like scanty urine with dropsical swelling. Acute form of Bright's disease. (*Colch.*). (7) In inflammation of kidneys with suppression of urine. (*Canth.* 1 hourly) (8) Dull pain in the kidneys, scanty urine charged with albumin and contains blood corpuscles. Suppression of urine and eruption of skin, feeling of suffocation. (*Apis*). (9) Albuminous, scanty and red urine, syphilitic complications. Dr. Leidlam considers it best remedy for nephritis of pregnancy and Dr. Baehr lauds in suppurative nephritis. (*Merc-c.*). See "Kidney affections" and "Nephritis".

Broodings—(*a*) Over one's condition, over disappointed affection. (*Acid-phos.*). (*b*) Over-imaginary bitter events and troubles (*Ig.*). See also "Melancholia", "Mania" and part(3) of "Insult—bad effects of insult and mortification".

Bronchitis and prevention of its attack in different weathers—*Calc-carbonica* in the autumn will often give a patient a winter free of cold. *Sulphur* can be another cold preventive in the hot weather. *Phosphorus* will prevent the usual cold in the thin, narrow chested and bright young man.

Bronchitis of different kinds—(1) Cough tickling and troublesome at night, free expectoration in morning ; thick yellow and sour mucus. Fat and flabby patient. (*Bry.*).

(2) Acute or chronic bronchitis where mucus is tough and stringy and difficult to raise. (*Kali-b. 3x.* 2 hourly.).

(3) Cough worse on lying down ; compels the patient to sit up in bed. (*Puls.* 2 hourly).

(4) Long standing bronchitis in old people, physical powers depressed, expectoration difficult to raise for want of power. (*Am-c.* 1 hourly).

(5) Painful spasmodic cough with difficulty in dislodging the sputum: shortness of breath on walking, dyspnoea and wheezing at night. (*Naphthaline*).

(6) Cough dry, loud, deep sounding and painful which makes the patient hold his chest. Accumulation of mucus in larynx useful in chronic bronchitis. (*Dros.*).

(7) Frequent fits of cough with thick, heavy yellowish, mucopurulent expectoration (*Antim-iod.*).

(8) Cough is tight, worse from evening to midnight, also from speaking, laughing, reading aloud, cold and lying on left side. The whole body trembles with the cough. The patient suppresses the cough with a moan just as long as he can because it hurts him. (*Phos.*).

(9) *Bronchitis* with continuous cough, frontal headache and coryza which has resisted many standard remedies will yield to *Narcissus*.

(10) Bronchitis with cough and cold. (*Bacill.*)

Bronchitis-children—Of young children. Suitable to pale and weak subject. (*Ferr-p.*)

Bronchitis-infants—(1) With chest loaded with mucus and rapid and wheezy breathing ; face pale or bluish, child becomes rigid and turns blue while coughing. While breathing a feeling of suffocation from accumulation of mucus. Nausea. (*Ip.*) (2) Wheezing, breathing, respiration superfical, vomiting of food. (*Ant-t.*). See "Pneumonia of infants".

Bronchitis-old people—Of old people (*Carbo-v.*). See also "Coryza" and "Cough" under different heads.

Bronchiectasis-dilation of bronchi due to an inflammatory process with sneezing—Hacking cough. Cough followed by sneezing. Difficult raising of tough, profuse mucus in the aged. (*Senega.*)

Broncho-pneumonia—*Kali-bich.*, *Squilla* and *Antimonium. tartaricum*. Compare *Calc-carb.* Dr. Tyler says that he has saved many children dying from this disease by giving them (*Ant. tart.*). See also "Pneumonia" under its different heads.

Bruise—Of skin ; acute stage : (*Arnica*).

Bruises-of bones—*Ruta*. It is the best remedy to relieve the pains in the bones. See "Dermatitis involving hands or face, scratching with weeping eczema".

Bruise-of cartilages—*Ruta*.

Bruise-fingers and spine—Specially fingers, toes and matrix of nails and injuries to the spinal cord. (*Hyper.* 3 hourly). See also "Spine injuries".

Bruise-skin with blacky blue appearance—Bruise of the skin, acute stage. Black and blue sore appearance on an injured part with intense soreness found about it. *Arnica* to be used until the soreness and bruise condition disappeared from the injured part. See "Slight injuries fester." "Contusion skin raptured".

Bruises-of tendons and insertions of tendons—*Ruta*. See "Contracture of tendons".

Bubo—Glands swelling *Badiaga* ; glands swollen painful in neck, axilla, groin and mammae. *Carbo. animals* 4 hours. See also "Glands" under different heads.

Bubo-syphilitic—Dr. Berjeau considers *Merc-cor.* and *Merc-iod.* are the most prominent remedies the former for acute bubo and the latter for indolent variety. See "Ulcers-syphilitic" and "Offensive".

Bugs—Bite of bugs. (*Hyper.*). See also "Bites".

Burns and scalds.—(1) Scalds. If the burns are deep, destroying the skin. (*Kali-bichr.* every 2 hours).

(2) If suppuration takes after burns then *Hep.*

(3) For after effects of scalds or burns *Causticum 6* internally every **15 to 30** minutes for pain and shock accompanying burns. If hurried breathing due to shock then give *Phosphorus* alternately with *Aconite* every hour.

(4) An excellent remedy for all stages of burn and scalds. It prevents blisters, pain in passing urine with passing of blood from the bladder. (*Cantharis*). Dr. Herring recommends it also externally 8 drops in half glass and cotton soaked applied.

(5) When gangrene is threatening. (*Ars-alb.*).

(6) (a) Acute, agonising pains in burn at the second stage when sensations like nettle rash. *Urtica urens* locally mother tincure in proportion of 1 to 15 drops of water. (b) *Capsicum* useful for relieving burning pains.

(7) In ulceration of duodenum and also in nervous patient when burnt (*Stramonium*). For immediate outer application use. *Tannic acid* 5% or *Cantharis* mixed with cold water in proportion of 1 dram to an oz. of water. The part burnt should be kept wet to avoid formation of blisters. Dressing with *Mullein oil* is also useful in burns. (*a*) *Succus calendula* one ounce in a pint of warm water is the best lotion to prevent suppuration. (*b*) One per cent solution of *Picric acid* applied on lint is the best outer application for burns until granulations begin to form.

(8) *Urtica-urens* is one of the best remedies for burns of the first degree and may be used locally and given internally. See also "Scalds injury by hot liquids".

Burns-causing contracture—Contracture of muscles and tendons due to an injury or burn of any septic process is usually removed by *Causticum* if given in high dose. See also "Contracture of muscles"

Burning-in anus—Burning and itching in anus preventing sleep which may be very great, driving him to desperation. He is compelled to bore with the finger into the anus ; so violent is the itching that the patient cannot let it alone. Cold application relieves whereas ointments increase the burning. (*Aloe*). Compare *Ratanhia*. See also "Itching-anus", and "Anus Itching."

Burnings-palm—Intense burning of palms. Patient cannot cover the hands. (*Phos.*). Compare *Sulf.* which has burning of feet and patient cannot cover feet. See also "Palms and head sweating" and "Feet burning" and" Sole burning with feet out".

Burning-sensation—(1) One of the chief characteristics of *Sulf.* is burning. It can burn as a matter of fact anywhere and everywhere of the body or over the whole body, either in the outer or in inner. Eyes burn, discharge from the nose burns, face burns, arm and soles burn, eruptions burn, throat burns, and stomach burns. Burning in rectum before or while passing stool. Burning in piles. Burning in urethra while passing urine. Nipples burning of *Arsenic, Phosphorus, Aconite* and *Bell.* (*Sulf.*).

(2) Chilly patient wants to be heavily covered. He feels better by application of heat (*Ars.*). See "Itching-scratching causing burning" and "Backache-burning sensation".

C

Calculus in kidney with agonising pain—(*a*) Stone in kindey-Agonising pain, twists about, screaming and groaning with red urine then *Ocimum canum*; writhing with crampy pains. *Diosc*. every 15 minutes. If violent pains in bladder extend from kidneys to urethra with urging to urinate then *Berberis* every 15 minutes. If no relief then give *Pareira brava* in tepid water, every half an hour in Mother Tincture when all other medicines fail. (*b*) *Galium aparine* acts on urinary organs as diuretic and of use in dropsies and gravel and calculi. See "Kidney-stone in".

Calculus-prevention of formation and dissolving of stone—(*a*) For preventing formation of stone and storing of uric acid in those who have gout and uric acid diathesis give *Urtica-urens*. (*b*) *Cardus marianus* will prevent further formation of stones. Similarly *Chionanthus virginica* will prevent formation of gallstones and discharge those already formed. See "Gravel prevention". (*c*) *Epigea Repens* MT—Dr. Bell says that this medicine is very effective in dissolving stones in kidney and urethra. Dose : 5 drops of Mother Tincture every 3 hours. See also "Stone in kidney".

Calculus-stone in liver or gall-bladder—*Calc-c*. every 15 minutes. If no relief within 3 hours then *Berberis vulgaris*. Try *Dioscorea* when pains radiate from gall-bladder. If pain felt in left lobe of liver then *Cardus marianus*. See also "Stone in bladder", "Stone in kidney" and "Gall-stone colic".

Cancer-breast—Of breast, ovaries and tumour. (*Lach.*).

Cancer-uterus—Of womb or uterus. They bleed easily (*Phos*). See also "Uterus-bleeding from."

Canine hunger also before epileptic fits—See "Appetite increased or ravenous" also "(2) of the same heading".

Carbuncles with pain and discharge—(*a*) Great intensity, redness, swelling and painfulness. *Bell.* is very often the first remedy. (*Bell*). See also "Boils-Carbuncles".

(*b*) When the patient is weakend by copious discharge and openings have run together and formed a large cavity, *Hep-s.* particularly when the voice is weak. (2) *Ars-a.* is chief remedy for carbuncles with burning as if coals of fire. Cutting and burning pain after midnight. (3) *Sil.* is particularly indicated for carbuncles between shoulders and nape of neck, specially when suppuration has set in. Fistulous opening with offensive discharge. During the process of ulceration it clears the wounds of its decaying masses and promotes healthy granulation. Give in high dilution of 200 or 1000 to be repeated weekly or monthly respectively. (4) *Myristica-sebifera* 3*x* is a homoeopathic knife, and is an almost specific drug for breaking open the carbuncle. It hastens suppuration and shortens its duration. It often does away with the use of knife.

(5) Repeated dose of *Arnica* will often abort a carbuncle.

(6) Intense pain and dark red swelling in the beginning, great restlessness. Pain revived by moving about. (*Rhus-t.*). See "Boils carbuncles".

(7) *Calendula* acts very quickly in stopping pain and fever in cases of carbuncles.

(8) For outer application on carbuncles, Dr. Moore recommends few drops of *Calendula M.T.* as compresses on carbuncles for rapid healing.

Carbuncles-dark blue colour—The dark blue colour must be present. (*Lach.*).

Carbuncles-hot compress for it—*Calendula* is used as hot compresses and gives great comfort where there is inflammation and redness with great deal of discomfort due to carbuncles.

Carbuncles-with diabetes with offensive discharge—Carbuncles with diabetes. Pus discharge with a very foul odour from several openings. Give *Carbolic-acid.* 200 dilution.

Carbuncles-with high fever—(*a*) *Anthracinum* in carbuncles is an excellent remedy. It has burning and high fever. Give in 1000 potency every fortnight. One dose will cure or generally improve the condition. (*b*) Paint the parts with *Echinacea* tincture for external use.

Carbuncles-in patient with some internal trouble—Unhealthy looking boils, appear in a patient with some internal trouble. *Ammon-carb.* is the remedy very often in such condition. (*Am-c.*).

Carbuncles-with marked toxemia with pain, fever and inflammation—Mottled bluish with intense knife-cutting and burning pain. The patient sick at night with delirium. Fever with a staring look, foul tongue and fetid breath. If an inflamed part is mottled bluish. (*Lach.*) Growing darker with burning pain *Tarentula cubensis* must be thought of. (*Lach., Tarent-cube.*).

Cardiac asthma or dyspnoea—The face is pale anxious. The pulse is small and irregular. Bronchitis of the aged or simple asthma when there is depression of the heart action. *Aspidosperma tincture* which acts as Digitalis of lungs increasing the oxygen in blood. See "No. 15 of Asthma of old person".

Caries of long bones;jaws, and palate—(1) Tearing and tension in long bones, worse at night, boring in bones, (*Bar-c.*).

(2) Caries of lower Jaw ; fistulous openings, (*Cistus-can.*). See "No. 5 of Teethaches."

(3) Caries syphilitic : Syphilitic caries, painful ulcers. (*Staphy.*).

(4) Caries of palate bones: In syphilitic patients after abuse of mercury. Caries of cervical bones and bones of the palate. There is offensive smell and discharge of small pieces

of bones. (*Aur-met.*). See "Syphilitics complications of nose, throat and palate."

(5) *Phosphorus* is the head remedy for caries of bones. May be tried when *Silicea* fails to cure completely or when progress is arrested.

(6) Caries of femur bone. (*Strontum nitricum.*).

Caries of bones-soft curvature and non-union of fractured bone—Bones, when they become soft or wasted away. Curvature and non-union of fractured bones. (*Calc-p.*). See also "Bones-curvature" and "Bones fracture."

Caries-of nasal bones with discharge and ulcer—(*a*) A horrible offensive may also come from the nose with ulcers inside. Caries of the bones of the nose. (Syphilitic ulceration of caries) (*Asaf.*).

(*b*) Caries of nasal, palate, mastoid bone ; they are tender to touch, soreness, and horrible odour from nose or mouth (*Aur. met.*). See "Nose syphilitic" and "Ozena".

Caries of teeth—prevention and pyorrhoea—See "Chapter V for details."

Caries-of vertebrae—Dr. Baehr claims that *Calc-c.* is superior to any remedy in caries of vertebrae, curvature of spine and rickets. Sour Sweat. See "Necrosis of bone."

Car-sickness—*Coccul.* Compare *Tabacum.* See "Sea sickness in car."

Cartilages bruised and injured—Bruised and injured cartilages and lingering pains thereon. (*Ruta.*). See also "Bruises-of cartilage."

Cat-bite—Bite of cat (whether mad or otherwise) lacerated wound, upper and lower leg swollen. (*Acetic acid.*). Apply it and also take externally. See "Bites" under its different heads.

Cat-bites-prevention of subsequent complications—Made safe by use of *Ledum* from its subsequent complications to tetanus or any other form of septic condition. There will be no trouble subsequently if *Ledum* can be given at once. (*Led.*). See "Bites-prevention of complications."

Cataract including myopia—(1) Drop into affected eye, 4 or 5 times a day *Succus Cineraria maritima* and keep it for months. Also effective in traumatic cases. (*Cinerar-mar.*).

(2) In incipient stages with a high degree of myopia. Constant inclination to touch and rub the eye in order to relieve a pressure in it. The cataract is arrested and sight improves. (*Caust. I M.* to be given every month.)

(3) In later stages. Stony cataract in arthritis subjects. Senile catatact. *Sulf.* should be given every fortnight in 200 dilution and no medicine before or after it for a day. For remaining days give *Calc-P. 30* thrice daily at 5 hours interval.

(4) The two most potent drugs for cataract are *Sep.* and *Nat-mur.* See "Eyes-cataract" and "Myopia."

Cataract-preventive—According to Biochemic exponent cataract is apt to develop when there is deficiency of salts. Dr. Oliver and Dr. P. Banerjee suggest the following salts for arresting the tendency of developing cataract: *Calc. fluor. 12X,* 4 tablets in the morning. *Calc. Phos 12X,* 4 tablets in the evening. *Net. mur.* and *Silicea 12X,* 4 tablets after principal meals ; while *Kali-phos. 12X,* be given at bed time. All these medicines are taken with warm water at least for three months. If there is diabetic tendency then *Nat.sulph.* should be added. *Tr. Cinerar mar.* drops may be droped in the eyes three times a day. Once preferably at bed time.

Catarrh—cold attended with discharge from mucous membrane of chest with consumption or sneezing—*Agar.* cures consumption, catarrhal condition of the chest, with night sweats and history of nervous symptoms. Violent cough in isolated attacks ending in sneezing. (*Agar.*). See also "Consumption-pulmonary" and "sneezing violent and excessive."

Catarrhal-chronic—*Sulph., Calc-Sil.,* in the order given one after another at the interval of a week is a useful method.

Catarrhal-deafness—Dr. Dewey thinks that *Kali-mur.* is the most valuable medicine for deafness following purulent or catarrhal otitis media. (*Kali-m.*). See "Ear deafness Catarrhal."

Catarrh nasal—cold attended with discharge from mucous membrane with herpes or bleeding scabs—(*a*) Nose red, harpes across the nose ; nose stuffed, chronic dry catarrh ; dry scabs readily bleeding. Discharge causing reddening of nose. (*Sulf.*).

(2) Nose completely closed so that the patient has to breathe through open mouth ; cronic dry catarrh of the nose. *Ammonium-carb.* and *Hepar-sulf.* according to symptom and *Lycopodium* which has strong influence in respiratory organs.

Catarrh-of nose blocks and breathing through mouth—Chronic, nose blocks on lying specially in night. Feeling of dryness. Discharge scanty and excoriating. Crusts and elastic plugs. Patient breathes through mouth. (*Lyco.*). See "Nose-block on lying" and "mouth open in sleep."

Catarrh-nose chronic dropping of mucus into throat—Constant dropping of mucus from back of nose into throat. (*Hydr.*). See "Nose" under its different heads.

Catarrh-of nose with blood—Chronic ; the patient frequently blows small quantities of blood. Bleeding from nose while blowing. (*Phos.*). See "Nose bleeding while blowing."

Catarrh-of nose with inflammation—Inflammation of an acute character with stringy discharges ; much pressure at the root of nose ; discharge of tough, green muscus, or hard plugs ; discharge dropping back into the throat and is stringy. *Kali bicromicum* is one sheet anchor in the treatment of disease of mucous membrane of the nose.

Catarrh-of nose thick-and large discharge with cough—Chronic nasal catarrh. Discharge thick, bland and in large quantity (*Kali-bi.* and *Puls.*). Yellowish saddle across nose ;

thick plug and crusts, pain at the root of the nose, cough must be hawked through mouth. (*Sep.*).

Catarrh-of the stomach—First give *Ipec.* and *Nux* if symptoms comes after eating but if there is much flatulence or rising of wind, *China* and then *Carbo-veg.*

Catarrh-with sneezing—Nasal discharge yellow and offensive ; tickling scraping cough; cold worse in the evening. On lying down the patient is forced to sit up to get rid of yellow mucous which accumulates; liking for sweet thing without thirst. Tendency for styes on upper lid. (*Pulsatilla.*).

Catarrh-of throat difficulty in swallowing—Bronchus of lungs inflamed ; inflammation of throat with stitches on swallowing ; better warm drinks. (*Lyco.*).

Catheter fever and avoiding its pain—(*a*) Its prophylactic is *Camphoric acid.* (*Camph-a*). (*b*) A dose of *Aconite* given shortly before passing a catheter will prevent pain, if there is any difficulty. (Dr. Clarke.) See "Stretches and remover of catheter Pain."

Cerebro-spinal meningitis—See "Chapter V for details".

Changeable symptoms—Pains wander from place to place and from joint to joint. (*Puls.*). See also "Pains wandering."

Changing disease—Changing of one so-called disease to another e.g. mumps to orchitis or mastitis (inflammation of the breast). (*Abrot.*) Compare *Carb-v.* and *Puls.* See "Metastasis."

Changing-position giving relief—Must change position constantly with relief for a short time by the change. Cannot lie on one position for long. In *Rhus-tox.* more the patient moves the better he feels. This relief from movements is a great characteristic of *Rhus-t.* Lying aggravates pain whereas walking about relieves the pain. This is just opposite of *Bry.* which is relieved by lying quietly. (*Rhus-tox.*). See also "Position changing".

Chapped hands and cracks in finger tips and palms perspiring—(1) Cracks at the ends of fingers and on the back of hands often much itching, skin rough and bleeding. (*Petr.*) (2) Dryness and cracking about finger nails, palms hot and perspiring. (*Nat-m*). See also "Finger-tips swollen", "Finger cracks" and "Palms and head perspiring."

Charcoal-fumes poisoning—*Ammon-carb*. See "Antidote" and "Poisoning charcoal-fumes."

Chest-violent cough with night sweat—Catarrhal condition of the chest, with night sweats and history of nervous symptoms. Violent cough in isolated attacks ending in sneezing. Cures consumption (*Agar.*). See "Night sweats."

Chest-weakness—With susceptibility to chills and colds, chronic catarrh, sore and septic throat, loss of weight, pallor, heavy perspiration at night, general weakness, temperature in the evening. (*Bacill.* and *Tuber* in high potencies.).

Chicken-pox—(1) *Variolinum* in *200* dilution one dose daily should be given at the commencement of treatment. Its administration is essential as it cuts short the disease.

(2) After 48 hours of administration of *Variolinum, Antimonium-tart.* should be given every 2 hours until fever lasts.

(3) *Bry.* should be given if there is fever and dry cough and the patient wants to lie quiet.

(4) *Merc-sol.* should be thought of after fever has left.

(5) Dr. Wadia suggests *Rhus-tox. 30* which will be very helpful in the cases of chicken-pox. As a preventive he suggests *Variolinum 200* one or two doses intercurrently.

Chicken pox-preventive—See "Chapter V for details."

Chilblains—(*a*) Sensation of coldness and warmth, pins and needles, stinging and burning where the sensation is feeble. The patient is extremely nervous and sensitive to cold. Itching and pricking. Burning of ears. (*Agar.*).

(*b*) Tips of fingers rough, cracked, fissured every winter; chilblains moist, itch and burn. Heels painfully swollen and red. Inflammation sets in every cold weather; Petrol. Parts deep red bluish, violent burning and itching, soles of feet particularly affected. *Puls* ; Chilblains in toes, foot sweat causing soreness in toes, patient loves fatty and saltish things (*Acid-n.*).

(*c*) Chilblains may be painted on the areas affected with *Tamus-communis* which will quickly remove the pain and gives great relief.

Child-frightened—*Aethusa-cynapium* is specially useful in children that rouse up in sleep frightened and in confusion like *Lycopodium*. See also "Fright-sleep", "Spasms of child during sleep" and "Crying of child" under its different heads.

Children's debilitating diseases—Difficulty in assimilation, difficulty in learning to walk or stand, difficult and delayed dentition. Sweating on head while asleep, vomiting and diarrhoea. Every thing smells sour. Abdomen enlarged. Body emaciated with large head. (*Calc.*). See also "Assimilation defective in children" and "Idiocy" and "Physically dwarf".

Children-late in learning to talking and walking—Compare *Natrum muriaticum* which has, "late learning to talk" and *Calcarea carb.* which has. "late learning to walk." These two features are combined in one remedy, *Agar.* In *Calcarea* it is due to defective bones. In *Agaricus* it is mental defect, a slowly developing mind. Children who cannot remember, make mistakes are slow in learning. The patient is sluggish aud stupid. (*Agar.*). See also "Walking delayed in fat children" under its different heads, also "Backward children" and "Under development in children".

Child-unmanageable—(1) Wild temper. Would fight with children and teachers in school. When angry would lock himself in lavatory. Easily frightened. Constitution thin and shiver. (*Phos.*).

(2) Difficult and bad tempered child. Kicks off the clothes and is rude to other children without any reason. Terrible

storm of temper. Violent rage and uncontrolled weeping. *Tuber. in* 30 *dilution,* one dose a week for about two months and repeat longer if necessary. See "Obstinate".

Chills-prevention against diseases due to chills—See "Chapter V for details".

Chilliness-must cover head, chilly patient—*Sil.* is a chilly patient. Must cover the head which relieves him. He lacks vital heat and is afraid to uncover the head or feet in cold weather. (*Sil.*). See "Vital force" and "Shivering-due to uncovering".

Chloroform-antidote—*Phosphorus* is the natural antidote to Chloroform. It will stop chloroform vomiting. (*Phos.*). See "Antidote".

Chloroform-its ill-effects—For bad effects of chloroform. (*Acet-ac.*). See also "ill-effects of chloroform".

Chloroform-nausea—ill-effects of chloroform. *Cham.* may be given for nausea and sickness after operation. (*Cham.*).

Chloroform-vomiting—Post-operative vomiting after chloroform anaesthesia. (*Phos.*). See "Vomiting due to morphine effect after operation."

Chlorosis-anaemia—Emaciated in cheeks and round the neck. General weakness. Nervous prostration or nervous irritability. Whether the anaemia is caused by loss of fluids, menstrual irregularity, loss of semen, grief or other mental diseases. Emaciation notwithstanding of what the patient eats. General Paleness, shortness of breath, palpitation. Loss of weight and throbbing headache. (*Nat-m.*). Dr. Nash recommends *Alumina* as a good medicine for chloratic condition. See "Anaemia-general weakness".

Choking—(1) If caused by copious mucus from posterior nose then give *Spigelia*.

(2) If choking due to heart-trouble. (*Cactus.*).

(3) Choking while eating and drinking. (*Mephitis.*). See "Breathlessness" and "Dyspnoea".

Cholera-with colic—With colic, agony, prostration and thirst. (*Ars-a.*). See "Cholera treatment".

Cholera infantum—Child with profuse, offensive and gushing stools lying prostrate with half closed eyes, perhaps moaning and rolling the head. The stool is offensive and at times, there may be prolapse of the rectum along with diarrhoea, with the aggravation in the morning, in hot weather and during dentition. The stools may be yellow or greenish-watery and when it is watery, it is always profuse. The child presses the gums together. Higher potency of *Podo.* has done the best in such cases. (*Podo.*).

Cholera infantum-sudden and extreme prostration—Vomiting and diarrhoea in children, extreme. prostration. It starts suddenly without notice in hot weather. The milk comes up partly in curds and partly liquid and accompanying the vomiting there is thin yellow greenish slimy stool. The child has the appearance as if it were dying, pale hippocratic face, there is a whitish-blue pallor around the lips, the eyes are sunken and there is sunken condition around the nose. The child sinks into an exhausted sleep. Death is stamped on the face from the beginning and if there is any medicine to save the life, it is this *Aethusa-c.* See also "Summer complaints of children during dentition".

Cholera infantum-worse by milk—Entero-colitis, always worse after taking milk (*Sep*). See "Entro-colitis of children" and "Milk-disagreeable".

Cholera-prophylactics—*Ars., Cupr-acet., Verat-a.,* (2) *Verat-a.* one dose daily is an excellent prophylactic according to Dr. Jahr. Some physicians prescribe *Verat-a,* and *Arsenic-a.* in alternation, *Verat-a.* one dose daily is given for 15 days, then *Arsenic-a.* is given in the same manner. All acids are prophylactics. Dr. Clarke recommends *Cuprum-aceticum 3X* to be given in little water night and morning for prevention. See "Prophylactics for other diseases".

Cholera-treatment—The four prominent symptoms of cholera are icy coldness of body, diarrhoea, vomiting and cramps. Against these four symptoms the remedies must be directed as follows :—(*a*) For coldness give *Camphor spirit* 2 to 5 drops in a little sugar every 5 to 10 minutes until warmth is restored 3 to 6 doses are sufficient. The patient must be well wrapped in blankets and hot water bottle placed around the limbs. Mustard plaster may be applied to the soles of feet. Enemas of warm saline solution (2 drops common salt to 20 ounces of water) should be given (*b*) For vomiting give *Ipec*. (*c*) For diarrhoea alternate *Ars*. and *Verat-a*. (S and V). In case of vomiting and diarrhoea alternate *Ipec*., *Ars*., *Verat-a* (I.S. and V.). For retention of urine give *Bell*. (*d*) For cramps give *Ars*. and *Cuprum-met*. The medicines may be given in the 3X or 6X potency. 2 or 3 drops may be given a dose in a little spoonful of water or a solution of each medicine may be prepared by mixing 5 to 10 drops in 4 ounces of water and of this medium spoonful given each time. Doses may be given every hour or every half an hour or oftener. Diet should consist of conjee water then arrow-root without milk, plain water. If there is vomiting do not give any food or drink. In convalescence great care in diet is required, else a relapse will take place. The above treatment has had great success in Father Mullers' Cholera camp. The Cholera chest should consist of *Camphor spirits, I* (=*Ipec. 2X*) *S* (=*Ars.3X*). *V* (*Virat-alba. 2X*) *Bell. 3X, Cup-met*. 6. Dr. Dass Gupta recommends *Hydrocyan-ac.* for sudden cessation of all discharges when respiration is irregular, and long standing faints, for suppression or retention of urine, absence of stool and vomiting Laurocerasus and for perfect picture of uraemia when urine is completely suppressed *Arum-triphyllum*. See "Asiatic cholera.

Cholera-rice water stool—Usual rice water stool ; vomiting and purging, stool profuse, gushing, prostrating. (*Verat*). Compare *Camphor* which has less profuse stool and the patient does not want to be covered.

Chorea—It is a nervous disorder characterised by irregular and involuntary action of the muscles : of the extremities and face. Numbness associated with pain (*Asaf.*).

Chorea in all parts of body-general—Twitching, tremblings, and jerkings ; quivering and tremors everywhere, these two are present in all parts of the body and limbs ; twitching of eye-lids. All jerkings ; twitching of eye-lids. All jerkings, twitchings subside during sleep. (*Agar.*).

Chronic-ulcers—Malignant chronic ulcers, bed-sores, carbuncles provided the dark blue colour is present. (*Lach.*). See also "Ulcers" under its different heads.

Cicatrix (scar or mark of wound)—A painful cicatrix with pain shooting up towards the centre of the body along the course of nerve always requires, *Hyper.* See also "Scar injured with pain" and "Tumours recurrent".

Cicatrin-scar with cold damp feet on left side of neck—On the left side of neck. Cold damp feet. Before the cicatrization could take place, the patient had a fistulous opening which was finally closed. As the *Calcarea carb* symptom of cold stocking was there, so by giving this medicine the cicatrix will suppurate and ultimately heal up without leaving any scar. (*Calc-c*).

Circumcision— *Staphy.* Give before the incision for circumcision, allays the pain following incision and prevents inflammation.

Cirrhosis of liver—(1) *Nasturt., Nat-chlo., Merc.* (2) Fatty infiltraion of liver and increase in soft fibrous tissue. Anaemia and absence of fever are characteristic. (*Kali-bi.*). See also "Liver" under its different heads.

(3) *Lyco.* is specially adapted for the treatment of liver cirrhosis.

(4) In the last stage of dropsy from Cirrhosis of liver. (*Mur-ac.*).

(5) For atrophic and hyperatrophic varieties of Cirrhosis of liver. (*Phos.*). See "Liver chronic and enlarged."

Clergyman's sore throat—loss of voice—Sudden loss of voice of singers and public speakers or of a lawyer, who is making his final efforts to sum up a case, speaking for hours, can be cured with *Arum-t.* enabling him to go on with his speech in a clear voice. It is specially suitable if the voice is uncertain and uncontrollable changing continually in its tone. (*Arum-t.*). Compare *Rhus-t.* and *Phos.* Also see "Voice lost suddenly."

Climacteric-headache—See "Headache at climacteric"

Climacteraic—Period of organic change—Cessation of menstrual function or menopause—(1) *Lachesis* is the head remedy for this period, severe headache beginning at the back and passing over to the front of the head. Flushing. Melancholic and irritable. It is suitable for haemorrhage, burning and vertigo. Fainting fit. Ustlilago often rivals *Lach.* in controlling the symptom.

(2) Rheumatism .or Rheumatic diathesis, muscles of the back and neck sore. Violent headache. (*Actea rac.*)

(3) Leucorrhoea, corrosive, fetid continued after menses cease. (*Sanguinaria.*)

(4) Mental diseases at the time of the change of the life. (*Fraxinus-am.*).

(5) The patient tried, wants to lie down, has a backache and vericose veins. (*Bellis--per.*).

(6) Facial neuralgia of the left side worse at bed time. Great nervous tension and unrest with propensity to work and worry of little things. (*Caulophyllum*). See "Menopause" under. different heads.

Coccyx-pain— See "Chapter V for details."

Coccyx-the last bone of the spinal column-injured—Injuries of coccyx from a fall are the most troublesome injuries on the spine at times. Many women sustain injuries of coccyx during labour and the soreness may remain for years thereafter. This little injury may make her quite nervous or hysterical. This can be cured by *Hyper.* See "Spine-injuries."

Coition—(1) Absence of spermatozoa in impotency ; chronic prostatic discharge (*Damiana*). (2) Want of energy in coition in impotency, emissions provoked by presence of women (*Conium.*). (3) Impotency due to masturbation. Penis relaxed with violent sexual desire. Erection when half sleep in the morning, ceasing when fully awake (*Caladium*). (4) Extreme sexual excitement (*Tarentula-h.*). See also "Impotency under its different heads."

Cold and its aborting— (*a*) *Calc.* causes grand cure in cold. Fat and flabby patient. Chilly. (*Calc.*). (*b*) *Ammon-carb.* will often abort a recent cold while *Cistus canadensis* aborts cold that centres in posterior nose. See "Prevention of cold."

(*c*) Dr. Blackie recommends *Ferr. phos. 12X* given quickly at the first sign of cold and then repeated for 3 or 4 doses every 10 minutes will often abort cold.

Cold-cold air causing sneezing—(*a*) Going out in cold air causes sneezing or running of nose. Nose stopped. Extremely sensitive to cold air. (*Hep.*). (*b*) *Nux-v.* 3 may prevent a cold if given early before the commencement of the running of nose. Compare *Acon.* See also "Sneezing-susceptible to cold."

Cold after exposure—Colds often exposure to wet, specially causing diarrhoea headache. Dry coryza. Complete stoppage of nose. Thick, yellow mucus, bloody crusts. Least cold stops the nose. Coryza of the new born. Hot days and cold nights towards the close of summer are specially favourable to the action of *Dulcamara*. See also "Exposure to cold" and "Nose stopped when going out."

Cold application and cold air relieves—*Puls.* Patient feels hot and is better in cool air and from cold application, locally.

Pains are better from cold application. The headache is better in cold air, and cool washing of head, etc. Relieved by cool open air, especially walking about slowly in open air, cold food and cold drinks. (*Puls.*).

Cold-from taking cold drink or cold food when one is hot—Drinking cold drink when the body is heated. Complaints due to cold food or drink when the body is heated and inffection due to cold wind or when cold water suddenly brought into contact with a heated body. (*Bellis-perennis*).

Cold-sneezing-immediate relief from it—Apply *Aconite* 6 or *Nat. mur.* 6 two or three drops on the tongue and sneezing stopped within two or three minutes. After it give *Bry. 30* or *Allium cepa. 6*.

Cold-aggravated in warm room—*All-c.* medicine is used principally for colds. Cold in the nose, throat, or larynx. Aggravated in a warm room. Worse in the evening. There must be rawness in the nose and rawness in the throat going down to chest. (*All-c.*).

Cold and cough-change of season—Cold and cough starting with getting wet or in the rainy season or change of season ; fever with cough. There must be restlessness, thirst and chilliness. (*Rhus-t.*). See "Periodicity."

Cold-common—Dry, tickling, cough, with only a little expectoration after a long paroxysm of coughing, mucus collects in the back of the throat and can't be easily dislodged and the patient may have to swallow it. Sneezing and blockage of nostrils in the morning. Urination frequent with the cold and sometimes incontinence on sneezing or coughing or blowing the nose. (*Causticum*).

Cold-loss of smell and taste—(1) Loss of smell with cold (*Sulf. 4* hrly.).

(2) Loss of taste with cold. (*Puls. 4* hrly.).

(3) Loss of taste and smell with cold. (*Mag-mur.*). See also "Smell sensitiveness and its loss"

Cold sensitiveness—(1) Sensitive to cold (*Agar.*).

(2) Very chilly and often worse in cold dry day. (*Ars-alb.*).

(3) Worse in cold dry weather and better in damp weather. (*Nitric acid*).

(4) Very sensitive to cold particularly to cold windy weather. (*Hepar-sulph*).

(5) Worse in dry cold weather but better on rainy days. (*Nux-v.*).

Cold air-extremely sensitive—Extremely sensitive to cold air. Wants to close all doors and windows and sit near the fire in cold weather ; cold air makes everything worse for *Hepar* patient locally as generally (*Hep.*). See "Wet weather-cold air and full moon causing aggravation."

Cold-draught sensitive—The patient is very sensitive to cold draught, light, touch and sound. (*Chin.*). See "Tendency to catch cold and aborting it."

Cold in dry weather—Sticking, sensation on the back of the throat and dry teasing cough at the beginning of the cold. The patient is chilly and will want to be covered up. Suffocations, croupy cough in the middle of the night. Give *Hepar-sulph*, which will stop developing of bronchitis.

Cold-ripe—(*a*)—The mucus assumes a thicker consistency instead of watery discharge. (*Puls.*). (*b*) The discharge from nose mucopurulent of yellowish green. (*Merc-sol.*). See also "Ripe cold."

Coldness in abdomen—The peculiar sensation of coldness in the abdomen as if the whole inside of abdomen was cold. (*Ambra.*).

Coldness of whole body with hiccough or cold sweat—Icy coldness of the body with cramps and obstinate hiccough, frequent vomiting, purging and cold sweat. (*Cupr-ars.*). (*b*) Coldness of the whole body of all internal parts such as heart, brain, lungs and kidneys, etc., even the breath is cold with paralysis and tremors, coldness of body with slow pulse and sinking. Give *Heloderma* 200 dilution. See "Sensation peculiar over the body."

Cold immunity from it—Recurring cold, congestion of the synuses, nasal obstruction, with discharge, burning nostrils. *Sulf.* will give immunity against such cold and coryza.

Colic—Gall-stone colic. (*Calc.*). See also "Gall-stone colic" under its different heads.

Colic-in babies—Wind colic in babies, making the little thing almost double up. Cutting and tearing pains. It screams with the violent cutting in the lower abdomen ; worse around the navel ; worse when sitting. (*All-c*). See also "Wind-trouble."

Colic-burning round navel—Soreness and burning round navel at every attempt to eat ; colicky pain in 'abdomen. (*Calc-ren*).

Colic of child in dysentery—Colic in acute dysentery. Specially in a child ; this abdominal colic occurs very often in which a child bends double in pain or draws legs. (*Coloc.*). See also "Dysentery-with colic."

Colic-with diarrhoea and vomiting—After eating or drinking accompanied by diarrhoea, dysentery and vomiting. Colic relieved by bending double or drawing the legs to abdomen. *Coloc.* is a supreme remedy for all severe abdominal colics. Specially in a child this abdominal colic occurs very often in which a child bends double in pain or draws legs. Such a colic is often found in acute dysentery. (*Coloc.*). Compare *Mag-p.* if relief is prompt from fomentation. Remember also *Staphy.*, *Dioscorea.*, *Stannum*, and *Mag-phos.* for colic pain. See also "Diarrhoea-with colic."

Colic-general with sharp pain and flatulence—Intestinal flatulent, forcing patient to bend double ; sharp and cramping pain ; often changing places. Pains relieved by warmth (*Mag-p.*). Compare *Chamomilla*.

Colic-infants—(*a*) Bending double, flatulent ; relieved by rubbing and warmth than by pressure. (*Mag-p.*). Compare *Coloc.* (*b*) When child seems to be full of wind ; liver enlarged and tender ; constipation with colic flatulence ; loss of appetite stool hard. (*Senna.*),

Colic-menstrual—Colic menstrual, hysterical or nervous. (*Cocculus.*). See "Menstruation with colic or diarrhoea."

Colic-pains in bowels—Abdominal colic round the navel. There are colicky pains in the bowels from eating or drinking when there is no diarrhoea, even when there is a state of constipation. The patient bends up like *Colocynth,* with abdominal colic round the navel. (*Aloe*).

Colic-pains at interval—Pains appear suddenly and intensively and disappears again very suddenly *i.e.* they come and go at intervals. (*Bell.*).

Colic-periodical—Colic at certain hour each day, periodical from gall-stone (*Chin.*). See "Periodicity."

Colic-renal (pertaining to kidney) difficult urination with stone in kidney—Violent paroxysms of cutting ; burning in whole renal region, with painful urging to urinate ; bloody urine by drops. Intolerable tenesmus. Cutting before, during and after urine. Constant desire to urinate. Urine scalds him and is passed drop by drop. Stone in kidney *Cantharis* to be given during attack. (*Canth*). See "Renal colic."

Colic-renal (pertaining to kidney) with gravel pain in right kidney—Urine scanty, slimy, flaky, sandy, bloody. Gravel renal colic ; severe, almost unbearable pain at conclusion or urination. Bladder distended and tender. Pain from right kidney downward, child screams before and while passing urine. (*Sars.*).

Colic-renal (pertaining to kidney) stone in kidney and its prevention—(1) Violent sticking pains in the bladder extending from kidney to urethra with urging to urinate *Berbaris vulgar.* This is head remedy for renal colic. (*Berb.*).

(2) Agonising pain, twists about, screams and groans, urine red with brick dust sediment. (*Ocimum-canum*).

(3) Writhing with crampy pains, must move about. (*Dioscorea*).

(4) Urine becomes turbid like clay water immediately after passing ; much pain at the end of urinating white sand, scanty, slimy, flaky urine. Teresmus of bladder (*Saras.*).

(5) When all remedies fail, then *Pareira brava* may be given in mother tincture in hot water in 4 drops doses every half hour. (*Pareir*).

(6) Preventives—gravelling urine pain back and loins- *Berbaris vulgar.* 6 hourly. Tendency to stone, uric acid in the tissue. (*Urtica urens*).

(*b*) (*i*) Dr. Jousset says that *Bell., Cham.*, are given in alternation when pains are violent regardless of the diseases which produced them in renal. (*ii*) Dr. Jahr says that *Puls., Cannabis., Sarasap.* and *Lyco.* have done wonders in his hands in alleviating renal colic and facilitating the passage of calculus through urethra. (*iii*) Dr. Preston used *Arg-nit.* when there is dull aching across the small of the back and also over the region of the bladder. (*iv*) *Ipomoea nil* has been used by Dr. Jacob Jeams for the passages of stone from kidney to bladder. Dr. Hempal records many cases of renal colic cured with *Coccus cacti.* (*v*) *Eupatorium purpureum* has to be used when there is a considerable amount of gravel deposit in the urine, dull pains in the renal regional and urine mixed with mucus, and also urinary tenesmus. (*vi*) *Nitric acid* should be though of when the urine contains oxalic acid and when that substance is principal ingredient of stone. See "Renal colic", "Gall-stone colic" and "Stone in kidney."

Colic-of pregnant women—Colic is as frequent in pregnancy as vomiting and anorexia (loss of appetite). Generally the trouble consists of abdominal spasms that set during the first months of pregnancy and not confounded with false labour pains. The best remedy is *Cham.* When there is wind in bowels; if this fails then *Nux-vomica* or *Colocynth* if the pains are extreme not allowing the patient to rest. See "Pregnancy—its affections."

Colic-stone with nausea—Renal colic is caused by a stone in the ureter. Colicy pains which urge to stool and urination ; pains extend towards rectum, with nausea from over-eating. (*Nux-v.*). See "Stone in kidney."

Colic-wind colic and diarrhoea corroding—Abdomen distended, wind colic ; stool green and watery corroding the anus, stool feels hot and smells like rotten egg. (*Cham.*). See "Diarrhoea—with colic."

Colic-due to indigestion—(1) *Nux-v.* is the head remedy for colic due to indigestion. It should be given in hot water. The pain may be in any part of abdomen.

(2) *Cuprum met.* is an excellent remedy for inflammatory colic, violent spasms of colic as if a knife was thrust into abdomen. (*Cupr met.*). See "Indigestion under its different heads".

Colic-radiating in all directions—Abdominal pain radiating in all directions, walls drawn in, cramps in legs and obstinate constipation but no flatulence ; stony hardness of abdomen. (*Plumbum*). See "Pains wandering".

Colitis and its treatment—(*a*) Treatment should be started with *Sulph.* 200. It would cure a large number of cases without any other remedy. (*i*) Membranous discharges, flatulence and constipation. (*Arg-n.* 30, 4 hourly.) (*ii*) Stools like scrapings of intestines, burning pains, thirst, nausea and vomiting (*Canth.*). (*iii*) *Thuj.* is an excellent remedy for colitis or amoebic dysentery to be given 1M potency. (*iv*) *Merc-c.* alternated with *Coloc.* are never failing remedies for such a trouble. See "Mucous colitis" or "Dysentery under its different heads".

(*b*) **Colitis-with pain and mucus**—Griping, cutting pains that cause the patient to writhe and bend double, press upon the abdomen, asks for hot application and made worse by eating and drinking. (*Coloc.*).

Collapse (general)—Hands and feet and surface of the body cold and blue ; patient lies motionless as if dying, breath cold, pulse thready and quick, cold sweat on the limbs ; voice lost, blueness of the finger tips ; feet icy cold up to the knees. (*Carbo-veg.*). Compare *Verat-a.* See "Serious conditions-collapse".

Collapse-Hahnemann's trio of collapse in cholera—(1) *Camphor,* collapse with scanty sweat, vomiting and purging or none of them at all-dry cholera.

(2) *Verat-a.* Collapse being the result of profuse draining discharge.

(3) *Cupr-met.* is indicated by the predominance of cramps.

Collapse-after operation—Collapse symptoms after surgical operations, great prostration, coldness of body, show oozing of the blood, cold breath and profuse perspiration will require *Strontiana carb.* It relieves shock at once and the patient gets warm and comfortable. (*Stron-c.*). See also "Shock of operation-collapse".

Collapse-cold sweats in cholera, measles, eruptive fevers—Rapid sinking of forces ; complete prostration, cold sweat and cold breath. Skin blue, purple, cold, wrinkled, face hippocratic (an appearance of the face indicative of rapid approach of dissolution ; the nose is pinched, the temples hollow, the eyes sunken, the ears leaden and cold, the lips relaxed and the skin livid). Whole body is icy cold, cramps in calves. "Cold sweat on face and forehead" such condition to be found in acute cases of cholera, pneumonia, typhoid, or intermittent fever, bronchitis or suppressed eruptive fever such as measles or scarlet fever or an eruption of skin, provided it is attended with profuse sweat. (*Verat.*) Compare *Ars.*, *Carb-v.* See also "Coma in diphtheria, measles, small-pox" and "Vital force exhausted and consequential collapse".

Collapse-in typhoid pneumonia and cholera—There *Carb-v.* may save life which is extinguishing ; hands, feet, surface of the body cold and blue, patient lies motionless as if dying ; breath cold, pulse thready and quick, cold sweats on the limbs; voice lost ; blueness of the finger tips ; feet icy cold up to the knees. (*Carb-v.*), Compare *Verat-a.* See also "Coma" under its different heads.

Collapse-with respiration trouble—The patient is pulseless, respiration is slow, deep, gasping or difficult and spasmodic. Pulse weak and irregular. Hysterical and epileptic convulsion, collapse in cholera, according to Dr. Sarkar *Hydrocyanic acid* will work as charm and would restore animation to a cropse.

Colour blindness—(1) There is every conceivable kind of deception in colours and vision. Various bodies fly before the eyes. The jerkings and twitching of the eye-lids. (*Agar.*). Compare (*Carb-sulf.*). (2) *Phosphorus* is another remedy for this disease. (*Phos.*). See also "Eye troubles", "Vision" and "Eyes-colour blindness".

Cool atmosphere-relieves—The patient wants to expose his body to the cool atmosphere. Open air relieves. Relief by open doors and windows. The patient kicks the feet out of cover. (*Sulf.*). Compare *Phos.* in which patient cannot cover hands. See "Feet burning".

Coma in apoplexy, typhoid and diabetes—(*i*) In apoplexy. (*Baryta-carbonica.*) (*ii*) Involuntary stool and urination, uraemic, pulse slow. (*Opium*). (*iii*) In typhoid fever, (*Baptisia-t., Phosphorus, Arnica.*) (*iv*) In diabetes (*Aluminium metallicum-200*). See also "Collapse" under its different heads and "Unconsciousness".

Coma-in diphtheria measles, small pox—The child is rapidly going into coma. Continued dreamy state while awake, pupils dilated. The child whines or cries all the time. Great prostration. The course of disease is usually sudden and goes into seriousness in diphtheria, measles ; small-pox, etc. (*Ailanthus*). See also "Collapse-cold sweat in typhoid-pneumonia".

Complaints-of anger—Colic or other complaints as a consequence of anger. (*Coloc.*). See "Anger complaints".

Complaints-one sided—See "One sided complaints".

Company aversion—(1) Of friends, tries to get away from them. (*Coloc.*).

(2) In hysteria. (*Cactus.*)

(3) In nervous patient. (*Ignatia*). See "Unsocial".

Company-desire for—(1) In heart diseases. (*Aurum-met.*)

(2) In hysteria. (*Conium*).

(3) In mania. (*Stramonium*).

Complexion-changing it into fair—(1) *Iodum* is an exellent remedy for changing complexion to fair colour. It should be used in 1000 potency every fortnight for about 6 months.

(2) *Caust.* and *Lyco.* to be tried in the given order when Iodum fails. Use in 200 potency every week.

Concussion of brain or spine :

(*i*) There is no medicine which equals *Arnica* in such cases. It is to be given in increasing potencies in repeated doses.

(*ii*) *Bry.* and *Hell.* should be tried.

(*iii*) If the trouble still persists *Cicuta* should be the next remedy and then *Bell.* and *Phos.*

(*iv*) For the chronic after effects of concussion *Cicuta* is the best remedy.

(*v*) *Rhus-tox.* and *Calc-c.* are most useful for spinal concussion. See "Brain concussion" and "Spine injuries".

Condylomata—(*a*) A wart like growth or tumour usually near anus or external genital organs specially of females, as a consequence of gonorrhoeal infection or otherwise all symptoms of suppressed gonnorrhoea. (*Thuj.*) See "Warts" under its different heads.

(*b*) Dr. Nash recommends the celebrated trio *Thuja, Stappisagric, Nitric Acid* for condylomala.

Confinement-abdomen pendulous—Pendulous abdomen after confinement. (*Podo.*) See "Abdomen pendulous after confinement"

Confinement-made easy—*Act-rac.* make confinement easy in hysterical and rheumatic patients. (*Act-rac.*). See also "Pregnancy-its affections" and "Pregnancy disorders".

Confusion of mind-in presence of others causing forgetfulness—Confusion of mind and embarrassment in presence of other presons. The toughts vanish in presence of other persons and strangers. Melancholy, sits weeping for days. Feebleness of mind, forgetfulness, which is common in old age, appear earlier. He asks one question and then moves to another without waiting for a reply ; or jumps from the stage to another without concluding the one. Alternation of depression with vehemence of temper. He gets up with confusion and dulness in mind. Hence aggravation in the morning and excitability in the evening. He cannot pass his stool in the presence of nurse. Music intolerable. (*Ambra.*) See also ',Mind confusion" under its different heads, and "Head".

Confusion-in diphtheria—*Lachesis.* See "Diphtheria followed by paralytic weakness".

Congestion of brain—Like *Bell., Gels.* has congestion of brain but neither the fever nor the congestion is so intense as in *Bell.* (*Gels.*). See also "Brain concussion" and "Brain-congestion".

Congestion of lungs—Burning pains, heat and oppression of chest ; tightness across chest ; sharp stitches in chest ; respiration quickened and oppressed. The cough is dry. Pain and distress under sternum (The breast bone). *Phosphorus* See "Lungs congestion due to lying down".

Congestion of lungs in dropsy—In dropsy ; congestion of lungs due to prolonged lying in bed compelling the patient to sit up. This hypostatic condition gradually creeps upwards so that a large portion of the breathing space is destroyed. It has a rattling breathing also. Difficult breathing. Gasping breath. Pulse small and irregular. (*Apoc-c*). See also "Hypostatic-congestion of lungs in Dropsy" and "Lungs congested in dropsy".

Conjunctiva—(1) Eyes red and congested. Red eyes at times ; eye-lids swollen. (*Bell.*).

(2) *Puls.* will be indicated where the discharge is thick and yellow glueing the lids. For profuse purulent discharge. *Arg-nit.* See also "Vision".

Conjunctivitis—(*a*) *Acon., Puls., Euphr., Guarea.* For lids closed, red, swollen, painful and photophobia. (*Calc-c.*)

(*b*) *Hepar* is one of the most important for conjunctivitis specially in cases that do not yield to *Acon.* or *Bell.* follows these remedies well. See "Eyes red".

(*c*) **Conjunctivitis with sharp pain**—Burning and stinging pain. Eye-lids swollen and red ; eyes feel better when washed with cold water. (*Apis-mel.*).

Conjunctivitis-watering and swelling with irritation—Watering of eyes, agglutinated lids in the morning. Margins of lids red swollen and burning. Discharge of acrid matter ; discharge thick and excoriating along with irritation of the eyes. (*Euphr.*)

(2) For oedamatous and swelling and acrid discharge (*Rhus-t.*).

(3) For pricking and itching sensation and profuse lachrymation. (*Zinc-sulph.*). See "Eyes watering with redness".

Consolation causing aggravation or weeping—(1) *Nat-m* patient is more irritated and disturbed by consolation. Weeping alternates with laughing. Consolation aggravates every mental symptom mainly the irritability and weeping, sad and joyless patient under even most cheerful circumstances. The prostration of mind as well as of body are the main features. (*Nat-m.*). · Compare it with *Puls.*

(2) Nothing pleases a *Puls*. patient more then consolation. She is immediately soothed by sympathy. *Puls*. girl often weeps while stating symptoms. (*Puls.*). Compare *Nat-m.* Patient is more disturbed and irritated by consolation. See also "Derangements at puberty" and "Weeping tendency in girls".

Constant-spitting—See (*b*) of "Saliva producing rawnes and constant spitting".

Constipation—(1) Constipation due to dryness of the intestinal tract and non-peri staltic action of the intestine, no desire for and no ability to pass stool until there is large accumulation. Great straining, must grasp the seat tightly, stool hard, knotty or soft adhering to the Parts. Stool like sheep dung. *Alumina*. Useful also for constipation of infants when stool green and rectum sore.

(2) Constipation due to the inaction of intestines. Stool hard, dry black balls. No urge for stool. (*Opium*).

(3) Loss of muscular activity and diminished secretion of intestinal glands. (*Plumbum*).

(4) Stool is hard to expel and causes bleeding, smarting and soreness in the rectum. (*Nat-mur.*).

(5) Constipation alternating with looseness of bowels with dull headache. Foul tongue, with piles and after abuse of purgatives. (*Hydrast.*).

(6) Diarrhoea of infants alternating with constipation. Difficult dentition with colicky pain. Fetid stool. (*Podophyllum*) (*b*) Whenever constipation is one of many symptoms of disordered health, the medicines directed to the chief disorder will usually remove the constipation. Also Spigelia in heart affections, Iris in migraine. *Gelsemium in* headaches, *Bry.*, *Calc-c.*, *Lyco.* and *Nux-v.* in typhoid. (*c*) Constipation caused by travelling ; (*Alumina* ; *Platina*.).

Constipation alternating with diarrhoea—The patient has never a clear motion and desires to go to stool several times without satisfaction but even a small quantity of stool relieves him for the time being. *Alternate constipation and diarrhoea in persons who have taken purgative all their lives.* (*Nux vomica*).

(*b*) Diarrhoea alternates with constipation ; often found in old people. The only remedy for this is *Antim crude.*

Constipation-since last confinement—Since puberty or last confinement, developing piles. Of infants with ineffectual urging, rectum contracts and protrudes during stool. (*Lyco.*)

Constipation-chronic with hard stool balls—Hard black balls ; chronic, stools large, stool recedes after being partially expelled, violent rectal pains. (*Thuj.*).

Constipation-chronic no stool for days—(*a*) *Aloe.* is useful in old chronic sufferers from this trouble who go many days without stool, but feel every little while (or several times in a day) that they must go to stool and then only a little wind passes. *Natrum-sulph.* will very commonly over-come that state. (*b*) Constipation of the most aggravated kind. No desire for stool for days. No ability to expel stool. Marble like masses pass but rectum still feels full. (*Alumina*).

Constipation-in all ages—Dr. Clarke recommends *Silica marina* for constipation for patients of all ages. This medicine is also useful in constipation always before and during menses.

Constipation-no desire for days together—Of long standing. Goes 4 to 6 days without desire. Large stools difficult to expel. Strains until covered with sweat to pass stool. (*Sanic.*).

Constipation-frequent unsuccessful desire—Frequent unsuccessful desire ; hard ; knotty, insufficient, itching and burning of anus. Child is afraid to have the stool on account of pain ; alternating with diarrhoea. (*Sulf.*).

Constipation-in old persons with ineffectual desire—Inveterate constipation in old persons. Frequent ineffectual desire for stool ; this makes patient very anxious ; at this time presence of other persons becomes unbearable. (*Ambra.*).

Constipation-obstinate, stool like sheep dung—An obstinate constipation with hard stools, unsatisfactory motions, sometimes stools in small balls like sheep-dungs. Anus is often cracked, bleeding and smarting after stool. (*Nat-m*).

Constipation-difficult expulsion—Difficult expulsion of even soft stool. Stool slips back again after protruding out. (*Sil.*).

(*b*) When faeces remain high up, or do not come down into the rectum and where enemas also do not act to excite desire. (*Hydr., Can.*).

Constipation-women during pregnancy—Habitual constipation of a very obstinate character especially in women and children. Sensation of weight and ball in the pelvis pressing on the rectum, not relieved by passing of the stool. Constipation during pregnancy, stool hard, knotty, in balls, insufficient; pain in rectum during and long after stool. (*Sep.*). See "No. 2 of pregnancy affections".

Constipation-causing rheumatism—Constipation causing rheumatism. Diarrhoea gives relief. (*Abrot.*). See "Rheumatism due to checked diarrhoea or constipation".

Constipation-rectum powerless—*Anac.* is of service when there is a great desire for stool but with the effort the desire passes away without any ejaculation. The rectum seems powerless as if paralyzed with a sensation as if pluggo-spasmodic condition of sphincter.

Constipation-stool like dog stool—Faeces slender, long, dry, tough like dog-stool. (*Phos*).

Constipation-stool hard—Stool hard, dry, as if burnt, inactive. No inclination. (*Bry.*).

Constipation-no urging—Offensive stool, inactivity, stool lies in rectum without urging, sensation of constriction of sphincter. (*Lach*). Remember *Nux., Sulph., Bry., Alumina* and *Lyco.* generally for constipation. See "Urging to stool."

Consumption-galloping—See "No. 12 of Tuberculosis."

Consumption-palliative—*Am-c.* is a good palliative in last stage of consumption. (*Am-c*). For hectic fever. (*Arsen-iod.*). For perspiration profuse and abundant. (*Stannum.*). See "Tuberculosis."

Consumption pulmonary—Pulmonary with night sweats. *Calc.* is one of the most effective agents in curing pulmonary consumption. (*Calc.*). *Calc.-c.* is recommended for fat subjects and *Calc-p.* for thin subjects. Both these remedies follow *Tuberculinum* and will cure the remnants of the disease. See also "Tuberculosis" and "Hectic fever".

Contracture of muscles—Contracture of muscles and tendons due to injury or burn or any septic process is usually removed *by Causticum* if given high. (*Caust*). See also "Injury-causing contracture" and "Burns-causing contracture."

Contracture of tendons—Contracture of tendons due to an injury or burn or any septic process is usually removed by *Causticum* if given high (*Caust.*). See "Burns-causing contracture" and "Bruises of tendons insertion of tendons."

Contusion-skin ruptured—Contusion or bruises where skin is in any way ruptured. *Arnica., Rhus-t* and *Calc-carb.* See "Skinslight-injuries fester" and "Bruise of skin."

Convalescence-after lingering disease—*Apoc-can.* is very useful in low form of disease such as typhoid and is useful after a lingering disease in the convalescent period. Patients who become generally prostrated, very chilly and anaemic and have great thirst with scanty urine and dry skin require *Apocynum.* very often for recouping their health. Dropsy also sets in very often at this stage. Under several circumstances *Apis.* would be indicated provided patient is hot, wants to be uncovered and wants cold things only and usually with scanty thirst. If patient has no appetite and has a good deal of thirst with chilliness and reluctance to uncover, he requires *Apocynum.* (*Apoc.*). *Psorinum* is very useful for weakness or debility during convalescene from severe acute diseases. See also "Prostration-at the end of a serious infectious disease."

C

Convulsion—(1) Convulsions with blue face and clenched fists. Jerking and twitching of the extremities. Rolling of the eye-balls. Vomiting. Also in whooping cough. (*Cupr-met*).

(2) Convulsions during dentition. Head hot with throbbing pain, eyes staring and pupils dilated, feet cold. *Bell. 200* to be repeated every 4th day till recovery.

(3) Convulsions due to the bad digestion. Chewing motion of the jaws. (*Nux-vomica*). See also "Dentition-inability to digest milk and convulsions." and "Convulsions, "in Chapter II of Homoeopathy in Paedriatic.

(4) Convulsions occuring after a fall or blow on the head ; the body becomes stiff and neck and back are bent backward or sideways. (*Cicuta-virosa*).

Convulsions-during fever of children—Starting from sleep during fever of children and jerking of muscles of fingers and toes. (*Bell*). See also "Dentition" under its different heads.

Convulsions-after child birth—After child-birth or after loss of blood. (*Chin*). See "No. 39 Pregnancy-disorder of."

Convulsions-child grinding teeth—Child bores the fingers in the nose and grinds teeth while asleep. Jumps and jerks in sleep. Very restless while asleep. The child is very ugly and cross like *Chamomila*. Kicks and strikes the nurse. It does not like to be touched. (*Cina.*). See "Grinding of teeth."

Convulsions-hysterical—Hysterical spasms and convulsions. Girls having pain in back of neck and headache. (*Actrac.*) See "Hysteria-convulsions."

Convulsions of epileptic type—(*a*) Convulsions from being scolded, from excitement and shock. More commonly the hysterioepileptic type with forthing of the mouth. Drawing of the muscles of the face. Muscles of the face will quiver and then stop and in another part of the face the similar condition. Eye-lids will quiver. The tongue quivers. (*Agar.*). (*b*) The patient becomes rigid. Jaws locked, bites tongue, forthing, at the mouth, unconsciousness. (*Cicuta-virosa*). See "Epilepsy" under its different head

Convulsions of child with sweat—In children with sleepiness and prostration, with clammy (sticky) hands, deathly countenance, and the sweat, exhaustion, and sleep. Eyes turned downwards. (*Aeth.*).

Convulsions due to tetanus—Convulsions with tetanic rigidity where injured parts are icy-cold and when spasms begin in the wounded part. *Ledum.* is the remedy. (*Led.*). See also "Tetanus" under its different heads.

Convulsions due to wounds—Convulsions with wounds in such parts as soles, fingers or palms need *Hypericum.* (*Belladonna, Ledum, Hypericum.*)

Convulsions-teething child—Of teething children. Also in night-mares. (*Acon.*). See "Dentition" under its different heads.

Corns-inflamed or burning—(1) *Thuj.* is head remedy.

(2) Inflamed or ulcerated. (*Nitr-acid*).

(3) With stinging and burning, the part becomes back ; feeble circulation in the skin. (*Ph-a.*).

(4) *Hypericum* is very useful for very painful corns and bunion.

(5) For local application, for painful corns a solution of *Salicylic acid* one in five to be painted on the corn at bed time, two or three nights, is often successful. See also "Warts."

Corn-soft and hard—*Sulf.* is the principal internal remedy for soft corns while *Antimon-crud.* is the principal internal remedy for hard corns.

Corns on soles—The feet are covered on the soles with corns and thickened patches of skin caused by friction or pressure and the patient can hardly stand on them on account of this tenderness. Pain in heels. Inflamed corn. (*Antimon crudu.*) See "Soles burning with feet out."

Corpulency—(1) Tendency to obesity particularly adapted to females who delay menstruation ; menses too late with constipation. Patients who are rather stout, of fair complexion with tendency to skin trouble. (*Graph.*).

(2) Persons who are fat, indolent, opposed to physical exertion, averse to go outside of their routine, get home-sick easily. Face red though cold. (*Caps*).

(3) *Thyr.* is a good remedy for reducing fat. See "Fat patient-tendency to obesity" and "Obesity."

Coronary-thrombosis with fever or palpitation—(1) Weakness of heart as if dying ; cardiac oppression. Palpitation with fever worse at night. (*Mercurius.*).

(2) Numbness, coldness of extremities, anginal pain and hypertension, boring in chest. (*Secale-cornutum.*). See also "Thrombosis."

Coryza-common cold—Common cold. *Ars-alb.* stands in the first rank for acute coryza ; it follows well after *Mercurius*.

Coryza-with thick discharge—Yellowish discharge from nose. (*Iodum.*). See also "Cough" under its different heads.

Coryza influenza—(1) Common cold with much sneezing, influenza. (*Acon.*).

(2) *Allium-cepa.* is useful when there is acrid discharge from nose and bland discharge from eyes. See "Influenza with cough.

Coryza-with irritating eyes—With irritating eyes and infection of throat. (*Euphr.*). See "Throat infection with running nose" and "Nose watering with irritation in eyes."

Coryza-with nausea—With stoppage of nose. Nausea to be present. (*Ip*).

Coryza-with sneezing—Throat feels as if it is burning. Sneezing and a hot fluid coryza. Anxious restlessness and fearfulness aggravated at night. If *Aconite* is taken frequently at the beginning the cold will clear up in twenty four hours.
(Dr. M.G. Blackie.)

Coryza-stopping of nose and sneezing—(*a*) (1) *Arum-t.* has most dreadful coryza. The nose is stopped up and more stopped up on the left side. Must breathe through mouth.

Sneezing worse during the night, fluent acrid. (*Arum-t.*).

(2) Dry cough with nose blocked with congestion in head. (*Bry.*). See "Nose stopping when going out" and "sneezing morning coryza."

(*b*) In coryza when nose has stopped give *Lyco. 30,* 4 times a day ; and sneezing takes place then *All-c.* in a similar way.

Cough-body trembles on account of coughing—Tedious cough ; worse from morning to midnight, from speaking, laughing, reading and also from lying on sides. The cough is also more by going from cold to a warm room. The whole body trembles with the cough. The patient suppresses the cough with a moan, just as long as he can, because it hurts him. (*Phos.*).

Cough-cardiac—(1) *Hydrocyanic acid* is head remedy for this and it should be tried first.

(2) Cough with difficult respiration, pulse irregular and face deadly pale.(*Dig.*)

(3) Irritating dry cough due to heart trouble with sense of choking. (*Naja.*).

(4) Spasmodic tickling cough especially in cardiac patients; cough with copious jelly like or bloody expectoration. Dyspnoea worse when sitting up. Small and feeble pulse. Gasping for breath *Laurocerasus* acts magically when the chosen remedy do not act.

(5) The dry, chronic, sympathetic cough of organic heart disease is oftener and more permanently relieved by *Capsicum*. See also "Dyspnoea with cardiac symptoms."

Cough-child, after exposure—Suddenly at night. The child, after exposure to dry cold wind, wakes up at midnight with hoarse, barking, clutches the *larynx*. Differentiate *Aur-met.* and compare *Hep-s.* (*Acon.*). See "Exposure to cold."

Cold child, with breathing difficulty—Difficulty in breathing. Spasmodic cough of all kinds when child becomes still and blue in the face. (*Ip.*). See also "Bronchitis."

Cough child, grasping larynx—A tearing pain in the middle of chest at every cough; coughing from licking in larynx specially when lying in a warm room. Cough of *Allium-cepa*. may be aggravated by cold air, but is always worse in a warm room. The cough is spasmodic severe, laryngeal cough completing the child to grasp the larynx. Feels as the cough would tear it. Differentiate it from *Aconite* "cough (*All-c.*). See "Whooping cough-child shakes and vomiting."

Cough-dry—Dry, tickling, worse at night, larynx sore and respiration oppressed. (*Bell.*). See "Whooping cough choking after midnight."

Cough-during day only with discharge—Cough during the day only and not at all at night. Nose dry. Tickling in throat pit causes cough. Copious mucous discharge. (*Rumex-crispus.*).

Cough-expectorations bloody and purulent—Tickling, expectorations grey, thick, bloody, purulent, salty. Raising mucus in large quantities affording little relief. (*Lyc.*).

Cough-with fever starting with chill—(1) Cough during chill-phase of fever is very characteristic, (*Rhus-t.*). It may be malaria, or it may be influenza starting with a chill, but the important thing about it is : if there is cough, it starts as soon as the chill-phase of the fever starts and the cough subsides more or less as soon as the heat phase starts, *i.e.* the temperature rises and the patient no longer feels the chill.

(2) Cough starting with getting wet or in the rainy season (*Rhus-t.*). See "Fever with cough and urticaria."

Cough-hacking with sweats of broken down persons—

(*a*) Hacking with night sweats of those broken down with sexual excesses. Despair, anxiety, fear and peevishness with suicidal thoughts due to above cause. (*Agar.*).

(*b*) Two or three drops of *Oleum-sant.* on a little sugar will frequently relieve the hacking cough, when, but a little sputum is expectorated.

Cough-morning, spasmodic with headache—Worse in the morning. The patient as soon as he wakes up early in the morning starts coughing spasmodically. This is a peculiar symptom of cough, coughing brings on bursting headache ; oppressed breathing. Tight dry cough at times with blood expectoration. (*Nux-v.*).

Cough of nervous origin with hoarseness—Violent spasmodic cough with frequent eructation and hoarseness. Whistling in chest during breathing ; a good deal of this cough is of nervous origin. (*Ambra-g.*). See "Nervous headache syphilitic."

Cough of old people—Chronic cough of old people with tendency to asthma. (*Ammon-c.*). See "Asthma of old people"

Cough oppressed breathing with prostration—*Am-c.* is full of catarrhal symptoms and cough with soreness in the air passage. Oppression of breathing. The main feature is great prostration. Short asthmatic cough. The complaints of this medicine come on at 3 O'clock. The patient is worse after sleep (*Am-c.*). See "Breathing oppressed."

Cough-pus-like mucus with sweat—Convulsive cough, with sweat, towards evening, with frequent pulse, expectoration of pus-like mucus ; worse in the morning and when lying on bed. (*Agar.*).

Cough-phthisic—Chronic hawking cough in sickly, pale persons, such as have inherited phthisis with oedema of extremities, diarrhoea and dyspnoea or night sweats (*Acet-ac.*). See "Tuberculosis" and "Phthisis."

Cough-rattling with breathing difficulty but no mucus coming out—Croupy or spasmodic, with breathing difficulty. The cough is loose and rattles but no mucus comes out, though it appears as if lot would come up. It may start when any part of body is exposed to cold air, even if hands or legs are exposed. Early morning cough. Suffocating cough of child. Begin with *Acon.* and follow with *Hepar.*

Cough-raw feeling in the chest—Burning and raw feeling in the chest while coughing, the raw feeling may be along the trachea and in chest. (*Arum-t.*).

Cough-respiration oppressed worse after eating and which hurts head—Dry at night with no expectoration, with soreness. Must sit up, worse after eating or drinking with vomiting. Coughing hurts the head and chest. The patient holds them with his hands. (*Bry.*). See "Respiration."

Cough of children during sleep—Child does not wake up when coughing ; cough dry. Quiet only by carrying. Fever also. (*Cham.*).

Cough-sour mucus—Tickling and troublesome at night, free expectoration in morning ; thick, yellow and sour mucus (*Calc.*).

Cough-unable to lie down and sitting for breath—Worse after twelve in night, springs out of bed, unable to lie down for fear of suffocation. Forthy expectoration. Must sit up to breathe. Respiration is wheezing. The air passage seems constricted. (*Ars-alb.*). See "Respiration."

Cough-urine escaping while coughing—Urine escaping involuntarily while patient is sitting. Sneezing or coughing. Loss of sensibility on passing urine. Frequent urination can be delayed while patient has to undergo a long journey or to sit for a long time in any meeting. The best constitutional remedy for bladder weakness. (*Causticum.*).

Cough-vomiting of mucus—Itching in larynx with gagging and vomiting of mucus. Wheezing and rattling of mucus, occasional spells of long coughing attacks. Hoarseness. (*Carb-v.*).

Cough with watering of eyes—Worse during the day, better at night with watering of eyes. This is important as most of the coughs are worse at night in children. (*Euphr.*). See also "Bronchitis" under its different heads and "Coryza."

Cramps in calves of legs and in other parts—(1) *Verat-a.* taken at midnight before going to bed for 2 or 3 nights will generally overcome the predisposition to cramps. *Sulph.* should be taken as an intercurrent remedy followed next day by *Verat-a.* as before. If this fails, then *Colocynth.* should be taken in the same manner.

(2) Cramps in toes, calves and soles ; (*Ferr-met* 6, 8 hourly.)

(3) Cramps in palms. (*Scrophul*).

(4) Cramps in legs and abdomen of pregnant women. (*Vib-o.*).

(5) Simple cramps in the muscles. (*Cholos Terrapinoe*).

(6) *Cuprum* 12th dilution never fails to give relief in cramps of calves.

Cramps of hysterical patient—Sometimes the hysterical patient gets cramps instead of faintings. (*Asaf.*). See "Hysteria-fainting."

Cravings for different things including lying down in bed—(1) Craving for alcohol or liquor. Give *Sterculia* M.T. 10 drops three times a day. If no improvement is noticed within reasonable period then increase one dram dose T.D.S.

(2) For craving for smoking give in 200 or 1000 dilution of *Tab.* See "Tobacco craving."

(3) Craving for always lying down in bed. He feels better by rest and his trouble and anxiety are aggravated by movements. (*Manganum.*)

(4) Wants to drink all the time morning till evening. (*Sulf*). See "Alcoholism.

(5) An individual steals money in order to buy liquor. (*Plumb.*).

(6) Irrestible craving to bite gums. (*Phyt.*). See "Gums biting".

(7) In order to take away craving for alcoholic drink a mixture of one part of *Sulphuric acid* and three parts of alcohol

may be given in doses of 10 to 15 drops 3 hours a day for 3 to 4 weeks.

Craving for acid and refreshing things—*Verat.*

Craving for opium—*Avena sativa* is a specific for removing morphine (opium) habit. Give 20 drops M.T. in hot water 4 times a day. A prolonged use will be necessary to completely get rid of the habit. See "Morphia-habit."

Craving for salt—*Nat-m.* is most useful remedy for abnormal craving for salt. These patients are in the habit of adding salt to their food before tasting it because they will never find the food too salty. (*Nat-m.*), See "Salt craving."

Creating-reaction—When carefully selected remedies fail to produce a favourable effect specially in acute diseases, due to depression of vital force or psora, *Sulf.* frequently serves to rouse the reactive powers of the system and clears up the case. It has power to meet and over-come certain obstacles to the usual action of drug. Give a dose of *Sulf.* wait for a few hours in an acute case and wait for a few days in a chronic case, then administer the indicated medicine. See also "Blocks" "Reaction creating reaction" and "Disease caused by suppression of eruption or other skin trouble.

Croup-loss of voice—When the child gets worse in sleep. A condition of larynx seen in children characterised by a harsh, brassy cough and crowing causing loss of voice *Lach.* is one of the best remedies in desperate case of croups. (*Lach*). See also "Voice loss of."

Cruel—Cruel, malicious and wicked at times and can inflict injuries on others without any sympathy or feeling. (*Anac.*). See "Perverted mind."

Crushing of nerve—Where a nerve has been crushed between hammer above and the bone below and nerve shows sign of inflammation and the pain then *Hypericum* is the remedy (*Hyper.*). See "inflammation of nerve injured" and "Nerve injury"

Crying of child-teathing trouble—Quiet only by carrying about. Crying or whining without cause or with fever, diarrhoea, teething or any other complaint, or if the child wants this or that thing, but throws them all away when offered. Child is very uneasy and tosses about *Cham.* is an excellent remedy for irritability and other symptoms of infants and children (*Cham.*). See also "screaming of children" and also "Dentition" under its different heads.

Crying of child before urinating—*Lyco.* Compare *Borax* also. See "urine-child crying".

Crying of child dentition-milk not digested—Troubles during dentition. Anguish, crying, and expression of uneasiness and discontent lead to *Aethusa, cynapium.* Most frequently indicated in diseases in children during dentition, summer complaints, when with diarrhoea there is marked inability to digest milk and poor circulation. Milk causes diarrhoea. (*Aeth.*). See "Milk not digested with diarrhoea".

Curvature of bones including curvature of hip joint and vertebra—(1) Curvature of bones, rickets and diseases of hip joint, offensive sweat may also be present, fistulous openings discharge offensive and parts around it hard and swollen (*Silicea.*).

(2) For caries of bones. (*Phos.*).

(3) Curvature hip diseases. (*Kali-carb.*).

(4) Curvature of spine due to caries of vertebra. (*Acid-phos.*).

(5) Another useful remedy in spinal curvature is *Baryta-mur.* See also "Bones-curvature" and "Rickets."

Cuts-sharp with knife—Sharp cuts with knife. (*Staphy.*). *Hypericum oil* and ointment be applied to cuts abrasions and wounds. See "Wounds incised and clear cut", "Knife cuts" and "Incised wound." Paint the cut with Calendula for outer applications See "Wounds infected."

Cyst-eyelids—Cyst on the eyelids. *Calcarea-fluorica 30.* If this fails then *Nitric-acid.* See "10 of Eye trouble" and "Wen."

Cystitis-inflammation of urinary bladder with burning pain in urethra and frequent urination—(1) Frequent desire to pass water which is natural or in increased quantity and slightly burning. (*Apis.*, 2 hourly.).

(2) Burning, cutting or stitching pain in urethra during and after urinating. (*Berberis-vulgaris.* 1/2 hourly.).

(3) Intolerable burnings pain in bladder, spasmodic pain along urethra, worse before and after urination specially arising from gonorrhoea or nephritis (*Canth.* to be given in large doses.).

(4) Cystitis of old people with constant desire to urinate. *Equisetum* will be useful when highly coloured and scanty urine passed with pain depositing mucus sediment.

(5) Involuntry passage of urine in sleep. (*Seneg.*).

(6) *Causticum* is one of the chief remedies for cystitis and is often given as a preventive to those who have a weak bladder and have to travel for long sight-seeing or attending functions lasting several hours. It will lessen the frequency of the urination during such trip. It is also useful for retention of urine after surgical operation. See "bladder" under its different heads.

Cyst-recurring round the eyelids—For recurring cysts give *Baryta carbonica.*

Cystitis-acute pain—See "Chapter V" for details.

D

Dandruff falling of hair and scalp itching—White scaly dandruff, hair dry and falling out. (*Thuj*).

(*i*) Sensibility in root of hair ; dandruff painful. (*Calc-c*.).

(*ii*) Abundant falling of hair when touched. White dandruff, alternating with catarrh or loss of smell. (*Nat-m*.).

(*iii*) Scalp with distressing itching. Falling out of hair. (*Graph*.).

(*iv*) In debilitated subjects with fair skin. (*Ars-a*.).

(*v*) When all remedies fail then take *Sulf. 30* twice a week and keep sclap clean. See "Hair under its different heads."

Dandruff-hair falls—Falls out in clouds. (*Lyco*.) ; hair falls out in bunches ; baldness of single spots. (*Phos*.). See "Hair" also.

Day blindness—Can hardly see her way after sunrise. (Both-*rops-lanciolatus*.). See "Blindness-also night blindness."

(2) Day blindness ; day light dazzles eyes due to which letters appear confused when reading. (*Sil*.).

Deafness due to different causes—(1) Due to over use of quinine. A buzzing sound in the ear. Taste of the mouth usually bitter. The patient desires fresh air and cannot stick in a closed room. Warm room aggravates. Walking in open air relieves. (*Sulf*.).

(2) General remedy for deafness is *Kali-muriaticum*.

(3) Of elderly people : Catarrhal deafness in elderly people in obstruction of eustachian tube. Worse in damp weather, (*Merc-d*.).

(4) Due to perforation of abscess in the ear. (*Hep-s*.).

(5) Deafness following purulent or catarrhal otitis media. Dr. Dewey says that *Kali-mur.* is the most valuable remedy in such cases.

(6) R.B. Bishambar Dass recommends *Mephitis* for deafness chronic or from birth. He starts treatment with 30 potency and goes higher. It should be given a long trial for 6 months or a year. A dose of *Tuberculinum 200* should be given every month as an intercurrent remedy. No other medicine is to be given two days before and after.

(7) Deafness after typhoid. *Petrol*; after measles *Puls*; after small-pox *Sulph.* and after influenza *Gels.* See also "Ear deafness" under different heads and "Otorrhoea."

(8) Deafness as a result of measles :(*Puls., Carb-v.*)

(9) Deafness as a result of small-pox :(*Mercury*; or *Sulf.*)

(10) Deafness as a result of intermittent fever. (*Carb-v., Calc., Puls.,*) See "Fever intermittent".

(11) Deafness as a result of fevers or nervous affection. (*Arn., Phos., Verat-v.*)

(12) Deafness as a result of enlarged tonsils. (*Bell., Merc., Calc.*) See "No. 3 of Hearing dulness." "Tonsillitis—hearing affected" and "Ear deafness-tonsils."

(13) When produced by a suppressed discharge from ear or nose.(*Hep-s., Lach., Bell.*)

(14) Syphilitic deafness. *Kreos.*

(15) Deafness—rheumatic—Absolute deafness of chronic type was cured by Dr. Cooper with single drop doses. (*Belladonna M.T.*) See "Rheumatic deafness."

Death-rattling—Such a rattling takes place in the throat before death. Dr. Anshutz says that such a rattling is eased by administering one or 2 doses of *Pulsatila 30.* and will ease the final departure.

Debility-due to excess—(*a*) The patient is normally weak; disinclined to move and does not want to be disturbed. The patient lies usually in a sleepy condition. *Ph-a.* is best suited to persons of strong constitutions who become debilitated by loss of vital fluids, sexual excesses, violent acute diseases or a long succession of moral emotions as grief, care and disappointed affections. (*Ph-a.*). (*b*) Slightest exertion brings great fatigue and weakness. Also after illness. (*Selenium.*) See also "Sexual desire irresistible" under its different heads. See "Typhoid debility" and "Weakness premature old ages with impaired functions."

Debility and prostration—due to loss of fluids—(*a*) Debilitated and broken down from exhausting discharge. Weakness in general and other complaints as a result of excessive loss of blood or other fluids, *e.g.*, diarrhoea. It is all the more indicated if the loss of blood has been sudden with faintness, (*Chin.*). (*b*) Prostration both physical and mental, headache and pain in limbs after exertion. (*Picric-acid*). (*c*) Debility of the aged and nervous debility from loss of fluid (*Baryta-carb.*). See "Weakness-due to loss of blood and fluids."

Debility-due to lack of digestive power—Debility from lack of digestive power in the stomach or general assimilative power. Tongue dirty white coat, there is nausea. Digestion is slow and the food remains in the stomach for a long time, undigested. Some time during meal time the patient has to leave his meal unfinished and to go to bathroom, (*Alstonia-constricta*)

Debility due to various causes—(1) Weakness of memory. Aversion to work. Weakening of all senses, sight, hearing. Depression and irritability. Nervous debility following seminal loss ; profound melancholy and hypochondriasis. Debility from overstudy. (*Anac.*).

(2) When every quick motion causes shortness of breath with perspiration about the neck. (*Samb.*).

(3) The patient is greatly prostrated after acute or violent diseases (*Psor.*). Compare *Selen.* which is useful for debility after typhoid.

(4) Debility from self abuse with sunken features, abashed facial expression, loss of memory, weakness of legs, back-ache, sexual sins and excesses. Stupifying headache. (*Staphy.*).

(5) Pallid as a corpse with flabby bloatedness, pale children who have swelling of cervical and other glands. (*Merc-dulcis*).

(6) *Kali Carb.* is one of the best remedies for debility. following labour. Combination of sweat and weakness. See "Vital force" or Naunasthena due to dibility for different causes.

Debility-of women—Wornout with hard work, mental or physical, muscles burn of ache which prevent her from sleep, albumen present in the urine, anaemia, lowness of the spirit and melancholy. (*Helonias dioicas*).

Decay of teeth of children—Specially in children. Teeth begin to decay at roots, crowns remain sound, crumble, turn yellow, Gums retract. (*Thuj.*). See also "Teeth decaying in children".

Deceiving including cheating—(1) Inclination to deceiving. (*Plumbum*).

(2) Desire for cheating with inclination to quarrel. Fussy (*Caust.*). See "Stealing."

Defective assimilation in children—(1) Children who sweat on head easily, emaciated and badly nourished children. Child may be hungry wanting food too often but not gaining weight due to bad assimilation. Large head, big belly, thin limbs, emaciated face, cannot walk or learning to walk late. Constipated. Does not grow according to age. Face looks old and creased as in monkey. (*Silicea.*). Compare *Calc-c.* and *Agar.* See also "Walking delayed in fat children" under its different heads. and "Assemilation defective in children".

Delayed—mental development—In children : compare *Natrum-muriaticum,* which has late learning to talk, and *Calc-c.* which has late learning to walk. These two features are combined in *Agar.* In *Calcarea* it is due to defective bones. In

Agaricus it is mental defect—a strong developing mind. Children who cannot remember, make mistakes and are slow in learning. The patient is sluggish and stupid. (*Agar.*). Compare *Silicea* and *Calc-c.* See also "Children late in learning to talking and walking."

Delirium—During fever, with spasms and jerks and twitching and starting from sleep. Laughs or screams. Gnashes teeth and becomes violent. Tries to bite or strike. Face is particularly red and eyes are red. The congestion of face and eyes main distinguishing feature from *Stramonium* (*Bell.*). Trio of delirium medicines : (1) *Bell.*, (2) *Hyos.* and (3) *Stram.* See also "Spasms of child during sleep" and "Talkativeness during fever"

Delirium-in child birth—Fever or puerperal delirium with convulsions. Eyes wild. (*Verat-v.*). See "Fever or puerperal."

Delirium-muttering in diphtheria measles, small-pox etc.—Muttering delirium with sleeplessness and restlessness. Great prostration. Child whines or cries all the time. Sees little animals *e.g.* rats or mice crawling up the limbs over the body. (*Ailanthus.*).

Delirium in typhoid—(1) Of mild type and is not violent in typhoid fever. Restlessness, thirst and chilliness *(Rhus-t.)*.

(2) Muttering delirium. (*Crot.*).

(3) Constant attempts to get out of bed and tremor of whole body *(Agaricus.)*. See also "Typhoid-delirium" under its different heads, and "Fever typhoid muttering delirium".

Delusion, also seeing snakes—It is an advanced stage of illusion. The patient hears voices dictating him. He has a controversy between two wills-the good and evil. (*Anac.*).

(1) See also "Hallucination" "Illusion" and "Will."

(2) Delusion about snakes. (*Lac-can.*).

Delivery-safe also for living birth, putting child right position and avoiding false pains—(1) *Actea-racemosa* may be given 3 or 4 months before delivery to ensure safe and painless delivery. It will help safe and painless even if it is given a few days before delivery. It also ensures living birth if given thrice daily for 6 or 7 months before delivery. It checks false labour pains also.

(2) False pains ; to avoid false labour pains and to ensure safe delivery in due time *Puls.* 100 dilution may be given every 15 minutes, 3 doses only at the time the delivery is expected. Never mind if the delivery takes place 2 or 3 days after but it will be safe. It also puts the child in right position if it has changed its position in the womb if given before the membranes are ruptured. See "False-labour pains."

(3) Pains after delivery. *Arn-m.* is an excellent remedy for such pains.

(4) Retention of urine after labour. (*Caust.*).

(5) Retention of placenta. (*Viscum-album*).

(6) *Puls., Nux., Bell.* 3x or 6x are issued in Father Mullers' Dispensary as delivery medicines. Give these during last few days of pregnancy each once a day. When labour pains commence prepare solution of 3 medicines 5 to 10 drops in 4oz. of water. Givc a medium spoonful alternately from these every 2 hours or every hour or half an hour. See "Pregnancy" under its different heads.

Dengue-fever—Sudden on-set with headache and bone breaking pain and sometimes an initial rash. Give repeated doses of *Acon.* to be followed by *Bry.* If bone pains are very severe then start *Eupatorium perfoliatum.*

Dengue fever-prevention—See "Chapter V" for details.

Dentition-diarrhoea—Diarrhoea during dentition. Green slimy, hot, sputtering, undigested with foetid flatus, (*Calc-p.*). If diarrhoea too long, then *Mercurius., Sulf.* or *Ipec.* See also "Diarrhoea-during dentition" under its different heads.

Dentition-difficulty—(1) Difficult dentition. Whole child smells sour, of frequent use in children with sour diarrhoea. (*Rheum.*).

(2) Dentition very difficult and painful. Gums spongy and painful. Restlessness, tossing about constipation and undigested diarrhoea. (*Kreosote*). See also under "Teething troubles incidental to dentition".

Dentition-difficult pressing gums swollen and teething irregular—(1) Difficult dentition, moaning, grinding the teeth at night ; intense desire to press gums together (*Phyt.*) ; head hot and rolling from side. (*Bell., Hell.*). Pressing of gums during an attack of acute diarrhoea. (*Podo*).

(2) If gums remain swollen and teeth do not break through or the teething takes place in an irregular manner then *Sulf. 30* and in about a week a dose of *Calc.* another dose of *Calc.* another week for avoiding lancing. See "Gums pressing".

Dentition-fever and diarrhoea—(1) Diarrhoea during dentition and fever, green stool, foul odour and colicky pain. Abdomen bloated. Child restless and uneasy and cries. Dry cough. Child quiet only by carrying about. (*Cham.*). See also "Eating dirty things by children".

(2) *Coffea* if fever accompanied by nervousness, weeping or crying. See "Summer complaints of children-during dentition and "Fever-during dentition."

Dentition-inability to digest milk and convulsions—

(1) Troubles during dentition. Anguish, crying and expression of uneasiness and discontent lead to *Aethusa cynapium* most frequently indicated in disease in children during dentition, summer complaints, when with diarrhoea there is marked inability to digest milk and poor circulation. Milk causes diarrhoea. (*Aeth.*)

(2) For convulsions during dentition give *Cham.*, or *Ignatia.*, *Bell.*, or *Stram.*, according to symptoms. See also "Convulsions" under its different heads and "Milk not digested with diarrhoea."

Denture-causing ulcer—Blisters on sides. (*Phytolacca*).

Depressed-in mind—*Psorinum* is very despressed in mind. Greatest despondency, making his own life and that of those almost intolerable. Such a state of mind follows acute diseases and it is especially beneficial remedy for such state of mind. See "Melancholia."

Depression-gloominess—Mental state of depression and gloominess alternate with physical state (*Act-rac.*). See "Mental shock-causing nervousness."

Depression-low spirited and unsocial—Low-spirited disheartened depressed, unsocial almost imbecile. (*Anac.*). See "Neurasthenia-with depression."

Depression-suicidal—Patient meditates always upon death, upon suicide, has no love for life which he thinks worthless. Like the victim of syphilis, mental states of great depression are produced by it. He is absolutely hopeless. (*Aur-met.*). See also "Suicide" and "Suicidal thought with broken down constitution".

Desire-of eating dirty things in pregnancy—For eating earth or lime (*Nitric-acid.*) sand and ashes-during pregnancy, (*Tarent-h.*) for indigestible things, chalk or charcoal (*Alumina.*) See also "Eating-dirty things by children". See "No. 15 of Pregnancy-its affection".

Derangements—at puberty—The girl often weeps while stating her symptoms. She is submissive and usually good natured. Menses usually late in time, scanty in flow, slightly, blackish in colour. Flow sometimes stops and flows again and so on. Menstrual trouble from wetting the feet just before menses. She feels hot too much ; intermittent flow with evening chilliness ; with intense pain and great restlessness and tossing about. Delayed first menstruation. Pain in the back. Nausea. Diarrhoea during or after menses. *Puls.* mental symptoms must be present, viz. quiet and of yielding disposition with a tearful mood. *Puls.* patient may be irritable. Breast sensitive in difficult young girls. Menses unduly delayed, menses do not start at proper age. (*Puls.*) See also "Consolation" and "Menstruation-scanty with weeping tendency". The following are a few troubles to which a girl at puberty falls a prey.

D

Alumina—chlorosis (Anemia): In chlorosis the patient desires strange foods and also a craving to eat strange articles, such as hair, dirt or sand. The menses are scanty, pale, and are followed by great exertion. There may be a leucorrhoea which is acrid, transparent and excoriates the genitals and extends down the limbs and feet during the day. Menses too early, short, scanty and pale. See "Anemia" and "Leucorrhoea acrid".

Actea-r—Chorea—(A nervous disorder, characterised by irregular and involuntary action of the muscles of the extremities and the face). This remedy is indicated in neuralgic and chorea disturbances in nervous hysterical patients. There is amenorrhoea. Pain in ovarian rigion. Pain immediately before menses. Also pain across pelvis, from hip to hip.

Ant-c—Melancholia—It is applicable to nervous and excitable, hysterical and peevish girls that are overcome by mellow lights, and as a result there is an outburst of affection, as is observed in the sick, and those who are suffering from the effects of disappointed affection.

Apis-m—Menses suppressed with cerebral and head symptoms, especially in young girls. There is more or less oedema about the privates. See "Menstruation, scanty late and suppressed".

Aquilegia—Dysmenorrhoea of young girls. Women at climaxis, with vomiting of green substances especially in the morning. See ' Dysmenorrhoea".

Artm-Abs—Epileptic conditions and convulsive diseases. Sudden and severe giddiness, delirium, and loss of consciousness. The Epilepsy is preceded by nervous trembling. See "Epilepsy"

Aurum-met—Heart palpitation of young girls.

Asafoetida—Mammae turgent (swollen) with milking the unimpregnated girls at puberty. See "Chorea."

D

Asterias-rub—Acne-removes tendency. Pimples on side of nose, chin and mouth. Disposition to pimples at adolesence. See "Acne".

Aurum-met—Foul breath in girls at puberty. Taste putrid or bitter. Ulceration of gums.

Baryta-carb—(Muscular atrophy)—Menses scanty. See "Muscles-different troubles including atrophy".

Bryonia—(Nose bleed instead of menses) See "Nose bleeding-instead of menses".

Cal-carb—Menses in little girls with itching and burning of parts. Milky leucorrhoea headache and colic before start of menses. Diathesis of tuberculosis at the age of fourteen.Hot swelling breast.

Calc-iod—(Hydrastis)—Goitre of puberty. Nipple retracted. See "Goitre of puberty".

Calc-phos—(Epistaxis) Schooling girls headache : use 12th and 30th. Menses too early, excessive and bright in girls. See "Headache-of school girls due to eye strain" and "Headache of anaemic girls".

Carb-ac—(Leucorrhoea in children)—Discharges always offensive. Erosions of cervix. See "Menstruation-in its place painful leucorrhoea".

Caulophyllum—(Chorea and nervous affections)—This is particularly a women medicine and is also used in discolouration of skin in women with menstural and uterine disorder. Sea "Chorea".

Causticum—(Chorea-epilepsy-convulsion)—Paralysis Burn ing desire for marriage.

Cimaphila-umbellata—Painful tumor of breast specially in young unmarried women. Women with very large breast and tumor in mammory with sharp pain through it.

Cimicifuga—Chorea-nervous affections ; disordered menses. uterine haemorrhage before puberty, facial blemishness, acne and rough skin. See "Facial blemishes".

D

Cyclamen—Acne in anaemic girls at puberty, with pruritus better scratching and appearance of menses. See "Acne".

Ferr-met—Copious urination, chlorosis. Retarded menses. Psoriasis in young girls, menses remit a day or two and then return, girls who are weak, delicate, chlorotic, yet have a firy red face.

Graphites—Large abdomen in girls at puberty also for menses too late with constipation. See "No. 2 of Abdomen pendulous after confinement".

Helleborus—Mania of melancholy type.

Helonias chamaelirium—Troubles of wombs, back and kidney. The menses are often suppressed and the kidney congested. Breast swollen, nipples painful and tender. Malposition of womb.

Kali-carb—Delayed start of menses in young girls with chest system or ascites, difficult first menses with backache.

Kali hydrodicum—Inflammatory condition of womb in young married girls, menses later profuse.

Lachesis—Large abdomen in girls, which is tympanitic, sensitive and painful. See "Tympanitis and dyspepsia in Typhoid."

Lycopodium—Amenorrhoea with non-development of breast, a girls reaches age of 15 to 18 without starting of menses. Breast do not develop and ovaries do not perform their function. Constipation from puberty.

Merc proto iod—Yellow leucorrhoea. Mammary tumour.

Merc sol—Mammae full of milk at menses in place of menses.

Nat mur—Melancholia.

Nux vom—At puberty, menses a few days before time and copious, continuing for several days.

Onosmodium—Restores diminutive or absent breasts to their normal size. Use in CM potency.

D

Penthorum—Post nasal-catarrh at puberty.

Petroleum—In young girls with or without ulceration of stomach. Genitals sore and moist. Itching and mealy coating of nipples.

Phosphorus—Epistaxis of tall slim girls. Chlorosis, anaemia with muscular debility. Profuse leucorrhoea instead of menses. Muscular debility.

Pituitary—Delayed puberty with defective development of breast.

Platinum—Masturbation before the age of puberty and its bad effects.

Polygonum—(Punctatum)—Amenorrhoea and metrorrhagia (uterine haemorrhage independent of the menstrual period) in young girls with shooting pain through the breasts.

Rhus tox—Breast very sensitive in sensitive and difficult girls. Menses early, profuse and prolonged.

Sabal Serrulata—Breasts shrunk due to menses or some other diseases of uterus, valuable for undeveloped mammary glands.

Senecio Aureus—Menses retarded, suppressed. Functional amenorrhoea of young girls with backache. Before menses, inflammatory conditions of throat, chest and bladder. Menses scanty or suppressed or they may be premature and profuse.

Sepia-Amenorrhoea at puberty from taking cold. Lentigo (freckle or spot on the skin) in young women.

Staphisagria—Ineffectual urging to urinate in newly married girls. Irritable bladder.

Sulph.—Large abdomen in girls at puberty. A tall awkward girl with an unhealthy skin has all the symptoms of approaching maturity. Vagina burns. Menses too late, short, scanty and difficult.

Turnera Aphradisiaca—Aids the establishment of normal menstrual flow in young girls.

Tuberculin—Cough in young girls with suppressed menses Benign mammary tumours.

Zincum Metallicum—Delayed puberty.

Dermatitis-toxic-inflammation of skin psoriasis—*Rhus-tox.* **Dermatitis involving hands and face, scratching with weeping eczema**—(1) (Inflammation of skin). Dermatitis badly involving hand and face. Extreme uneasiness. Scratching of affected parts leading to bleeding and causing bruises. Bruises turned into weeping eczema. (*Sulf.* 30 first day, *Graph.* 30, 3 doses next day ; 3rd day *Sulf.* 30, and later on weekly dose of *Graph.* 200 for 4 weeks only). See "Eczema", "Eruptions" under different heads. and "Bruise and skin with black and blue appearance".

(2) When due to external injuries of ulcerated nature. Destruction of skin resulting in ulcers. *Calend.* 30 internally ; *Calend. M.T.* mixed with 8 parts of boiled water to be applied locally.

(3) Dermatitis-solar : due to sensivity of skin to the rays of sun. (*Sulf.*).

(4) Washermen, dyers or miners handling mercury or carbolic acid. (*Rhus-t.*).

(5) Caloric or toxic dermatitis which may be due to cold or heat. Redness and swelling of skin. It may be due to handling mercury or carbolic acid. (*Apis-m*).

(6) Skin inflammation due to contused wounds. (*Arn-m.* 1000 potency internally and *Arn-m. M.T.* locally. To be repeated 8 hourly). See "Contusion-skin rupture."

Despondent and sad—*Stannum.* patients are generally very sad and despondent crying all the time. (*Nat-m. ; Puls. ; Sepia.; Stannum.*). 12 ; 30, 200 or 500 potency.

Diabetes with swollen ankle and acidosis (an abnormal production of acid in body and its defective elimination)—(1) With or without sugar in the urine , where there is great thirst ; weakness and pallor and loss of flesh (*Acet-ac.*).

(2) Excessive urination with sugar (*Argentum.nit.*).

(3) Diabetes accompanied with swollen ankles. (*Argentum-met.*).

(4) Diabetic, acidosis : *Soda-bicarb.* and *Lithi.-carb.*

Diabetic-coma—(1) Acetomea, complete loss of consciousness ; delirious, talking with wide open eyes, drowsy, stupor, stertorous breathing, sweating skin, apopletic state. (*Opium.*).

(2) Drowsiness, incapable of recognising people or answering question, constipation but passing urine involuntarily. (*Aluminum-met.*). *S*ee "Coma" and Collapse".

Diabetes-mellitus— (1) A proper and planned diet plays an important role in the treatment and control of diabetes. Many factors have to be considered in the planning of a diabetic diet *e.g.* type of diabetes, age and sex of the patient, his weight, height, the type of work that he does etc. Most patients with Diabetes mellitius are obese and usually beyond 40-50 yrs. of age *i.e.* late onset obese type of diabetes ,the following remarks concerning the diet are more relevant for this group of patients. The diet prescribed should aim at :—

(1) Reduction of weight to the optimum level depending upon age, sex, and height of the patient.

(2) To provide enough energy for the bodies requirement, this depends upon the patients' type of work *i.e.* sedentary, medium work or heavy work.

(3) To provide enough carbohydrate to prevent any acidosis or ketosis.

(4) Enough to provide enough proteins, vitamins and minerals necessary for the body.

In the planning of diabetic diets the following are kept in mind *e.g.* caloric requirements, amount of protein, carbohydrate, fats, minerals and vitamins that a patient should take. A diabetic diet should supply half the calories as carbohydrates, the rest by proteins and fats. 1 gm. of protein per kg. of ideal weight is enough. If these considerations are kept in mind the diet for a man whose ideal weight should be 70 kg. and who is a sedentry worker and is not over weight should require about 2250 cal. a day. (See Table I.)

Table I

Nutrition expert group of the Indian Council of Medical Research in 1968 has recommended the caloric and protein needs for different age and sex groups of normal individuals as follows :

	Calories	Proteins
Man :		
Sedentary work	2400	
Moderate work	2800	55 gm.
Heavy work	3900	
Women :		
Sedentary work	1900	
Moderate work	2200	45 gm.
Heavy work	3000	
Pregnancy (2nd half)	+300	+10 gm.
Lactation (upto 1 year)	+700	+20 gm.
Infants		
0—6 months	120 kg. of body weight.	
7—12 months	100 kg. of body weight.	
Children		
1—3 years	1200	17—20 gm.
4—6 years	1500	22 gm.
7—9 years	1800	33 gm.
10—12 years	2100	41 gm.

Adolescents :	Calories	Proteins
13—15 years boys	2500	55 gm.
,, gitls	2200	50 gm.
16—18 years boys	3000	60 gm.
,, girls	2200	50 gm.

—For caloric and protein requirements of different categories of peoples, pamphlets on diabetic diets should be consulted for details about formation of diabetic diet to suit individual patient. Food that a diabetic patient can take without measuring, and the foods he should avoid are given in (Table II).

Table II

Diabetic can have the following without measuring :

1. Salad—raw vegetables, clear vegetable soups.
2. Vinegar, chutney, spices, Achars without oil.
3. Black tea and coffee, plain soda, nimboo pani. without sugar.

Avoid :
1. Sugar, gurh, honey, sweets, ice-creams, cakes, pastries, chocalates.
2. Fried foods.
3. Alcoholic and sweet soft drinks, fruit juice.
4. Nuts and dry fruits.
5. (*a*) Potatoes, Arbi, Yam, Plantain, Beetroot.
   (*b*) Mangoes, Bananas, and grapes, Chicken.

Diabetes-dyspepsia—Profuse urination. Unable to retain urine. Excessive thirst ; debility. Diabetes of the dyspeptic and caused by derangement of assimilation. (*Uranium-nitricum.*) It is undoubtedly the best remedy.

Diabetes-gangrene—Diabetes and diabetic gangrene, (*Ars-alb.*). See "Gangrene", "(*a*) of Boils-Carbuncles" and Carbuncles with diabetes milk offensive discharge."

Diabetes-insipidus—Profuse flow of colourless urine containing no sugar. (1) If during night and day. *(Scilla.)*.

(2) If chiefly in the night. (*Phos-ac. and Murex.*)

Diabetic-itching—Itching without eruptions. Dr. Dewey says the *Dolichos* will control diabetic itching and is specially useful in senile pruritus. Worse at night. Worse across the shoulders. (*Dolichos.*) See 'Itch' and "No. 3 of Eczema general at different places."

Diabetic-complication—For every kind of complication in diabetes use. (*Graphites.*).

Diabetic-hypoglycaemia due to insulin —This occurs due to insulin reaction when urine is free from sugar. The symptoms are weakness, faintness, dizziness, palpitation, nervousness and confusion. This reaction may progress unconsciousness and convulsion. The treatment is very simple, a few lumps of sugar, syrup, sweatmeat or sweat drinks should be immediately taken. Avoid any delay.

Diabetes-mellitus of various types—(1) Useful in diabetic of tuberculous or rheumatic diathesis, sudden extreme dryness of mouth. Tendency to skin eruption, losing weight. Ability to exercise steadly diminishing. Sleepless night. Copious perspiration on slight exertion. Brick-dust urine but not always. Passes urine once or twice in night. Thirst much for cold water. (*Phos*).

(2) Diabetes complicated with albuminaria. (*Canth.*)

(3) Voracious appetite, and costive bowels. Thirst, nausea, dry skin, dry tongue, urinates copiously. (*Lactic acid*).

(4) Diabetes with constipation, albumin, and casts in urine (*Plumbum*).

(b) (1) Awkwardness inclined to drop things from hands; chronic urticaria, diarrhoea before and during menses, great weakness of joints and weariness; intolerable itching at the tip of coccyx. (*Bor.*).

(2) Lips dry, great thirst, emaciation irritable and melancholy; urine profuse clear, containing sugar, rheumatic symptoms, abluminous and phosphatic urine, feet feel numb when sitting, burning sensation in top. (*Helon.*).

(3) Melancholy, afraid to remain alone. Irritable, constipated, red sand in urine, abdomen bloated, flatulence, impotence, haemorrhoids and great falling of hair. (*Lyco.*). Both the lower and the highest potencies are credited with excellent result.

(4) Weak memory, melancholia with suicidal thoughts, tongue coated and blistered, chronic nasal catarrh, ravenous hunger soon after eating, very thirsty, rests more comfortably on abdomen, intense itching of anus, enlarged and painful, prostate with frequent urging and painful urination. (*Med. 200*).

(5) Copious urine with sugar, diabetes with grief, anxiety restlessness and weakness with emaciation. Patients impulsive violent, irritable, hysterical, feigns sickness. Patients who feel sore all over the body. Consolation causes weeping. (*Tarent-h. 30-200*).

(6) Slightest injury causes suppuration, over-sensitive physically and mentally, peevish, and unreasonably anxious; extremely sensitive to cold air, urine voided slowly, without force drops vertically, baldder weak, stool sour, while undigested and fetid, itching of glans ; menses late, scanty, profuse sweat. (*Hep-s.*).

(7) Intense thirst though the tongue looks moist, frequent urging to urinate, trembling of hands, excessive perspiration, quantity of urine more than the water drunk. Large flabby tongue with imprints of teeth. (*Merc. 6-200*).

(8) Urine frequent, ineffectual tenesmus, albuminous, low specific gravity, excessive and rapid emaciation, weakness, loss of memory, obstructed flatus with intense colic., paralysis of lower limbs; mental depression. Constipated, cardiac weakness, gastralgia, constant vomiting, chronic intestinal nephritis. (*Plumbum. 6-200*).

(9) Patients who have suffered with syphilis, herpetic eruptions, glandular tumours, itching over the entire body; relieves the pruritus of diabetic patients, mouth dry. (*Ars-b.*).

(10) For various complications of diabetes when cause not known. (*Graph.*).

(11) Diabetes of nervous origin; frequent urging to urinate, pain in loins, emaciation and prostration. (*Acid-phos.*).

(12) It reduces the quantity and frequency of urine and by its continued use the quantity of sugar will be lessened. (Give 2 or 3 grains of 3rd trituration *Uranium nitricum* in the morning and at night). Alongwith this *Uranium nit. 3x* give alternately, *Syzygium Q,* T.D.S. which will reduce the sugar in a fortnight.

(13) *Cephalandra Indica* is a grand homoeopathic medicine for diabetes mellitus. Its power to lessen sugar is unquestionably great and this disease is radically cured by this drug.

(Dr. S.C. Ghose, M.D.)

(14) Legs tremble; give way on walking; debility of the aged, debility; great thirst, sugar in urine. *Glycosuria* with motor paralysis, (Curare 4th dilution for diabetes mellitus).

(15) Diabetes with "Carbuncles"—See "Carbuncles with diabetes".

Diabetes mellitus-with thirst and of nervous origin—(*a*) great thirst, weakness, emaciation. Urine in very large quantities. Specific gravity high, small red pimples itch violenty. Diabetic ulceration. (*Syzygium Jambolanum*). It is a most useful remedy in diabetes mellitus. No other remedy causes in so marked degree the diminution and disappearance of sugar in the urine. 10 drops to be taken thrice daily. It will prove more useful when alternated with *Ars-a.* (*b*) Diabetes of nervous origin when due to worry, mental over-work and sexual excess.(*Phos-a.*).

Diabetic-neuritis with fidgetiness and involuntary urination—Brain and spinal symptoms, tremblings convulsive twiching and fidgety feet. Involuntary urination when walking, coughing or sneezing. Nervous motion on feet when asleep. (*Zinc-m*)

D

Diabetic-sugar contents in urine—In a diabetic patient the fasting blood sugar should not normally exceed 100 mg%, while after meals 110 mg%. It is the appex limit of the normal. An excessive eating will lead to unassimilated glucose in blood and will appear as sugar in urine. Very low intake of food is equally harmful as it may lead to very low lavels of blood glucose. And obese diabetic must never overeat and a lean one should not fast unduly.

Diabetes with rheumatism—See "Rheumatism with Diabetes."

Diarrhoea and its treatment—For acute diarrhoea Dr. Dass Gupta begins treatment with *Acon*. If 2 or 3 doses fail, then he gives *Ip*. If this also fails, then he prescribes Puls. and *Nux-vom*. alternately. If still the diarrhoea, persists, he gives *Phos* ; when all these fail, then *Ars-a*. should be tried, and then *Verat-alba*. For chronic diarrhoea, he suggests *Sulph.*, *Cal-c*. and *Phos*. See also "Bilious diarrhoea".

Diarrhoea-chronic—According to Dr. Nash *Nitric acid* is one of the best medicines in diarrhoea. Diarrhoea slimy and offensive. After stools irritable aud exhausted.

Dr. P. Banerjee recommends *Chapparo 30*, *Nitric acid* and *Aloe 30* altenately four times daily as very effective.

Diarrhoea-due to indiscretion in dieting—(1) Acute diarrhoea on the first day. Intense thirst. (*Acon.*).

(2) If due to indiscretion in dieting or over-eating, *Nux-vom*. to be followed by Puls. See "Diarrhoea-due to indiscretion in food".

Diarrhoea-after measles—Diarrhoea after measles which is very common is often cured with *Puls*. Try this always. (*Puls.*). See "Measles not coming out properly No (i)".

Diarrhoea-alternating with constipation—(*a*) Alternating with constipation in patients addicted to purgatives. Frequent in effectual desire of passing of small quantity of stool which give relief immediately after passing it though for short time. (*Nux-v*). (*b*) Diarrhoea of infants alternating with constipation. Difficult dentition with colic pain, fetid stool, (*Podo.*). (*c*) *Alumina* is useful for constipation of infants when stool green and rectum sore.

Diarrhoea-alternating with constipation with old people—There is a form of diarrhoea which alternates with constipation, oftenest found with old people where *Antimonium Crudum* is the only remedy.

Diarrhoea after eating or drinking with burning pain and restlessness—After eating or drinking, stool offensive followed by great prostration. After decayed food or animals matter or alcoholic drinks. But it should have burning pain, restlessness, and thirst for little quantity and often. Warm drinks are preferred. (*Ars-alb.*). See "Pain abdominal burning".

Diarrhoea-cadaverous smelling stools of old people—Of old people with frequent, involuntary, cadaverous smelling stools followed by burning, itching and gnawing in rectum from which a glutionus and acrid moisture exudes. Bluish burning piles, pains after stool. (*Carb-v.*).

Diarrhoea bilious with colic after eating or drinking—(*a*) comes after eating or drinking accommpanied by colic (*Coloc.*) (*b*) For bilious diarrhoea *Cham.* is the best remedy. It has green stools like chopped eggs. *Cham.* should be followed by *Merc-s.* and *Sulf.* See "Colic-with diarrhoea and vomiting." and "Bilious diarrhoea."

Diarrhoea-during dentition—(1) Green, slimy, hot supttering, undigested with flatus. Teeth develop slowly. Troubles incident to dentition. Remedies the whole constitional defect during dentition. Compare *Chamomilla.*, which is good for acute troubles of this period. Sweating on head. (*Calc-p.*).

(2) Difficult dentition, child peevish and restless, child smells sour. (*Rheum.*).

Diarrhoea during dentition with green stool and foul odour—Green stool, foul odour and colicky pain. Abdomen bloated ; stool green, watery corroding the anus like stirred egg ; stool feels hot and smells like a rotten egg. (*Cham.*) Compare *Calc-p.* See also "Dentition" under its different heads.

Diarrhoea-discharge draining the patient—Very painful, watery, copious, and forcibly evacuated, followed by great prostration with sweat. Profuse draining discharge (*Verat-a.*).

Diarrhoea-in dropsy—Dropsy alternating with diarrhoea. Diarrhoea is copious and watery often involuntary. (*Apoc-can.*) See "Dropsy-with diarrhoea".

Diarrhoea-due to indiscretion in food—The patient has diarrhoea from the slightest indigestion or indiscretion in food. It has painful, watery diarrhoea with disgusting smell. (*Asaf.*). See "Diarrhoea due to indiscretion in dieting".

Diarrhoea-green stool—Thin green dysenteric stool (*Bell.*).

Diarrhoea-of marching soldiers—Soldiers have to undergo long marches, have to sleep on ground usually damp and have to eat all sorts of food in such circumstances. (*Silicea.*)

Diarrhoea-after midnight—After midnight ; painless, driving patient out of bed as if the bowels were too much to retain their contents. Weak, empty sinking sensation. (*Sulf.*)

Diarrhoea-milk upsets—In children when milk upsets and causes diarrhoea accompanied with thrush.(*Nat-c.*). See "Milk not digested with diarrhoea" and "Aversion to milk and other things".

Diarrhoea-in menses—A copious diarrhoea during the first day of menses and exhaustion coming on every menstrual period .(*Am-c.*). See "Menstruation-with colic and diarrhoea".

Diarrhoea-nervous—Of nervous type from emotional excitement, fright and bad news. (*Gels.*). See "Nervous diarrhoea".

Diarrhoea-due to over-eating in summer—Worse in the morning on first movement on rising and often occurs as an effect of over-eating in the summer (constipation is its general character). If often occurs as a result of dietetic errors specially when warm weather sets in after cold. Compare it with *Nux-vomica* diarrhoea which is also worse in the morning, is mostly caused by over-eating and is apt to put in the dysenteric type. It is caused from continued over-eating and inactivity, the abuse of drugs, coffee, tobacco or alcohol. The *Pulsatilla* diarrhoea, is more apt to occur in the night from over-eating, is attended with great rumbling of the bowels. It is caused from too rich foods, pastries, fat foods and ice-cream in excess. (*Bry.*) See "Summer diarrhoea-due to over eating".

Diarrhoea-during pregnancy—*Nux-mosch*. Compare *Cham.* and *Puls.* See also "Pregnancy-disorders of" No. 31.

Diarrhoea-after eating and drinking with rumbling stool escaping with flatus—There is lot of rumbling which may be so loud that others may hear it. The stool may gurgle out of flatus. There is leakage of stool even with flatus, uncertain whether gas or stool will come out. The patient holds the stool with difficulty and the stool may escape if the mind is off the sphincter. Every mouthful of food and even drinking water will hurry the patient to stool ; weakness after stool may be great. Lumpy stool mixed with water. The stool is offensive and hot which burns like fire and makes the anus sore. Pains about the navel shooting down towards rectum. (*Aloe*). Compare *Oleander* for chronic diarrhoea, stool undigested; passes stool with the least emission of flatus. See "Stool-involutary in children."

Diarrhoea unable to wait with tenesmus :—Morning diarrhoea with great deal of hot flatus (*Aloe*), with burning in rectum, straining before, during and after stool. Tenesmus after stool. Violent, sudden pains ; can't wait (*Agar*). Compare *Merc.* and *Sulf.*

Diarrhoea-in tuberculosis :—Dr. Hughes recommends, *Ipec.*, *Dros.*, *Kreosote* and *Ars-a.* See "No. 14 of Tuberculosis".

Diarrhoea-in early stage of typhoid :—There is often diarrhoea in the early stage of typhoid in which *Rhus-tox* is indicated. Restlessness, thirst, chilliness ; tongue has triangular tip with the rest of tongue coated. The patient from the very beginning a little stupefied, the brain is more or less cloudy with slight and mild delirium (not violent.) (*Rhus-tox.*). See also "Typhoid diarrhoea."

Diarrhoea-in typhoid watery and acrid :—*Arum-triphyllum* has a diarrhoea which is asscciated with typhoid fever. It is like the yellow corn-meal and musky. The faeces are also acrid and make the anus and adjoining parts raw and burning. The rawness may extend to adjoining parts even if the stool touches those parts. The typhoid patient picking the nose and the lips until they bleed. (*Arum-t.*). See "Typhoid-diarrhoea" and "Fever typhoid with drowsiness and diarrhoea".

Diarrhoea-small pox :—The most useful remedies are *An-t.*, *Ars-a.*, *Merc-sol.* and *Rhus-tox.* Compare Thuj. See. "(g)of small-pox."

Diarrhoea sour of undigested food with vomiting :—Diarrhoea of undigested food, fetid with ravenous appetite. Everything from mouth to anus turns sour. Eructations, vomiting and stool smell sour. Worse in afternoon. (*Calc.*). See "Sour every thing".

Diarrhoea-after vaccination-and chronic :—Chronic diarrhoea worse after breakfast : discharge forcibly expelled ; gurgling sound : flatulence ; diarrhoea specially from the effect of vaccination and after vaccination. (*Thuj.*). See "Vaccination".

Diarrhoea with draining discharge :—Very painful, watery, copious and forcibly evacuated followed by great prostration with sweat ; profuse draining discharge (*Verat-alba.*).

Diarrhoea with mucus and bleeding with watery stool and thirst :—Stools profuse, watery, pouring away as from a hydrant with lumps of white mucus like grain of sago and tallow. Stools involuntarily oozing from open anus. Thirst for iced cold water during diarrhoea. Burning in rectum, stomach and intestines. Bleeding from piles. (*Phos.*).

Diarrhoea painless with watery white stool without exhaustion :—Stool white in colour and watery in consistency, without much pain. It can be both chronic or acute but the patient does not feel any exhaustion or weakness after diarrhoea, on the contrary he feels a little better. The diarrhoea is painless and there is a lot of rumbling noise and the abdomen. The stools are gushing. The diarrhoea does not produce any marked debility or exhaustion. The exhaustion is primary of nervous exhaustion. (*Ph-a.*).

Diarrhoea-of children with changeful colour :—(*a*) The stools are constantly changing in colour and character. No stools are alike. They are green, yellow, white, watery, or slimy. Enterocolitis of children in hot weather. (*Puls.*). (*b*) Rheum after every motion if the motions are 'frothy. *Iris.* for bilious diarrhoea. See "Bilious diarrhoea".

Diarrhoea-children, offensive :—Of children particularly when loose stool offensive ; eructations. (*Bap.*).

Diarrhoea-frothy of child ; periodical :—Painless, stool undigested, frothy and yellow. In children the abdomen is bloated with lot of flatus. Child is weak and pale with dark rim along the eyes. Diarrhoea may be periodical. There is tendency to diarrhoea either in the evening or after eating fruits.

(*Chin.*) Compare *Podo.*

(2) During dentition with desire to bite gum. (*Phyt.*). See "Periodicity".

Diarrhoea-of children sour smelling :—The whole child seems to smell sour, and the child longing for sour things. Though ordinarily the child dislikes sour things. (*Hep.*). Compare *Calc-c.* See "Sour-everything".

Diarrhoea-of children involuntary stool without knowing :—Involuntary stool even solid in little children who may drop the stool all over the carpet without knowing that they have done so. (*Aloe*). See "Involuntary-stool of children".

Diarrhoea-in children with vomiting of milk :–Vomiting diarrhoea in infants with extreme prostration during dentition when with diarrhoea there is a marked inability to digest milk and poor circulation. (*Aeth.*). See "Milk-not digested with diarrhoea".

Diarrhoea-of vomiting children in summer ; starting suddenly :—Vomiting diarrhoea in children with extreme prostration during summer when with diarrhoea there is a marked inability to digest milk and poor circulation. It starts suddenly without notice in hot weather. The milk comes up partly in curds and partly in liquid and accompanying the vomiting there is a thin yellow, greenish ; slimy stool. The child has the appearance as if it were dying with pale hippocratic face. Death is stamped on the face from the beginning and if there is any medicine to save the life it is this *Aeth-c.* See "Vomiting-starting suddenly in children with serious symptoms".

Diarrhoea foamy-of children with nausea especially in summer—Of children specially during summer as a consequence of over-eating or wrong eating. Stool fermented or frothy or foamy or like green grass ; stool with mucus or watery or dysentery-like stool with or without blood. But nausea must be present and abdominal colic. A dose of Ip. 200 may often set the matters right. (*Ip.*). See "Summer diarrhoea due to overeating".

Diarrhoea-of children after every meal ; draining the patient and causing weakness :– Particularly of children. Must be characterised by :—

(1) The profuseness of stool.

(2) The stool is gushing.

(3) The offensiveness of stool.

(4) Extreme weakness and prostration after very stool.

(5) The aggravation in the morning, hot weather and during dentition. There is often present prolapsus ani ; sleep

with eyes half closed and rolling the head from side to side and moaning : frequent gagging (retching) or empty retching. The profuse stools are so much that they seem to drain the patient dry, and the patient feels extreme weakness and prostration from stool. The stools may be yellow or greenish, watery and when watery always profuse ; comes out as if it is coming out of tap. The child presses the gums together. Diarrhoea after every meal. Hardly any thirst inspite of so much drainage (*Podo.*). Campare *Ph-a.* in which the patient does not feel exhaustion in spite of so much drainage.

Digestion with heart-burn, bitter taste and flatulent colic :—(1) Imparied digestion, inspidity of food, yellowish tongue, bitter taste, heartburn, acidity, flatulence, distension of stomach, inability to sleep, (*Nux vom. 3* times a day).

(2) Sufferings caused by over-loading the stomach with fat, of greasy things, unwholesome meat, nausea sometimes diarrhoea. *Puls.* a dose every 4 to 6 hrs. (Particularly for females and children.).

(3) After food, oppression, nausea, and sour risings ; complete loss of appetite (*Hydr.* every three hrs.) See "Dyspepsia" under its different heads and also "Indigestion".

(4) Least food causes distress. Flatulent Colic. Marked anaemia. The patient is tired all the time. (*Tr. Aletris farinosa 30.* Five drops thrice a day).

Digestion disorder-flatulence of whole adbdomen :—Disorders of digestion. *China* is a great flatulence remedy, *i.e.*, it cures flatulence and distension in abdomen. Distension of whole abdomen. Patient feels uncomfortable and oppressed and can hardly breathe. (*Chin.*). Compare *Carbo-v.*, *Lyco.* See "Flatulent dyspepsia", See "Indigestion-chronic and atonic".

Digestive troubles-after eating decayed food :—After decayed food or animal matter or alcoholic drinks and chewing tobacco. But it should have (1) Burning pain, (2) Restlessness and (3) Thirst for little quantity of water and often, warm drinks are preferred. (*Ars-alb.*). See also "Food poisoning".

Digestive trouble-due to different troubles :—According to Dr. Laurie *Nux-vom. 6x,* one dose twice daily after meals and *Ars alb 6x.* one dose at bed time will give strength to stomach.

Digestive trouble with bloating of lower part of abdomen due to liver disturbance :—Failure of digestive powers when function of liver is seriously disturbed. Bloating is confined mostly to the lower part of abdomen below navel. Relieved by belching wind or by passing flatus. (*Lyco.*). Compare *Carb-v.* and *China.* See "Liver-bilious and deranged digestion."

Digestion-mouth ulcerated :—*Nat-m.* has a good action in the whole of the digestive system starting from mouth to the anus. The lips and mouth are dry with lips and corners of the mouth ulcerated or cracked. (*Nat-m.*). See also "Ulcers in mouth".

Digestion-weak after typhoid:—Weak after typhoid, flatulence, eructations give temporary relief. Simplest food disagrees specially fatty foods, (*Carb-v.*) Compare *Puls.* See "Weak-digestion after typhoid" .

Dilation of cervix :— *Staphysagria*

Dilation of heart (hypertrophy) :—Hypertrophy :—*Arsenic, Plumbum, Sulphur* and *Petroleum.* See "Heart" under its different heads.

Diphtheria-causing gland :—After recovery causing suppurating and inflamed glands on both sides of neck. Emaciation. No power in legs. Saliva from mouth and discharge from nose. Give *Bacillin 200* and later on *Silica.* This treatment will open the abscesses and will heal them rapidly.

Diphtheria laryngeal false membrane :—False membrane in the throat. Laryngeal (*Acet-ac.*).

D

Diphtheria followed by paralytic condition, food not swallowed :—Inflammatory condition of throat after diphtheria followed by paralytic condition of throat when on account of inflammation; liquid or food is not swallowed. (*Arum-t.*). See "Paralytic weakness of throat muscle after diphtheria" and "Confusion in Diphtheria".

Diphtheria-left sided—Left sided ; membrane dusky and bluish; pain aggravated by hot drinks. (*Lach.*)

Diphtheria-paralysis of heart :—*Naja Tripudians* is to be administered when there is impending paralysis of the heart. The patient is blue and awakens from sleep gasping.

(Dr. Farrington)

Diphtheria-preventives :—*Diphtherinum 200 ; Mercurius cynatus 30* to be given in water. See "No. 7 of Preventives".

Diphtheria-prophylactics-*Apis. 30 ; Diph. 30.*

Diphtheria-right sided :—The disease begins in the nose or right tonsil and extends to left. Worse cold drinks. (*Lyco.*).

Diphtheria tonic after its attack :—For subsequent weakness after attack of diphtheria give *Calc. Phos.* as a tonic.

Diphtheria-swollen with ulcers treatment :—(1) Throat livid and swollen. Tonsils studded with deep ulcers. Great prostration. (*Ail.*).

(2) In very bad cases of malignancy of diphtheria with suddenness of attack, extreme prostration and threatening collapse. Membrane is greenish and spreads through, nose bleeds, flow of saliva. Dr. Carter recommends *Mercurius cynatus* as a very successful remedy for this disease. (*Merc-cy.*). *Diphtherinum* 200 should be used as an intercurrent remedy. The treatment may start with this remedy.

(3) Pulse weak, breath and discharge very offensive ; collapse almost at the beginning. Swallows without pain : but fluids returned by nose. Dr. Carter of Children's Hospital; Paris thinks that both *Mercuris cynatus* and *Diptherinum* are also useful in post diphtheritic paralysis.

(4) Pseudo-membrane suffocating, hoarse, whistling cough having a croupy sound. *Bromine* is decidedly a remedy for such a trouble according to Dr. Dewey. (*Brom.*).

(5) Oedema of throat is the first indication. The throat has a glossy red appearance. Membrane forms on either tonsils and is grayish dirty looking and tough. Blisters on the border of the tongue., Drowsiness. Enlarged uvula, suffocation from actual closure of throat and larynx and patient in imminent danger of death. (*Apis-mellifica.*).

(6) Highly inflamed throat which is much swollen; coated tongue, swollen glands. Difficult to swallow ; dark red membrane. Pain from throat to ears when swallowing. (*Phyt.*).

(7) Confusion of mind in diphtheria. (*Lach.*).

(8) Delirium, headache, green stools, suppression of urine with chilliness and high fever, putrid throat. Dr. Slough did not lose a single case after he commenced using *Ignatia 200th* trituration persistently, a tea spoonful every hour or two.

Diphtheria suffocating :—Diphtheria in which the whole throat fills right up with oedematus swelling and the patient is in imminent danger of death by suffocation from actual closure of the throat and larynx. (*Apis melli.*). (Dr. Nash)

Diphtheria-weak heart :—Diphtheria where there is impending heart failure or paralysis (*Nux-vom.*).

Diphtheria-when patient progressing :—The nose is stopped, the child starts from sleep gasping for breath. Throat purple, swollen, ulcerated accompained by great exhaustion, with enlarged tonsils and glands. The patient is worse after sleep. When patient is getting along very nicely but dies of heart failure. In great instances if *Ammonium carb* were given in time it would save life. (*Am-c.*).

Diplopia-double vision :—(1) Seeing double with both eyes but normal when seeing with one eye. (*Senega.*).

(2) Letters or objects appear doubles (*Stram.*).

(3) Every things seems double so that one object represents to him merged with another with voilent tension in the eyes. (*Aurum foliatum*). See also "Eyes" under its different heads.

(4) Double vision on turning the eyes to the right and also double vision when seeing with both eyes but normal when seeing with one eye. (*Plumbum.*).

(5) Double vision associated with both eyes. (*Verat-v.*).

Discharge bloody :—Bloody discharge from nose or mouth. Great prostration. Face dark (*Ail*). See "Nose bleeding"

Discharge offensive :—*Asaf.* is a medicine for discharges from everywhere possible *e.g.* catarrhal discharges, copious discharges from uterus, watery stool. These discharges are horribly offensive and acrid. A horribly offensive discharge comes from the nose with ulcers inside. (*Asaf.*). (See "Nose dripping while eating" and "Ulcers syphilitic and offensive").

Diseases caused by suppression of eruption or skin troubles :—*Sulf.* acts from within outward and pushes every thing deep-seated of internally, out on the skin especially if there be suppression or retrocession of some eruption or skin trouble at the back or chronic ailments, rousing the sunken reactive forces of the body, itself clearing up the case and curing when indicated medicines fail to produce favourable effects or by helping them to cure. See "Suppressed skin trouble" and "Creating reaction".

Discolouration-of skin :—(1) Blackish or bluish spots on skin. (*Ars-alb.*).

(2) Yellow or brown patches on the abdomen (*Phos*).

(3) Red lines extending upto the arm or leg (*Hyper.*).

(4) Green skin (*Conium*).

(5) Skin looks dirty (*Sulf*).

(6) Greasy skin. (*Nat-mur.*).

(7) When skin becomes blue after dysentery. (*Iris-ver*).

(8) Discolouration of the skin after psoriasis. (*Kali-ars.*).

(9) Skin blue after being beaten or after fever skin purple (*Lach.*).

(10) Skin becomes black in cholera. (*Ars-iod.*).

Disfigurement of face :—If disfigurement is due to small-pox then give *Variolinum* every fortnight and *Sarracenia purpurea 6* thrice daily for a considerable period.

(2) If acne or scars left by ulcers and boils have disfigured the face then give *Silicea* and *Calc. flour.* See "Small-pox preventive and for disfigurement".

Disinfectant and germicide—Oil of *Cinnamon.* in aqueous solution is best local disinfectant. 3 or 4 drops in two quarts of water as a douche, wherever a germicide and disinfectant is needed. 3 drops on sugar for hiccough. According to Mr. Chamberland no disease germ can long resist the antiseptic power of essence of *Cinnamon* which is as effective to destroy microbes as corrosive sublimate.

Dislocation :—(1) *Arnica* for redness and excessive inflammation and pain after dislocation—a dose every 2 hours. *Aconite* should follow *Arnica* after 2 hours, if the pain continues.

(2) If the pains don't subside after the dislocation is reduced then give *Tr Rhus-t.* two tea spoonful in half a drachm of water, 3 such doses each day until the pain entirely disappears. See "Fracture pains".

(3) **Dislocation of patella while going upstairs** :—*Can. sat.*

Distension :—After meal to loosen clothes. (*Puls.*) Flatulence, distension passing upwards (*Carb-v.*); flatulence passing downwards. (*Lyco.*) See also "Flatulence under its different heads, and "Bloating stomach".

Distension-in drospy :—In dropsical conditions. Abdomen very much distended. The stomach is inflamed. The blood vessels are distended. The patient's stomach is distended and he must vomit ; and with distension of his whole body he drinks and vomits. It is with difficulty that he can eat ; he will drink and not digest. Sense of pressure in the epigastrium in the chest. (*Apoc-can.*) See "Dropsy flautlence".

Diuretic—A hydrogogue diuretic in the treatment of dropsies. Albuminaria, uraemia and diabetes. (*Urea. 10* grains every *6* hrs.) and *Argent-phos.* which is an excellent diuretic in dropsy, also *Galium aparine* acts on urinary organ, is a diuretic, of use in dropsies, gravel and calculi.

Dog bite-its complications :—Made safe by use of Ledum from its subsequent complication of tetanus or any other form of septic condition. *Ledum* will prevent not only subsequent inflammatory complication but also prevent shooting pains. (*Led.*). See also "Rabies".

Dog bite wound :—Bite of dog, burning better by hot steam, headache due to dog bite. Peculiar sensations at seat or in the adjacent parts, pricking sensation, boring and burning proceeding from wound. *Lyssin=Hydrophobinum* (saliva of rabid dog). See No. 3 of "Bites".

Dose—(*a*) The subject is rather puzzling and has been already briefly dealt with under "Administration of Medicines" and the reader is advised to go through it first. It is only by experience and keen observation that a practitioner can be able to determine what dilution (strength) is to be given of a particular medicine and at what intervals. The very high potencies seldom require repetition if clearly indicated, to produce a long curative action in chronic cases. But in severe acute sickness several doses in quick succession are most useful. When medicine is given at interval, the curative power is increased and may be safe if it is discontinued with judgement. When a positive effect has been obtained, the medicine should always be discontinued and the greatest mischief may come from continuing to give it. In chronic diseases for the first prescription the single dose will be found even the best. Higher dilutions should not be repeated more frequently than once a week. It is always better to begin low and go higher and higher. Each change of potency brings new and deeper curative action. A deep acting chronic remedy should seldom be given in the midst of paroxysms but at the close of it. When symptoms change, the remedy must be discontinued but not changed at once. The repetition of the dose to intensify the action of the remedy must not he considered as the rule but the exception. See also "Administration of medicine"

(b) Please read first "Administration of medicine", "Potencies and of medicines and "the first part of heading 'Dose' in order to have a clear idea of what potencies are to be used. I have been flooded with inquiries in this respect mostly from new lay practitioners. I have already stated that it is only by experience and keen observation that a practitioner can be able to determine what potency is to be given and at what intervals.

It is obvious that two constitutions are not equal in all respects. In homoeopathy remedies are considered first and foremost in relation to individuals and not to disease. The stage of disease and phase of symptoms, the age and sex of the patient, the nature of disease whether chronic or acute and susceptibility of the patient, his temperament and environments have to be taken into consideration when determining this question. Every Practitioners' experience is his best guide. A given number of repetitions more or less according to the serverity of case will serve to place the patient under the influence of the medicine. In affections of mild type the invervals may vary from 6 to 12 hours. It is, therefore, unethical to bind the hands of the Prescriber. In the revised edition of this Prescriber I have indicated in certain cases the potency of the drug either based on the experience of eminent physicians or of my own but the Prescriber is free to vary it according to the circumstances even in such cases.

I describe my own practice which I have found very successful. I generally start with 30 potency which can safely be repeated and gradually go higher up to 200. I usually give complementary or supplementary medicine of 30 potencies in alternation with principal remedy daily, according to symptoms, repeating in all 4 times a day. When principal remedy reaches up to 200 then I make it a weekly affair according to change of symptoms. With this procedure I invariably give intercurrent medicines such as *Tuberculinum, Sulphur Baciltinum, Thuja, Nux-vomica* and nosodes suited to the condition and nature of trouble. These intercurrent medicines are usually given in 1 M. potencies or higher if need be. No other medicine is to be given that day and also for a week at least. This time may be varied according to the condition of the patient.

Then again, if need be the same procedure is coutinued either with change of remedies or with same medicines as the situation demands.

I rarely use decimal scale potencies.

Below I will quote the method of selection of potencies by some of the celebrated Homoeopaths :—

(i) Give the higher potency to those accustomed to the low or to allopathic treatment.
To those accustomed to high potency give still higner or much lower i.e., change the potency for the patient. After improvement stops, change the potency if the same remedy is indicated. (Dr. Cas)

(ii) The low potency fits the simple case. It may require repetition. Higher may be demanded for complete cure. (Dr. T. Hutchinson., M.D.)

(iii) In digestive complaints use lower potencies. It is for this reason nutritive medicines like *Calc. Phos* or *Nut-mur.* are most efficacious in low potencies. In acute diarrhoea and vomiting low potencies are similarly preferable and should be taken in dry form which is indeed important. The indicated remedies taken in dry form act like smoothing oil upon temptuous waves, in any case, much surer and quicker than taken in water. (Dr. C. Cotta)

(iv) Low potencies for the recent and high for the chronic. (Dr. G. Royal, M.D.).

(v) Very high potencies such as *C.M.* may over-shoot the mark. It is better to drop back and try the 30th you may be surprised. However I think 200th. is a fine potency to start with. (Dr. W.K. Bond, M.D.)

(vi) It frequently happens that high will relieve most effectively, otherwise they would have never come into use, but it also happens now and then that low potencies succeed when high have failed. (Dr. Wheeler.).

(vii) For mental distress and diseases of psychic origin the high potencies (10 M and upwards) would be employed, other things being equal, and that for grossly material conditions such as marked organic and pathological changes the lower or the medium potencies would be selected. (Dr. E. Wright, M.D.)

(viii) Every homoeopathic physician who is able to select the right medicine and who avoids the great fault of precipitation which is always injurious, will soon perceive that the high dynamization when given at long intervals and without repetition, are generally preferable to large doses which are repeated or changed too frequently. (Dr. Boenninghausen).

(ix) Dr. Thomas Reed, an experienced homoeopath, was very famous for his cures in appendicitis, gall-stones and renal colic. He often commenced a case with one dose of *C.M.*, then followed with lower potencies from tincture to 6th potencies.

(x) Hahnemann taught that the right remedy will act in almost any strength or potency but that the wrong remedy will be impossible whatever strength is selected.

Dread of loneliness and animals—Of being alone, *Conium* ; of dogs and other animals, *China. off.* ; of trifles *Ignatia*. See also "Fear" under different heads and "Fright."

Dreams of different types like crying and dreams causing insomnia—(1) When due to indiscretion in diet. (*Nux-v*).

(2) When talking and crying out during sleep ; anxious dreams. (*Magnesia-muriatica.*).

(3) Of weeping with tears : fearful dreams, (*Glonoine*).

(4) Sexual dreams with emission every 3rd or 4th day. (*Nux-v.*). See "Emission".

(5) When not traceable to obvious cause. (*Kali-bromatum,* Gr. V. at bed time.) ,(b) **Dreams causing insomnia :—**

Dreams causing insomnia :—

(1) Dr. Jahr thinks that *Nux-v.* and *Lachesis* are useful when arising from excessive mental exertion. Dr. Farrington and Dr. Dewey think *Ambra grisea* is suitable for sleeplessness arising from worried mind.

(2) *Avena-sativa* 10 or 15 drops will induce sleep in nervous and exhausted people.

(3) Dr. Dewey says that *Passiflora,* 30 to 60 drops repeated when necessary will induce sleep when mental irritation or pain is the cause of wakefulness.

(4) For children the best remedy is *Cham.*, if this is not sufficient, try *Ant t.* or *Puls.* See also "Insomnia" and "Sleeplessness" under their different heads.

(5) Starts up frightened for too frequent and vivid dreams. (*Hyos.*).

(6) Dreams of snakes, of urinating and on waking must hurry to prevent the accident (*Lac-c.*),

(7) Dreams of animals. (*Merc.*).

(8) Dreams of thieves entering the house and thus disturbing the sleep. (*Sil.*).

(9) Dreams of fire. (*Bell.*).

(10) Dreams of passing stools. (*Aloe.*).

(11) Dreams of ghosts, imaginative of misfortunes. (*Kali-c.*)

(12) Dreams of funerals. (*Chel.*).

(13) Dreams of dead people ; of falling from height. (*Thuja.*

Dreams of dreadful animals and ghosts—The patient imagines to see ghosts and dreadful animals. Child starts up from sleep very often and gnashes his teeth. (*Bell.*). See "Teeth-gnashing by a child".

Dribbling of urine due to paralytic condition of sphincter and bladder—(*i*) Constant dribbling of urine after labour which is due the paralytic condition of sphincter, bladder, on account of the contusion, is always removed by *Arnica*. See "Urine dribbling after labour ordinary", "Labour retention of urine" and "Stricture of urethra."

(b) *Bell, Cina, Cannabis-sativa* and *Cantharis* may be used according to symptoms.

(2) Urine dribbles out involuntarily due to paralysis of bladder. It is retained and then dribbles out. (*Alumina*).

(3) There is irritability at the neck of bladder and the same symptom is found here as with rectum. There is vesical torpor or paralysis. There my be dribbling of urine or retention. The urine is dark with a red brick sadiment or bloody or mixed with a tenacious mucus. (*Nux-v.*).

(4) When wetting the bed without tangible cause except habit. *Equisetum* is a good remedy for involuntary discharge of urine or for suppression or difficulty in discharging urine.

(5) An intercurrent remedy when other well selected remedies fail is *Psorinum*.

(6) Nocturnal enuresis passing large quantities of pungent smelling urine, or scanty or high cloured or copious pale urine ; with pungent odour ; worse during menstruation, dribbling of urine : painful tenesmus of bladder, severe pain at the conclusion of urination. (*Medorrhinum.*).

(7) Vertigo when trying to rise ; objects whirl before the eyes, eyes sunken with contracted pupils. Paralysis of bladder hence involuntary urine. (*Cicuta virosa*).

(8) For constant dribbling (*Verbasc-t.* 3 or 4 hourly).

(9) Unconscious of passing of urine. (*Arg. n.*).

(0) Dribbling of urine night and day. *Turnera-aphrodisiaca 2x* in water four times a day.

Dribbling of urine due to partial paralysis of bladder of woman and leaky bladder of man—In the partial paralysis of the bladder in old woman when there is a constant dribbling of urine which cannot be controlled, then give her *Nux-vom.* 3 times a day.

(2) In the leaky bladder of old man who cannot hold the urine but it dribles on the clothes and there is a constant desire to urinate while the act does not give relief give *Equisetum* 10 drops in half a wine glass of water every two hours. See "Urine" under different heads.

Dropsical effusion (pouring out of fluid)—The dropsical effusion may be general or local, it is found in the thoracic (belonging to the throat) cavity, in ovaries, in abdomen cavity, scrotum and genital of females. There is an absolute absence of thirst (*Apis-mell.*). If there is thirst in such cases then *Acetic acid, Arsenic* and *Apocy*.

Dropsy-due to liver—Due to hepatic disease (*Lyco*). See No.(12)of Liver and its various troubles.

Dropsy-flatulence—Weakness, trembling, aversion to work. Great flatulence or wind ; distension as if abdomen would burst. (*Chin.*). See "Distension in drospy".

Dropsy-of chest—*Hydrothorax* (dropsy of chest) with general dropsy aggravation at 3 A.M. (*Kali Carb 200*).

Dropsy-general swelling—Oedema every where, general anasarca, abdomen with pain. (*Apis-mell.*).

Dropsy-swelling of feet—Swelling of feet and leg. (*Merc-sol.*). See also "Hydrothorax dropsy of chest".

Dropsy-with diarrhoea—Anasarca with dropsical condition. Dropsy alternating with diarrhoeal condition, is great key symptom to *Apocynum*. Diarrhoea is copious and watery and often involuntary. Functions of all vital organs namely skin, kidney, bowels, uterus, all tend to stop their functions, causing formation of dropsy. (*Apoc-can*). Compare *Apis*. which is hot while *Apoc*. is chilly and is sensitive to cold air and to cold drinks. See also "Hypostatic-congestion of lungs in dropsy" and "Diarrhoea in dropsy".

Dropsy-due to liver kidney or heart—(1) Dropsy from liver diseases, lower extremities, afternoon fever with no thirst, difficult breathing on lying down ; urine scanty and high coloured, bowels constipated. Give *Lyco. 30*. After 3 or 4 doses if there is no improvement then *Apis*. should be given. If still trouble persists then *Ars-a*. should be given.

(2) Jelly like diarrhoea, urine dark and scanty, sudden dropsies and actual dropsies. *Helleborus* is very useful in many forms of dropsy. (*Hell.*).

(3) Dropsy-kidney : Dropsy from congestion to the kidney, dull aching in renal region, dark smoky urine. (*Terebinthina.*).

(4) Dropsy heart—Due to disorders of heart and lungs. Puffiness of the face with oedema about eyelids, thirst, vomiting. In dropsy oozing of serum is also a symptom. (*Arsneicum.*). It is suitable in all forms of dropsy and is an important diuretic. Compare *Rhus*. and *Lyco*. for oozing of serum.

(5) Dropsy-abdomen :—Dropsy of abdomen with gastric disturbances. Belching and diarrhoea. Profuse sweating (*Acetic-acid*).

(6) For dropsy with enlargement of liver and spleen R.B. Bishamber Das recommends *Liatris-spicata M.T*. in 10 drops doses.

(7) An excellent diuretic in dropsy. (*Argent.phosph.*)

(8) *Prymula veris* is very good in the case of dropsy. See also "Ascites-dropsy of abdomen" and "Congestion of lungs in dropsy".

Drowsiness—The patient lies usually in a sleepy condition and does not like to be disturbed. Sometimes unconscious ; indisposed to move or to talk. The patient is normally weak, due to loss of vital fluid, sexual excesses and violent acute diseases. (*Ph-a*). See "Sleepiness".

Drunkenness—If a person has taken a little too much wine and feels ill therefrom, give him *Nux-vom*. If the smallest quantity of wine affects the head then give him *Zincum*. See "Alcoholism". See "Nos. 1 and 4 of cravings".

Dryness of mucous membranes causing dry stool or dry caugh—Stools hard and dry as if burnt. Thirst for large quantities water at longer intervals. Mouth and lips are parched. The same condition of dryness obtained in the lungs and bronchi which causes hard dry cough with no expectoration. Dry cough hurts the head in headache. (*Bry.*).

Duodenal-ulcer—(1) Vomiting of food and mucus mixed with bile and blood. Dr. Jahr recommends *Phos.* as most essential aid. (*Phos.*).

(2) Great burning in stomach. Vomiting immediately after eating or drinking. (*Ars-a*).

(3) Dr. Pope recommends *Kali bi.* when the ulcer is at the cardiac end of stomach (*Kali-bi.*).

(4) *Uranium nitricum* is said to arrest the tendency to formation of uclers. (*Uran*). See also "Gastric ulcer" and "Ulcer of stomach".

(5) Tarry stool with bloody vomiting. (*Ham*).

(6) When there is a considerable haemorrhage and collapse and heart weakness is threatened due to haemorrhage, then give *Trillium*. If haemorrhage, does not stop then *Secale* is a valuable medicine to stop it.

(7) Old duodenal ulcer with intolerable burning, epigastric pain with much flatulence. (*Arg-n.*).

(8) Gastric and duodenal ulcer. The patient feels severe pain when stomach is empty. 2 or 3 hours after meals the pain begins in the stomach. *Anac.* is a valuable remedy in such cases.

(9) For persistent scarring in duodenal ulcer. (*Graph.*).

(10) Heart-burn, pain or pressure or eructations in duodenal ulcer. (*Lyco.* in higher potencies).

(11) *Anacardium* is a most wonderful remedy for duodenal and gastric ulcer, as soon as the complaint of violent

pain appears two or three hours after meal, *Anac. 3x* may be given.

(12) For constipation, sinking in the stomach region palpitation of the heart, vomiting often of blood, general weakness and frontal headache (*Hydrast.*). See "Peptic ulcers".

Duodenal ulcer-perforation—For ulceration, perforation and catarrh of the duodenal and gastric ulcers, with jaundice, thickly coated tonque and discharge from the bowels stringy mucus (*Kali-bich.*). stands second to no other remedy. (Dr. G. Royal)

Duodenal ulcer preventing its development—Lean and lively young man worried about business suffering greatly from anticipation, minds active that he cannot relax at night *Lycopodium* will prevent the development of duodenal ulcer as a result business or family worries If stresses recur then the same medicine may be given again.

Dwarfishness-hand and legs short—The teatment should begin by giving *Tuberculinum* not lower than 200 in dilution but should not be repeated frequently. One week after this *Baryta-carb 200.* should be given. (ii) *Tuberculinum* and *Syphilinum 200,* or 1000 dilution given alternately every week or fortnightly will cure the dwarfishness. (iii) For dwarfish children who are small, weak, pale, very large head, fontanelles large and bulging out bones of skull, thin and cracking under pressure, thin like tissue paper give *Calc-phos.* (iv) Deformity due to structural changes in spinal cord. The hands and legs do not grow. They also drop out as in senile gangrene. (*Secale-cor.*). (R.B.B. Dass) See "Short stature".

Dysentery with griping and fever—Give *Merc-c.* and *Ipecac.* in ordinary cases. If there is severe griping *Colocynth.* also *Ars.* is to be given when there is burning pain cold extremities, thirst and prostration. *Acon.* If there is fever. (Father Muller) See also "Colitis".

Dysentry-its after effect—Patient never being well since the attack of dysentery (*Dysentery-co. 30*).

Dysentery-amoebic—With tenesmus while straining, pain so great that it nauseates. Worse around navel, little thirst. Stool with mucus or with or without blood. (*Ip.*).

Dysentery with blood—In the first stage with good deal of blood in discharge and with temperature. (*Ferr-p*). It is very valuable and often cures in a very short time. (Dr. Nash). See "Blood dysentery".

Dysentery-blood with urging for urination and tenesmus of rectum—Bloody dysentery, tenesmus not relieved by passing of stool. Stool hot bloody, slimy (muddy), offensive with cutting pains and shreds of mucous membrane. But there must be tenesmus or urging of the bladder and rectum at the same time and urine passing in drops with much pain along with the stool, i.e. the tenesmus of the rectum must extend to bladder area also in order that *Merc-c.* may act or vice versa i.e. along with the symptoms of the bladder the constant urging for urination there should be urging to stool. It has more intense symptoms which appear suddenly and vehemently. (*Merc c.*). Compare *Nux-v.* which must have absolute relief for some time after stool. "Blood dysentery".

Dysentery-with bloody motion—Three or four bloody motions daily with more or less pain. (*Chaparro amargosa*).

Dysentery after eating or drinking, with colic—Comes after eating or drinking accompanied by colic and vomiting. Such a colic occurs in acute dysentery. (*Coloc.*). See also "Colic-of child in dysentery".

Dysentery-amoebic and it prevention of recurrence—After cure of this kind of dysentery some time it recurs and causes colites, hepatic disturbances or diarrhoea. Dr. C.L.W. Greman suggests *Merc. cor. 6, Ipec, 3, Aloe. 4,* and *Colocynth 6.* according to indication to be used for two months.

Dysentery-chronic with constipation, diarrhoea and mucus—Chronic. In dysentery there is violent tenesmus heat in rectum, prostation even to fainting and profuse clammy sweats. Pains about the navel shooting down towards rectum. There must be absolute constipation with stool but the urging with flatus continues throughout the day in chronic dysentery patient. (*Aloe*).

(2) R.B. Bhishambeı Das recommeds *Chaparro-amargoso* in chronic or acute dysentery or diarrhoea where everything has failed.

(3) In dysentery when *Cantharis* has removed mucous stool like scraping of intestines there *Kali-bichromicum* will often complete the cure when stool is gelatinous with periodic constipation.

(4) Bloody stool after eating and drinking with pain in the abdomen. (*Trombidium 6.*)

To prevent the dehydration specially in chidren, glucose in water is given at regular intervals.

(5) *Sulf. 200* is the head remedy for colitis and chronic dysentery. Compare *Staphylocein* which cures this disease quickly. (Dr. Sukartee)

Dysentery-with gripping, with repeated desire to go to stool—The patient has intense griping pain with repeated desire to go to stool but there must be relief even though for a short time after every stool. (*Nux-v.*) Compare *Merc-sol.* and *Merc-c. Merc-sol.* has no relief after stool. *Merc-sol.* will suit when mucus is present, *Merc-c.* where blood is preminent.

Dysentery-malignant with cold extremities and paralysis of sphincters—*Phos,* is indicated in advanced and grave cases where there are cold extremities and paralysis of sphincters.

Dysentery-of old people—Of old people. (*Bapt*).

Dysentery-bloody with tenesmus and its treatment—There is a great tenesmus (inclination to urge repeatedly for stool and a sensation of "cannot finish"). Offensive odour of mouth. The patient has slight difficulty in passing urine. Greenish bloody, slimy and whitish grey stool. Aggravation at night. Compare *Nux-v.* also useful in dysentery of summer weather.

Give a few doses of *Aconite* first and follow it with *Merc sol.* A dose of *Sulf.* is needed to support *Merc-sol.* when dysenteric symptoms are practically cured.

Dysentery-bloody of summer weather—There is a great tenesmus, offensive odour of mouth. The patient has slight difficulty in passing urine. Greenish, bloody, slimy and whitish grey stool. Aggravation at night. (*Merc-sol.*) Give a few doses of *Aconite* first and follow it with *Merc-sol.* A dose of *Sulf.* is needed to support *Merc-sol.* when dysenteric symptoms are practically cured. Compare *Nux-v.* which is also useful in dysentery of summer weather. See "Summer diarrhoea-due to over-eating".

Dysentery-amoebic and its prevention of recurrence—After cure of this kind of dysentery sometimes it recurs and causes colitis hepatic disturbances or diarrhoea. Dr. C.L.W Graeman suggest *Merc-cor. 6, Ipec. 3, Aloe 4,* and *Colocynth 6,* according to indication to be used for two month.

Dysentery-with fever—See "Fever with dysentery".

Dysmenorrhoea irregular with leucorrhoea, with pain (difficult or painful menstruation)—(1) Colic. Menses too early too copious and last too long ; Colic with crampy pain at the navel, violent abdominal cramps. Discharge fetid and itching. (*Kreosotum*).

(2) Menstrual irregularities at the critical age. Violent colic, has to lie down in consequence of uneasiness, sleeplessness, at night, violent frontal headache, watery and milky leucorrhoea, nose bleed, toothache. (*Sep.*).

(3) Pains are of agonising, burning extending down to thighs, Menstruation profuse with pain, headache before menses, Dr. Hale recommends *Xanthoxylum*.

(4) Menses are too early. Pain in the sides, groin. stomach ache, nausea, coryza with stoppage of nose, violent colic, pain in the knees ; itching, at the parts. (*Magnesia-carbonica*).

(5) According to Dr. Conard Wesselhoeft the most useful remedy in dysmenorrhoea with scanty, irregular menstruation, uterine cramps, profuse clotted blood discharge is *Cocculus*.

(6) Dymenorrhoea where there is excruciating pain through the uterus and lower part of the abdomen. The pain precedes the menstrual flow. Pains from back to loins. Dr. W. Boericke recommends tincture Viburnum *opulus 20* drops in a small glass of water. Teaspoonful doses should be frequently given.

Dysmenorrhoea-or difficult-or painful menstruation in hysterics—Severe pain all through the flow. The more the flow and greater the pain. Irregularity of menstrual flow in the hysterical and rheumatic constitutions. (*Act-rac*). See "Rheumatic dysmenorrhoea".

Dysmenorrhoea-too early with painful dark flow (painful menstruation) of neuralgic type—Of neuralgic variety. Menses too early, flow dark, stringy, worse before pain but better when flow begins. Swelling of external parts. Relieved by warmth and slight pressure of hand or a hot water bottle. (*Mag-p.*).

Dyspepsia with flatulence also acid dyspepsia—(1) Chronic, longing for acid things. (*Hep*).

(2) Flatulence very marked with great relief from belching. Belching after every meal, pain of ulcerative type. Gastralgia in delicate nervous women (*Argentum nitric.*).

(3) Pain in stomach immediately after eating. Regurgitation of food after eating and nausea. Alternate constipation and diarrhoea. (*Amon-mur.*). See "Pancreatic troubles".

(4) Dr. Jousset recommends the alternation of *Nux-v.* and *Graphites* in most cases of dyspepsia. He gives *Nux-v. 12* one hour before meals and *Graphites* 12 one hour after meals and claims that this is all sufficient in most cases of dyspepsia. This is continued for 8 days and resumed after an interval of rest.

(5) Food lies like a load, pressure and heaviness immediately after eating. Tympanitic abdomen ; cutting pain in stomach soon after eating. (*Kali-bich* 200) See "Digestion" under its different heads and also "Indigestion and gastric trouble".

(6) *Acid dyspepsia*. The gastric symptoms with most pronounced acidity, sour eructations ; great distension of stomach and flatulence. Flatulent Colic (*Rob.*).

(7) Flatulent distension of abdomen and oppressive feeling about the heart. (*Slag.*), or *Silco-Sulpho Calcite or Alumina 3x* trituration in 5 grain doses. (Dr. Meridith). See "Acidity with wind" and "Gastritis chronic acid stage."

Dyspepsia-with bad taste with, rich food and vomiting—Indigestion and digestive disorders. Indigestion with bad taste in mouth, nothing tasting well, not even water. Dryness of mouth without thirst caused by rich greasy food and these rich and greasy food, e.g. cakes, pastry and heavy sweets upsetting the stomach. Weight as from stone. Great tightness after a meal. Vomiting of food eaten long before. Water - brash with foul taste in morning. *Puls.* patient does not tolerate fat. (*Puls.*). See "Taste-nothing tastes well during digestive trouble" and "Indigestion with bad taste in mouth".

Dyspepsia-of adults from brain trouble and constant eating—When digestion has absolutely ceased from brain trouble and from excitement. *Aeth.* has cured dyspepsia from constant feeding in those nibblers, those hungry fellows who are always eating, always nibbling, always taking crackers in their pockets until the time comes when the stomach ceases to act. (*Aeth*). See "Nervous-dyspepsia from excitement" and "Indigestion of adults from constant eating".

Dyspepsia-of old people—Great distention in abdomen immediately after eating a little. Abdomen distended with wind after eating. *Kali-carb.* is specially adapted to broken down aged people who are anaemic.

Dyspepsia-due to fermentable food with flatulence in lower abdomen—Due to fermentable food, cabbage, beans etc. Desire for sweet things. Food tastes sour, eructations. Great weakness of digestion. After eating pressure in stomach with bitter taste in mouth. Eating even so little creates fulness. Rolling of flatulence. Failure of digestive powers when function of liver is seriously disturbed. Bloating is confined most to the lower part of the abdomen below navel. Relieved by belching wind or passing flatus (*Lyco.*). Compare *Carb-v.* and *China*.

Dyspepsia-with acidity due to incompatible food—Acute abdominal disorders caused by incompatible food. After eating sour taste in the mouth. Pressure in the stomach for one or two hours after eating. Tightness about the waist. Cannot do mental work after food for three or four hours. Bloating of stomach with a stony weight in stomach. Never happy after food but happy after stool. Colic ; liver enlarged. (*Nux-v.*). Compare *Puls.* (b) Stomach digestion perverted. Gastric symptoms with most pronounced acidity. Acrid eructations. Distension of stomach and bowels and obstinate flatus. (*Robinia.*). See "Acidity-with wind".

Dyspepsia-of old also with heart trouble—Old dyspeptics with brain fag. The stomach refuses to do its work. The food remains in the stomach. Sour vomiting. Sinking sensation in the abdomen after a normal stool. (*Phos-a.*), (b) In dyspeptic trouble of the aged with functional heart symptoms and associated with gastric disturbances. (*Abies nigra.*) See "Heart-burn" and "Heart-flatulence pressing."

Dyspepsia-nervous—Of nervous type. The main symptom in the sphere of stomach is a pain, which is sometimes removed by eating. (*Anac.*). See "Nervous dyspepsia from excitement."

Dyspepsia-with wind trouble after typhoid—Digestion weak after typhoid, flatulence ; eructations give temporary relief. The simplest food disagrees specially fatty foods. Excessive wind in the upper portion of the abdomen, pressing upwards in the chest and causing distress in the heart. Relieved by belching wind or passing flatus. (*Carb-v.*). Compare

Puls., *Lyco* and *China*. See "Tympanitis in typhoid including digestion weak after typhoid" and "Digestion weak after typhoid".

Dyspepsia-wind—Abdomen distended with wind after eating (*Kali-c.*). See "Wind trouble".

Dyspnoea with cold sweat and palpitation—Dyspnoea that we have in this medicine (*Am-c.*) is due to heart and is not asthmatic. The dyspnoea increases in warm room and cold air usually relieves but the body feels cold. The complaints of this come on at 3 o'clock in the morning with palpitation, cold sweats. (*Am-c.*). During attack give *Cactus 200* five drops in water and follow it with *Arsenic 30* in water one teaspoonful every 5 minutes. When every cold spell brings on catarrh of the chest of old people with thick mucus and he must sit up and fanned and cannot lie down because of difficult breathing and filling up of the chest then *Ant-t.* will ward off such attacks of catarrh of long standing. If expectoration is yellow then give him *Ammoniacum*. See "Breathlessness", "Breathing oppressed" or "Respiration" and "Choking".

Dyspnoea-with cardiac symptoms—Due to nervous excitement with cardiac symptoms. Difficult breathing of asthma type on slightest exertion in nervous people. (*Ambra.*) See "Heart with suffocation" and "Cough cardiac"

Dyspnoea-hysterical—Hysterical. Attacks after coition as *Ambra*. Nightly aggravation. (*Asaf.*).

(1) Oppression of chest with choking and obstruction of breathing. (*Naja-tripudians*).

(2) On taking slightest food. (*Phos.*) See "Hypostatic-congestion of lungs in dropsy".

Dysponea-of pregnant females with swollen legs—It is accompanied by digestive derangements. It is generally after a meal that females are attacked by the distress of breath, with anguish, congestion of the head ; red face. Dr. Jahr recommends *Nux-v.* Two globules on dry tongue as the best remedy for this trouble, in some cases if there is flatulence and distension then *China* is an excellent remedy, and for swelling of legs with puffed face *Arsenic*. is recommended. See "Pregnancy disorder No. 15".

Dysuria (painful urination including involuntary stool and urine)—Pain and feeling of bladder not relieved by urinating. Urine flows only drop by drop. Incontinence (involuntary evacution) in old women also with involuntary stools. Involuntary urination. (*Equisetum tincture,* 6th potency.). See "Incontinence-involuntary evacuation of urine".

(2) Patient driven almost mad with painful micturition, the burning and straining truly awful. *Triticum repens*. M.T. 10 drops in a little water.

(Dr. Burnett)

E

Earache—Throbbing and heating pain (*Bell*). See No.(2)of "Boils"

Ear-boils on it—Boils are extremely painful throbbing. Eruption on auditory canal *Calc. picrata* 30th or 200 potency. *Belladonna 30* in hourly alternation with *Merc. sol.* will prevent the development or suppuration of boil.

Earache-inflammation spreading during cold—In coryza the inflammation soon spreads to the ear, throat and the larynx. Violent earache even to the discharge of pus from the ear. Ringing in the ear. (*All-c.*). Compare *Puls., Cham.,* for earaches in children, also *Kali-m.* for such troubles.

Ear discharge offensive in children—Both chronic and acute troubles particularly in children. Pus may be thick and greenish. Thirstlessness, feeling of heat and restlessness, relieved by slowly walking about in cold air. Hearing difficult as if the ears were stuffed. Discharge offensive. Dimnishes acuteness of hearing. Otorrhoea. (*Puls.*). See "Otorrhoea" under different heads.

Ear-deafness also perforation—(*a*) *Kali-m.* is the general remedy for deafness. (*b*) Due to perforation or abscess in the ear. (*Hep-s.*). See also "Deafness".

Ear-deafness catarrhal in old people—Catarrhal deafness in elderly people and by obstruction of eustachian tube. Worse in damp weather (*Merc-d.*) See "Catarrhal deafness"

Ear-deafness chronic or from birth—Deafness chronic or from birth is cured by *Mephitis.* Start treatment with 30 potency and go higher. It should be given a long trial say for 6 months or a year. A dose of *Tuberculinum 200* should be given every month as an intercurrent remedy. No other medicine is to be given 2 days before or after. (R.B.B. Das)..

Ear-deafness due to obstruction—Deafness due to obstruction in the ear. (*Verbascum*).

Ear deafness after-measles—*Puls.* twice a week. If it fails then *Carbo-v.,* every 4th day, See "G (ii) Of Measles not coming out properly"

Ear deafness-tonsils—Deafness associated with swelling of tonsils (*Bar-c.*). See also "Tonsil" and "Tonsillitis hearing affected" and No. 12 of "Deafness due to different causes."

Ear discharge fetid—Discharge of fetid pus. (*Hep.*). See "Ear discharge purulent"

Ear-drops—Sticking pains in ears. Neuralgic earache. *Plantago* M.T. may be dropped in the painful ear.

Ear-hardness of hearing—Almost deaf, sensation of plug in the throat and ear, chilly, sexual, and sensation of plug in rectum. *Anac. 200* and higher if need be. See "Hearing dulness."

Ear-hearing—Dulness of hearing without any organic affection of the ear. Hearing music aggravates many bodily symptoms. (*Ambra.*). See also "Hearing dulness."

Ear inflammation *i.e.* **Otitis and discharge**—When the external ear is swollen, red, violent pain and itching in the external canal and sometimes closure of the whole external canal. Dr. Jousset and Dr. Farrington recommend. (1) *Puls.* and if this fails then *Merc-s.*

(2) When the pus is thin, offensive, long lasting and the canal is sensitive to touch. *Tellurium.*

(3) Great soreness of mastoid portion, chronic suppuration of ear with bursting headache, the pain goes to the throat and the drum is perforated. Threatened mastoid abscess. (*Caps*).

(4) Inflammation of external and internal ear with discharge of pus. Stinging in behind the ear. (*Bell.*).

(5) Chronic persistent discharge. Dr. Dewey recommends *Silicea*.

(6) Horribly offensive discharge (*Psor.*).

(7) Discharge with pain and dryness after measles. (*Colch.*)

(8) Inflammation of internal and external ear. (*Kali-b.*). See "Glands-ear swollen", "Otitis" and "Otorrhoea".

Ear mastoid—Caries of the bones of ear, caries of mastoid process ; obstinate otorrhoea. (*Aur-met.*). See also "Mastoid abscess".

Ear pain of various types—(1) *a.* Ringing in ears. Earache, with soreness swelling and heat, driving patient frantic. Ears feel stopped. (*Cham*). *b.* With swelling of ear gland creaking noises in ear when swallowing. (*Kali-mur.*).

(2) When pain starts from ear to teeth. (*Manganum acet.*).

(3) When snapping creeping pain is associated with hiccough. (*Tarent-h.*).

(4) Tearing pain in left ear. Pains often end in a stitch specially in head. Worse cold and wet weather. (*Guaiacum*).

(5) Pain in right ear extending to teeth and face. Coldness, creeping and numbness in whole right side of face. (*Plant.*).

Ear pain-earache of infant—(1) Digging and tearing pain. (*Bell.*).

(2) Infantile earache. The pains are violent and the patient is restless. *Cham.* is specific.

(3) Darting and maddening pain in the ears, itching of external ear, discharge of fetid pus. (*Hep-s.*).

Ear discharge-purulent—Discharge purulent like putrid meat from ear ; granulations. Polypi creaking when swallowing; chronic otitis (inflammation of ear). (*Thuja*). See "Ear discharge fetid".

E

Ear discharge-causing redness—Discharge from the ears. Wheezing in ear. Catarrhal deafness. Discharge causing redness of ear (*Sulf.*). See "Catarrhal-deafness".

Ear discharge-syphilitic—Burning in the ear with discharge of fetid pus and stitching in the ear from within out, of syphilitic origin. (*Asaf.*).

Ear-wax—Accumulation of wax. (*Conium*).

Eating-dirty things by children—Eating dirty and indigestible things particularly in children is a great symptom of (*Calc.*). See No. 15 of "Pregnancy its affections".

Eczema-all over body—Eruption is almost all over the body. Wet patches sticking to the garment with irritation at night. *Bacillinum* in frequent doses.

Eczema-external application—*Hydra.*, *Skookum chuck*, *Hamamelis*, *Calendula* and *Echinacea*, in form of cerate or in olive oil (one part to ten) recommended for external application.

Eczema-general at different places—(1) Eczema alternating with asthma. Asthma worse in winter. Vomits during attack and is better after that. Frequent colds and cough. Vaccinated more than once. Asthma alternating with eczema, *Thuja 200-3* doses to be given 4 hrs. apart. Next day *Ip.* in repeated doses. According to symptoms give *Sil. 30* and finish with *Sulf. 200*—only 3 doses and after a month follow it with. *Sulf. 1000* (only once). See "b (1) Asthma of old persons". (Dr. Wadia).

(2) **Eczema-blood purifier**—*Gunp.* is a great antipsoric remedy and is a great blood purifier. It helps to clear up many skin troubles. Should be given for a long time in 3x potency. See "Blood purifier".

(3) **Eczema-of diabetics**—Itching wihout eruption. *Dolichos* will control diabetic itching and is specially useful in senile pruritis. Worse at night. Worse across the shoulders, also about elbows, knees and hairy parts. (*Dol.*) (1) Dr. Dewey. See "Diabetic itching".

(4) **Eczema-ankles**—Itching about ankles joints, and folds of skin, between fingers and palms. Vesicular eruption between fingers. (*Sel.*).

(5) **Eczema around anus**—Soreness in anus, wiping it. (*Graphites*).

(6) **Eczema-entire body**—Eczema over the entire body, itching worse at night, intense when undressing. The patient is despondent and morose, takes cold easily. *Tuberculinum* as an inter-current remedy when well selected remedies fail. It is almost important medicine in all skin troubles. Similar case is with *Syphilinum* for each has its special field and symptoms.

(7) **Eczema of gouty persons**—Excessively irritating, itch like eruption with redness, specially in a person with tendency to gout and a teasing cough. (*Led.*)

(8) **Eczema-margin of hair**—The skin is rough and coarse ; much soreness in the folds of skin ; intense itching specially at night, wetting makes it burn ; dryness and heat of scalp. Dr. Dearborn says *Sulf.* 6 will cure more pruritis than any other thing. It is great antiseptic. See "Eruptions in hair of forehead" and "Hair eruptions on the root."

(9) **Eczema-in the folds of neck**—Eruptions like variola. Eczema that dries into crusts and burns like fire, worse from washing. *Hydras.* a dose night and morning with the application every night of one part of *Hydras.* and 10 of glycerine. (Dr. Laurie).

(10) **Eczema-on genitals**—Intense itching ; but scratching is painful. Pustular eruption specially on face, genitals and testes : with fearful itching followed by pain and burning. According to Dr. Hughes *Croton* relieves the itching of eczema rapidly and permanently. See "Eruptions on genitals" and "Itching-female organ."

(11) **Eczema-pustular**—Vesicles, and pustules, eczema with purulent or watery secretion followed by formation of scabs and crusts which are inflamed during the increasing and become dry during the decreasing moon ; itches terribly, worse

washing in cold water ; worse face and hands and scalp around occiput. Worse at night and warmth of bed. Suitable for gonorrhoeal and syphilitic patients. (*Clem*). (Dr. Boericke).

(12) **Eczema-red blotches**—Itching worse by scratching Red and sore blotches here and there. The hairy portions of the body itch more. Useful also in blind boils and for itching of hands, knees and elbows. (*Fragopyrum*.) See "Eruptions scarlet."

(13) **Eczema-on scalp**—Eczema dry and scaly, on the scalp and face, crusts over the scalp, the hairs fall out, oozing lifts up the crusts and exposes new vesicles, worse at night and from the warmth of bed. Eczema more on the sides of the head and face, cheeks and ears. Sebaceous glands secrete excessively. (*Psor*.). If the whole scalp is covered with eczema like a cap *Cicuta 200* See "Milk crusts on "scalp".

(14) **Eczema-with swelling of glands**—Swelling of glands and lymphathic vessels, of the body, face and limbs ; soreness or itching of skin : excoriation of joint of the hands : (*Sep*)., See "Neck gland swelling".

(15) Dr. Dewey says that the most important remedies in all skin affections are *Tuberculinum* and *Syphilinum* as each has its special field and symptoms and we should not forget them when treating such cases. Vesicles surrounded by red areola with, itching, chiefly about nose, neck, shoulders, and back of the ear, with nausea and cough. (*Antimonium tart.*). See "Dermatitis involving hands or face, scratching with weeping eczema" and "No. 3 of this head for sun's rays causing skin trouble. "*Hydrastis*, *Sookum chuck*, *Hamamelis* and *Echinacea* in the form of cerate are recommended.

(16) Itching vesicles, rapidly, becoming pustular, large, and later confluent, discharging a yellowish fluid, spreading from right to left and affecting fingers, eyelids, face and scrotum, chest and neck ; unbearable itching. (*Anacardium*).

(17) Eczema of hands and wrists, one attack hardly subsiding before another sets in ; oozing out when using hand

intolerable itching and soreness with dyspepsia and cough with swelling of glands. (*Juglans cinerea)*.

(18) Dry chronic eczema ; skin of arms thicker and rougher than natural, itching and tingling when getting warm (*Kali-arsen*.).

Eczema-blister like—Both chronic and acute. The eczema being of vesicular type, *i.e.* there are small blister like eruptions. Lot of itching. The patient scratches without much relief. Three cardinal symptoms present viz. restlessness, thirst and chilliness. (*Rhus-t.*). See "Eruptions with blisters spreading redness."

Eczema-ears—(1) Moist oozing behind ears. (*Lyco.*).

(2) Eczema weeping, fluid comes out on scratching. Give *Graphites* 200 to 1000, in chronic cases and lower 6 times in acute cases. (*Graph*.). Externally in all cases of eczema *Graphites cerate* be applied.

Eczema-on face—Obstinate eczema on the face and head of small children. (*Kali-m*).

Eczema-hands and weeping eczema—(1) Eruptions on back of hands and wrists half way upto elbows ; itching, aggravated by scratching. Eruptions moist after scratching. Eruptions worse from washing. (*Mezereum*)

(2) Eczema weeping ; fluid comes out on scratching ; give *Graphites* 200 to 1000 in chronic cases and lower dilution in acute cases. See "Dermatitis...with weeping eczema."

Eczema-on back of hand—Moist eczema on the back of hands. Baker's eczema, also in the bend of knees. (*Bovista*.).

Eczema-on hands, fingers—On hands and fingers. (*Carb-v., Merc-s., Sulph,* and *Sep.*).

Eczema-hair follicle—(1) Raw and inflamed and specially wrose at the edges of hair. Crusty eruption in bends of limbs, margin of scalp behind ears. Affects hair follicle. (*Nat-m.*).

(2) Little pimples on the hair which bleed when scratched. (*Calc-c.*). See also "Hair-eruption on the root" and "Pimples".

Eczema-on anus—*Graphites* is one of best anal remedy. There is often eczema around the anus and it is one of the best remedies for fissure-ani. (Dr. Boericke).

Eczema-of head—Eczema of head. Discharge is corrosive and excoriates the parts it touches. (*Arum-t.*). See "Eruption on head".

Eczema-on lids—*Graphites* leads all the remedies for eczematous affections of the lids, and *Staphisagria* stands second.

Eczema-on nose—Eczema on nose and lips. (*Alum., Kali-c.,* and *Phos*). See also "Itching of nose".

Eczema-oozing—Oozing of pus or clear fluid ; patches burn after scratching ; eruption on lips, about mouth and nose (*Sep.*). See "Eczema wet."

Eczema-on hairy parts—On hairy parts, intolerable itching, copious exudation, head covered with thick leather like crusts under which pus collects, hair are glued together. Pus becomes offensive. (*Mezereum*). See "Hair eruption on the root."

Eczema-inveterate—Severe eruption on the skin of many years duration. (*Bacillinum*).

Eczema-on external ear and meatus—Eczema of outer ear and meatus, the surface of which is oozing, shiny, and in part scaly ; the discharge from wound *dries* up into scab ; also with throat trouble, *Med 1000* and *Bacill. 1000* and *CC*.

Eczema-itching and recurring—(1) Intense itching eczema. (*Anac.*).

(2) Repeated recurrence of eczema with bleeding cracks and patient feels pleasure while scratching. Give *Streptoccocin 1M. or* C.M. dilution. See "Reappearance of skin trouble."

Eczema-on palms—(*a*) whole palm of the hand covered with eruption, itching and pain, palm covered with thick scabs. Dr. Runwel cured this case with *Petrol. 200* in 4 weeks.

(b) Blister like eruptions (eczema) in the palms of han[illegible] (*Ranunculus-bul.*). (Dr. Nash).

Eczema scalp—(1) With crusts specially on the scalp. Itching of the scalp specially in the morning on rising. (*Agar.*).

(2) Eczema on scalp of children with offensive secretions tending to form scabs. Give *Rhus-t.* 200 every week and then 1000 potency every month. If the scalp is covered with eczema with a cap. (*Cicuta 200*). See "Milk crusts on scalp."

Eczema and other skin troubles—Skin cold, flabby and sweaty. (*Calc.*).

Eczema-of vesicular type—Vesicular eczema. Vesicles filled with thin yellow fluid. Copious on inside of hands and fingers. Sensitive to heat and warm room. Fond of open air. Periods too soon with copious flow. (*Kali-s.*). See also "Vesicles-yellow" and "Eruptions Vesicles".

Eczema-of long duration—Eczema inveterate with severe eruption on the skins extending to penis or prepuce and eyelids and cojunctiva. Begin treatment with 6 grams of *Aurum met.* *3* times a day to be followed by *Merc. sol.* in a low trituration and ultimately with *Kali chlor.* For opthalmia and eye trouble give. *Tr. Jequirity 3x,* drops in water night and morning. (Burnett).

Eczema drugs for external use—(1) *Tr. Alnus* Q. or according to Dr, Jahr oil of *Lavendar* is most efficacious of all external application.

(2) Tr. *Adrenalin chloride* (one-one thousand solution).

(3) The affected portion may de sponged with solution of *Bicarbonate of soda* in a little warm water.

Eczema wet—Wet eczema oozing sticky matter. (*Graph. 200*). See "Eczema oozing."

Eczema-on wrist—Eczema from wrist extending to forearms. hands papular and excoriated. Purple blotches on back of hands. (*Primula obconia*).

Elephantiasis—(1) The chief remedy for this obstinate trouble is *Myristica-sebifera* to be tried for a long time in increasing potencies. It is amenable to treatment only in the beginning of the onset of disease.

(2) The skin is thickened, hardened and itches (*Elaeis guineensis* tincture 5 to 20 drops. (Dr. Blackwood).

(3) The skin is covered with a dry eruption, often showing great thickening with exfoliation of the scabs, which is most characteristic. *Hydrocotyle Asiatica* of tincture 8 drops.

Emaciation—*Sil.* patient is weak and emaciated with a skin that is pale and muscles are lax. Thin limbs and big belly. Large head, emaciated face, constipated. Does not grow according to age. (*Sil.*). See "Rickets including curvature".

Emaciation due to anaemia—Due to deficiency of blood. (*Plumbum*). See "Anaemia under different heads".

Emaciation with sweating in head of children—In children with sweating head, slow growth, slow closing of fontonelles in emaciated children. (*Calc-p.*). See also "Face child creased like monkey", "Anaemia-in infants", "Sweat on head and hands in sleep" and "Slow development with sweating head".

Emaciation-extending down-ward—Emaciation while eating well. Emaciation extending downward, *i.e.* most emaciation in the face and round the neck. (*Nat-m.*). See also "Marasmus" under its different heads "Hunger canine" and "Chlorosis anaemia."

Emaciation after measles—Emaciation after measles. (*Hydrastis*). See also "Measles" and part "(iii) of Measles not coming out properly".

Emaciation-in T.B.—*Agar.* fattens up emaciated T.B. patients. (*Agar.*). See also "Weakness anaemia" and (*c*) "of Tuberculosis".

Embolism—a state of plugged condition or obstruction of the vessels—*Cactus g.*, *Zincum phos.* and *Colchicum* may be given according to symptoms.

Emissions—Emission and prostatic discharge at stool. Has morning erections but no more. History of repeated gonorrhoeas. The patient has lived in excess and now suffers from relaxed and cold genitalia. (*Agn.*). See "Sexual excitement ineffective", "Impotence--sexual excess" and "Prostate discharge."

Emission-nightly—(*a*) Nightly pollutions with great exhaustion. Sexual weakness ; immediately after every erection, discharge of prostatic fluid (*Ph-a*). (*b*) If *Thuja M.T.* is given in 5 to 7 drops, it controls nocturnal seminal emission better than any other remedy. See also "Spermattorrhoea." (Dr. Robert).

Emphysema (In this disease there is a condition in which the normal air spaces in the lungs are increased ,or there is abnormal presence of air or gas in the body tissues)—In this disease there are respiratory troubles. Cyanosis (blue discolouration of skin) and dyspnoea ; worse sitting up. Exercise causes pain around heart. Tickling dry cough. Patient puts hands on heart. Gasping for breath. *Laurocerasus*. See "Dyspnoea", "No. 3 of Angina pectoris", "No. 9 of Heart", and "Breathlessness". (Dr Boericke).

Encephalitis-inflammation of brain—Vertigo, heaviness of head, with heavyness of eyelid, headache preceded by blindness. (*Gels*).

Endocarditis-rheumatic heart—Cardiac weakness or inflammation of the lining membrane of the heart or its valves or enlargement of the heart. The condition of heart may be a sequence or rheumatic state which has been removed by suppressed methods (*Aur-met.*). See also "Rheumatic heart".

Entero-coitis (inflammation of intestines and colon.) of children—Of children, Inflammation of intestines and colon. The stools are constantly changing in colour and character. They are green, yellow, white, watery slimy during hot weather. (*Puls.*). See also "Colitis", "Cholera infantum-worse by milk" and "Milk disagreeable".

Enteric fever—The chief medicines are *Bapt., Bry., Bell., Ars, Rhus., Phos., Ip,* according to symptoms. See "Fever typhoid".

Enuresis-incontinence urine of child—Urine white, quickly becomes turbid. Ravenous hunger or diarrhoea, child cross, irritable, kicks and strikes. Does not like to be touched. *(Cina)*. See "Incontinence—involuntary evacuation of urine".

Enuresis-involuntary discharge of urine—Poor sleepers, eat too much, increased desire ; burning in orifice of urethra, during and after micturition. Involuntary micturition in night while coughing passing flatus. According to Dr. M.G. Blackie *Pulsatilla* is one of the best remedies for this disease. See "Incontinence involuntary evacuation of urine".

Epilepsy—(a) Epileptic spasms followed by nausea and vomiting, night epileptic fits. *Hyoscyamus 30* to be given 4 hourly. (Dr. Schubert).

(b) Attacks of even chronic epilepsy which only occur after mortification or similar vexation and not from any other cause may always be prevented by timely administration of *Ignatia* (Hahnemann).

(*c*) Give *Tanacetum* in drop doses 4 times a day in every case of epilepsy. (Dr. Pierson).

(*d*) *Cuprum* is an excellent remedy for stopping the frequency of epileptic attacks in obstinate cases than any other medicine. (Dr. Schwart).

(*e*) When the fit comes at the new moon and headache follows the fit, caused by sexual abuse or excess in men. Fits occur during or near the menstrual period in women. (*Kali-brom*). Most authors recognise this medicine as best prophylactic ; next comes *Glon.*

(*f*) When due to masturbation or sexual excesses, the fit may return during coition. Before attack, irritability, incoherent talks. Attacks may occur during sleep. Pupils largely dilated and unaffected by light before the attack. (*Bufo.*).

(*g*) With syphilitic history. Fit occurs after mid-night (*Nit-ac.*)

(*h*) Sudden rigidity followed by jerks and violent distortions, oppression of the breathing, lock-jaw, face dark red, frothing at the mouth, great prostration after attack. (*Cic-v.*).

(*i*) Recurring attacks of epilepsy. When the fit is preceded by trembling, vertigo and giddiness. Loss of memory after the attack. Give *Asinthinum in M.T.*

(*j*) *Sulf.* and *Psorinum* are to be used as intercurrent remedies for epilepsy almost by all.

(*k*) After severe attack give *Bell. 200.* (Dr. J. H. Karshaw)

(*l*) According to Dr. Hering for attacks occurring in rapid succession, give *Absthium*.

(*m*) Epilepsy without aura.(*Zincum valerian*). (Dr. D. Gupta)

(*n*), Attaok during full moon : epilepsy aggravated around full moon generally needs *Silica*.

(*o*) If several epileptic spasms occur during the menstrual period and the patient has no realisation until told ; she needs. *Bufo*. (Dr. Kent)

(*p*) Along with *Ignatia* Dr. Nash recommends *Amyl nitrite*. It has good reputation for arresting paroxysms of epilepsy and resuscitating patients under anaesthetics. It may be sprinkled in tincture form of 30 potency for smelling. These two medicines may be kept as stand by the patient for using them before attack.

Epidermolysis—(A rare skin disease by which blister forms on the skin on slightest pressure)—*Ranunculus* is the only remedy for the so called incurable disease. (R.B.B. Das)

Epilepsy-preventing its attacks—See "Chapter V for details."

Epilepsy and convulsions.—More commonly the hysterio-epileptic type with frothing of the mouth Drawing of the muscles of the face. Muscles of the face will quiver and then stop and then in another part of the face the same thing. Eye-lids will quiver. Teeth feel too long. The tongue quivers. (*Agar.*). Compare *Saccharum-off.* See also "Convulsions of epileptic type".

Epilepsy-recent—(1) Falls insensible, turns blue, violent convulsions. (*Kali-c*).

(2) Violent convulsions, rigidity, foaming at the mouth or contortions, *Bell.* every night for a week, then *Opium* for a week followed by *Hydrastis* twice a day for a week.

Epileptic-spasms of children :— *Sil. 200.*

Epistaxis (nose bleed)—(1) Bright red blood with nausea (*Ip.*).

(2) *Millefolium* is a general remedy for this without knowing the cause if *Bry.* fails.

(3) Dr. Cartor advises *Trillium* as an excellent remedy. The mother tincture to be applied locally for arresting bleeding.

(4) For stopping nose-bleed *Natrum-nit. 30* has been found very useful. See "Nose bleeding".

Eructations-the act of belching with distension-(1) Loud, copious and painless belching. (*Arg-n.*).

(2) Distension of the stomach, eructations with tasting of food, taken with or with-out heartburn. (*Carb-v*).

(3) During the attack *Chamomilla* mother tincture 1 drop in hot water 1/2 hour for 3 or 4 hours will often give relief, if other indicated medicines fail according to Dr. Clarke. See also "Stomach eructations".

Eruptions right sided—(*a*) With swellings start on right side, travel across to left side. (*Lyco.*). See "Swelling on right side."

(*b*) All kinds of eruptions cured by *Jug-c.*

Eruption-in measles retarded—(1) Bry., and *Sulph* are the best remedies but on their failing Dr. Jahr recommends *Verat.*

(2) In small-pox eruptions retarded. If the erptions are not well out in spite of *Variolinum, try Sulphur.* If the result is not

satisfactroy, *Bry*. should be given in repeated doses. After *Bry*., a dose of *Sulphur* may help to bring out the eruptions.

(3) Eruptions and itching worse by scratching until burning comes and then bleeding relieves. (*Petr*.).

(4) Chronic form of urticaria. Nettle rash on whole body, itching. (*Astac*.)

(5) Violent itching of the scalp as form lice. Smarting after scratching; eruptions offensive smelling. Eruption violent, itching, bleeding and oozing. (*Oleander*).

(6) Vesicular eruptions with intense itching, burning and multitude of small vesicles in close contact. Eruptions and itching about the eyes, scalp and specially genitals, scrotum and penis. (*Crot-t*). See "Measles-not coming out properly" and "Small-pox also haemorrhage small-pox no regular rash".

Eruptions-with swelling blisters spreading redness—Eruption with spreading redness and swelling. There are small blister like eruptions. There is a lot of itching and the patient constantly scratches without much relief. But there must be (*i*) Restlessness, temporarily relieved by changing position. (*ii*) Thirst for large quantity of water and (*iii*) Chilliness relieved by cover or warm application. (*Rhus-t*). See also "Itching causing burning", "Eczema-blister like", and "Rash on childs body".

Eruptions-on covered parts—Eruption only on covered part; worse after scratching (*Thuja-occ*.).

Eruptions on genitals with small vesicles and large blebs—Eruptions both on male or female gentitals. (*Petrol* is meant for small vesicles while *Rhus-tox* is meant for large blebs,) See "No. 9 of Eczema general".

Eruptions-on face—Pustules which run together forming thick yellow on face, head covering the whole scalp, solid like a cap, and other parts of body. (*Cicuta virosa 200*). See "Ringworm on face."

Eruptions in hair on forehead—Itching eruptions on the face. Specially at the margin of the hair on forehead. Crusty eruption in bends of limbs, margin of scalp behind ears. Affects hair follicle. (*Nat-m*). Sea "Eczema on face".

Eruption like eczema on head—*Arum-t.*, has some skin eruption specially on the head like eczema. Specially when the discharge is corrosive and excoriates the parts it touches. (*Arum-t.*). See "Eczema on head".

Eruptions-itching—Itching and burning ; worse scratching and washing. Pimple eruption, pustules, (*Sulf.*). See "Eczema itching and recurring".

Eruptions-moist—Eruptions moist, itching or dry, increasing at the margins of hair (*Nat-mur.*).

Eruptions on scalp-life long—Coppery eruption of scalp ; breath foul ; chronic insomnia (*Syp. cc.*) and later on spiritus glandium.

Eruption-scarlet on whole body—Whole body is red as if covered with scarlet eruptions. Flat ulcers, a pungent burning sensation.(*Am-c.*).

Eruption tendency—Tendency towards skin eruptions on the chin, neck, and elsewhere. (*Silica*).

Eruption-thick and large—Thick like pocks often pustular, as large as a pea. (*Ant-tar.*).

Eruptions-vesicles—All over. Yellow vesicles are common. Itching of eruptions. (*Anac.*). Compare *Rhus-t.* See "Eczema of vesicular type".

Eruptive fevers-rash failing—Eruptive fevers *e.g.* scarlet fever, measles, small-pox, the eruptions are usually of bluish tinge instead of bright red. The regular rash dose not come out, but in its place red spots, (roseola like) make their appearance ; the usual uniform spread of the eruption has failed or has been suppressed. Bleeding from gum and nose. Great prostration and stupefaction. (*Ail*). "Stupor-sudden in eruptive fevers", "Measles not coming out properly" and "Fever eruptive with irregular rash".

Erysipelas—High fever. Intense redness of erysipelas spot, which may start from a small boil or so. The patient is very thirsty. Skin red, smooth and shiny and at times with little blisters on it. Patient delirious with high fever. (*Rhus-t*).

Erysipelas-prophylactic—*Graph. 30.*

Eosinophilia—It is a disease which shows increase above the normal number of eosinophis in the circulating blood or tissue. The symptoms of the disease are that the patient would take a deep breath, resembling a long sigh, belaboured inspiration, the chest is constricted and the aggravation takes place during day time. It is an occult syndrome often allergic in nature. Laboured, respiration, asthmatic bronchial suffocations, frequent remission are there. *Lachesis* is a sure cure for such a tropical eosinophilia.

Escape—(1) Desire to escape in fever, *opium*.

(2) Desire to escape in hysteria The other medicines are *Belladonna, Verat alba.*, and *Lyco.* which may be given according to symptoms of the case.

Examination-fear—(1) Fear or fright of examination in students. (*Anac*).

(2) Specific for examination funk. Terror of anticipation. (*Arg-n.*). See also "Fear" under its different heads and "Fright of examination".

Examination-fussy children—For fussy children who are fussy about examination in their schools. (*Gels.*).

Examination-nervousness—(1) Weak hearted. Irritable ; lacks stamina and gives up hopes. Over-nervous in school examination. (*Sil.*).

(2) Depression about passing examination (*Lyc*). See "Brain-fag" and "Depression gloominess".

Excessive sexual desire—Phos. excites the sexual appetite in both sexes. It is almost irresistible and leads the patient into a mania in which he will expose himself. This is succeeded by the opposite extreme of importence though the desire remains after the ability to perform is gone. (*Phos.*). See also "Sexual desire irresistible".

Excoriation-due to walking—See "Chapter V for details."

Exposure to cold—Any disease from exposure to dry cold weather or cold air has mostly *Aconite* in its early stage. It is indicated in complaints from very hot wheather specially gastro-intestinal disturbances ; coryza and much sneezing as well as night-mares and nightly ravings. (*Acon.*), See "Cold after exposure".

Expulsion of foreign bodies—Promotes expulsion of foreign bodies from the tissues *e.g.* fish bones, needles, thorns, bone splinter. (*Sil*). See also "Foreign bodies":

External Homoeopathic medicines—These are marked with M.T., after them *e.g.* (*Aconitum M.T.*) to distinguish them from the internal mother tinctures which are marked with (*e.g. Aconitum Q*). The external medicines are used locally, to aid the action of internal medicines. Usually the medicine which is used externally is also administered internally thus for injuries *Arnica M.T.* is used externally and at the same time *Arnica 3x* is given internally. The external remedies are used in the following ways : On wounds, cuts bruises, etc., where the skin is abraded or injured, the pure tincture should not be used, but lotions, prepared by adding one part of medicine to 9 parts of boiled water should be used for washing or in compresses (*i.e.* lint or cloth moistened with the lotions). For ulcers and old wounds, ointments prepared by mixing the medicine with glycerine or oil may be applied. On parts where the skin is not injured, the tinctures may be applied pure, or diluted in compresses, or they may be mixed with some lubricants, glycerine, olive oil, or coconut oil and rubbed in (massaged). The addition of lubricant prevents injury by friction.

(1) *Aconitum M.T.* is used in cases of local inflammation arising from suppressed perspiration. Use in compresses, 1 in

9 parts of water. For neuralgia rub it mixed with a little glycerine or oil on the painful part.

(2) *Apis. M.T.* :—Is to be used for stings of bees, wasps, etc., Rub a little undiluted on and around the place of sting.

(3) *Arnica. M.T.* :—For bruises, contusions, sprains, blisters on the feet after walking, much soreness caused by riding on horse back or walking, soreness caused by lying on side in bed, itching, chilblains, corns and bunions ; fresh wounds inflicted either by sharp or blunt instruments. In the case of domestic animals it can be used in same way, the lotion may be stronger 1 in 3.

(4) *Belladonna M.T.* :—Sore throat, hoarseness, loss of voice, hard dry cough. Rub externally throat and neck with the tincture pure or mixed with glycerine or oil. Also rub on enlarged glands mumps and painful abdomen.

(5) *Bellis M.T.* :—Used undiluted for painting on moles, twice a day.

(6) *Bryonia M.T.* :—Stiff neck, rheumatism, lumbago, stiffness and pain in the joints. Rub the painful or stiff part with the tincture, pure or mixed with glycerine oil.

(7) *Calendula M.T.* :—To be employed in deep cuts, ulcerated wounds, boils, and open sores. To be used in compresses I part of *Calendula* mixed with 9 parts of water.

(8) *Cantheries M.T.* :—and *Causticum M.T.*—These tinctures are useful in cases of burns and sclads ; compresses of 1 part with 9 parts of boiled water.

(9) *Ceanothus M.T.*—To be rubbed on region of liver and spleen for enlargement of these organs especially after malarial fever, pure or mixed with glycerine or oil.

(10) *Euphrasia. M.T.* :—5 drops in an ounce of tepid boiled water to wash the eyes in cases of discharge.

(11) *Glycerine* :—It is to be rubbed on sore hands, cracks in the feet. It is added to other external tinctures for lubrication.

(12) *Hamamelis. M.T.* :—To be used for compresses in bleeding from wounds on any part of the body, in bleeding piles swollen painful veins, 1 part of the tincture should be mixed with 9 parts of boiled cooled water. Also for bleeding gums.

(13) *Hydrastis. M.T.* :—To be used in cancerous sores, and sloughing and gangrenous wounds and pox and for injections in leucorrhoea and gonorrhoea 5 to 10 drops in an ounce of boiled water.

(14) *Hypericum M.T.* :—This red tincture obtained from *Hypericum perforatum* is a very ancient and popular remedy for wounds arising from punctures, cuts, bruises and lacerations causing violent pain. A characteristic for the use of this tincture is the pain spreading upwards from the wound (according to the position of the limb). It is applied in the same manner as the tincture of *Arnica*. (One part of the tincture mixed with 9 parts of luke warm boiled water); simultaneously *Hypericum 3x* should be given internally.

(15) *Iodum M.T.* :—To be used in swelling of the throat, chest, heart, liver, testicles, legs and other parts of the body. Apply the pure tincture on the swollen or painful parts once in every three days. Diluted with 1 or 2 parts of water, it should be applied to fresh wounds after removing all dirt with soap and water.

(16) *Ledum M. T.* :—Joints swollen and stiff on account of rheumatism and gout should be gently rubbed with the tincture mixed with glycerine or oil. It is also good in cases of bites of cats, dogs, etc., or stings of insects, and other poisonous wounds, such as by fish bones, oyster shells, etc., the pure tincture may be applied.

(17) *Phytolacca. M. T.* :—To be rubbed pure or diluted with glycerine or oil or used in compresses (1 part with 9 parts water) on inflamed and enlarged glands, parotid, sub-maxillary tonsils, breasts, etc.

(18) *Rhus tox M. T.* :—To be used in rheumatic pains in the joints or the small of back, in sprains or strains of the wrists, muscles and tendons, mixed with glycerine or oil.

E

(19) *Ruta. M. T.* :—*Ruta graveolens* is like, *Arnica* and *Calendula*, one of the best remedies of the homoeopathic medical treasury and absolutely indispensable. It is used in case of sorness to thighs by walking and riding injuries to periosteum and to the nails as well as for ingrown nails with suppuration. Also for bed-sore. Mix 10 drops in an ounce of water. In case of sprains and dislocations of the wrists, and ankle joints, the pure tincture or mixed with glycerine or oil may be rubded. After over-exertion of the eyes, wash them with a lotion 1 or 2 drops in 1 ounce of boiled and cooled water. In all these cases *Ruta.* 3x may be given internally.

(20) *Astyrax Balsam* :—Cures itch and destroys the itch insect (scabies). It should be rubbed into the boils and not to the whole skin. After about 10 hours wash with soap and warm water. Apply for 3 or 4 days. As this Balsam is inflammable, it should not brought near fire.

(21) *Symphytum M. T.* :—In fractures of bones and injury to the periosteum, place compresses of the tincture mixed with 5 parts of water. The fracture must be previously set and put in splints. If suppuration has taken place *Symphytum* is no more applicable.

(22) *Thuja, M. T.* :—For warts specially soft warts, also for in-growing toe-noils. Rub pure or mixed with glycerine or oil, internally give *Thuja 3x.*

(23) *Urtica tincture* :—Undiluted or mixed with an equal part of boiled water, for burns of the first degree (with or without formation of blisters) in compresses. At the same time *Urtica 3x* is to be taken internally.

(24) *Vaseline* :—For lubrication on any part, to be mixed with other medicines for preparing ointments.

(25) In skin diseases specially in ring worms, psoriasis, herpes tonsurans, acne rosacea, use locally as a cerate 4/8 grains to the ounce Vaseline *Chrysarobinum.* It should be used with caution on account of its ability to produce inflammation.

Internally 3rd to 6th potency. (From Guide to Health of the Homoeopathic Dispensary Kankanady, Mangalore).

(26) For sprains, wounds, haemorrhage apply *Ferrum phos.* (Schuslar.)

(27) For eczema *Hydrastis, Skookum, Chuck, Hamemelis, Calendula* and *Echinacea* in the form of create are recommended for application.

(28) For fistula in anus wash with *Calendula* lotion after every stool and apply *Calendula ointment* lotion to be prepared with one part of M.T. and 9 parts of boiled water.

(29) For scorpion bite apply *Ledum M.T.* externally. Liquor ammonium is also an efflectative external application.

(30) For bites of centepeds, spiders etc. Mother tincture *Apis Mellufica* is one of the best external medicines for local application.

(31) For bleeding anal fissure apply *Hamemelis M.T.* soaked on cotton.

(32) For ulcers in anus paint with *Tr. Paeonia*. It is also useful for bed sores.

(33) For bed sores paint *Tr. Calendula* thrice a day after washing them twice daily with equal parts of *Tr. Arnica* and boiled water.

(34) For washing eyes. 15 drops of *Calendula M.T.* in a tea cup of boiled but tepid water.

(35) For burns or scalds. If skin broken *Cantharis* ointment. If skin raw, *Urtica urens* ointment.

(36) For chafing and chapped skin. Paint *Calendula M.T.* also apply *Tamus cerate*.

(37) For Toothache : Paint with *Plantago M.T.*

(38) Pimples on face. *Arnica* or *Ledum* lotion M.T.—one part drug 10 parts boiled water.

(39) For Ring-worms : Apply *Phytolacca M.T.* or *Chrnarobonim* in oil or as a *cerate* 4 to 8 grains in vaseline. The latter

causes inflammation sometimes and it is to be used with caution. *Phytolacca* can also be applied for inflammation of the breast also.

(40) For *styes* : Hot compresses with *Calendula M.T.* lotion with absorbent cotton provides great relief.

(41) According to Dr. Anshutz, dressing wounds with *Calendula lotion* will prevent scars, gangrene or even tetanus.

Eyes burning—Burning in the eyes but the tears are not acrid. Eyes cannot stand light. (*All-c.*) See "Tears".

Eyes-affections—All possible affections of the eyes, acute or chronic, conjunctivitis, iritis, spots, vesicles, *Euphrasia* should be called to mind.

Eyes-colour blindness—There is every conceivable kind of deception in colours and vision. Various bodies fly before the eyes. The jerkings and twitching of the eye-lids (*Agar.*). Another excellent medicine for colour blindness is *Phosphours*. See "Colour blindness".

Eyes cataract-its prevention—(1) Cataract soft. (*Colchicum.*)

(2) *Cineraria* for cure of cataract one drop 4 or 5 times a day. To be continued for several months is effective in traumatic cases.

(3) Dr. A. B. Norton found *Causticum* most useful in checking acute cataract. See "Cataract".

Eye-ball removal—A horrible sensation of coldness in the eye socket from which eyeball has been removed. Ciliary neuralgia following excision of eyeball *Mezereum* gives enormous relief.

Eyes detachment of retina—Detachment of retina. Patches upon retina, opacity of cornea. Soft cataract. (*Napthaline*). See also "Retina".

Eyes-lids-drooping swollen, itching and ulcers along lids—(*a*) Heaviness of eye-lids. Cannot keep them open. The eye-lids droop in acute condition. The patient is drowsy. (*Gels*) See "Ptosis".

(*b*) (1) Eye-lids swollen often. Completely closing eye, corrosive tears making lids and cheeks sore. (*Ars.*).

(2) Eye-lids itch in day time and stick together at night, edges covered with sticky mucus. (*Euphr.*).

(3) When the eye-lids are swollen and are glued together in the morning with yellowish secretion. (*Cham.*)

(4) When there is redness in the eyes and eyelids, and there are small yellowish ulcers along the margins of lids with a discharge yellwish matter. (*Merc-s.*) See "Blepharitis".

Eyes dimness—Dulness and dimness of vision without any ostensible cause. (*Ambra.*). See "Vision-dim".

Eyes dissimilar—Both eyes are not similar in shape. Left eye is much smaller and lid does not open so wide as the lid of right eye. Give *Scilla 1 M* repeated each month for 3 months. Later on *Scilla 45 M*. Eyes will match with each other.

Eye-lotion—5 drops of *Euphrasia* in an eye. Glass of water be prepared and use as a lotion for sensation of dust or sand in the eyes and eye pain.

Eyes-red—Red eyes at times, blood shot. Mouth and throat very red and dry inside (*Bell.*). See "Conjunctivitis".

Eye-strain with headache—Eye-strain followed by headache. Eye red, hot and painful from sewing or reading fine prints. Weary pain while reading. (*Ruta*). See "Headache of school girls due to eye-strain".

Eyes syphilitic—(a) Syphilitic eye complaints with ulcers on the eye-ball, ulcers on the cornea, which are ameliorated in open air, with a sensation of numbness in the eyes. Inflammation of eyes with severe sharp pains that come from within out. The discharge from the eye is acrid, bloody and offensive. (*Asaf.*). See "Syphilitic iritis eyes".

(b) Eye-lids thickened, covered with pustules, inflamed, pale, red, swollen and oozing. (*Tell.*) (2) Small pustules like acne on the margin of lids. (*Sep.*). (3) With syphilis an copious lachrymation. (*Nit-ac.*). See "(b) of Eye-lids droopings".

Eye-foreign body in it—Insect or any small foreign body will be immediately expeled and the conjunctival will be relieved by *Coccus cacti*. It will be also useful in sensation of foreign body between upper lid and the eyeball. See "Foreign bodies".

Eyes-reading causing pain :—Little reading causing pain at the back of both eyes with pain at the back of the head. *Conium 30 and* a lotion of *Ruta M. T.*

Eye troubles and troubles after operation on the eye—(1) Acute trouble wlth dislike for looking into light and watering of eyes. Will cure almost all possible affections of the eyes both chronic and acute if with irritation of eye. (*Euphr.*).

(2) Corneal abscess. (*Calcarea muriatica*). See "Ulcer corneal".

(3) Loss of eye lashes. *(Petroleum)*. Compare *Ac-phos.*

(4) Eye-lids red and swollen ; eruptions on lids which become red and covered with scabs or crusts. *(Graph.)*.

(5) Eczema of the lids characterised by hard crusts. (*Mezereum*).

(6) Night blindness with or without glaucoma. *(Physostigma.)*.

(7) Night blindness. (*Lyco.*).

(8) During pregnancy night and day blindness. (*Ranunculus bulbosus*).

(9) Intense pain both in and around the eyes. (*Mercurius-c.*).

(10) Cyst on the eyelids. Give *Calcarea flour.* If it fails, then *Nitric acid.* See "Cyst-eyes-lids".

(11) Glaucoma :—Eserinum in several cases acted like a charm and the pains subdued almost at once. Dr. Jahr recom-

mends *Phos.* while Dr. Fellows speaks of favourable result with *Gels.* and *Spigelia. Phos.* will diminish neuralgic pains. See also "Glaucoma".

(12) For granular lids try *Hepar-sulph.* and later on *Graphites*.

(13) Granular lids when lashes turn inwards towards the eye and inflame it. Lower lids entirely inverted. (*Borax.*).

(14) Falling of hair from eyebrows. *Kali-c.* If it fails then *Anatherum* may be tried for falling of hair from eye-brows.

(15) Swelling of lids with stinging and shooting pain. (*Apis.*).

(16) (*a*) Injury. In all eye troubles due to injury give *Arnica. 2 M.* in the beginning 2 or 3 doses at 24 hours interval. If there is no improvement by this, give *Hyper.* 30 every 12 hours. (*b*) Blunt article thrust into eyes. *Tr. Symphytum* both internally and externally.

(17) (*a*) Ingrowing eye lashes. First *Borax*; if it fails then *Puls.* (*b*) For myopia or short-sightedness, *Phy. 3x.* 4 hourly.

(18) Great intolerance of light so much so that eyes cannot be opened in night. Oedematous swellings of the eyes with redness, acrid discharge. (*Rhus-t.*).

(19) Haemorrhages into the retina. *Lachesis*. By its use the haemorrhage disappears along with inflammation. See also "Retina".

(20) Styes :—*Puls.* In R. S. Bishambar Das's experience, *Staphy.* is an excellent remedy for styes which is normally given by him when *Puls.* fails. In his experience this remedy proved effecfive in all cases of eyes whether chronic or otherwise or whether on lower or upper lids. *Hep.-s.*, when there is a tendency for recurrence.

(21) For night blindness. (*physostigma.*).

(22) Sudden loss of vision. (*Iodum*). Compare *Acon.*

(23) Black spots before eyes. (*Sulph.*).

(24) (*a*) Oedematous swellings, redness, and acrid discharges, gush of tears on separating lids. *Rhus-t.* is one of the most important opthalmic remedies for such troubles. (*b*) Neuralgia of left eye with soreness of head. (*Kali. iodatum*).

(25) *Mercurius* has been found useful in styes, glandular affections and rheumatic trouble of the eyes.

(26) *Jaborandi* is an excellent internal remedy in iritis ; it allays inflammation, controls the spasms of muscles and will absorb adhesions.

(27) For burning pains above the eye-brows. *(Asaf)*. See "Photophobia".

(c) After operations on the eyes :—(i) Principal remedy. (*Aconite*). (ii) Violent pains in temples. (*Ignatia*). (iii) Pains shooting into head (*Rhus-t.*). (iv) Jerking pain with vomiting and diarrhoea. (*Asarum.*). (v) Promotes the absorption of lens debris, (*Senega.*). (vi) Especially after removal of eyeball, pains radiate and shoot downward with cold feeling and stiffness of bones. *(Mezereum.)*. (vii) Objects appear as if tinged with blood. (*Strontium*). (viii) Hammering and jerking in the eyes. (*Crocus.*). (Dr. Dewey). (28) Objects look smaller then they are. (*Platina.*). See also "Diplopia-double vision", "Vision", and 'Optic sclersosis" and "Optic neuritis". (29) Bloating of upper lids which hang down like bag of water*(Kali-c.)* while for bloating of lower lids, *(Apis,)* *Phos.* for bloating all round the eyes and the whole, face. See "Anaemia-face bloated".

Eye-upper half invisible—Hemianopia. Upper half of objects invisible. (*Aur-met.*).

Eyes watering with redness and with pain—Great redness of the eyes, with lachrymation ; burning eye-balls and vascular appearance (Vascular-consisting of vessels). Sharp shooting pains in the eyes. Engorgement left after an acute inflammation. (*Aesc.*). See also "Watering from eyes", Nose watering with irritation in eyes" and "Tears or watering from eyes with swollen lids".

F

Face- acne—*Asterias rub.* and *Kali-brom.,* these two remedies are almost specific for pimples on the face. If they fail then *Rad-brom.* 30 might be tried. In inveterate cases of severe type *Ars-iod* and *Sulphur-iod.* may be tried. See also "Acne" and "Pimples".

Face-hair on lips and chin of women—Give *Thuja 200* every month and *Oleum-jeç.* 3x thrice daily except on the day when *Thuja.* is taken. Wax should be obtained from the chemist who deals in allopathic drugs. The wax in the container should be melted and the tolerably melted wax should be applied like a layer, on portion containing hair. It should be kept till it becomes cool. After this the layer of wax should be removed by finger and the hair will automatically stick to the layer without causing pain. This procedure may be repeated without any harm if hair again appear. They can also be removed (electrolyses)in a beauty parlour. See Portion (b) "of Hair".

Face-ulcers on lips—*Silicea* and *Nitric-acid.* See also "Ulcer" under its different heads and ' Lips crack".

Face-ringworm on—See "Ring worm on face,chest".

Face-swelling of upper lip—*Hepar-sulph.* and *Apis.* See also "Swelling of upper lips".

Face-child creased like monkey and does not grow—The child has thin limbs with a pinched emaciated face and the face looks old and creased as in monkey. The child has a big belly and does not grow according to his age (*Sil.*). See "Defective assimilation in children".

Facial blemishes—In young women. (*Act-r.*).

Facial-discolouration with urine trouble—Due to menstrual irregularities or uterine trouble discolouration of the skin takes place in women. (*Caul.*).

F

Facial-paralysis with neuralgia—(1) Paralysis from exposure to cold wind or draught. (*Caust.*).

(2) Neuralgia, twitching and numbness paralysis. *Cocc. indicus.* See "Paralysis face of left and right". "Neuralgia of face pain in nerve due to exposure".

Fainting due to causes like sight of blood etc.—Persons who easily faint away (i) from standing (ii) from sight of blood (iii) from trying dress and (iv) while evacuating. (*Nux-m.*).

Fainting-easily—Frequent fainting and nervous trembling faints when eating. (*Moschus.*).

Fainting on excitement and fright—(*b*) On slightest excitement. (*Moschus.*). (2) When frightened. (*Opium.*).

Fainting-from exertion with sweat on forehead—Attacks of fainting from least exertion with sweat on forehead. (*Verat.*).

Fainting-fits with depression—She weeps and has fainting fits with uneasiness and exhaustion. It has depression of spirits. (*Am-c.*).

Fainting of hysteric women—The woman patient faints easily and is of hysteric disposition. She is sensitive both to heat and cold. She is weak and lean and is easily exhausted after exertion. But even then she is fond of walking very fast. Flashes of heat ; hands and feet are hot. (*Sep.*). See "Hysterical disposition".

Fainting-hysterical with grinding of teeth—All the patients go off in fainting from no cause whatsoever or from a closed room. From excitement or any other type of mental disturbance. Hysteria is a common feature of *Asaf.* but fainting is the common feature. They get stitching pain suddenly from bone to surface, *i e.* from within out. Lump in the throat or suffocation is a sort of hysterical spasm of oesophagus. Grinding of teeth at night. (*Asaf.*). See "Hysteria" under its different heads.

Fainting-in pregnancy while riding or nursing—From extreme of cold and heat, after getting wet, from riding in carriage. Sense of sinking faintness in pregnancy, child-bed or during lactation. Hysteric (*Sepia.*). See "(C) Pregnancy disorder of".

Fainting-with pain—*Hepar*

Fainting-due to loss of fluids—Due to loss of fluid, blackness before eyes and ringing in ears. More indicated if the loss of blood has been sudden with faintness. (*Chin.*). See "Debility-due to loss of fluids".

Fall-to prevent consequential ills—A person falls down the stair-case, he strikes his head against a step causing great soreness to spine. *Hypericum* must be given at once to prevent any complication due to inflammatory changes with either to spine or the cord. (*Hyper.*). See "Spine-injuries".

Falling out of hair—(1) From general debility. (*Phos acid*) ; hair falls when combed. (*Nat-mur.*). Bald spots on head. (*Phos.*).

(2) Falling with great itching. (*Vinca-minor.*). See "Hair" under its different heads, "Baldness" and "Nursing with falling of hair".

False-labour pains—*Caulophyllum* is specific specially during the last week of pregnancy. *Act-rac.* is recommended by Dr. 'Hering'. See "Pregnancy-its affections", "Pregnancy disorder" and "Labour pains-distinction between true pain and false pains".

Fat patient with puffiness of face—The patients of *Asaf.* look fat, flabby and purple on the face. It is a veinous purple face with puffiness. Asaf. is a remedy of fat persons and will hardly be applicable to lean persons. The patients look purple when out in the cold or when excited. (*Asaf*).

Fatty degeneration of heart—Dr. Burnett recommends *Vanadium* and *Bellis. perennis* as an alternate remedy See "Heart" under its different heads.

Fat patient-tendency to obesity—*Calc-carb.* is usually fat and flabby patient. The patient is normally sluggish and slow movement. It is very often indicated in children. Tendency to obesity specially in children, and young people is characteristic of *Clac-carb*. Abdomen looks enlarged and inflated specially in children. The body is emaciated with large head in children. (*Calc-c.*). See also "Obesity general".

Fatigue-corporeal or mental causing pain, headache or confusion—(1) For removing pains in the joints from lifting heavy weights or from violent physical exertion. (*Rhus-tox* 6 hourly).

(2) Headache, restless, nervous excitability. unrefreshing sleep, lassitude, *Nux-vom*. 3 hrly. (Dr. Laurie).

(3) Fatigue with great debility or after any exertion producing exhaustion. (*Ars-a.*).

(4) Fatigue due to taking no food for a long time. (*Coff.*).

(5) Distracted and incapable of mental exertion from much mental work of different kinds in rapid succession. (*Aeth-c.*)

(6) *Arnica* should be administered whenever there is muscular fatigue from whatever cause. Its power to aid the restoration of exhausted muscle is wonderful.

(7) Confusion, pain in the fore-head, langour, feeling of sinking and sleeplessness. (*Chin.*). See "Over-strain and over work". and "Air traveller fatigue".

Fear :—(1) When fear causes diarrhoea. (*Op.*).

(2) Fear of animals. (*Bell.*).

(3) Fear of being scolded, of water, of people, of being poisoned. (*Hyos.*).

(4) Fear that something terrible or sad will happen. Fear of shadow or of insanity. (*Calc-c.*).

Fear-of remaining alone—The patient fears to be left alone. (*Phos.*). See "Dread" and "Loneliness",

Fear of crowds—Fear of crowds and scene in cinema inspiring fear. (*Acon-1M* single dose.).

Fear-of darkness—The patient is afraid of the dark, in a thunder-storm etc. (*Phos.*). Compare *Sepia.* See "Loneliness fear of darkness".

Fear-of examination—Fear or fright of examination in students. (*Anac.*). See also "Examination" under its different heads. "Anxiety".

Fear-of loneliness—Afraid of being alone. (*Sep.*). Compare *Phosphorus.* See "Loneliness".

Fear-loneliness and thunder-storm—The patient fears to be left alone ; is afraid of the dark, in thunder storm, etc. (*Phos.*) Compare Sepia. See also "Dread" and "Thunder storm".

Feet burning, kicking feet out of cover—Burning of soles so much so that the patient kicks the feet out of the cover, (*Sulf*), Compare, *Phos.* in which patient cannot cover hands. Apply *Graphites M.T.*—in olive oil, externally. See "Burning palms and soles burning with feet out" and "Cool atmosphere relieves".

Feet-moving when asleep and automatic movements—Nervous motion of feet while asleep. Cries out during sleep. Automatic motion of feet and hands. Bores head into pillow. (*Zinc-m.*).

Feet-offensive—Offensive foot sweat, of axillae ; intolerable ; sour carrion like odour of the feet without perspiration every evening. Diseases from suppressed foot sweat, of palm and head specially of children. (*Sil.*) Compare *Calc-carb.* See "Odour-offensive of body" and "Offensive foot sweat".

Feet-out with burning soles—The patient puts feet out of bed. Burning soles at night. (*Cham.*). Compare *Sulf.* See soles burning with feet out.

Felons-its aborting—See "Chapter V for details".

Fever-blisters :—*Nat-mur.* is an excellent remedy for blisters and can be given at any stage. See also "Blisters" its different heads.

Fever-chill with sweat over head—Chill at 2 p.m. ; chilliness and heat, fever with sweat. Pulse full and frequent.

Sweat over head in children so that pillow becomes wet. (*Calc.*) See "Chilliness must cover head" and "Fever-malaria with shaking chill".

Fever-chilly with thirst—No other remedy except *Ignatia* has the thirst during the chill and at no other stage.

Fever-colicky with sweat—Light chill, colicky pains, cold sweat on forehead. Paleness around mouth or lips, dark bluish rings around the eyes. Face is cold and hands warm. (*China*).

Fever-consumptive—With hectic fever or drenching night sweat with no thirst in fever. (*Acet-ac.*). See also "Consumption palliative" and "Hectic fever (the protracted fever of phthisis)".

Fever-with cough and urticaria—With chill. Thirst only during chill, for large quantity of water. *Urticaria.* The burning and itching intense. Cough during chill phase. The cough starts as soon as the chill phase of the fever starts and the cough subsides more or less as the heat phase starts. Aching of bones both during chill and fever. Gushing diarrhoea. Great restlessness day and night. (*Rhus-t.*). See "Cough-with fever".

Fever-child with trembling and startling—Child in acute fever condition startles, grasps the nurse and screams as if he is afraid of falling. All the tremblings from weakness of nervous system specially in acute febrile cases should attract the notice of *Gels.* If in addition to these there is light thirst *Gels.* is most probably the remedy. (*Gels.*). Compare *Borax.* See "Startling of child".

Fever-delirium—High, burning steaming heat and no thirst. Feet icy cold. Chill. Child starts up from sleep. Delirious condition. Very often face red. *Bell.* Compare *Acon.* and *Bry.* See also "Delirium".

Fever-of children with foul smelling stool—Of children, child lies half dozing and half confused, mouth ulcerated at times foul smelling, loose motions, with foul smelling stools, great prostration. The tongue is dry. (*Bapt.*), See "Toxemia of children".

Fever-during dentition—High, with one cheek red and hot, the other pale and cold. Child restless and uneasy and cries. Quiet only by carrying about. Dry cough and diarrhoea, (*Cham.*). See also "Dentition fever and diarrhoea".

Fever-eruptive with irregular rash—Eruptive fevers, *e.g.* scarlet fever, measles, small-pox. The eruptions are usually of bluish tinge instead of bright red. The regular rash does not come out, but in its place red spots, roseola like, make their appearance, the usual uniform spread of the eruption has failed or has been suppressed. Bleeding from gum and nose. Great prostration and stupefaction. (*Ail.*). See also "Measles-not coming out properly", "Small-pox" under their different heads and "Eruptive fevers-rash failing".

Fever-glandular due to swollen and enlarged tonsils—Due to the swelling of tonsils or joints of neck or nose.

(1) Tonsils enlarged, tearing pain in middle and external ear, throat feels constricted, feels cold, no thirst with fever. (*Bell 30*. Compare *Calc.*).

(2) If swelling of gland still exists when fever has left. Tonsils swollen, shooting pain into ears. (*Phyt. 30*),

(3) The other medicines which are useful are *Bar-c., Calc-iod., Kali-iod.* and *Bacill.* according to symptoms. See "Tonsillitis" and "Glands swelling."

Fever-influenza—(1) *Ars-a.* is the head remedy for influenza. It cures 95% cases with restlessness, thirst for small quantities of water, sneezing, and running from nose.

(2) *Sulphur* should not be forgotten as an intercurrent remedy. If the temperature does not subside within 48 hours, then *Sulphur 200* be given on empty stomach. No other medicine to be given at least for 12 hours.

(3) *Gelsemium* should be thought of in early stage of flu with sneezing chilliness, watery discharge from nose, and aching pain in the muscles.

(4) Fever with chill followed by vomiting bile and pain deep in the bones. (*Eupat-perf.*)

(5) High fever, flushed face ; nose stopped Hoarseness. (*Caust.*). See "Influenza" under its different heads and also "Influenza with fever".

Fever-pernicious intermittent—Intermittent fever which is pernicious or congestive with an extreme coldness, thirst, face and forehead cold and deathly pallor on face. (*Verat.*). See "Intermittent fever" and see also "No. 10 of Deafness"

Fever-malaria with cough and chill—Restlessness, thirst and chilliness. Cough during the chill phase of fever. Fever starting with a chill but the important thing about it is, there is cough, it starts as soon as the chill-phase of fever starts and cough subsides more or less as soon as the heat phase starts, *i.e.* the temperature rises and the patient no longer feels the chill. (*Rhus-t.*). See "Malaria" and "Ague".

Fever-malaria intermittent—Intermittent or malaria. Chill between 9 and 11 a.m. ; heat ; violent thirst increases with fever. Dryness in the mouth with the lot of thirst. Drinks good deal of water. A deep crack in the middle of the lower or upper lips. Small pearl like blisters near the corner of the mouth during the attack of fever. The tongue mapped with red islands. The fever returns at intervals or on alternate days round about 10 a.m. with sleepiness during the heat and a lot of thirst. Symptoms relieved by sweating. Numbness and tingling in fingers and toes. A dose of *Nat-m. 200* be given after the fever attack is over and another next morning 4 or 6 hours before the expected attack. *Nat-m.* should never be given during fever attack. (*Nat-m.*). See "Malaria"

Fever-malaria with nausea—With (i) consent nausea, (ii) splitting headache and (iii) thirst during the period of heat. (*Ip.*) See "Tongue coated".

Fever-malaria periodical—Chronic. Chills every six weeks. The patient has aches all over the body. Feeling of chilliness in the afternoon and evening and heat all night. Burning pains in the intestines. Very restless during fever. More sensitive to cold than heat. (*Sulph.*).

(2) Fever returning at clock-like periodically. (*Cedron*.). See "Periodicity" and "Fever-periodic."

Fever-malaria with shaking chill—The paroxysm comes at 10 or 11 a.m. or at 3 and 10 p.m. Strong shaking chill with thirst. The heat stage is very violent and is frequently associated with yawning and sneezing. The sweat is exhausting, thirst present. (*Chininum-sulphur.*). See "Fever chill".

Fever-milk—Best results are obtained by giving freely *Bell.* If this fails, then according to Dr. Farrington *Bry.* should be given in repeated doses. See "Milk fever."

Fever-puerperal—(1) Dr. Jahr says that a dose of *Sulphur* followed by a dose of *Nux-v.* acts like magic.

(2) If there are stitching pains in such a fever than *Kali carbonicum has* achieved signal success in such cases. See also "Pregnancy—disorder of No. 34" and "Puerperal mania".

Fever-remittent with chilliness—Frequent flushes of heat, violent chilliness of heat throughout entire body. Night sweat ; remittent type with coated tongue with red tip and border ; bright red colour of lips ; heat on crown of head with flush of heat ; burning in feet but feels cold. (*Sulph.*).

Fever-with dysentery—Dysentery sets in with violent fever intense thirst, drinks and vomits. (*Aconite*).

Fever-with rigour, ache and with sore throat—Burning heat. The face is red and hot like *Belladonna* yet the patient covers himself well and cannot have even a part of cover removed. He feels very chilly then. The fever may be accompanied with sore throat, rheumatism or any other trouble with gastric symptoms. Aching in limbs and back. Excessive rigour with blueness of finger nails. Perspiration sour, only on the one side of body. The patient cannot move or uncover in the least without feeling chilly. Cold stage predominates. (*Nux-v.*)

Fever-seasonal malaria or influenza—Ordinary or it may be malaria or influenza or of a change of season fever with restlessness, thirst and chilliness. Fever with cough. Cough starts as soon as the chill phase of fever starts, it subsides when temperature rises. (*Rhus-t.*). See "Periodicity."

Fever-remittent of children drowsy with trembling—Child lies drowsy and does not want to move on account of weakness. No thirst. There is trembling of limbs when attempting to move. The tongue trembles also. The child does not speak and resents to be spoken to or asked questions. *Gels.* is useful in the remittent type fever in children. This fever usually milder in nature as opposed to active and violent from calling for *Acon.* and *Bry.* (*Gels.*).

Fever-rheumatic—See "Rheumatic fever with various complaints."

Fever-septic—(1) *Pyrogen* is an excellent remedy for septic fever. Great restlessness, tongue flabby.

(2) Great prostration and restlessness. (*Ars-a.*).

(3) Sepsis due to injury (*Echinacea*).

(4) *Rhus-tox* is the best prophylactic for cases of surgery to be given in dilution of 30 every 3 hours. It will prevent sepsis. See also "Septic infection" Septicemia " blood poisoning for relieving fever" and "Antibiotic".

Fever-simple—For simple fever give A, B, C, S (*Acon. Bry. China Ars.*) alternately every 2 hours or every hour. Prepare solution of each medicine 5 to 10 drops in 4 ounce water in separate glasses.

Fever-patient talkative with intermittent fever—Intermittent fever. The patient becomes very talkative during fever. The higher the fever more is talkativeness. The patient usually sleeps during perspiration after the fever is over. The chills are very violent and are followed by intense fever. Pains in knees, ankles, wrists. (*Podo.*). See also "Talkativeness during fever" and "Delirium".

Fever-without thirst and with bad taste—Chilliness without thirst, headache, diarrhoea and nausea. Heat in parts of body. One sided sweat. Chill at about 4 p.m. Bad taste in the mouth and nothing tastes well not even water. Pains and fever in acute conditions are usually attended with chilliness and aggravated by warmth. (*Puls.*). See "Thirst complete absence".

Fever-with thirst—Thirst for large quantities of water and restlessness. Impatience and anxiety ; cold stage most marked ; coldness and heat alternate. High temperature. Child unappeasable and tossing about. Temperature worse in the evening or at night. (*Acon.*). See "Thirst—large quantities of water".

Fever-typhoid and its treatment—(1) If given in the beginning when nervous prostration begins (*Gels.*) makes the course of fever easier and shorter. Compare *Bapt.*, *Bell.*

(2) Rai Bahadur Bishamber Dass says that he has secured great success in treating typhoid cases beginning the treatment with *Ars-a.* He gives 3 drops doses every 2 hours 6 doses daily. If temperature does not abate then he gives *Sulph. 200* one dose on empty stomach. No other remedy that day. Starts again with *Ars. 30* following days. If no improvement is seen during next four days he gives *Psorinum 200* in the morning on empty stomach. No other remedy that day. Starts again with *Ars. 30* from the following day. If this also fails during the next 4 days then he gives *Tuberculinum 200 or 1000* in the morning empty stomach in the same way as *Sulph. or Psor.* Waits for 2 days then again starts with *Ars 30*. The normal symptoms for *Ars-a.* are restlessness, thirst for small quantities of water at short interval, prostration.

(3) *Phosphorus* is used when typhoid complicated with pneumonia.

(4) *Baptisia* is indicated when fever complicated with diarrhoea.

(5) *Acid muriatic* in intestinal haemorrhage.

(6) For sleeplessness in typhoid. (*Absinthium*).

(7) For typhoid fever with unconsciousness, suppression of urine, loss of pulse, tympanitic, abdomen, great prostration

and nervous excitability. *Cuprum metallicum 200* every 12 hours.

(8) Weakness and prostration following typhoid. (*Acid-phos.*).

(9) Tympanitis. *Carb-v.* the main remedy, then *Lyco.*, *Asaf.*, *Ter.*, and also *Agar*.

(B) **Fever-typhoid**—Haemorrhage-*Secale* in very bad cases when the patient is on the verge of death. See "Typhoid" under its different heads.

Fever-typhoid with delirium and diarrhoea—The typhoid patient picking the nose and lips until they bleed. Delirium, excitement, and manifestations. The urine is scanty and even some times suppressed. Diarrhoea associated with typhoid; stool like yellow corn-meal and musky. (*Arum-t.*). See "Delirium" and "Typhoid diarrhoea."

Fever-typhoid with drowsiness and diarrhoea—Restless-ness, thirst and chilliness. The patient from the very beginning a little stupified, *i.e.* the brain is more or less cloudy with slight and mild delirium (not violent). Tongue has triangular tip with the rest of tongue coated. Diarrhoea in the early stage of typhoid is also indicative of *Rhus-t.* (*Rhus-t.*). See "Drowsiness" and "Diarrhoea in typhoid, watery and acrid".

Fever-typhoid high temperature—High temperature, intermittent septic fever, worse after midnight, intermittent typhoid fever. Best remedy for fever of typhoid character and should be given after *Rhus.* (*Ars alb*)

Fever-typhoid with ear and lung complications—(*a*) Typhoid with lung complications: stupor and low muttering delirium; better after sleep. Thirst for large quantity of water which must be icy cold. Burning in palms. Vomiting in the morning. Fidgetiness all over the body. (*Phos.*). (*b*) Deaf-ness after typhoid. (*Petr*). See "Typhoid with pneumonia".

Fever-typhoid-muttering delirium—Typhoid, typhus, stupor or muttering delirium, sunken countenance, falling of lower jaw. Tongue dry, black, trembles, in protruding ; perspiration cold ; lung complications, (*Lach*). See "Delirium in typhoid".

Fever-typhoid relapse—Due to indiscretion of diet *Antimonium-crudum* is best then comes *Ip*. See "Relapse of typhoid fever" and "Typhoid-relapse".

Fever typhoid with stupor and haemorrhage (1) *Ph-a* has strongly depressing effect on the sensorium and nerves The patient lies in a stupor or in a sleep, unconscious of all that is going on around him, but when aroused is fully conscious Intestinal haemorrhage, blood dark. (*Ph-a*.) Compare *Baptisia* in which stool is offensive. *Baptisia* is applicable more in early stage of typhoid than *Ph-a*. which comes at a much later stage.

(2) *Acid-muriatic* is indicated in haemorrhage from intestine. The evacuations are constant with unconsciousness. In fact the patient is on the very brink of grave. See also "Haemorrhages" under their different heads and "B" of "Fever typhoid"

Fever-periodic—Intermittent, sweats profusely on being covered or during sleep. Thirst before chill. Returns chill generally in forenoon but never at night. Periodic fever. (*Chin*). See "Periodicity" and "Fever malaria-periodical".

Fever-stage early—Early stage of febrile condition but suitable to pale and weak subjects. An acute fever remedy like *Aconite* and *Belladonna*. (*Ferr-p.*).

Fever-with throat trouble—Gastric or bilious. Profuse perspiration without corresponding relief. Tongue is flabby and swollen with imprints of teeth all around it. The patient is very chilly but does not very much want to cover it. The whole mouth is offensive in look and odour. Creeping chilliness. With throat trouble like tonsillitis or bronchitis etc. Heat and shuddering alternately *i.e.* chilliness and heat alternating. Intense thirst though tongue and mouth are moist. (*Merc-sol.*). See "Throat sore" and "Tongue swollen with offensive mouth."

F

Fever-with vomiting—Pulse quick, mouth and lips are parched and thirst for large quantity of water though taken at longer interval. White and thickly coated tongue. Chill with external coldness. Dry cough. Profuse perspiration. Constipation and vomiting of water and bile. (*Bry.*). See also "Vomiting- gastric disturbance periodical".

Fever-due to vaccination—Give *Merc-sol.* 30 two doses, follow it with *Hep-sulph.* 30 two doses. Ultimately *Thuja* 30 two doses. (Dr. B.C. Guha). See "Vaccination fever".

Feverishness-of children—Hot, dry skin, restlessness, thirst and quick pulse. (*Acon.* every half an hour.).

Fibroma or fibroid tumour—(*i*) Profuse haemorrhage. *Epiph.* 30 once or twice a week. (*ii*) In women with tendency to enlarged thyroid. *Thyroidine* 3*x* gr. v. ; T.D.S. (*iii*) Intractable bleeding ; (*a*) *Ficus-r.* 3*x*, 4 hourly ; (b) *Thlaspi bursa pastoris* 5 drops, 4 hourly. (*c*) *Hydrastinum mur.* 2*x* gr. *ii*, (*iv*) Pain from sacrum to pubes. Flow bright but intermittent. *Sabina* 3, 2 hourly. (*v*) (*a*), Dark flow but painless. (*Ham.* 3, 2 hourly.). (Dr. Clarke), (*b*) Fibroid tumour in uterus near fundus. (*Puls.*) (*ii*) Womb packed with fibroid tumour, burning feet and sometimes shivering. (*Kali-iod.*). (*iii*) For fibroid tumour with painful menses. *Frax-Am.* to be given at bed-time in 10 drops of mother tincture and *Verat-alb.* in 30 dilution every morning (*c*) Dr. Boericke recommends *Calc-iod.* for fibroids and *Trillium, Ergot* and *Lapis* for fibroma (benign tumour) while Dr. Nash suggests *Phos.* for growths like fibroids and other fungus growths. (*d*) Fibrous bodies : *Calc, Plat-met., Staphy* and *Thuja.* according to symptoms. See also "Uterine tumour or fibroid with consequential haemorrhage" under its different heads and "Tumours at different places."

Fidgetiness including constantly moving legs—(*a*) *Phos.* has peculiar fidgetiness all over the body. He cannot sit or stand still for a moment. The child must be moving or doing something he may be moving this or that part of body. (*Phos.*) See "Restlessness-moving his body".

(*b*) Nervous and hysterical persons keep legs constantly moving or jerking. (*Valerian of Zinc.*). See "Movements".

Filariasis—A diseased state due to the presence of filaria which burrows in the skin producing irritation and swelling—(*a*) Swelling of parts which become hard, it affects the general health of patient. (*Merc. sulphuricus* in various potencies up to M.M.) Dr. T.S. Iyer says that this remedy is specific in this particular disease and may be used safely in all such cases.

According to Dr. Robinson *Capsicum* cured a number of cases.

(*b*) According to Dr. P. Banerjee *Calc-flour 30x* and *Fer. phos. 30x*, 3 tablets of each may be given twice a day.

Finger boring and grinding teeth during sleep—Bores finger in the nose, grinds teeth while asleep. Jumps and jerks during sleep. (*Cina.*). See "Boring into nose" and "Nose child boring fingers in worms".

Finger-cracks—Cracks at the ends of fingers and on the back of hands, skin rough or bleeding often much itching (*Petroleum.*). See "Chapped hands and cracks in finger tips". "Nostrils-cracked" and "Nail-skin cracking".

Finger-fractured, immobile—Immobility and stiffness in fingers and other small joints like toes and ankles after fracture or surgery. (*Caul-t 3x T.D.S.*). See "(*b*) portion of fracture union, stiffness and lameness".

Finger-end or toe-ends or nails injured—When nerve-rich area, as fingers ends or toe ends are injured or nail has been torn off or nerve has been crushed between hammer above and the bone below and nerve shows sign of inflammation and the pain can be traced up to nerve. *Hypericum* is the remedy. (*Hyper.*). See "Nails of finger hurt".

Fingers dropping things and not holding things properly—Fingers fly open when holding things. Clumsy motion of hands and fingers. Dropping of things. The patient is continually breaking the dishes. (*Agar.*) See "also "Incoordination of muscles".

Fingers rheumatic—Rheumatic affections of joints. Involuntary contractions of fingers, partial paralysis of fore-arm. Writer cramp (*Argentum metallicum*). See 'No. 5 of Rheumatism'.

Finger-feels dead and tips swollen—Tips of fingers swollen, red, feel dead. (*Thuja.*). See also "Chapped hands and cracks in finger tips".

Fingers-warts on—

(*i*) Index finger-right : *Caust., Lyco.*
Index finger left : *Thuja.*

(*ii*) Little finger :*Caust., Lac-c.*

(*iii*) Middle finger : *Berb., Lach.*

(*iv*) Back of finger : *Lach.*

(*v*) Ring finger : *Nat., Sulph.*

(*vi*) Back of ring finger : *Dulc.; Lach.*

(*vii*) Side of finger : *Calc-c., Sep., Thuja.*

(*viii*) Tips of finger : *Caust., Thuja.*

(*ix*) Around joints of finger : *Sars.*

(*x*) Thumb : *Lach., Ran.-b., Thuja.*

(*xi*) Left hand : *Psor.* (M.E. Douglas)

Fissure—(1) Constipation, when fissures are caused by large and hard faeces covered with mucus. The anus is extremely sore. (*Graph.* 6-30.).

(2) Much pain with constant oozing of fetid matter. There is much tenesmus. (*Nit-ac. 6.*).

(3) The anus burns after stool, cutting pain, constipation or diarrhoea. (*Rat. 3 to 6.*).

(4) When anus smarts all the time, much oozing. (*Paen. 3.*).

(5) With crawling and itching sensation in anus. (*Platina 6th trituration to 30.*)

(6) Dr. Boericke recommends *Led.*, *Graph.* and *Petrol.* according to symptoms.

(7) *Calendula* cerate for fissures between toes. See "Anus fissure".

Fissures-with warts—In anus, painful to touch, surrounded with flat warts or moist mucous condylomata. Movements as of something living. (*Crocus*). Without pain. (*Thuja.*). Externally *Hamumelis M.T.* if it bleeds.

Fistula—(1) With one or two small openings and either internal or external. (*Hydrastis, Nit-ac.*).

(2) Lachrymal. (*Sil.*).

(3) In tuberculous subjects. (*Bacillium testium*).

(4) Great itching, soreness in anus with burning pain. (*Berb-v.*).

(5) Externally apply cerate of *Thuja* or *Silicea M.T.*

(*b*) (1) *Nit-ac.* is the head remedy for fistula. It should be given in 200 dilution every week.

(2) In the beginning when the abscess has just appeared and is throbbing with headache. *Bell. 3x* or *Merc-sol. 6x.*

(3) *Calc-f. 12x* and *Sulf.* are to be given inveterate cases.

(4) Try also *Aesc. 6, Caust. 6, Chin 30* and *Rat. 6* according to symptoms.

(5) When there is ulceration of rectum with discharge of blood. (*Phos.* 30.).

(6) *Berb.* has suffering and pain in persons who have been operated up for fistula in anus and when the fistula has been closed.

Fistula-of the anus—*Merc., Graph., Calc., Silicea.* Wash the part with *Calendula* lotion and apply *Calendula* ointment. See "Eczema—on Anus", "Anus-fissure and fibroma". After every stool wash the part with *Calendula* lotion and apply *Calendula* ointment.

Fistula-at the root of teeth--Lachrymal fistula. (*Fl-ac.*) See "Teeth-aches". No. 5.

Fistula-of the glands—*Phos. Sil., Merc.,* See "Glands-glandular or bony ulceration".

Fistula-of the eyes—*Sulph., Puls., Hepar-s.* Externally *Calend.* lotion.

Fistula-lachrymal of eyes wih itching corner—Sensation as if wind blowing through eyes. Violent itching of inner corner of eyes. (*Fl-ac.* 6-30.). See "Lachrymation".

Fistula-with piles—In anus. Fissures and haemorrhoid also. (*Sil.*). See "Haemorrhoids with ulceration".

Fistula-of vagina—*Puls., Asa-c., Nit-ac , Petrs., Thuja., Lach.* and *Antimonium* according to symptoms. See "Vagina bleeding".

Flatus-offensive and gurgling—Distressing belching, rumblings ; turmoil in abdomen. Offensive flatus ; rumbling and, gurgling in belly ; pinching colic. (*Agar.*).

(*b*) *Rhus-glabra* will disinfect the bowels that the flatus and stools will be free from odour. See "Wind trouble".

Flatulence-after rich food ; with foetid eructation and painful distension—*Pulsatilla* is recommended when flatulence occurs due to rich and greasy food. *Arsenic* is required for a patient who gets foetid eructions after consuming cold drinks and food while *Colocynth* is a prominent remedy for painful distension of abdomen with grip ping pain.

Flatulence-in children—Lot of loud rumbling in the abdomen like croaking of frog. Abdomen puffed up and big specially in children. (*Thuja.*).

Flatulent distension-at climateric—Flatulent distension of the stomach with foetid, offensive leucorrhoea, the menses are profuse and offensive. There is burning of hand and feet. *Sanguin. canades.*

Flatulent-dyspepsia—(1) Flatulent dyspepsia where anything turns into wind. (*Nux-mosch.*).

(2) *Fucus-ves.* By this remedy the flatulency is diminished and ultimately disappears. Use mother tincure in **3** drops doses. See "Distention" "Dyspepsia" and "Digestion disorder flatulence".

Flatulence-lower region—Great flatulence with rumbling. Gas passing downward in the lower region. Belching relieves, passing flatus relieves. (*Lyco*). Compare, *Carbo-v.* and *China.* See "No. 6 of Bilious attacks" and "Wind trouble."

Flatulence-remover—According to Ringer **10** to **15** minims of *Tr. Sulphuric Acid* of 3rd attenuation if taken before each meal will remedy (stomach affected with burning and eructation).

Flatulence-with loud eructations—In the abdomen there is wind coming up in volumes with hiccough like contractions of the diaphragm. Expulsion of the wind like the sound of pop gun. Loud eructations of wind from stomach. (*Asaf.*).

Flatulence-in the upper portion—Excessive wind in the upper portion of the abdomen pressing upwards in the chest and causing distress in heart. Whatever he eats becomes wind. The simplest food disagrees. Relieved by belching wind or passing flatus. (*Carb-v.*). Compare *Lyco.* and *China.*

Flatulence in whole abdomen—Wind not relieved by passing flatus. Indigestion. *China* cures flatulence and distension in abdomen. The patients say that whatever they eat turns into gas. Distension of whole abdomen, patient feels uncomfortable and oppressed and can hardly breathe properly. (*Chin.*). Compare *Carb veg.*, *Lyco.*, and *China* which are trio of homoeopathic flatulence remedies. See also "Distension" and "Wind-trouble".

Fluids absorption in joints and swellings—Fluids anywhere in the body like the enlargement of the joints and rheumatism, exudations into serous sacs, pleura, meningeal membrane, perito membrane. After the acute symptoms are over the swellings persist. A dose of *Sulphur* will often help the absorption. (*Sulf.*). See also "Power of absorption-of fluids".

F

Flying pains—Tearing pains flying from one part to another. Scarcely more than skin deep. Sometimes flying along the course of nerve. Flying gout. (*Aesc.*). See "Pains flying along nerve," "Wandering joint-pains" and "Gout pains flying".

Flying-gout pains—In all the joints, gouty rheumatic affections ; neuralgic affections. Especially this rheumatism tendency is found from the elbows to the hands, in fore-arms and hands. Tearing pains flying hither and thither without any particular order ; relieved by heat. (*Aesc.*). See also "Gout pains flying" and "Wandering joint-pains".

Food poisoning—(1) Vomiting, pain in stomach, diarrhoea, (*Nux-vom.*).

(2) After eating ice-cream or over-ripe fruits. (*Ars-a.*).

(3) After eating spoiled and tainted meat. (*Carb-v.*).

(4) Convulsions during food poisoning. (*Hyoscyamus.*). See "Ptomaine-poisoning" and "Digestive trouble after eating decayed food".

Food smell-causing nausea—Cannot bear the smell or sight of food. It causes nausea. (*Ars-alb.*). Compare *Sep.* and *Colch.* See also "Smell-senstiveness".

Foreign bodies—Promotes expulsion of foreign bodies from the tissue *e.g.* of fish bones, needles, thorns, bone, splinters. (*Sil*).

Foriegn body in the eye—Take the *Calendula lotion* in a small cup and dip the eye in the lotion and move the eyelid so that lotion will splash over the eyeball and the inner walls of the lids. (*Calendula*). See "Eye-foreign body in it". and also "Expulsion of foreign bodies".

Forgetfulness-with absent mindedness and loss of memory—(1) Absent minded, forgetful, buys things in market and walks away without them. (*Lac. caninum.*).

(2) Old people where age has taken the keenness out of all mental faculties. (*Baryta-carb.*).

(3) Even things spoken of a moment ago are forgotten, constant loss of memory. (*Ailanthus-glandulosa.*).

(4) Weak memory and forgetfulness with slowness of perception. (*Oleander*). See also "Memory loss-due to excesses" under its different heads, "Senile decay" and "Absent mindedness"

Fracture-no union, swelling pain sepsis and compound fracture—(1) Broken bones do not unite quickly. (*Calc-p.*).

(2) To help the reunion of bones. *Symphytum* is very useful. Externally lotion of *M.T. Symphytum.*

(3) As soon as a fracture has been set right by a surgeon *Arn.* in 1000 dilution should be given every 4th hrs. at least for 12 hrs.

(4) Great anxiety, uneasy with restlessness. Sleeplessness Inflammation of parts bluish and purpulish in appearance *Lach.* should be given.

(5) For swelling and discolouration and unhealthy suppuration and sepsis *Crotalus* may be given. Compare *Anthrac.*

(6) For compound fracture. (*Hyper.*). See "Bones fracture".

Fracture compound getting suppurated—Sometimes such fractures become suppurated and lacerations of soft part takes place and the injured person gets septic fever. In such cases give *Arnica 30*X, 4 to 5 drops every hr. internally and apply compresses moistened with same dilution. It will alleviate the pain and the suppuration is reduced almost to nothing and a favourable condition is established. Dr. Von Grauvogl has tried this treatment with great success in hospital.

Fracture, green stick of children—For green stick fracture *i.e* an incomplete fracture of long bone seen in children ; the bone is bent only on the convex side (*Calc-c.* 200).

Fracture-pains and formation of callus—(1) Relieves pains of fractured bones. *Rhus-t. 30* to be given alternately with *Bry.* 30 every 2 hours for throbbing pains and restlessness.

(2) According to Dr. Lilienthal "*Ruta* aids in forming callus after fracture when there is much pain in the part injured" See "Bones pains".

F

Fracture-sleepless patient—The patient complains of sleeplessness after accident. Give a dose of *Slicta pulmonaria 200* and repeat it and the victim of fracture will go to sleep. It is better than morphine in inducing sleep. See "Sleeplessness due to pain or yawning".

Fracture-union stiffness lameness—(*a*) For formation of bone or conversion of tissue into bone. For early union of bone. (*Calc.*). Give *Calc-c. 200* in 4 doses, 1 dose every 4th day. See "Bones-fracture".

(*b*) **Stiffness and lameness after reunion of bone**—After reunion in fracture *Ruta* is very valuable for stiffness and lameness. It may be given 1x dilution and may be alternated with *Rhus-t. 30*. Each may be given for a week. See "Finger fractured immobile".

Freckles (a yellowish or brownish yellow spot on the skin.) on different parts—(1) Dark freckles on chest. (*Nit-ac.*).

(2) On face (*Kali-c.*).

(3) On cheeks. (*Sep.*).

(4) For pale pigmentation of the skin give *Sepia 6x* and *Kali-mur. 6x* alternately for several days and apply externally following lotion. *Tr. Sepia* and *Tr. Oleum santali* in equal quantity with 30 ml. of distilled water. This mixture may be applied at least twice a day on the affected portion. See "Spots brown and yellow saddle on face" or "Birth marks".

Frequent urine—See "Urine polyuria".

Fretfulness—(*Calc-br.*). See "Peevish".

Fried things-fond of—*Calc-p.* is fond of fried and highly seasoned meat. (*Calc-p.*)

Fright due to noise, lightning causing involuntary evacuations—(1) If the frightened patient becomes very cold and gets diarrhoea with involuntary evacuations. (*Verat-a.*).

(2) Immediately after being frightened by sudden noise or any other shocking disturbance and fright followed by great

heat in head and cold "sweat or fainting" and fits of children due to fright followed by screaming and trembling. (*Op.*). See "Noise frightening".

(3) Fear of lightning, incessant screaming after thunder-clap ; diarrhoea and abortion after fright. Nervous dread (of singers and speakers.) from appearing in public (*Gels.*). See "Fear" and "Dread".

Fright of examinations—Fear or fright of examination in students. (*Anac.*).

Fright-of interview and stage—Take *Ignatia 30* every 2 or 3 hours before interview or appearing on stage and one dose just before interview or appearing on stage either for play or delivering a speech. This removes nervousness, shivering or sweating. See "Examination fear" and "Examination nervousness".

Fright rousing child in sleep—*Aesc.* is specially useful in children that rouse up in sleep frightened and confusion like *Lyco.* (*Aesc.*). See "Fear" under its different heads, "Child frightened" and "Weak children waking with irritablity".

Fright stage—A few doses on the day of performance may be given prophylactically of *Ignatia*.

Frost bite stinging and itching—Sensation of coldness and warmth, pins and needles ; stinging and burning where the sensation is feeble. The patient is extremely nervous and sensitive to cold. Itching and pricking. Burning of ears. (*Agar.*).

Fungus-a spongy morbid excrescence—(1) *Lachesis* is a remedy of great value in fungus, haematodes, black measles, small-pox, malignant boils, carbuncles, chronic ulcer and bed sores, the characteristic dark blue colour must be present.

(2) Slight wounds bleed much. The same tendency to bleed extends to fungoid growths like fibroids fungoids (resembling fungus) is very dangerous, and troublesome. (*Phosphorus*).

G

Gall-stone colic and prevention of formation of stone—(1) *Calc.* (*a*) *Chionanthus virginica* prevents the formation of gall-stones and promotes the discharge of those already formed.

(2) (*a*) *Cholesterinum* to be tried in gall-stone colic. It removes congestion and cures fever due to upsetting of gall-bladder. (*b*) *Carduus marianus* has the reputation of preventing further formation of stones. (*c*) Dr. G.W. Boericke gives combinations of *Chelidonium, Chionanthus* and *Hydrastis* in equal parts in drop doses for relief of pain. He also recommends *Dioscorea* as helpful and curative. *Cholesterinum* is a specific for gall-stone colic and relieves the distress at once. See "colic-renal-stone in kidney" and "Renal colic-severe pain caused by efforts to pass a stone locked up in ureter."

Gall-stone-colic bilious—(1) Headache and vomiting bile. Pain relieved by heat, very nervous. Startles easily. Feet cold in bed. Menstrual flow clotted, flow thick and dark. Inclination to commit suicide. (*Net-sulf.*).

(2) Nausea vomiting, violent contractions of abdominal muscles, cold extremities and perspiration, (*Nux-vom.* every half hour.). See also "Biliary colic".

Gall-stone-colic with liver trouble—Gall colic. Distension. Fermentation and sluggish bowels. Liver enlarged. Gall-stone. Jaundice due to hepatic and gall-bladder obstruction. Constant pain under angle of right scapula. *Chelidonium majus.* is a prominent liver remedy covering many of the direct and reflex symptoms of diseased condition of that organ. (*Chel.*). During attack it may be repeated half hourly. See "Bladder" under its different heads and "Liver" under its djfferent heads.

Gall-stone-colic periodical—At certain hour each day, periodical from gall-stone. (*Chin.*). See "Periodicity".

G

Gall-stone-prevention of formation of stone—*Chionanthus* is said to prevent the formation of gall-stone and their discharge.

Gall-stone-pain—See "Chapter V for details".

Gall-stone-prevention of formation of stone—See "Chapter V for details."

Gall-stone-shifting—Pain from gall-bladder to chest, back and arms, pain suddenly shifts to different parts ; renal colic better walking about. Hurried desire for stool. (*Dioscorea.*) See "Pains wandering" and "Renal colic severe pain caused by efforts to pass a stone locked up in ureter".

Ganglion—(*a*) *Ruta*; *Benz-ac.* Give *Ruta 50M.* and it will without fail remove ganglion. (*b*) *Benz-a.* may be given internally in the dilution of 30 while ointment of *Benz-a.* if applied externally will reduce the size of ganglion.

Gangrene of different parts due to carbuncles etc. and after operation—(1) Of wounds ; traumatic gangrene. *Lachesis* is eminently curative of gangrenous affection. (*Lach.*).

(2) Dry gangrene of toes and fingers thrown away. (*Secale-cor.*).

(3) Carbuncles and boils become gangrenous. (*Carbo-v.*).

(4) Bluish, moist gangrene, the limb being covered with black blister, burning and much swollen, emitting foul odour. (*Crotalus.*).

(5). After operation when gangrene sets in, tissues are not strong enough to reproduce healing inflammation ; there is sort of blackness and stitches break open. Give *Sulphuric acid* which is a wonderful remedy in such cases. See "Wounds unhealthy no tendency to heal" and "Diabetes gangrene".

Gastralgia—Gnawing or burning pain in the stomach. Loss of appetite. (*Nux-v.*). See "Burning pain sensation" and "Hunger gnawing-relief by eating."

Gastritis chronic-acid stage—*Hepar sulph.* is benefical when there is great desire for acids, vinegar and spices, and highly seasoned food, nausea in the morning and acid eructation.

The patient is peevish, easily angered and very sensitive to all impressions. See "Dyspepsia with flatulence," also "Acid dyspepsia".

Gastritis-chronic with eructation—*Lyco.* is an important remedy during the acid stage of chronic gastritis. Sensation of burning in the stomach with sour eructations. Mental depression. Bowels constipated.

Gastritis stomach rejecting food eaten with hiccough—Inflammation of the stomach attended by heat, constrictive pain, vomiting and nausea. Smallest quantity of food or drink immediately rejected. Thirsty. Hiccough and feverishness. (*Veratrum-viride.*). See "Vomiting of all things".

Gastro-enteritis—(1) Much griping, cutting and fainting pains in bowels ; trembling, cold limbs and irregular pulse. (*Narcissus poeticus*).

(2) Attack with heavy stool, vomiting and cold perspiration. (*Verat-alba.*).

(3) Diarrhoea immediately after eating or drinking ; pain at the pit of abdomen and the patient is nervous. (*Argen-n.*).

Gastro-intestinal disturbances—(1) Pertaining to the stomach and intestines *e.g.* Vomiting, motions, distension. Intense thirst. (*Acon.*).

(2) *Vanadium* is true digestive tonic after an acute attack of irritation. It is also useful for absence of appetite. See "Appetite absence."

Gastro-intestinal trouble-due to much travelling—Due to much travelling abroad ; travellers can pick up exotic germs which usually upset the bowels causing diarrhoea or dysentery *Dysentery co* or *Morgan* which are nosodes can prevent and clear the trouble completely. (Dr. Norton).

Gastric (pertaining to stomach) trouble of different types—(1) From dietetic error such as pastry, ice cream, pork and heavy fatty food. With persistent nausea. (*Ip.*) is indicated after the food is out of stomach and the stomach feels more or less light. (*Ip.*). Compare *Puls.* which is indicated while the food is still in stomach and lies in it.

(2) For heartburn give *Puls.*

(3) Nausea with flow of sour water from mouth. (*Calc-c.*)

(4) For acidity, slow digestion, flatulence. (*Carbo-v.*). See "Acidity".

(5) Everything tastes, bitter. Sour eructations. (*China.*).

(6) Heartburn, appetite lost, distress immediately after eating. (*Lyco.*). See "Heartburn".

(7) Cannot bear milk in any form. Sudden violent vomiting or curdled milk. (*Aethu.*).

(8) Gnawing, grinding pain, relieved by eating. Bilious eructations, jaundice, constipation. (*Chelidonium.*).

(9) Dyspepsia of the aged or weak anaemic exhausted patients. After meals there is an undue flatulent distension. (*Kali carbonicum*).

(10) In dyspeptic trouble of the aged with functional heart symptoms. (*Abies-nigra.*). See also "Dyspepsia" under its different heads. "Digestion" and "Debility due to lack of digestive power".

Gastric and duodenal ulcers-distinction between the two—*In Gastric ulcer* when food is taken, there is comfort for a while and then pain appears but disappears later as the stomach empties

In duodenal ulcer, when food is taken, there is comfort for a while then pain, but the pain does not disappear until more food is taken. The "Pain in gastric ulcer." (Dr. Tytler).

Gastric and duodenal ulcer with haemorrhage and its cure—Agonizing feeling in the stomach. Gastric ulceration even with haemorrhage. Patient absolutely blanched from loss of blood. *Ornithogalum* will clear up the case and can cure gastric and duodenal ulcer.

Gastric ulcer and arresting its formation—(1) Gastric ulcer with much burning. (*Mezereum*).

(2) Round ulcer of stomach. Gastric symptoms are relieved after eating. Vomiting of bright yellow water. (*Kali-bi*).

(3) Ulceration of stomach, vomiting of blood and food taken, gnawing pain, distension of stomach. (*Acetic-acid.*). Dr. Jahr recommends *Phos.*

(4) *Uranium nitr.* is said to arrest the tendency of formation of ulcers.

(5) Ulceration, pain in left side under ribs. Radiating pain. Enormous distension. Craving for sweets, *Argentum nitricum* in form of tincture 2 or 3 drops doses. See also "Duodenal ulcer", "Ulcer of stomach" and "Peptic ulcer."

Genitals and touching it by hands- (*a*) Bearing down in genitals worse from riding in carriage. (*Asaf.*).

(*b)* Hands constantly kept on genitals—*Stram. 30.* Three times a day. See

"(6) of Herpes Zoster for herpes of genital organ".

Genital-females itching with swelling—Horrible itching of genitals with swelling of labia during menses. (*Ambra.*). See also "Itching female organ" and "Pruritus with burning urine".

Giddiness—(1) Tends to spread from neck to head and is worse while looking upward. (*Sil.*).

(2) Giddiness on rising from bed or seat, on moving about, nausea. (*Selenium.*).

(3) Vertigo on turning over bed or on rising from lying down. (*Bell.*).

(4) Vertigo whilst lying down. Constipation, (*Nat-m.*).

(5) Giddiness on lifting or moving the head, relieved by reclining. (*China 3* times a day). See also "Vertigo" under its different heads.

Girls having no menses—Young girl having no menses ; without periods for nine months, one breast smaller than the other, and undeveloped mammary glands. (*Sabina.*). See "Menstruation suppressed for months together".

Glands at different parts chronic enlarged—(1) (*a*) *Aur-met.* wonderfully affects the glands, the parotid glands, the glands about the groin, the lymphatics in the abdomen, in fact the glands everywhere. The mammary glands, the testes and ovaries are involved and undergo state of hardness and infiltration (passing of fluids into tissue spaces or cells). *Arum-met.* cures chronic enlargement of the testes and lumps in the mammary glands and tumours in these glands. See (*Aur-met.*). "Testes atrophic".

(*b*) Enlargement and induration of gland especially of neck. Glands have a certain elasticity and pliability about them rather than the stony hardness. (*Lapis albus.*). See "Neck gland enlarged".

Glands-ear swollen—Parotid glands swollen. Sharp pain shooting from ear into the glands. Dr. Farrington recommends *Kali-bichromicum.* See "Parotid gland" and "Ear imflammation"

Glands-enlarged-neck—Enlargement of laymphatic glands in the neck, under-developed body. (*Calc.*). Compare *Merc-sol.* See "Neck glands enlarged".

Gland-of-neck enlarged under right ear—Gland as enlarged as the size of a nut for several years. First give *Bacillin 100* every eighth day and later on *Calc-phos. 30* T.D.S. and finish it with *Bacil.* as given previously.

Glands-of-neck caused by a blow—Gland enlarged causing suppuration First give *Bacil 200.* Follow it with *Hepar-sulf.*

Glands-glandular or bony ulceration—Prevents inflammation tending to form pus or ulcers not healing quickly. Every little wound tends to form pus. (*Sil.*). See "Ulcer delayed healing", "Fistula of glands" and "Wound forming pus".

Glands-in both axillae—Inflammation of both the armpits with abscesses. Constipation. *Hepar-sulf 6* four times a day will open the abscesses and heal them. Follow it with *Sulf.* 30 which will arrest the boils and ultimately give *Nit.-acid* 30.

Glands and surface of bone inflamed—Inflammation of glands due to syphilis. indurations and inflammations of membrane covering the surface of bone. (*Asaf.*).

Glands-outside neck—Outside the throat and neck glands are enlarged and felt as lumps. (*Am-c.*). Compare also *Bufo.* See "Neck-gland swelling".

Glands-swelling also with suppuration—(1) Acute swelling with inflammation of glands, *e.g.* neck etc. The patient should be thirsty, restless and chilly. (*Rhus-t.*). Compare *Merc-sol.* where the patient somewhat restless, will not usually keep cover and will perspire porfusely without much relief.

(2) For suppuration and inflammation of the glands. Nodosities in the breasts. (*Scrophularia.*).

(3) Swelling of glands with pain. Hard and red. (*Merc-iod.*). It follows *Bell.* well.

(4) Enlargement of glands of axilla, groin and neck with skin symptoms. The abdomen is large and hard. (*Jug-r.*). See "Axilla different complaints" and "Swelling with inflamed glands".

Glands-swollen and inflamed—Swelling and inflammation of glands which are inclined to form pus. The patient is somewhat restless, will not usually keep the cover and will perspire profusely without much relief. (*Merc-sol.*). Compare *Rhus-t.* See "Swelling with inflamed glands".

Glands-swelling-due to discharge from nose—Alongwith excoriating discharge from nose the glands of the neck and even the parotid (situated near the ear) may be inflamed and are sore, (*Arum-t*). See "Parotid glands swollen after measles", "Catarrh of nose with blood" and "Neck-glands with discharge from nose".

Glands and ulcer on neck-tubercular—(*a*) Enlaiged and of tubercular nature. Easily tired. Takes cold from wet feet usually. Menses every three weeks, profuse and very bright red flow. *Tuberculinum* in very high doses.

(*b*) *Drosera* is another good medicine for tubercular glands. See "Neck glands enlarged".

(*c*) When there is drawing of pus and suppuration has already taken place with emaciation and loss of appetite. *Insulin* in potencies from 30th to 200th is very efficacious.

(*d*) For tubercular ulcers and sinuses. *Bacill.* in very high potencies ; also *Ol-j.* in high potencies.

(*e*) *Bacill. 30* may be given once a week for tubercular glands. See "Neck gland enlarged".

Gleet—Chronic stage of gonorrhoea in the male with muco-purulent discharge. There is not much discharge but a few drops which glue up the orifice of urethra in the morning. It is persistent. Emissions thin and watery (*Kali-iodatum* for thick discharge of long standing and for smarting and burning on urinating, try *Capsicum*) (*Sep.*). See also "Gonorrhoea".

Glaucoma and its checking (1) (*a*) Increased intra-occular tension with severe sudden pain in the eyes with rapid failure of sight. *Eserine* in several cases acted like a charm, the pains were subdued almost at once. Dr. Jahr says that *Phos.* is the surest remedy for this and *Phos.* is useful in glaucoma beginning with neuralgic pains. It will check the pain and check the degeneration. If *Phos.* cannot cure the whole trouble, *Lyco.* and *Sil.*, says Dr. Jahr, will be indispensable. Dr. D. C. Dass Gupta has treated this trouble successfully by *Osmium 200* giving it once a week for 4 or 5 weeks while Dr. Dewey recommends *Spigelia* and *Phos.* See "Eye-trouble" and "Part 13 of vision" also.

(*b*) *Gels.* is one of the most valuable remedies in glaucoma, often palliating the severe pains and improving the neurotic symptoms of disease. *Gels.* dilates the pupil through its paralysing effect on the third nerve.

(2) *Bry.* may be thought of in rheumatism of the eyes with violent pains shooting through the eye-balls into the back of the head or up, towards vertex, worse by moving eyes.

(3) Severe shooting pains which appear at the same fixed time. (*Cedr.*).

(4) For glaucoma with sciatica pains and flatulence ; severe burning pains relieved by pressure ; worse from rest at night and from stopping when it feels as if it would fall out. (*Coloc*).

(5) (*a*) When there is dim vision try *Sulf.*

(*b*) Glaucoma pains. Relief from pain is spasmodic and is relieved by heat and pressure. (*Coloc.*).

Glaucoma threatened—For this trouble besides dropping *Pilocarpine* drops in the eyes give *Ledum* as an internal constitutional remedy.

Glossitis—(1) Inflammation of tongues. *Merc.* is the main remedy and seldom fails to cure. (Dr. Curtis).

(2) If there is oedema then *Apis.* seems to be the best general remedy and is often followed by astonishing results.

Glycosuria—Glycosuria with motor-paralysis (trembling of legs which give away while walking) *Curare* 4th dilution.

Goitre (Exopthalmic)—(1) Abnormal protusion of the eye-ball from the orbit on account of goitre. Patient very sensitive to heat. Desires hot food. Aggravation in warm room ; must have fresh air. Diarrhoea after heavy meal. Menstruation irregular or profuse and painful ; very sensitive mentally. Likes sweets. Depressed usually. (*Lyco.*).

(2) Dr. Zopfy of Germany who had much experience claims that *Calc-c.* will cure in most simple cases within a very few weeks. *Calcarea jodide* is also a very useful remedy—a dose every night for a week then wait for a week.

(3) Painful goitre, pain on swallowing. Goitre in inhabitants of valleys with cardiac symptoms. *Spongia*—a dose night and morning for 6 days, then pause for a week and then repeat.

(4) *Iodine* is a classical remedy for exopthalmic variety.

(5) *Thuja* is particularly indicated when superficial veins of the swelling are distended and painful. A dose every 6 hours for 4 days then pause for 4 days after which proceed with like doses at intervals of 12 hours for 4 days, then pause again for 6 days and so on. (Dr. J. Laurie).

(*b*) Suitable for fat persons. Acts better with pale patients who are debilitated and anaemic, who suffer from muscular weakness and palpitation from least exertion. *Thyr. 3x* two or 3 doses per day. It is to be repeated at intervals. The pulse should be watched. *Thyr.* re-inforces the action of *Lycopus* and is complemented by *Fucus vesiculosus*.

(2) Hard, goitre of the size of hen's egg with enlargement of thyroid gland. (*Brom.*).

(3) Many observers speak highly of *Lycopus virginicus* as a remedy for exopthalmic goitre. Its chief indications seem to be constriction of chest, weak pulse which is remittent and rapid.

(4) *Ferrum phosphoricum* is also useful in exopthalmic variety.

(5) Goitre due to water of valleys. Simple goitre of soft doughy type rather than hard indurated variety. (*Lapis albus.*). Dr. J.H. Kanopp recommends *Fucus vesiculosus* as specific for exopthalmic goitre, as for dose he says that a tea-spoonful of the tincture be given twice or thrice daily in an advanced case.

Goitre of puberty—*Hydrastis.*

Gonitis-inflammation of knee joints—See "Knee grating and weakness with swelling".

Gonorrhoea—(1) In the second stage when greenish discharge has set in and the burning and tenesmus continues. Urine hot, burning, scanty, or suppressed ; in drops with great pain. (*Merc-c.*).

(2) Gonorrhoea of long standing complicated with syphillis. (*Cinnabaris.*). Compare *Thuja*.

(3) Chronic gonorrhoea with biting and burning at the back of bladder and in urethra before and after micturition. (*Copaiva.*)

(4) Gonorrhoea extremely violent with yellow and white thick discharge, crawling in urethra and jerking in testicles. (*Tussilago pet.*).

Gonorrhoea after effects causing constitutional diseases *Thuja* is an antidote to the constitutional disease resulting from the after effect of gonorrhoea and having its most characteristics manifestation excrescences like warts etc.

Gonorrhoral arthritis—See "Arthritis-due to gonorrhoea."

Gonorrhoea-chronic and painful—Cold, gleety discharge. *Agar.* comes in the cure of old discharge from urethra, chronic gonorrhoea after all sorts of local treatment have been used. The penis is cold and shrunken ; excessively painful retraction in testes ; continued itching tingling in the urethra and the last drop will remain discharging for long time. (*Agar.*). Compare *Petroleum.*

Gonorrhoea-gleety discharge—Chronic gonorrhoea. Slight painless yellowish discharge glueing the meatus. Night sweats ; bone pain ; worse during perspiration. *Sepia* and then *Merc-sol.* See also "Gleet".

Gonorrhoea-painful with inflammation—Inflammation of prepuce and glands ; pain in penis. Bad effects of suppressed or maltreated gonorrhoea *e.g.* warts or condylomata on genitals specially of females. (*Thuja.*) See "Condylomata".

Gonorrhoea-repeated—History of repeated gonorrhoeas. The patient has lived in excess and now suffers from relaxed and cold genitalia, emissions, prostatic discharge at stool. Despair, anxiety, fear, peevishness and suicidal thought from above cause. (*Agn.*).

Gonorrhoea-swollen prepuce—Green discharge ; worse at night ; urging to urinate ; intolerable burning in fore-part of urethra when passing last few drop ; prepuce hot and swollen (*Merc-sol.*). See "Urethritis" and "Prepuce".

Gout-acute pain—*Gultheria oil* in 10 to 20 drop doses never fails to arrest the pain of acute gout arthritis and rheumatism. Similarly *Urtica urens* M.T. be given 10 drop doses 2 or 3 times a day.

Gout-in different parts including arthritis deformans—(1) Since uric acid in joints mostly responsible for gout so administer *Urtica urens* M.T. at least 5 to 10 drops in boiled water for removal of deposits first. This remedy is said to cure more cases of gout than any other. Under its use pain and swelling subside and quantities of sand passed.

(2) Gout engrafted on gonorrhoeal or syphilitic constitution. Chronic case with wandering pains. Specially useful when there are urinary symptoms—the urine smells strong like that of the horse. Swelling and pain of right knee : tearing pain in great toe. Cures symptoms of uric diathesis (constitutional tendency to rheumatism) (*Benz-a.*).

(3) Pain in ankles and bones of feet ; border of foot and soles as if gouty. Chronic rheumatism due to uric acid. (*Lith-c.*).

(4) The ball of great toe is swollen, sore, and painful on stepping ; cold remedy worse from warmth and better by cold application. Gouty nodosities. Pains in the extremities, pain and swelling proceed upwards and heart becomes affected. Specially useful for gouty inflammation affecting the knee joint. (*Led.*).

(5) Constitutional gout when there are nodosities in the joints. Chronic cases where there are deposits of urate of soda concretions in the joints and hands become twisted. (*Ammonium-phos.*)

(6) Dr. Herbert mentions that *Picric acid* is useful in arthritis deformnas (a general term sometimes used to mean chronic rheumatoid or degenerative arthritis) and thinks that treating

the disease from homoeopathic stand point will yield best results.

(7) Joints swollen, rheumatic tearing in all limbs specially right side. Worse before or during thunder storm ; cold, or wet or unsettled weather. Cannot sleep unless legs are crossed. Enlargement of joints not due to gouty deposits. (*Rhododendron.*).

(8) Pains in heels relieved by putting most of the weight on them. Gouty and rheumatic states are associated with kidney and liver distrubance. Urine cloudy, grayish, depositing sediment renal (pertaining to kindey) or biliary (pertaining to fluid from liver) calculi. (*Berb-v. 200*).

(9) Rheumatism in sycotic persons due to suppressed gonorrhoea. (*Sars. 200*).

(10) *Colchicum autumnale* is indicated in those of robust constitution who suffer from rheumatic and gouty complaints and in the diseases of aged. See "Arthritis" and "Rheumatism" under their different heads.

Gout-long bones—Old gouty constitution, Pain in the hip joint. Pain in the bones between joints ; better by motion. (*Ph-a.*). See "Bones an abnormal out-growth".

Gout-in all joints—In all the joints, gouty, rheumatic tendency. (*Staphy.*).

Gout-preventing—*Colchicum* in strong Tr. if given in drop doses prevents an immediately threatened or arrests attack of gout.

Gout-swollen joints—(1) Pain in limbs joints. Joints swollen hard pressure relieves. (*Chin*).

(2) Pain in soles of feet and heels. (*Acid-tartaricum.*).

(3) Pain in wrists and ankles with fever. (*Trimethylaminum.*).

(4) Tonic spasms of the toe of right foot very painful. (*Cuprum-acet.*).

(5) Rheumatism attacking joints particularly elbow and knee joints with great swelling, redness and high fever. (*Salicylic-acid.*).

(6) For gout accompained with diabetes. (*Phaseolus.*).

Gout-pains flying—In all joints, when there is gouty and rheumatic affections, neuralgic affections, especially rheumatism tendency is found from the elbows to the hands. Tearing pains flying hither and thither without any order, relieved by heat. (*Aesc.*). See "Knee grating and weakness with swelling", "Flying pains" and "Wandering joint pains".

Gout-nervous—In nervous constitutions *Asaf.* is full of rheumatism and gouty symptoms ; gouty and rheumatic symptoms improve the general symptoms. (*Asaf.*). See "Rheumatism of nervous patients".

Gout of toe and heel—Acute attack of gout, terrific pain, joints stiff and feverish. Inflammation of great toe, gout in heel. Swelling and coldness of legs and feet. (*Colchicum.*). Allopaths give it under the name of Clochicine and Probenecid to control high uric acid to prevent recurrence after *Colchicine* has brought down the acute condition. (Readers' Digest, November 1959). See also "Arthritis hypertension" and "Rheumatism" under its different heads.

Granulations after operation of abdomen—If the abdominal cavtiy has been opened and the walls of the abdomen take an unhealthy look and there are stinging burning pain, *Staphysagria* is the remedy that will make the granulations healthy. (*Staphy.*). See "Abdomen-cavity opened".

Gravel—*Sarsaparilla* is the remedy which has excruciating neuralgia of kidneys. Renal colic and passage of gravel and formation of vesical calculi. This remedy relieves the suffering attendant on gravel specially with rheumatic symptoms. (*Sars.*) See also "Calculus in kidney" and "Stone in kidney".

Gravel-prevention—(1) Gravely urine, pain in back and loins. (*Berb.*).

(2) Tendency to stone ; uric acid in the tissues in gouty subjects. (*Urt-u.*). See also "Calculus-prevention of formation of stone."

G

Grayness of hair and its prevention—(1) Hair gray in early life ; falls out. *Phos. ac., Hydrastis.* (*Asparagus.*). See "Hair" under its different heads.

(2) To prevent hair growing gray and to restore them to natural colour. (Begin giving *Thyroidin 30* daily at least for one month or longer if necessary and thereafter use this medicine in 200 potency once a week for one month.). See "Premature gray hair".

Grief-ailment due to—(1) *Aurum-met.* has ailments from grief, disappointed love, fright or anger and mortification. (*Aur-met.*). Dr. Jahr recommends *Ignatia* for nervous women burdened with grief and chronic, long standing effects of grief. (*Phos-ac.*). See "Anger-complaints" and "Suicide" under their different heads.

(2) When the patient is irritable, cross and uneasy, fearful and anticipates danger and grieves constantly. (*Staphy.*).

(3) Chronic complaints from long lasting grief and sorrows ; great sadness and sorrows. (*Lach.*).

(4) Depressed and joyless, disposition to cry and weep. (*Coloc.*). See "Widows remedy".

(5) Unhappy love if accompained by a good deal of jealousy. (*Hyos.*). See "Melancholia".

Grinding of teeth—While asleep. Restlessness during sleep. (*Cina.*). See "Convulsion-child grinding teeth" and "Teeth grinding by child".

Groin-abscess in it—Old abscess in left groin with pain. (*Silica. 30 T.D.S.*).

Gums-swollen, ulcerated with decayed teeth etc.—(1) Gums and teeth swollen. Spongy and swollen gums with slight bleeding. The whole mouth is offensive in look and odour ; flabby tongue with imprints of teeth on the sides. Secretion of too much saliva. (*Merc-sol.*). This may be given in alternation with *Bell.* See "Mouth-offensive odour and swollen gums."

(2) For gum, many abscesses with decayed teeth. Give *Hekla-lava*.

(3) For bleeding gums *Phos.* and if it fails, then *Merc-sol.* See "Pyorrhoea".

(4) Gums tender and bleed easily. Pain in sound teeth. Gums swollen and bleed when touched. (*Arg-n.*).

(5) Swelling of gums with no loose teeth. Sour taste. Bloody saliva. (*Mag-c.*).

(6) When there is deficiency of calcium and loss of enamel on teeth. (*Calc-f.*).

(7) Very rapid dacay of teeth, with spongy bleeding gums ; teeth dark and crumbling. (*Staphy.*). Compare *Kreos*.

(8) Consider *Hyper.*, *Nux-v.* and *Hyos.* for gums painful after extraction of teeth. First *Phos.* should be tried. See "Teeth aches", and "Tooth" under their different head.

Gums-biting Irrestible inclination to bite gums and teeth. (*Phyt.*). See "No. 6 of Cravings".

Gums-pressing—In children during dentition period. (*Podo.*). Has desire to press the gums together. When this symptom is very clear and the child always presses the gums together, *Podo*, will be useful if there is diarrhoea. If this symptom is present during the attack of acute diarrhoea, think of *Podo*, See "Dentition-difficult, pressing gums, gums swollen".

Gums-receding with loose teeth—(1) Gums settle away from the teeth and bleed. Teeth become loose, a general condition. (*Am-c.*).

(2) Gums recede, spongy, and bleed easily. Teeth loose, sour, pain on touch and from chewing. Fetid odour from mouth. (*Merc-s.*).

(3) When teeth get loose and separated from gums. Bleeding from teeth when cleansing. Pain both from hot, cold or saltish food. (*Carb-v.*). See "Teeth" under its different heads.

Gum-boil-pus formed—When pus has formed or there is watery offensive pus ; gums sensitive to cold air ; fistulous opening which heals slowly. (*Sil.*). See "Pus-formation" and "Pyorrhoea".

Gum-boil-throbbing—(1) Throbbing pain in teeth. (*Bell.*). See also "Teeth-aches" under their different heads and "Boils throbbing".

(2) Swelling of cheek and whole left side of face. Gum-boil painful. Mouth hot and tender. (*Bor.*).

(3) Gum-boil inflamed, bleeding and painful, pains cutting and burning ; gums scurvy. (*Carb-a.*).

(4) *Merc.* and *Bell.* in alternation when there is extensive, bright, inflammatory redness and swelling, the gums and roof of mouth participating. A dose every 3 hrs.

Gum-paint—(*a*) Teethache and are sensitive and sore to touch. Toothache, with reflex neuralgia of eyelids. Toothache with salivation. *Plantago* mother tincture may be painted on gums and hollow teeth which will relieve pain like a charm. The gums may also be massaged with it. See "Toothache" under its different heads.

(*b*) Dr. P. Banerjee recommends the following gum paint for swelling of the gums or gum boil which he found very efficacious. Tinc. *Aconite* 15 drops, Tr. *Echinecea* 20 drops and Tr. *Plantago* 25 drops to be mixed together and to be applied to the painful portion of the gum or teeth after gurgling with warm water.

Gun shot wounds—(1) *Hyper.* or *Symph.* according to indications.

(2) According to Dr. Jahr if such gun shot would be treated with *Calendula* then the injured limb can be saved.

H

Haematemesis (the vomiting of blood from stomach)—
(1) Dark blood (*Ham.*, every 15 minutes.).

(2) Bright blood. (*Ip.*, every 15 minutes.).

(3) From mechanical injury. (*Arnica*, every 15 minutes.).

(4) *Ipecac* in repeated doses.

(5) When convulsions have set in. (*Secale.*).

(6) When signs of collapse.(*Verat-a*).

Haematuria (bloody urine)—(*a*) *Canth.*, *Ham.*, *Tereb.*, *Nit-ac.* *Millefolium* is specific with painfulness of kidneys.

(*b*) (1) Dr. Jahr advises to give (*Cann-i*) if no other remedy is specifically indicated and if this does not give relief then *Canth.* may be given. If these two remedies have no effect then *Nux-v.* may be tried.

(2) Urine bloody. Burning soreness when urinating. Stinging in urethra (*Apis.*).

(3) With pain in kidneys, with dark bloody urine (*Ham.*).

(4) Due to mechanical injury, emission of blood from urethra. (*Arn.*).

(5) Chronic catarrh of bladder with cutting pain in bladder, pain in back before urinating ; ceases after flow ; slow in coming ; must strain. Heavy red sediment. *Lyco.* a few drops of tincture 3 times a day have proved efficacious.

(6) Difficult urination with burning in bladder. Difficulty, accompanied by heat and pain in passing the urine which escapes drop by drop and is bloody ; much blood with very little urine with coffee ground sediment. (*Ter.*).

(7) The urine is high-coloured, bloody and albuminous, flow of bloody mucus from bladder, emission of blood drop by

drop. (*Canth.*). Where the exciting cause of disorder is not known, then a recourse in almost all cases of haematuria may be had by giving *Cantharis.* (Dr. Laurie).

(8) Urine bloody, scanty slimy and sandy. Blood in urine towards the end of urination. Great pain near neck of bladder (*Sars.*).

(9) When there is continued nausea, oppressed breathing, cutting pain in the abdomen, along with the passage of bloody urine. (*Ip.*).

(10) Intractable cases or those which are not well understood. Mother tinctures of *Thlaspi bursa* or *Senecio* or *Arsenicum-hydrogenisatum* 3 may be tried according to symptoms. See "Urine" under its different heads and "Bloody urine".

(11) In haematuria with painfulness of kidneys *Millefolum* is a specific remedy in such cases. See "Urine" under its different heads and "Bloody urine".

Haemoglobin-its shortage—Vanadium increases the amount of haemoglobin, also combines its oxygen which destroys their virulence.

Haemopbilia- a sex-linked disease transmitted by females—A sex-linked hereditary disease occurring in males with abnormal bleeding.' Patient bleeding since birth ; every cut or scratch would keep on bleeding until he is exsanguited. Rheumatic pain in knees and elbows. Swelling of knees. Pale from haemorrhage, constant bleeding from the gums. Small wounds bleed too much. Small bruises make him black and blue. Great thirst for water. (*Lach.*).

Haemoptysis-blood spitting from lungs—(*a*) Dr. Jousst relies on *Ipec.* and *Millefolium* alternately, while Dr. Thomas has successfully treated pulmonary cases with *Abclypha Indica.* (*b*) Slight bright haemorrhage. The patient has tendency to phthisis and suffers from bronchial catarrh, headache and epistaxis. (*Ferr-p.*). (Blackwood). See also "Blood spitting", "Bleeding from lungs" and "No. 15 of Tuberculosis". (Dr. Baehr).

Haemorrhages under different conditions. (1) The control of Ipecacuanha over haemorrhages deserves honourable mention. Bright red, profuse, with heavy breathing and nausea. It has haemorrhages from the nose, stomach, rectum, womb, lungs and bladder, from all the orifices of the body. (*Ip. 200*). Compare *Cortalus* and *Secale*.

(2) Active, bright, with great fear and anxiety. (*Acon.*).

(3) From injuries, bodily fatigue and exertion. (*Arnica.*).

(4) Blood hot, throbbing carotid, congestion to head. (*Bell.*).

(5) Almost entire collapse, pale face ; wants to be fanned. (*Carbo-veg.*).

(6) Great loss of blood, ringing in ears, faintness (*China.*).

(7) Delirium, and jerking and twitching of muscles. (*Hyos.*).

(8) Blood decomposed, sediments like charred straw. (*Lach.*).

(9) Active haemorrhages of bright blood. (*Nitric-acid*).

(10) Profuse and persistent, even from small wounds and tumours. (*Phos.*).

(11) Partly fluid and partly hard black clots. (*Platinum.*).

(12) Intermittent haemorrhages. (*Puls.*). See also "Bleeding" under its different heads.

Haemorrhage-bright blood—Blood bright and red colour from any out-let. *Ferr-p.* is good haemorrhage remedy, *i.e.* it stops bleeding. (*Ferr-p.*). See "Bleeding-bright".

Haemorrhage dark-blood—Of mouth, nose, bowels or uterus ; blood dark with faintness ; loss of sight and ringing in the ears. Sudden. *China* to be given in repeated doses. See also "Discharge" and "Bleeding dark."

Haemorrhage-from uterus in dropsy—From uterus in dropsy. Though it has amenorrhoea with dropsy, it has also copious menstrual flow which may be frequent and lasting too long.

From copious menstrual flow, the patient becomes anaemic and then dropsical. (*Apoc-can.*). See also "Menorrhagia in dropsy".

Haemorrhage-from any orifice—From any orifice of the body. It may be from nose, wound, rectum, stomach, uterus, lungs or bladder. Nausea must be present with bleeding which must be of bright red colour. (*Ip.*) See "Bleeding tendency."

Haemorrhage-during pregnancy if abortion apprehended and also haemorrhage continuous—(*a*) *Sabina, Crocus, Kreosotum* and *Secale.* (Dr. Nash.). See also "Abortion", "Miscarriage" under their different heads and "Bleeding during pregnancy".

(*b*) Haemorrhage continuous—*Ip., Sabina, Arn.* and *Cinnamon* ; haemorrhage intermittent ; *Puls* ; haemorrhage with bright red blood ; *Ip., Arn.,* with dark blood ; *Sabina., Cham. Secale* ; for convulsions ; *Ip., Hyos., Plat., Cinnamon.,* for blows on abdomen : *Arn., Stram : Rhus., Cinnamon.,* when there is no peculiar symptom indicating the remedy then *Mill.*

Haemorrhage-in typhoid—Haemorrhage from any mucous membrane, bleeding from nose, lungs, bowels ; eyes sunken. discoloured lips ; hippocratic countenance : gradually approaching unconsciousness (*Ph-a.*). Nitric acid is another remedy for haemorrhage in typhoid if blood is bright red.

Haemorrhage-in typhoid from bowels—(1) From bowels of decomposed blood which occurs during exhausting diseases like typhoid. (*Lach.*).

(2) If the blood comes in large clots then according to Dr. Nash *Alumina* is one of the best remedies for haemorrhages of the bowels in typhoid fever. See also "Typhoid, haemorrhage intestinal".

Haemorrhage-of any kind—For haemorrhage when there is no peculiar sysmptom, indicating any other remedy give *Millefolium* which is an invaluable remedy for various types of haemorrhages; blood bright red.

Haemorrhage-uterine—Chronic illness of uterine haemorrhage. Menorrhagia, large clots mixed with bright red liquid.

Feet always damp and cold, stockings become damp. Constipation. Sore throat. If any severe shock or mental disturbance brings on uterine haemorrhage. *Calc-carb*. See also "Uterine haemorrhage" and "Menorrhagia excessive menstruation."

Haemorrhage-veinous from any organ and blackish blood—Veinous bleeding from any organ, *e.g.* lungs, stomach bowels, uterus, nose, etc., blackish blood and not the red arterial blood. In the weakened conditions when the blood oozes from the surface, *China* and *Carb-v.* are complementary medicines. In these cases of haemorrhages *China* is good for the after-effects of the haemorrhages. See also "Veinous stasis" and "Veinous bleeding".

Haemorrhoids-bleeding—One drop of *Mucuna* mother tincture is specific for bleeding piles, 2 or 3 doses a day will arrest in 2 or 3 days. See also "Piles" under their different heads.

Haemorrhoids-blind or bleeding—Bleeding or blind. Haemorrhoids protrude, become constricted, purplish, Stitches in them on sneezing or coughing. Constant urging in them on sneezing or coughing. Constant urging in rectum, not for stool. Constricted feeling in anus and a throbbing pain as if little hammers are striking in painful piles. (*Lach.*). See "Piles-throbbing pains in both types of piles", "Piles both blind and bleeding" and "Piles inflamed" for local application.

Haemorrhoids-of- both types—*Aesc.* cures both blind and bleeding piles. Chronic constipation. Pile is purple. The rectum seems full of sticks with liver engorgement. The stool becomes jammed into the rectum against these distended veins and then ulceration takes place. Great piles remedy. Pain in back and hips. (*Aesc-h.*). See "Piles with distended veins in rectum", "Haemorrhoids" and "Piles".

Haemorrhoids like bunch of grapes round the anus with itching—(*a*) Specific for haemorrhoids, which look like bunch of grapes round the anus. There is relaxation about rectum with protrusion of anus and bleeding piles. Itching and burning in anus preventing sleep, which may be very great driving him to desperation. Cold application relieves itching. (*Aloe.*). (*b*) For itching and redness of children. (*Sulf.*). See "Piles itching".

Haemorrhoids painful—Bleeding and painful. Intestinal mentation and mental despondency. (*Lyco.*).

Haemorrhoids-pregnancy—With prolapse during pregnancy or after child birth. (*Podo.*). See "No. 4 Pregnancy-disorders of."

Haemorrhoids with ulceration— Haemorrhoids with ulceration, the anus and surrounding parts are purple and covered with crusts, ulcers within the anus very painful ; the whole mucous membrance studded with ulcers and cracks. (*Paeonia.*). See "Piles with pain and ulcerated pimples" and "Fistula with piles".

Hair different complaints—(1) Falling of hair. (*Am-c.*).

(2) The hair will fall and not grow. Baldness due to syphilis. (*Ustilago mydis.*). A near specific as is possible in *Flouric acid.*

(3) Falling off hair due to dry white scaly dandruff (*Thuja*).

(4) Falling off with dryness. (*Kali-c.*).

(5) Senile whitening of hair. Start treatment with *Thyroidine 30,* next *Jaborandi.* C.M. potency should be tried every fortnight for about 4 months. If this also fails then try *Lycopodium* and *Acid-phos.* for grey hair in given order one after the other in dilutions of 30. If no result is achieved within 3 months, these 2 remedies may be given alternately in 1000 dilution every fortnight. (*b*) For hair on lips and chin of women, give *Thuja.* 200 every month and *Ol-j* 3x thrice daily except on the day when Thuja. is taken.

(6) Bald spot on the side of head. The head sweats easily. The most important remedy is *Graphites.*

(7) Falling of hair from general debility. (*Phos-acid.*).

(8) Falling of the hair with great itching of the scalp. (*Vinca-minor.*).

(9) Falling of hair after child birth or severe illness. (*Carbo-v.*). (*b*) For grey hair in early life, falls out. *Ph-a., Hydr., Aspar.*

(10) Losing of hair after chronic headache. *Sepia.* See also "Baldness", "Beard", "Face-hair on lips and chin of women", "Grayness of hair". See "Premature gray hair".

(11) For abnormal growth of hair. (*Ol-J*).

Hair falling after disease and in pregnancy—Great falling of the hair at the climacteric or after chronic headaches. (*Sep.* and *Nat-mur.*). See "Falling out of hair" and "(*e*) of Pregnancy disorders of."

Hair-eruption on the root—Itching eruptions on the face, specially at the margin of the hairs on forehead. Affects hair follicles (*Nat-m.*). See also "Eczema hair follicles," and "Eczema on the hairy part."

Hair-falling—(1) Falling out of hair. (*Thuja*).

(2) Falling of hair from head, eye-brows, eye-lashes and genitals. (*Acidphos*).

(3) Falling of hair of anaemic persons. *Ferr-p. 6x* internally and rub Tr. *Geranium Robertianum* externally.

(4) Excessive perspiration on head causing baldness. Alopecia following acute exhausting disease. (*Thalium.*). See "Falling out of hair" and "Baldness".

Hair-for growing rapidly with dark colour—The hair will grow rapidly and become darker. (*Wiesbaden*). See also "Face-hair on lips and chin of women".

Hair-gray—Dr. Blackwood says that *Jaborandi* if used continuously for a long period it will restore the original colour of gray hair. This medicine has favourable influence in Alopecia. *Jaborandi M.T. 30* ml. and coconut oil 100 ml. should be used for external application. While Dr. Dass says that grey hair will become darker rapidly in cases of falling of hair. (*Wiesbaden.*).

Hair-lips chin—See "Face hair on lips and chin of women".

Hair-loss of moustache—*Bacillinum 30* in frequent doses has great influence in loss of hair.

Hairless patches on chin—Roundish hairless patches on either side of chin. *Thuja 30* to be taken three times per day.

Half-sided headache with stinging pain and nausea—Half sided headaches of women of *Sep.* temperament and who are suffering from uterine troubles. Pain comes in terrific shocks so as to jerk the head inspite of the patient. Stinging pain from within outwards and upwards. Mostly on left or in forehead with nausea, vomiting, worse indoors and when lying on painful side. During menstrual period. (*Sep.*) See also "Headache half-sided".

Hallucinations seeing ghosts and dreadful animals—See monsters and hideous faces. The patient imagines to see ghosts, dreadful animals. Child starts up from sleep often and gnashes his teeth. (*Bell.*). Compare *Stram.* See also "Delusion", "Dreams of dreadful animals, "Ghosts" and "Voice hearing".

Hands-warts upon back—(1) *Ars., Nat.-c, Nit.-ac.*

(2) Left hand : *Ferr-ma.*

(3) Right hand : *Ars.*

(4) Inside of hand : *Ruta.*

Hand-sore—Extremely sore, cracked and bleeding and often oozing a thick yellow discharge. (*Graphites 6*).

Hands-pain—See "Chapter V for details."

Hay-fever—Dr. Allen recommends *Arundo mauritanica 3rd* potency, while Dr. Merch suggests *Chromic sulphuricum 3rd* trituration, both as a prophylactic and curative drug for this fever while the third Dr. Monis Weiner always found *Acidum succinicum 3x* trituration more effective for such a kind of fever. Patient has frequent running nose (*Coryza*) and violent spasmodic sneezing accompanied by watering eyes and a bewildered feeling in the head. (*Sabadilla*).

Head confused-convulsive movement—Confused : (*Athamantha*) : nodding of head : (*Aurum sulphuratium*), numbness in head ; (*Ostrya.*) : empty sensation in head ; *Kali bromatum* convulsive movement of head : (*Lyco.- Nux-m*) ; rush of blood to head : (*Paeonia, Sulf.*). See "Numbness of head".

Head-constant nodding—Constant nodding of the head ; paralysis agitans. (*Aur. Sulph.*).

Head of children large—Large in children. Eating dirty and undigestible things. Enlarged lymphatic glands, abdomen enlarged and inflated. (*Calc.*). See "Eating dirty things by children" and "Abdomen children".

Head-drawn back—Head drawn back from contraction of muscle of neck. (*Act-rac.*). See also "Rheumatic pains-in back and neck", "Wry neck" and "Headache of nape-head drawn back."

Headache-of anaemic girls—Headache of anaemic school girls after school hours. (*Calc-p.*) Compare *Nat-m.* According to Dr. Nash, *Natrum-m.* is one of the best remedies for chronic headaches when they come in paroxysms with intense throbbing. See "Head-ache of school girls due to eye strain".

Headache-bursting—As if the skull would burst and face flushed. (*Chin.*).

Headache-bursting from motion and coughing—Bursting and splitting, worse from motion, stooping and coughing and relieved by lying still. The patient holds the head and chest with hands while coughing. Worse by moving the eyes, walking about and relieved by lying still. (*Bry.*). See "Cough child grasping larynx".

Headache-at the base of brain—With dull pain at the base of brain. Heaviness of eye lids. Better by compression and lying with head high. The headache is aggravated by mental work, lying with the head low or heat of room or sun. It is relieved by hard pressure and by profuse flow of urine. The patient wants to lie with the head resting upon high pillow and lie perfectly still. (*Gels.*). See "Mental shock causing nervousness".

Headache-boring pain in right temple—Boring pains in the temple, scalp sensitive and sore. (*Hep.*).

Headache-at climacteric—Nausea, drowsiness, vertigo, blurred vision and prostration, palpitation of the heart, pale face. Complaint worse after sleep. The distress is removed by profuse menstruation. (*Lach.*) "See Menopause".

Headache-chronic—Chronic headache between scalp and brain. Sensation of opening and shutting of occiput (the back part of the head). Pain as if head would burst. (*Cocculus.*).

Headache-before menses with constipation—Headache on vertex, throbbing as with little hammers. Headache comes before menses. Chronic constipation, with no urging for stool for a week, then a painful difficult stool. (*Sep.*).

Headache-cutting—Pressing headache starting from both temples, drawing and tearing in the head to and fro. Shooting through the head, lancinating, cutting pains, worse on exertion, better from quiet lying. Headache when blowing nose. Pressing pain in the left frontal eminence and in the eyelids. (*Ambra-g.*).

Headache-from mental exertion—(1) From mental exertion with nausea ; head feels hot and heavy. (*Calc.*).

(2) Headache from mental strain, loss of sleep, worry, aching of vertex, occiput and eye-balls. (*Act-rac.*). See "Mental faculties dull".

Headache-after exertion, physical—Severe attacks of headache specially after physical exertion round about 10 a.m. Aches as if thousand little hammers were knocking on brain in the morning on awaking ; after menstruation. From sunrise to sun-set : with pale face, nausea, vomiting periodically. (*Nat-m.*). See "sun-headache".

Headache-congestive—See "Chapter V for details".

Headache-due to exposure to sun—(1) Sun-headache due to exposure to sun-heat. Very pale face. Patient sleeps into the headache. The patient is distressed with a headache every time he is exposed to the sun heat for some time. (*Lach.*).

(2) Intolerance of light and sound. (*Phellandrium*). See also "Sun-headache".

Headache-of school girls due to eye strains—Caused by strain of the eye by long continued study or by using fine needles in stitching or sewing. Anaemia. (*Calc-phos.*). or (*Nat-m.*). See "Eye strain" and "Headache of anaemic girls."

Headache-extending to eyes—(1) Beginning in the nape of neck and running forward over head to the eyes. Better by covering the head and lying on left side or washing it with warm water. (*Sil.*).

(2) Over left eye with acidity. (*Carb-v*).

(3) Headache over right eye. (*Kali-bich.*).

Headache-frontal—Frontal headaches, worse stooping, lying on back and moving eye-lids. (*Coloc.*).

Headache-gastric—Headache in occiput (the back part of the head) or over the eyes. Aggravations are from mental exertions, from sound or in open cold air. The headache is more on walking in the morning, after eating and from abuse, from stimulants. Such headaches occur in conjunction with gastric, hepatic, abdominal and haemorrhoidal affections. (*Nux-v.*).

Headache half sided—Half-sided headaches of women of *Sep.* temprament and who are suffering from uterine troubles. Pain comes in terrific shocks so as to jerk the head. Stinging pain from within outwards and upwards. Mostly on left or in forehead with nausea, vomiting ; worse indoors and when lying on painful side. During menstrual period. (*Sep.*). See "Half sided headaches."

Headache-hard pressure relieves—Bursting headache better by hard pressure. Cracking sensation in head. (*Nux moschata.*).

Headache-migraine—(1) Nervous sick headache caused by excitement and over-exertion. (*Scutellaria*).

(2) Migraine due to acidity and sluggishness of liver. (*Chionanthus*).

(3) Periodical nervous sick headache. The patient vomits a bitter bilious substance, which gives relief. Migraine of the eye with constipation. (*Iris-versicolor.*). If this fails, then *Cyclamen.*

(4) Damiana is an excellent remedy for migraine. It should be given in mother tincture in 15 to 20 drops doses every 2 hours and in severe cases every half hour and the patient will sleep after two doses.

(5) Pressive pains, intolerance of light. (*Kali-carb.* 1/2 hourly. during attack). See "Migrain" also.

Headache-of different types and relief from it—(1) *Tr. Passiflora* M.T. 15 drops.

(2)*Glonoine 30,* 5 drops. These medicines may be given alternately every 15 or 30 minutes interval and they will work marvellously in relieving pain like allopathic Saridon or Anacin. Dr. P. Banerjee also suggests *Glonoine 30* for quick relief.

Headache-of nape-head drawn back—Which is relieved from cold washing. Head drawn back from contraction of the muscles of the nape. (*Act-rac.*) See "Neck-stiff" and "Head drawn back".

Headache-with nausea—With nausea and with a bruised feeling of the bones of the head and extending down to the root of the tongue. The nausea must be there with headache. (*Ip.*). See "Nausea persistent" and "No. 3 of Specific for different diseases"

Headache-nervous—Nervous headache with nausea, vomiting ; diarrhoea, pale face ; cold sweat on forehead. (*Verat.*). See "Nervous headache-syphilitic".

Headache-periodical increasing with sun—The periodical sick headache ; begins in morning, increases during the day lasts untill evening ; head feels as if it would burst or as if the eyes would be pressed out ; relieved by sleep. Burning in eyes. Pain begins in occiput (back part of the head), spreads upwards, and settles over eyes specially right ; headache returns at climacteric every seventh day. (*Sang.*). See "Sun headache".

Headache-periodical—Periodical. (*Puls.*). Compare *Niccolum sulphuricum*. See "Periodicity".

Headache-pains from right to left—Dull aching pain, it seems that the brain would be pressed out. Pains felt in the back of head. Dull frontal headache from right to left. "Shooting in left parietal bone (one of the bones of skull) later in right". (*Aesc.*).

Headache-severe frontal left to right—Dull frontal headache. Headache very severe and the eyes cannot stand the light. Trouble goes from left to rightside. (*All-c.*). Compare *Lachesis*.

Headache-of school girls growing too fast and strain Headache of school girls from eye strain or overuse of eyes of students who are growing too fast and too tall. (*Ph-a.*). See "Headache of school girls due to eye strain".

Headache-during small-pox—Dr. Jahr recommends *Bell.*, *Bry.* and *Rhus-tox*. See Sub-head 'h' of "Small-pox" also "Haemorrhagic small-pox,no regular rash and its stages".

Headache-syphilitic or hysterical—Old syphilitic bone pains in the head. These pains in the head are sometimes very distressing. These bone-pains of the head usually called "Nervous headache" are either syphilitic, hysterical or scrofulous. They aggravate at night and pains extend from within out. (*Asaf.*). See "Syphilis pain in bones" and "Nervous headache syphilitic".

Headache-due to not urinating—Due to not attending the desire to urinate. (*Agar.*). See "Urine-headache-due to not attending it".

Headache-wandering—Wandering stitches about head; pains extend to face and teeth. Frontal and forehead pains. Neuralgic pains commencing in right temporal region. The headache is better in cold air and from cold washing of head The patient is worse in warm and closed room and feels relieved from cold applications ; tying up head tightly with a band relieves the headache. (*Puls.*). See "Pains wandering."

Head-lice—Hair to be bathed in lotion of *Sabadilla*. Internally. *Nat-m.* See "Lice"

Hearing-dulness—(1) Dulness of hearing without any organic affection of the ear. Hearing music aggravates many bodily symptoms. (*Ambr.*). See "Deafness" and "Ear-hardness of hearing".

(2) Hearing defect when due to blows, concussion, when blood is discharged from nose and ears. (*Arn.*).

(3) When hearing is associated with swelling of tonsils or enlargement of tonsils, also noises in the ears from arteriosclerotic conditions. (*Bar-c*). Compare *Nit-ac.* See "No. 12 of Deafness".

(4) Hearing better for high pitched sounds. Has deafness to low tones, while higher ones are heard distinctly, comparative deafness to sound of voice but great sensitiveness to sound as of passing vehicles and also a shrinking from low tone. Enlargement of tonsils. Buzzing in ears. Vertigo due to hearing. (*Chenopodium-a*). (Dr. Boericke)

Heart—(1) Palpitation from indigestion. (*Nux., Puls., Carbo-veg.*).

(2) Nervous palpitation. (*Mosch., Ign.*).

(3) With tightness across the chest. (*Cactus.*).

(4) With pain. (*Spig.*).

(5) With throbbing headache, flushed face and sensibility to noise. (*Bell.*).

(6) With great anxiety, burning in the body with cold extremities. (*Ars-a.*).

(7) For fatty degeneration of heart, Dr. Burnett recommends *Vanadium* and *Bellis perennis* as an alternate remedy.

(8) Pains about the heart followed by palpitation, sinking at the pit of stomach. (*Act-r.*).

(9) Palpitation on the slightest movement, breathlessness, pallor and faintness on sitting up. (*Dig.* 3 *gr. or v.* 4 hrly.).

(10) Anginal pain and hypertension, numbness and coldness of extremities. (*Secale-cornutum.*).

(11) Difficulty of breathing due to oppression of chest, palpitation on slightest exercise, sharp pains in heart. (*Medorrhinum.*).

(12) Hypertrophy of the heart with insufficiency of mitral valves, gasping for breath, low vitality, out of breath in walking. (*Laurocerasus.*).

(13) Tobacco heart when due to cigarettes. Palpitation from the least exertion. Increases energy of heart's action, renders it more regular. (*Convallaria Majalis* Tincture 5 to 15 drops in water of wine glass).

(14) Palpitation with vertigo and choking in throat. Wakes with palpitation at about 2 a.m. Darting pains through heart. Cardiac dyspnoea ; dropsy with enlarged heart ; cardiac. debility after influenza. (*Iberis* 1x-2 or 3 drops of tincture, T.D.S.). See "Palpitation of heart, with sweating and breathlessness", "Angina pectoris palpitation." and "Emphysema".

Heart-angina pectoris—Palpitation, pain, dyspnoea, angina pectoris. (*Ars-alb.*) See also "Angina pectoris palpitation." and "Palpitation-violent and with congestion".

Heart-block—(1) Great weakness and sinking of strength. faintness, coldness of skin and irregular respiration. Dilated heart, tired, irregular with slow and feeble pulse. (*Dig.*).

(2) For heart failure. Sensation as if heart ceased beating, then starting very suddenly. (*Convalaria Majalis* Tr. 15 drops.). See "Palpitation from noise and heart failure of the aged." and "No. X of Angina pectoris palpitation and pain."

Heart-burn—With a loaded tongue, flat taste, bowels loose. (*Puls.*). Also *Carbo-v.*, *Nux.* and *Sulph.* See also "Acidity with wind" and "Gastric trouble".

Heart-carditis (inflammation of the heart)—Pericarditis (inflammation of membranous sac which envelops the heart) *Aconite* 30th in watery solution. (Dr. Jahr.)

Heart-coronary (arteries and veins around the heart)—insufficiency—Dr. D.M. Forest suggest *Cholesterinum* 30 to 200 for patient suffering from this disease. It is useful when other remedies fail.

Heart-degeneration—Degeneration, fatty heart, liver and kidneys with anaemic condition, anxious mind, the patient fears to be left alone. (*Phos.*).

Heart-flatulence pressing—Excessive flatulence mainly in the upper portion of the abdomen pressing upwards to the chest and causing distress in the heart. (*Carb-v.*). See "Flatulence" under its different heads and "Dyspepsia-of old with heart trouble".

Heart failure-after infectious disease—Great lassitude and prostration at the end of acute, serious infectious disease. Usually in the case of such patients, they say, that the patient progressed nicely and finally died of heart failure, *e g.* recovery after diphtheria. In many such cases, *Ammon-carb.* will save such lives. (*Am-c.*) See "Diphtheria—when patient progressing".

Heart-noise disturbs—Shock felt in the heart from sudden noise. Aggravation lying on left side or back. (*Agar.*). See "Palpitation from noise and heart failure of the aged".

Heart-palpitation and pain—Violent palpitation. Frequent attacks of palpitation, specially with foul odour from mouth. Pulse weak and Irregular. Pericardial pain with breathlessness and aggravation from movement. *Spigelia* is an important remedy in pericarditis and other diseases of the heart. See also "Palpitation" under its different heads.

Heart-palpitation increased by walking—Palpitation and bad feeling in heart increased by walking. Chronic weakness of heart. (*Naja-tripudians*).

Heart-pulsation audible—Audible pulsation from the heart in the ear. (*Aesc.*).

Heart-cardiac-failure—Dr. M.G. Blackie suggests *Ammon. caust.* for quick relief.

Heart-audible respiration—Palpitation with anxiety and rapid audible respiration. Profuse sweat. Pulse is irregular and feeble. Intermittent action of heart. *Verat.* is one of the best heart stimulants in homoeopathic doses and acts better than many stimulants like Brandy. (*Verat*). Compare *Arsenic* and *Carb-v.* See "Respiration".

Heart patient fainting—When the patient faints away without apparent cause then give *Linaria-vul.* which may be serviceable in fainting of cardiac origin according to Dr. Boericke.

Heart-trouble tubercular—See "No. 17 of "Tuberculosis".

Heart-weakness due to jaundice—Slow weak heart with excessive jaundice. Ashy white stools. (*Digitalis.*).

Heart-weakness due to rheumatism—Cardiac weakness or inflammation of the lining membrane of the heart or its valves or enlargement of the heart. The condition of heart may be a sequence of rheumatic state which has been removed by suppressed methods. (*Aur-met.*) See also "Rheumatic heart" and "Endocarditis-rheumatic heart".

Heart-with suffocation—Troubles acute or chronic, the peculiar suffocation, cough and aggravation from constriction. (*Lach.*) See "Dyspnoea—with cardiac symptoms".

Heart-weak—*Am-c.* is a good remedy for cases with weak heart and emaciation. A single dose given high usually suffices to stop the palpitation. *Am-c.* Compare *Crataegus M.T.* Give *Crataegus M.T.* 5 drops in water 3 times a day for sometimes in order to get good results. See "palpitation of heart with sweating and breathlessness".

Heart-trembling and fainting—Trembling round heart. Palpitation weak pulse and fainting. According to Dr. P. Banerjee *M.T. Moschus* 5 drops per dose or *Carbo. veg* 200 acts like coramine of the allopathy.

Heart-worse lying down—Fluttering of the heart with weak faint feeling, worse lying down. Irregular intermission of beats of heart and pulse, worse on lying left side. Violent pulsation of the heart which shakes the body. (*Nat-m.*). See also "Angina pectoris".

Hectic fever (the protracted fever of) phthisis—(1) Fever of phthisis. Fever with sweat. Chilliness, heat, sweat over head in children, so that pillow becomes wet. (*Calc.*).

(2) In consumption with moist coated tongue. (*Baptis.*).

(3) In consumption with dry tongue. (*Ars.*). See also "Tuberculosis" and "Consumption pulmonary" and "Fever consumptive".

Heels—According to Dr. Clarke (1) If there is tearing in the heels, sprained pains in the ankles then give *Silica*.

(2) Cramps in the feet tearing in the instep and great toe. (*Colchi.*)

(3) Rheumatic pains in legs and feet. Pain as if ulcerated on standing. Dr. Boericke says there is numbness, weariness and lameness of legs after walking distance. Pain in balls of feet on stepping (*Berb.*).

(4) Aching of heels, relieved by elevating feet ; pain in legs patient tried to get up ; feet puffed up. Pain on ankles and feet. Neuralgia in toes (*Phytolacca*).(Dr. Boericke)

Heels-painful—(1) Pain in the heels like pricking of nails. Menstrual flow black and clotted. Puts feet out of bed to cool them. Open air is greatfull. Warm room is oppressive. Constipation. No appetite. Sleepless. (*Puls.*). See also "Gout of the heels" and "Rheumatism" under their different heads.

(2) Ulcers on heels from friction. (*All-c.*).

(3) *All-c* may be used when there are blisters in feet.

(4) Pain in the heels. (*Cyclamen* 30. B.D.). See "Blisters in feet".

Hemicrania—A severe pain affecting one side of the head. If the pain is on the right side of head then give *Sanguinaria*

200 twice and if the pain on left side then give *Spigelia* 200 twice and if the pain comes at the fixed time then give *Cedron* 30 four times daily. Comapre *Sepia* which is regarded by Dr. Baehar as an excellent remedy for such a trouble. (Dr. P. Banerjee)

Hemianopia—(1) Upper half of objects invisible. (*Aur-met.*).

(2) Vanishing of left half. (*Lyc.*).

(3) Vanishing of either vertical half. (*Mur-ac.*). See also "Eye-troubles" and "Vision".

Hepatitis-inflammation—(1) Inflammation of liver. Degeneration of liver with anaemic condition. (*Phos.).*

(2) Dr. Jahr begins treatment with *Acon.* and for remaining symptoms he uses *Bry., Bell.* and *Merc-sol.* See also "Liver" under its different heads.

Hepatitis-liver enlarged—Liver enlarged when there are painful sharp pains in the hepatic region which prevent taking breath. The abdomen is distended with gas and, the patient lies on the right. (*Merc-sol.*). See "Liver-chronic enlarged."

Hernia—Right-sided, specially in children. (*Lyco.*). (*b*) *Cocculus* is said to prevent when a weak feeling in the abdomen indicates that a hernia may take place, though the symptom is probably of purely nervous character. See "Bowels-intussusception."

Hernia-prevention—See "Chapter V"for details .

Hernia-infants—(*a*) Umbilical (navel) hernia of infants. (*Nux-v.*).

(*b*) *Plumbum* relieves, strangulated hernia when *Aconite, Belladonna,* or *Nux. v.* fail in many cases.

Hernia-pain—If *M.T.* of *Lyco.* mixed with a small quantity of water be rubbed on painful part it gives relief to pain of hernia.

Hernia-threatened strangulation—(1) Pain in old hernia (*Nux*).

(2) Threatened strangulations.(*Nux-v.* every ten minutes.).

(3) Strangulated and sloughing (*Lach.*). In fat children (*Calc.*). In thin children. (*Sil.*).

(4) In strangulated hernia of old people with severe gripping and aching pain. (*Pituitary* in 30th potency). See "Strangulated hernia."

Hernia-weakness of abdominal muscles—If it seems that hernia may take place due to weakness of abdominal muscles. (*Cocculus*).

Herpes-zoster—(*a*) (1) A routine medicine is *Rhus-tox.* which will cure most of the cases.

(2) The chief remedy according to Dr. Jahr is *Ars-a.* He says that eruptions as well as pains will disappear after 10 days use. The clusters are large and deep which bleed when removed. Thirst for small quantities of water at short intervals.

(3) Herpes with burning, bruised and stitching pains, much itching as the eruptions dry up ; the eruption with tendency to form large blisters. Acrid exudation which makes surrounding parts sore. *Ranunculus bulbosus 30* to be given 3 times a day has been found to be most efficacious. It cuts short the course which is from 14 to 20 days.

(4) Another efficacious medicine is *Iris-v.*

(5) Baehr thinks *Mezereum* as the principal remedy.

(6) For herpes of genital organ like prepuce give *Merc-sol.*, *Nitric-acid* and *Natrum-mur.* according to symptoms.

(*b*) (1) Locally in all cases a lotion of *Canth. 3x.* 10 drops to the ounce may be kept applied on linen. Another useful application is a mixture of *Zinc oxide* and *Castor oil* in sufficient proportion to make a paste, or the eruption may be painted with Collodion.

(2) When the eruption has disappeared and the pain persists or when there is pain without eruption, *Plantago M.T.* may be painted on all parts.

(3) On genital organs *Phytolacca* may be applied.

(4) Dr. Moore recommends a few drops of *Calendula* on a compress on ulceration of herpes zoster.

Hiccough—(*a*) In hysterical cases ; *Moschus* every ten minutes. In chronic cases : *Cyclamen.* every ten minutes, also during pregnancy. In obstinate cases ; *Hydrocy-ac., Sulphuricum-acidum* and *Kali bromatum.*

(*b*) *Magnesia phosphorica* is said to be specific for hiccough. Give it in 12x doses, or give tincture *Ginseng* which is also useful for indigestion which is supposed to be the cause for hiccough.

(*c*) Three drops of oil *Cinnamonum* with sugar if given stops hiccough.

(*d*) Severe and rapid hiccough. Give *Scutellaria M.T.* every two hours.

Hiccough of infants—*Nux-v.* or *Chamomilla* according to symptoms.

High blood pressure—(1) Due to disturbed function of nervous mechanism. Arteriosclerosis. (*Aurum-muriaticum natronatum.*).

(2) *Lachesis* a head remedy for high blood pressure.

(3) For high blood pressure and its consequences give *Adrehalin 200* to 10 M.

(4) Dr. W. Lang recommends daily dose of combination of *Crataegus, Glonoine* and *Passiflora* where symptoms are not clearcut. In his experience, the daily dose of above combination will make the patient comfortable and prevent further deterioration in the general condition of such patients.

(5) When there is high blood pressure with heart-trouble, heart feels distended, fills whole chest. Worse lying down on left side. Alternating moods. Aching and itching in the eyes. *Cenchris contortrix* which is a wonderful restorative and deep-acting remedy. See "Blood pressure high and low".

(6) *Tinctures Crataegus* 5 drops, *Passiflor. M.T.* 5 drops, and *Tincture-Glonoine 6x* to be given respectively of two

drops each at two hours interval give wonderful result, as the pressure comes down within a short time.

High blood pressure or Hypertension—(*a*) (1) When due to suppressed anger or resentment, violent headache, vertigo. (*Aurum-met.*).

(2) Vertigo and noises in the ears. Arterio-sclerosis. Icy cold body. Thickening of arteries with cardiac dilation. (*Baryta-muriaticum.*).

(3) Irritability and excitement by opposition and headache. Constipation, with itching piles. (*Glonoine.*).

(4) When due to shock produced by bad news. (*Gels.*, M. dilution.).

(*b*) Low blood pressure—(1) Exhausted, fast growing persons. (*Calc-phos.*).

(2) Dizziness, fainting. Noises in the ears, loss of vital fluids. (*China-off.*). See "Blood pressure high and low".

(3) With low vitality and flatulence in the upper part of abdomen. (*Carb-v.*).

(4) *Tuberculinum* should be administered as an intercurrent remedy when the patient is wasting in health.

(5) Worse in winter and cold stormy weather ; persistent vertigo ; rheumatism and gout and sciatica, buzzing and stopped feeling in ears. (*Viscum-a.*). See "Blood pressure high and low".

High blood pressure valvular—Valvular lesions of arterio-sclerotic nature. (*Aur-met. 30.*)

Hip disease-chronic inflammation of bones—(1) Sharp pain from hip to knee. (*Kali-carb.*).

(2) Much pain on movement and heat in the joint. (*Bry. 6* hourly).

(3) The distress is excessive, the patient cannot rest. specially at night, cries continually. (*Cham.* every 1 or 2 hours).

(4) When the swelling and puffiness of the joint resists all other measures. (*Merc. iod.*).

(5) Very severe, heavy or digging pain, aching pains around the hips. *Conium* 4 to 6 hours.). See "Bones curvature" and "Caries of bones-soft .

(6) Rheumatism of hip. (*All-s.*).

(7) Pain in left hip. (*Ovi gallinae pellicula*).

Hips-pain—See "Chapter V"for details".

Hoarseness-clergyman's sore throat—Patient can hardly make loud noise. The *Phos.* voice becomes clear by clearing the throat *i.e.* by removing the mucus from the vocal cord. Clergyman's sore throat. Apt to be worse in the evening or fore-part of night. Pain in the larynx ; cannot talk on account of pain. Burning in throat. (*Phos.*). Compare *Arum-t.* See "Voice hoarse", "Clergyman's sore throat-loss of voice." and "Voice lost suddenly".

Hoarseness-catarrhal with expectoration of mucus—Acute complaints of the voice ; catarrhal hoarseness ; copious expectoration of mucus from larynx. (*All-c.*). See "Voice hoarse".

Hoarseness-damp air—Which is worse in the damp air and in the evening. (*Carb-v.*). See "Sore throat extending to wind pipe".

Hoarseness-sudden—The sudden loss of voice of singers and public speakers or of a lawyer. Clergyman's sore throat. *Arum-t.* enabling him to go on with his speech in a clear voice. It is specially suitable if the voice is uncertain and uncontrollable, changing continually in its tone. (*Arum-t.*). Compare *Rhus-tox.* and *Phos.* See "Voice-lost suddenly".

Hoarseness-weakness of vocal cord—*Rhus-tox*, hoarseness is more weakness of the vocal cord and the initial stiffness is removed by continued use of the vocal cord *i.e.* by warming up the organ by its use. (*Rhus-tox.*). Compare *Arum-triphyllum* hoarseness.

Home-sickness—(1) If the patient is apathetic, listless or indifferent. (*Phos-a.*).

(*ii*) If silently brooding and not communicative. (*Ig.*). See "Broodings".

(*iii*) *Capsicum 200* is the head remedy for home-sickness. Sleeplessness.

Hormone-its deficiency causing grey hair, baldness and diabetes—Is a specific product of an organ or of certain cells of an organ, transported by the blood or other body fluids, and having a specific regulatory effect upon cells remote from its origin. This term is used for internal secretions from ductless glands giving *Adrenaline, Thyrodine, Insulin* etc. When these ductless glands become deficient, certain diseases are caused which can only be cured by making the glands efficient by the use of homoeopathic medicines. For instance, premature grey hair and baldness are caused by the deficiency of Thyroid glands. The use of *Thyrodine 30* or *200* dilution will not only prevent grey hair, but help in restoring natural colour. Similarly, *Insulin 30* or *200* should be used as an inter-current medicine in diabetes to make efficient the glands which produce insulin.

Hot patient—*Lyco.* is a hot patient and wants open air and craves everything warm. Wants food hot rather than cold.(*Lyco*).

Hot weather complaints—*Acon.* is indicated in complaints from very hot weather specially gastro-intestinal disturbances. (*Acon.*). See "Summer complaints" and "Summer diarrhoea".

Hunger without appetite—Without appetite. (*China.*).

Hunger canine—There is a canine hunger but even then emaciation continues. After eating, *Nat-m.* patient is tired and sleepy. He has not got a nice feeling after eating, he feels dull, lethargic, and wants to lie down with a feeling of discomfort in the stomach and liver region. (*Nat-m.*). See "Emaciation extending downward" and "Appetite increased or ravenous."

Hunger-in children satiety soon—There may be want of appetite in *Lyco.* or there may be a strong feeling of hunger with the peculiarity that the patient sits down hungry to the table but a few mouth-fuls will fill him and he rather feels distressingly full. This alternate condition of hunger and fulness is most prominent in *Lyco.* particularly in children. Easy sense of satiety. (*Lyco.*). See also "Appetite of child" and "Appetite absence".

Hunger emaciated child—The child is very hungry and even then goes on emaciating and growing weaker due to bad assimilation. Emaciated and badly nourished children. Large head, big belly, thin limbs, emaciated face. Cannot walk or learns to walk late. Constipated. (*Sil.*). Compare *Calc-carb.* See "Emaciation-Children".

Hunger-gets up at night to eat—Fainting feeling in stomach and must eat then. Gets up at night to eat. (*Phos.*). See "Stomach fainting feeling at night to eat".

Hunger gnawing-relief by eating—Gnawing hunger. The important symptom regarding the stomach is a peculiarly empty feeling or sensation of gnawing hunger and the patient wants to eat something immediately the gnawing starts. It is known as "All-gone sensation in the stomach". (*Sep.*). See "Stomach pain-relief by eating" "Stomach -gnawing hunger and forcing patient to eat".

Hunger-lost—(1) Complete loss of appetite for food, drink or tobacco. (*Ign.*).

(2) Loss of appetite for everything. (*Rhus-tox*).

(3) Fulness after a few mouthfuls as if too much has been eaten. (*Prunus-spinosa.*).

(4) Simple loss of appetite or after acute illness. (*Gentiana-lutea.*). See "Appetite-absence".

Hunger—Increased or ravenous yet emaciation. See "Appetite increased or ravenous".

Hunger-sinking sensation eating every 3 or 4 hours—(1) Weak empty sinking sensation in the stomach with hunger at 11 a.m. (*Sulf.*).

(2) Feels faint if he does not eat every 3 or 4 hours. (*Iod.*) See "Stomach sinking sensation".

Hydrocele of boys— (*Abrot.*).

Hydrocele-chronic—(1) (a) The testes are involved and undergo state of hardness and infiltration (passing of fluids into tissue spaces or cells). *Aur-met* cures chronic enlargement of the testes. (*Aur-met.*).

(*b*) Left-sided hydrocele of long standing. Testicles swollen, painful ond drawn up. Apparently no cause found. Useful in acute condition. (*Rhododendron*).

(2) Burning and aching of testicles with or without swelling. Of congenital form. Pains wander from one part to another. Head remedy. (*Puls.*).

(3) Aids absorption of fluid. Herpetic eruption on organs. Dropsical swelling of scrotum. (*Graph.*).

(4) Testicles swollen and indurated cause absorption of fluid. Loss of sexual power ; offensive sweat of genitals ; atrophied testicles. (*Iodum.*).

(5) When hydrocele is due to injury accompanied by soreness. (*Arn.*).

(6) Neuralgia of testicles and spermatic cord. (*Oleum animale*).

Hydrocele-congenital—It may yield to *Bryonia.* Compare *Puls.*

Hydrocele-indurated testes—(1) *Calcarea-flourica.* For local application compresses of *Hamamellis M.T.* to be applied in warm water.

(2) The enlarged testicles may be rubbed gently with *Mullion oil* as liniment. See also "Testicles".

Hydrocele-congenital by birth—*Bryonia.*

Hydrocephalic children-birth prevention—See "Chapter V" for details .

Hydrocephalus-increase of fluid in skull—(a) The little one has chills and fever along with it and his skull is beginning to distend with it. The last stage of it is hydrocephalus with great stupor, when there is great prostration, loss of flesh, stiffness of limbs with dropsical swelling. Then it is that such remedies as *Apis.*, *Calc-carb* and *Apocynum* take hold with wonderful depth. The first sign of this remedy *Apoc-can* as well as of *Apis.* working in a case is that it increases the flow of urine which has been scanty before. (*Apoc-can.*). For Hydrocephalus think of *Tuberculinum* also. See also "Meningitis".

(*b*) (1) Delirum and chronic convulsions in hydrocephalus. *Hedera helix* is an effective remedy. Give one drop dose of this tincture. Next morning there will be a clear flow of fluid from nose. Second dose may be administered if there is danger of recurrence.

(2) In hydrocephalus, cerebrospinal meningitis, inflammation of membranes of brain, much prostration, bores head into pillow and screams out ; lids swollen. (*Apis.*).

(3) Child begins to roll its head, throws it back and cries out in sleep or awake ; boring pain, headache with coldness and trembling, passes urine unconsciously, watery stool with flatulence. (*Arg-n.*).

Hydrothorax-dropsy of the chest—*Lactuca.*, *Ran-bulb.*, *Kali-carb.*, *Merc.*, *Sulf.*, *Fluor-ac.*, *Adonis*, according to symptoms. See "Lungs-congested is dropsy" and "Dropsy of Chest". Compare *Ars-alb.*

Hyper-acidity—A most effective sour medicine with (1) acidity and frontal headache is *Robina* 3x.

(2) Yellow coating at the base of the tongue. Sour eructation and sour taste with vomiting. (*Natrum-phos. 6.*).

(3) For those who are accustom to high living and rich ood with results in gasses. Aversion for milk. (*Carbo-veg. 30.*)

(4) Bilious eructaion take place in the evening and the patient has absolutely no thirst. (*Puls. 200*). See "Acidity under their different heads.

H

Hyperaemia of the brain—(1) Head-hot with intense congestion ; pain from nape of neck. Pulse soft and slow. (*Veratrum-viride*).

(2) Dull, heavy ache with heaviness of eyelid bruised sensation and better compression and lying with headhigh. Pain in temple. Scalp sore to touch. Wants to have head raised on pillow. (*Gelsemium*.). See "Inflammation of brain".

Hyper-sensitiveness—Of pain. For adults, *Cham.* is the leading remedy for pain and the peculiarity about this is that the sensation of pain is far in excess of the actual cause of pain. The patient must be peevish and snappish, which is the peculiar mental condition of *Cham.* (*Cham.*). See "Over-sensitiveness".

Hyper-sensitivity in homoeopathy—Very often one will find patients who are sensitive to the rightly selected remedy that even a single dose will create enormous reaction. This condition one could almost call an "allergic" condition in homoeopathy. In these cases, one would usually find in the history of antecedents of some acute infectious disease which has sensitized the system to this extent. Hypersensitivity is usually removed by giving proper nosode and then the selected remedy can be easily applied without causing any unpleasant aggravation. This aggravation has often marred a cure for the simple reason that the hyper-sensitivity has not been removed. The difference between "Hyper-sensitivity" and "Block" is that the block causes lack of sensitivity to the homoeopathic drugs. The patient does not react even to the right remedy, whereas "hypersensitivity" creates over-sensitiveness to the drugs.

Hypertension-hypotension—See "Blood pressure high and low."

Hypochondrium-the hepatic region—Fullness, pain and burning in the hepatic region. *Aloe* will serve as a palliative to be followed by *Sulf, Sulphuricum acidum, Kali-nit.* or *Sepia, Aloe. Kali-nitricum* is often indicated in asthma, also valuable in cardiac asthma.

Hypostatic congestion of lungs in dropsy—Congestion of lungs in dropsy. Congestion of lungs due to prolonged lying in bed compelling the patient to sit up. This hypostatic condition gradually creeps upwards so that a large portion of the breathing space is destroyed. It has a rattling breathing also. Difficult breathing. Gasping breath. Pulse is small and irregular. (*Apoc-can.*). See "Congestion of lungs in dropsy" and "Lungs congested in dropsy".

Hypotension-low blood pressure—See "Low blood pressure."

Hysteria—(1) The patient faints readily. Nervous palpitation and excitement when there is no organic disease of heart. From least excitement violently angry, or scolds till she faints. Wants a deep breath. Constrictive feeling in throat. *Moschus* rapidly dissipates an hysterical attack even when it has gone so far as unconsciousness.

(2) Patient haughty and contemptuous. Looks down upon others ; fits preceded and followed by a sort of asthma. The patient suffers either from excessive menses or has suppressed menses. (*Platina 30.*).

(3) Excessive loquacity ; terrifying hallucination, sees ghosts, hears voices and talks with spirits. Devout, earnest, beseeching and ceaseless talking. *Delirium* with desire to escape. Convulsions without loss of consciousness. (*Stram.*).

(4) Hysterical fits with pain in abdomen. Pains that come and go gradually. Colic relieved by pressure. (*Stam.*).

(5) Hysteria when preceded by oedema of limbs and face. Attacks coming at the time of menses. (*Thyroidinum.*).

(6) On cure the tendency to attack of hysteria the following medicines are suggested by R. B. Bishamber Das—

Zincum-v. 3, Nux mosch. 30, Sepia 30, Platina 200 , Moschus. 6, Kali-phos. 30, and Scutellaria tincture of 1st dilution. See "Fainting-hysterical" and "Fainting with pain".

Hysteria-attacks to prevent it—*Camphor-mono-bromata* in invalueable during attacks and may be given on a lump of sugar every 5 to 10 minutes.

Hysteria-consolation aggravates—(1) Weeping alternates with laughing ; consolation aggravates every mental symptom mainly the irritability and weeping. Sad and joyless even under most cheerful circumstances. Unaffected by the surrounding impression and grieves on everything. The prostration of the mind as well as the body is main feature. (*Nat-m.*).

(2) *Pothos.* given in 10 drops of mother tincture is specific for hysteria. See also "Consolation".

Hysterical-disposition—(1) Fainting from extreme of cold and heat after getting wet from riding in carriage. Sense of thinking of faintness in pregnancy, child bed or during lactation. Hysteric. (*Sep.*).

(2) *Ignatia* is specially adapted to women of sensitive and easily excited nature ; effects of grief and worry end menses irregular. See "Fainting hysteric women".

Hysterical-convulsion—Hysterical spasms and convulsions. Mental state of depression and gloominess alternate with physical state. Girls have pain in the back and headache. (*Act-rac.*). See "Convulsion-hysterical".

Hysterical-fainting and also for cerebro spinal meningitis—(1) Hysteria is a common feature of Asafoetida. All the patients go off in fainting from no cause whatsoever or from a closed room, from excitement or any other type of mental disturbance. Sometimes they get cramps instead of fainting. But fainting is the commonest feature. They get stitching pain suddenly from bone to the surface *i.e.* from within out. Lump in the throat or suffocation is a sort of hysterical spasm of oesophagus. Grinding of teeth at night. (*Asaf.*).

(2) Loss of consciousness accompanied by involuntary jerking of muscles. (*Cicuta-virosa.*). It is also useful in cerebrospinal meningitis when head turned or twisted to one

side. See "Throat-hysterical lump", "Cramps of hysterical patient" and "Meningitis-iflammation of covering membrane of brain".

Hysterical-fits after intercourse—In women after intercourse. (*Agar.*). See "Coition".

Hysterical-joints—*Cotyledon.* See "Teeth-grinding hysterical".

Hysterical-laughing—The attacks are feigned. The patient has immoderate attack of uncontrollable laughter. (*Terent-h.*). See "Laughter".

Hysterical-shivering—Hysterical shivering in the first stage of labour. (*Act-rac.*). See "Shivering" under its different heads. and "Pregnancy of hysterical women-changing symptoms".

Hysterical-vomiting—*Kreosotum* hourly. See "Vomiting in dropsy and hysterical vomiting".

Hysteria-weeping—She weeps and has fainting fits with uneasiness and exhaustion. It has a depression of spirits. (*Am-c.*). See "Weeping tendency in girls" and "Weeping tendency-indifference."

I

Idiocy-physically dwarf—Children are mentally and physically dwarfish and do not grow. Swollen tonsils and swollen abdomen. *Baryta-carb.* is head remedy. It may be alternated with *Tuberculinum. 1M.* dilution once every fortnignt. See also "Children-late in learning to talk and walking" and "Dwarfishness".

Ill-effects of carbon-monoxide gas—*Nat-m.* is preventive against bad effects due to exposure to this gas.

Ill-effects of chlorofom—*Cham.* may be given for nausea and sickness after operation. (*Cham.*). See "Chloroform antidote" under its different heads.

Ill-effects of high altitude—(*a*) For mountaineers. Useful in various complaints incidental to mountain climbing, such as palpitation, dyspnoea, anxiety and insomnia. Exhausted nervous system from physical and mental strain. Loss of voice. Headache of high altitude. Distension of abdomen. (*Coca-erythroxylon.*).

(*b*) (i) Ill-effects of nuclear explosion : *Phosphorus* and *Strontian carb.*

(ii) For protection against effects of exploding atomic and hydrogen bombs. (*Bioflavin.*).

(iii) For ill-effects of sulphonamide group of drugs (*Sulphapyridine.*).

(iv) For ill-effects of carbon-monoxide. (*Acet-ac.*).

(v) For ill-effects of charcoal fumes, (*Am-c.*). Compare *Bovista.*

(vi) For ill-effects of hair dyes. (*Tuber. 200.*).

Ill-effects of stretches—Where coldness, congestion of head and receding tearing pain occur from stretching sphincter or tearing of a sensitive part takes place, *Staphysagria* is the remedy. "Stretching" and "Tearing" are the key words here. (*Staphy*). See also "Stretches."

Ill-effects of radiation, explosions and other such things—See "(b) of Ill-effects of high altitude".

Illusion—(1) When the intellect is slightly effected, it is an illusion and what he sees, he knows is not so. Low spirited, fears he is pursused, looks for thieves and expects enemies. (*Anac.*) See also "Delusion" and "Hallucination".

(2) Delusion about snakes. (*Lac., Can.*). See also "Insanity".

Impetigo-an acute inflammation of skin disease with boils—Eczema with drastic derangement. Pimples, and vesicles and pustules. Eruption with burning and itching, worse at night. (*Antim-crum*).

Impotency-desire but inability—(1) (a) The sexual desire remains after the ability to perform is gone. (*Phos.*).

(b) Seminal emissions without dreams. Loss of confidence ; afraid to marry for fear of impotency. Senile dementia. Impotence after gonorrhoea. (*Thuja.*).

(2) Dribbling of semen during sleep. Semen thin, odourless. Erections slow, insufficient, too rapid with long-continued thrill. On attempting coition penis relaxes. Dr. Herbert thinks that mental condition of inability is more of a leading symptom than that of timidity. (*Sel.*). If *Sel.* fails then *Agnus castus* 3 followed by *China* and *Lyco.* makes the victim a different man.

(3) Want of sensation during coitus with no discharge of semen. (*Graph.*) See "Sterility-barreness in females and in males".

Impotency-emisson premature—No erectile power. Premature emisson. Penis small, cold and relaxed. Ill-effects of onanism (masturbation) or sexual excesses. Strong desire but unable to perform. *Lyco.* high single doses at intervals of a week or more. *Lyco.* is one of the best medicines for impotency. See "Sterility in males" under "Sterility b (1)" and also "Sexual desire irresistible" under its different heads.

1motency-due to masturbation—**(1)** Great emaciation with dark rings under eyes, shyness and gloomy. (*Staphy.*).

(2) Headache, frequent involuntary emissions at night. Digestion weak.(*Nux-vomica*). See also "Masturbation" and "Emission"

Impotency-no orgasm—Organs seem larger, puffed and relaxed and cold. Erection when half-asleep, Ceases when fully awake. Relaxation of penis during excitement. No emission and no orgasm during embraces. *Caladium-saguinum* has a marked action on the genital organs and pruritus of this region (*Calad.*).

Impotency-sexual excess—The patient has lived in excesses and now suffers from relaxed and cold genitalia ; emission ; prostatic discharge at stool. Has morning erection but no more. History of repeated gonorrhoeas. (*Agn.*). See also "Coition", "Sex-weakness" and "Emissions".

Improperly-fed babies—Indigestion of improperly fed babies. The bowels become relaxed. The mother feeds the baby every time it cries at short intervals. Digestion absolutely fails. (*Aeth.*). See "Indigestion of babies due to over-feeding and intolerance of milk".

Incontinence-involuntary evacuation of urine-dribbing due to prostrate—**(1)** (*a*) Drs. Jahr and Hering first resort *Sulph.* giving 2 or 3 doses within 8 days. If this fails then Dr. Jahr gives *Sep.*, *Bell.* and *Puls.* and in case of small fat children *Calc-c.*, *Sil.* may be useful after *Bell.* while *Causticum* has inability to retain urine during first sleep in winter. See also "Wetting the bed", "Urine-escape involuntary", "Dysuria" and "Enuresis incontinence of child".

(*b*) Constant dribbling of urine ; noctural enuresis of long standing resisting treatment. (*Verb.* 3rd attenuation). See "Dribbling of urine".

(2) Involuntary urination. Frequent urination, children pass a great deal of urine flooding the bed. Adults suffering from this trouble due to sexual excess or self pollution. (*Ph-a*).

(3) Dreams of urinating. Enuresis in the first part of night. Must hurry when desire come to urinate. (*Kreos*).

(4) Old persons frequently urinating at night and sometime urine cannot be retained and passes involuntarily. The flow stops suddenly and again flows. (*Con.*).

(5) In old men with enlarged prostrate. (*Aloe.*).

(6) A few drops are passed with every fit or coughing in women. (*Rumex*).

(7) Constant dribbling of urine from bladder, enuresis, mostly noctural. (*Verbascum 3rd attenuation.*).

Indigestion-chronic and atomic—Solid food causes great pain, there is slowness of digestion, great accumulation of flatus and at times the vomiting of undigested food long after it has been eaten. (*Lyco.*). Blackwood (Digestion disorders-flactulence of whole abdomen).

Incised wound—Clear-cut incised wound with a sharp instrument even if it is done with surgeons' scalpel. (*Staphy.*). See also "Wound incised and clear-cut" and "Cuts-sharp with knife".

In-coordination of muscles—Clumsy motion of hands and fingers. Dropping of things. Fingers fly open when holding things. The patient is continually breaking the dishes. (*Agar.*). See also "Fingers-not holding things properly".

Indifference—Indifference towards all things, to joy, to grief, to people. (*Ambra-g.*). See "Grief-ailments due to".

Indigestion of adults-from constant eating—When digestion has absolutely ceased from brain trouble and from excitement. *Aeth.* has cured dyspepsia from constant feeding in those nibblers, those hungry fellows who are always eating, always nibbling, always taking crackers in their pockets until the time comes when the stomach ceases to act. (*Aeth.*). See "Dyspepsia of adults from brain troubles and constant eating".

Incontinence of urine due to paralytic bladder—There are violent straining and ineffectual efforts in passing urine, with a scanty discharge ; also dribbling of urine in old men from enlarged prostrate.(*Nux-v.*). See "Dribbling of urine due to paralytic condition of sphincter and bladder"

Indigestion-acid dyspepsia—Eructations sour, sour taste, and sour bitter vomiting. (*Mag-carb.*). See "Sour every thing" and "(6) of Dyspepsia—also acid dyspepsia".

Indigestion-hysterical women—Dyspepsia of hysterical women specially during pregnancy. Hiccough and weak digestion. (*Nux-v.*). See "Hiccough".

Indigestion of aged—Dyspepsia of aged or weak anaemic subject, broken down by long illness, heartburn. Jaundice and diarrhoea. (*Kali-carb.*). See "Dyspepsia-of old".

Indigestion-of babies due to overfeeding and intolerance of milk—Indigestion of improperly fed babies. A certain class of infants come down sick in hot weather, in hot nights, and they get brain trouble and from that time the stomach quits business, the bowels become relaxed and everything put into the stomach either comes up or goes right through. Such children are those whom the mother puts to the breast or feeds every time the baby cries at shorter intervals ; so they are improperly fed babies. *Aethusa.* is at the head of the list of medicines for that condition, that is, when digestion has absolutely ceased from brain trouble. (*Aeth.*).

(2) Also *Aethusa* is useful in cases where milk cannot be tolerated in any form and vomiting of curdled milk. See "Overfeeding of children" and "Improperly feed babies" and "Milk not digested with diarrhoea".

Indigestion-with bad taste in mouth—An indigestion with bad taste in the mouth, nothing tasting well, not even water, dryness of mouth without thirst caused by rich, greasy food will be a good indicator for *Puls.* during digestive disorders. *Puls.* patient has no liking for fat nor does he tolerate fat ;

with *Puls.* cold things agree. (*Puls.*). See "Taste" under its different heads, also "Dyspepsia with bad taste with rich food" and "Taste—nothing tastes well during digestive trouble".

Indigestion-from brain trouble or excitement—When digestion has absolutely ceased from brain trouble and from excitement. The characteristic symptoms relate mainly to the brain and nervous system connected with gastro-intestinal disturbances. (*Aeth.*). See also "Nervous diarrhoea" and "Dyspepsia of adults from brain trouble and constant eating".

Indigestion-dyspepsia—Chronic dyspepsia. Loss of appetite. Aversion to food ; hungry without appetite. (*Cocculus*). Dr. Jouset recommends the alternation of. *Nux.* and *Graphites. Nux. 12* one hour before meal and *Graphites.* 12, one hour after meal. See "No. 4 of Ayspepsia."

Indigestion-flatulence, ulcers—Flatulence very marked. Belching after every meal. The least plain food makes pain worse. Gastric ulcer. (*Argent-nit.*). See also "Gastric ulcers" and "Flatulence".

Indulgences—A helpless victim of indulgence like wine and women. Irritable, nervous and dyspeptic. Constipation with ineffectual urging. Sleepless. *Nux-v.* T.D.S. one dose daily at bed time.

Infantile-liver—(1) Enlarged liver and spleen in children (*Calc-ars.*).

(2) Slow fever with night sweats, chronic constipation, diarrhoea with swelling of legs and feet. (*Acetic-acid*).

(3) Gastric disorders of disease, throws out milk as soon as taken, eats and vomits again, intolerance of milk. (*Aeth-c.*).

(4) Uneasiness with dull pain in liver and stool soon after a meal. Jaundice but no fever. Involuntary stool with passing of urine or wind. (*Aloe.*).

(5) Liver pains, obstinate constipation, useful in the early stage of disease (*Alumina.*).

(6) Dr. D.N. Ray applauds, *Calc-ars.* as a sheet anchor for infantile liver of malarial origin.

(7) Jaundice with dull headache, bitter taste, tongue white in centre, lips and edges red. Nausea with vomiting with pasty stool. *Card-m.* highly recommended by Dr. D. C. Das Gupta.

(8) Jaundice with soreness of liver, yellow urine in hypertrophic (increased size of liver) stage. (*Chionanthus.*).

(9) Liver atrophied, marasmus, jaundice, prostration and obstinate constipation. (*Hydrastis.*).

(10) When the child seems to be full of wind, liver enlarged and tender. Constipation with colic. Loss of appetite. Stool hard. Oxaluria. (*Senna.*). See "Liver" under its different heads and "Jaundice".

Infantile liver-congenital—The mother due to some metabolic defects gives birth to child who in infancy suffers from infantile liver ; then *Medorrhinum* will rectify if mother is administered this medicine even during pregnancy.

Infants-nose blocked—Exposure to colds and draughts. Sniffles. Loose choking cough. Cannot expire. (*Sambucus.*, night and morning). See "Nose-block on lying" and "Snuffle-stuffing, nose of infants".

Infançy-baby dying in infancy and grown up child in early-age—(*a*) If babies die in infancy give to the mother during pregnancy *Sulf. 6* and *Chlc-p* 6 alternately daily one dose. (*b*) Children or grown up boys, who are otherwise strong dying at an early age by wasting out, be treated by giving *Alfalfa* with material doses (5-10) drops of tincture several times daily for about six months. See "Pregnancy-giving birth to dead babies".

Inflammation-acute—Acute in various organs. (*Merc-sol.*). See "Mouth inflamed".

Inflammation-compresses hot—Hot compresses of *Calendula* give great comfort where there is inflammation and redness with great deal of discomfort.

Inflammation-of brain—(1) Cerebral congestion from sudden emotional excitement. Worse by noise or light. (*Aconite-n.*).

(2) Congestion and cerebral irritation with head hot; throbbing carotid and headache. *Vertigo.* with falling to left side or backward ; Headache from suppressed catarrhal flow ; pain : fullness specially in forehead. (*Belladonna.*).

(3) Congestive headaches, hyperamia of the brain from heat or cold. Throbbing headache, shocks in head, headache in place of menses. (*Glonoine.*).

(4) Inflammation of brain, with unconsciousness ; brain feel loose. (*Hyoscyamus*).

Inflammation-of cord—*Hypericum* to be given at once to prevent any complications due to inflammatory changes. (*Hyper.*). See "Spine injuries" and "Poliomyelitis–inflammation of gray matters of spinal cord and its preventure".

Inflammation-due to eruption on skin—Painful swelling of eruption on the skin. The patient cannot bear to have it touched when pus has formed or is about to form. *Hep.* follows *Merc-sol.* very often very well, specially in cases of boils and inflammatory swellings. (*Hep.*). See also "Boils", under different head and "Over-sensitiveness".

Inflammation-of eye-lids, loss of lashes and eczema—*Petroleum,* also for loss of eye lashes. Eyelids swollen and red. (*Graph.*). Swelling with eczema of eyelids with hard crusts (*Mez.*). See also "eyes" and "Hair falling".

Inflammation of kidney—(1) Uraemia with unconsciousness ; pupils dilated, convulsions. *Helleborus* 30 every 2 hours.

(2) Granular degeneration of kidneys, gouty kidney. (*Plumbum.*). See also "Uraemia", "Pyelitis" "Nephritis inflammation of kidney", and "Kidney affections".

Inflammation localised—In localised inflammation *Belladonna* is the first remedy where there is great redness and swelling. It does not matter where the inflammation lies *i.e.* whether in the throat, head or elsewhere, slightest jar or even shaking of the bed causes pain in inflamed parts. *Bell.* has more localised inflammation. *Bell.* Compare *Aconite.* See "Swelling-localised" and "Jar".

Inflammation-of bone—See "Bone inflammation".

Influenza-old nasal catarrh—(1) Recurrent fever and sweat, general prostration. Headache. Loss of appetite *Ar., Iod., Gels.* and *Euper. perf.* each in 30th potency may be give in alternation 3 or 4 times a day when other medicines fail, useful at any stage.

(2) With gastric symptoms, sore throat, vomiting with greas. Alternate doses of *Cinnamon* and *Cadmium sulf.* each 3 to 30 every two hours. Nash says *Cad. sulf. 30* and *Cinnamon.* 30 in alternate doses every 2 hours (Dr. Iskander Guy and Rohilah Guy of California.)

Inflammation-of nerve injured—When nerve rich area, such as finger ends or toe ends are injured or a nail has been torn off or nerve has been crushed between hammer above and the bone below and nerve shows sign of inflammation and the pain can be traced up to the nerve, *Hypericum* is the remedy (*Hyper.*). See "Nerve injury" and "Crushing of nerve".

Inflammation tending to pus—*Sil.* prevents inflammation tending to form pus. Inflammation of bones, tissues and glands. *Sil.* prevents formation of pus and is usually given after *Hepar-s.* for healing the discharge of ulcer that has taken place after *Hepar-s.* has formed and burst open the abscess (*Sil.*). According to Nash, *Sil.* ranks as the first of remedies for inflammation ending in suppuration. See also 'Pus-prevents formation".

Inflammatory complication in the wounds—*Ledum.* will prevent not only the subsequent inflammatory complications in the wounds but will also prevent the shooting pains that naturally come when nerves are involved in the injury. (*Led.*). See also "Wound unhealthy no tendency to heal".

Influenza-with cough—With much cough and expectoration along with irritation of eyes. (*Euphr.*)

Influenza-with fever—(1) Fever with cough ; cough starts as soon as the chill phase of fever starts ; it subsides when temperature rises. (*Rhus-tox.*). See "Cough with fever".

(2) Fever with chill followed by vomiting and pain in bones. (*Eupatorium-perf.*).

(3) High fever, nose stopped, dry cough. (*Causticum. 1 M*).

(4) Watery discharge from nose, muscles, headache. (*Gels.*).

(5) *Sulphur 200* to be given as intercurrent medicine empty stomach. See also "Rheumatic pain in influenza" and "Fever influenza".

(6) Confusion of mind, breath foul, restless, throat painful, right ear painful, toxic, thirsty ; intense pain all over body. (*Bor.*).

(7) Does not want to be disturbed, motion aggravates pain, thickly coated white tongue, headache relieved by pressure. Constipation ; lack of appetite ; pain in the chest in coughing. (*Bry.*).

(8) Fever slowly progressing ; restless, relief by constant movement and change of position ; disturbed sleep, bright red tongue ; attacks of sneezing, racking cough ; violent abdominal pain. (*Rhus-t.*).

(9) Fairly high temperature. Sleeplessness. Feels hot but sensitive to draught ; aches from head to feet ; dry mouth with good deal of thirst for cold water ; nasal discharge thick ; ringing in ear, pain in eyes, digestive disturbance, pains starting in legs and going upwards ; marked discrepancy between the pulse rate and temperature. (*Pyrog.*). See "Fever-influenza".

(10) Sudden onset of influenza fever with chilliness, throbbing headache and great restlessness. (*Aconite*).

(11) The fever of influenza with excessive sneezing which shakes the whole body. The throat is swollen with headache. (*Sabadilla.*).

Influenza-with running of nose—Running of nose. Thin watery excoriating discharge. Nose feels stopped up. Sneezing without relief. Prophylactic for influenza. (*Ars-alb.*). See "Nose watering causing rawness".

Influenza-post , weakness—Dr. Dewey recommends *Phos.* as tonic. See "Weakness-after influenza".

Influenza-preventive—Dr. Guha prescribed *Thuja. 200* once a week and *Gels. 30* thrice daily as a prophylactic dose during influenza epidemic. During attack, *Gels. 200* may be given three times a day. Noel Pudephatt recommends Ars. 3. night and morning as a preventive. For treatment of influenza the following medicines according to symptoms be given. Begin with *Aconite* alternate with Merc-sol. 30. *Rhus-tox.* and *Bell.* are other remedies indicated for influenza. In Hindustan Times during influenza epidemic, the following advice was published. Preventive : *Arsenicum 200.* Curative : *Influenzinum. 30.* Other remedies suggested being Eupatorium perfoliatum *All-c., Gels.* and *Bapt.*

Influenza prophylactic—*Thuja 200* once a week. With one daily dose of *Gels. 30* throughout the epidemic. acts as prophylactic (*Thuja* and *Gels.*). *Bapt.* 3x and 30. See "Probhylactic-influenza".

Injury—(1) *Arnica* is good remedy in the first stage of injury where much bruisinghas been done and the pain is intense but diffused and not running the nerve course as Hypericum. (*Arn.*).

(2) Nerves injured in soft parts while treading on nails, needles and pins, also in bites of insect and animals.(*Hyper.*).

(3) Paralysis of extremities caused by a fall when chair is withdrawn when a man tries to sit. (*Rhus-tox.*).

(4) Pregnant woman falling and feeling pain. (*Arnica*). If the pains become violent then *Chamomilla* after *Arnica.*

(5) Over-lifting; strain of mis-step. (*Arnica* and *Rhus-tox.*).

(6) Swelling, of foot after sprain : Dr. Herring says that *Bovista* is good for oedematous swelling of foot even after sprain.

(7) Fracture pains. When pains become unbearable give *Cham.* first then *Hypericum.* For subsequent pains *Ruta., Colch.* and *Merc-s.,* are useful.

(8) To help the bones to reunite give *Symphytum* and *Calcarea phosphorica* to promote the growth of callus.

(9) For lameness after sprain specially of ankles and wrists. (*Ruta*).

(10) Burns; Dr. Herring says that *Cantharis* tincture for external use in proportion of 5 to 8 drops of tincture to a half tumbler of water is most effecatious for burns. Internally *Cantharis* and *Capsicum*, are best remedies to relieve burning. (*Cal-c.*) If hands and feet or the whole body becomes much swollen. *Causticum* is very useful for old burns. See also "Pain in injuries" and "Burns".

Injury-children tending to form pus—Slight injury tending to form pus mostly in children. (*Hep.*). Compare *Silicea, Calcarea*. See "Skin-slight injuries fester".

Injury-causing contracture—Contracture of muscles and tendons due to an injury or any septic process is usually removed by *Causticum* if given high. (*Caust.*). See also "Contracture" under its different heads.

Injury-eyes—Injuries from blunt articles thrust into eyes. (*Symphytum.*). No remedy equals this. Tincture dose. Both internally and externally. See "(b) of eye troubles".

Injury to finger-causing inflammation in armpit—Injured finger causing swelling and tender lump in the armpit of the size of pigeons egg. Great restlessness and pain *Hepar-sulf. 6* every two hours and *Aconite* 3 at bed time.

Injury-fracture—Also for formation of callus and always allays the irritability often found at the point of fracture preventing the knitting of the bone. (*Spmphytum.*). See "Bones fracture" and "Fracture".

Injury head-caused by accident—(*a*) Headache which varied in severety ; patient unable to concentrate or to do any paper work and to travel. *Natrum sulf.* is one of the best of the after injury remedies

(*b*) Head pains after a head injury. *Opium* frequently given for such injury.

(*c*) Patient having fractured his skull in an accident, severe headache after it but without any pressure from the fracture. (*Natrum sulf.*).

Injury-preventing from putrefication—*Calendula* makes lacerated or suppurating wounds impregnable against putrefication and restores the vitality of the injured part, particularly where the part is broken as suggested by Dr. M.G. Blackie.

Injury-stump—Also useful in irritable stump after amputation. (*Symphytum.*) (Dewey.). See "Amputation neuritis".

Injury to finger causing inflammation in armpit—Injured finger causing inflammation and tender lump in the armpit of the size of pigeon's egg. Great restlessness and pain. *Hepar sulf. 6* every 2 hours and *Aconite* 3 at bed time.

Insanity—(1) *Aur-met.* is an insanity medicine and the insanity that starts in the perversion of affection proceeds on to the intellect. The cause of this type of insanity is either prolonged anxiety or unusual responsibility or great loss of property and finally inherited syphilis. Over-use of mercury is also one of the causes. (*Aur-met.*). *Anacardium, Hyoscyamus, Stramonium* and *Bell.* are four pillars which bring illusioned mind to the sphere of intelligence and reasoning. See also "Delusion" and "Hallucinations".

(2) Wants to destroy things, tear up his clothes, puerperal mania and convulsions with coldness and cold sweat. (*Veratrum-alb.*). According to Dr. Hahnemann *Verat-a.* promotes a cure of almost one-third of the insane in launatic assignment. See "Puerperal mania".

(3) The patient is talkative, quarrelsome, restless and wants to uncover, foolish laughter, inclined to uncover the body and expose sexual organs and sings obscene songs. (*Hyos*). See also "Perverted mind" and "Mania".

(4) Any form of mania which increases sexual desire. (*Baryta-mur.*). See "Mania-amorous or religious" and "Mania marked by extreme uncleanliness".

(5) The patient likes to run away, wants to kill himself, threatens to kill others, mania to escape. (*Melilotus.*). See also "Illusion".

(6) Insanity when it is connected with disorder menstruation in young girls. (*Thyr.*).

(7) Insanity due to masturbation. Wants to curse and abuse every body approaching him (*Staphy.*). See "Masturbation".

(8) Violent on hearing some particular name and seeing any particular object. (*Kali-brom.*).

(9) Violent out-burst of rage to kill his dearest friend or relative and immediately thereafter will repent. (*Crocus.*). See "Jealousy".

(10) The patient keeps washing hands and feet very frequently. (*Syphil. C.M.*). If the patient likes frequent cold bath then either *Puls.*, *Asar* and *Arg.-n* . be given.

Insects bites or stings—(1) Great oedema and swelling after bites, sore and sensitive. (*Apis.*).

(2) Stings of venomous insects. (*Arsenic.*).

(3) Insect or mosquito bite intense pain. Tetanus due to injuries. (*Ledum.*). See also "Stings" and "Bites".

Insertion of joints—*Ruta.*

Insomnia—(1) Sleeplessness. The child cries at night (*Cypripedium.*).

(2) Restless and wakeful, resulting from exhaustion. Especially in the feeble infants and aged. Produces normal sleep. Insomnia of the infants and the aged, and the mentally worried and overworked, with tendency to convulsions. *Passiflora incarnata.* Mother tincture 30 to 60 drops repeated several times.

(3) Wakeful, sleeps till 3 a.m. after which only dozing. Sleep disturbed by dreams. Sleepless on account of mental activity. Disturbed by itching of anus. (*Coffea cruda.*).

(4) Entire inability to sleep. Dreams with nightmare. Startling on falling to sleep with chilliness. (*Daphne Indica.*).

(5) Hysterical people who get easily excited,have stomach problem and worries. (*Ambr-grisea.*).

(6) For nervous people, being exhausted from a previous disease. (*China-ars. 6 or 200.*).

(7) Those depressed and in pain. *Kali-phos. 200* and *Mag-phos. 200* alternately.

(8) For those addicted to tea drinking. *Valerianicum 30* and *Aqua-regia 30* alternately.

(9) The patient should take *Gels. 1x* a dose half an hour before retiring and a dose on retiring. If he wakes in the night, he should take this *Gels.* every half an hour until he sleeps again. See alse "Dreams" and "Sleeplessness" under their different heads and "Sleep-cat nap type."

Insomnia-sleep impossible—Restless, impossible to get sleep. Abdomen tense, relieved somewhat by evacuation and passing of mind. Nervous bowel spasm. Difficult breathing. (*Tr. Lactuca-virosa*) 5 times daily.

Insult-bad effects of insult and mortification—(1) Melancholy and loss of memory in consequence of mortification ; takes every thing in bad part and becomes violent and uses profane language. (*Anac.*).

(2) Disposition to cry and weep ; anger ; extreme irritability ; violent abdominal pain ; diarrhoea and vomiting every time food is taken. Sleeplessness. (*Coloc.*).

(3) Brooding over imaginary troubles, prefers, to be alone ; sits quietly and gazes into vacancy. Late sleep and restlessness. No desire for food. (*Ig.*). See "Broodings".

(4) Pride and over-estimation of one's self ; fault finding. (*Platina.*).

(5) After wounded pride ; not getting praise she expected from others ; inclined to use strong language and violent expressions. (*Paladium.*).

Intestinal-tuberculosis—See (b) of "Tuberculosis".

Intermittent fever—(1) Periodicity. Chill towards evening with slight or violent thirst and after the sweat there is much prostration. (*Chininum sulphuricum*.).

(2) For malarial conditions in children. The chill starts from the feet. The patient wants to be held during the chill to prevent his shaking ; the characteristic time for the chill is about the middle of the day. Drowsiness, dizziness, dulness. Thirst is not marked. (*Gels*.).

(3) Spleen and liver enlarged. Chill commencing about 10 o' clock in the morning, beginning in the back and full of great thirst, pains in the bones, pains in the back, headache and debility, shortness of the breath ; fever blisters on the lips ; white coated tongue, sleepy in the day time and sleepless at night. (*Nat-m*.).

(4) Chill prevails, intense thirst, drinking causes an aggravation. Thirst is wanting during hot stage. (*Capsicum*.). (Dewey.). See also "Fever intermittent" and "Fever malaria" under their different heads.

Intermittent-fever prophylactic—*Ars.* or *Chin-s.* to be taken night and morning and continued at longer interval.

Intermittent fever-tertian or quotidian type—*Chin-o.* is of service in intermittent fever. It may be of the tertian (returning every other day) or double tertian; quotidian (an intermittent fever, the paroxysms of which recur daily or double quotidian (a fever having two paroxysms a day usually differing in characters) type or the paroxysm may return every 7th or 14th day anticipating several hours each succeeding chill. (*China*). See "Chapter V" also.

Intolerance of milk—Cannot bear milk in any form ; it is vomited in large curds as soon as taken, then weakness causes drowsiness. (*Aeth.*), Compare *Mag-c.* and *Naturm-carb.* See "Milk-not digested with diarrhoea".

Involuntary stool of children—Involuntary stool even solid in little children who may drop the stool all over the carpet without knowing that they may have done so. (*Aloe.*), See Diarrhoea-of children (involuntary stool) and "Stool involuntary in children".

Iritis—Acute and chronic conjunctivitis, paralysis of accommodation, hyperemia of retina with weakness of accommodation. Pain over eye, between it and brow. (*Duboisia*).

Irregularity-of menstrual flow—It may be copious, suppressed or scanty. Severe pain all through the flow. The more the flow the greater the pain. (*Act-rac.*). See "Menstruation irregularities".

Irritability of child—Crying or whining without cause or with fever, diarrhoea, teething or any other complaint, or if the child wants this or that thing but throws all of them away when offered and, above all, the child is consoled by being carried about. Child is very uneasy and tosses about. *Cham.* is an excellent remedy for irritability and other symptoms of infants and children. (*Cham.*). See "Weak children-waking with irritability" and "Crying of child" under its different heads.

Itch in different parts of body—(1) Intense itching of skin, worse in warmth of bed. (*Psorinum*).

(2) Pimples of the size of a pea in different parts of body. The slightest scratch or injury inclines to ulceration. (*Hepar*, a dose night and morning.)

(3) Small itching pimples that ulcerate. (*Mercurius.*, a dose night and morning).

(4) Itching in the folds of the skin about the joints particularly the ankle joints. (*Selenium.*).

(5) Violent itching of the scalp as from lice. Smarting after scratching. (*Oleander.*).

(6) Eruptions, itching on palms of hands. (*Anagallis.*).

(7) Vesicular eruptions with intense itching and burning and multitude of small vesicles in close contact. Eruptions and itching about the eyes, and specially genitals, scrotum and penis. (*Croton-tig.*). See also "Barbers' itch", "Eruption". "Scabies", and "Diabetic itching."

Itch-application external—*Calendula* in olive oil one to ten parts to be applied.

Itching-anus—(*a*) Itching and burning in anus preventing sleep which may be very great driving him to desperation. He is compelled to bore with the finger the anus ; so violent is the itching that the patient cannot leave it alone. Cold application relieves the itching whereas ointments may increase the burning. (*Aloe*). Apply externally lotion of *Hydrargyrum.* See "Anus itching".

(*b*) For itching and redness of rectum of children. (*Sulph.*) See "Burning in anus" and "Anus-itching".

Itching-changing—Without eruption, changing places on scratching. (*Agar.*). See "Changing disease" and "Changing symptoms".

Itching-distressing extremely—*Sulphuric acid* is an excellent remedy for relieving the distressing itching, tingling and formication of chronic inflammatory disease of the skin characterised by small pale papules and severe itching and also for lesions of the skin which consist of solid papules with exaggerated skin markings. Such papules are deeply seated and are most prominent on the extensor surface of limbs. This medicine is to be internally given. It is also useful for itching of chronic urticaria.

Itching-female organ—Horrible itching of genitals with swelling of labia during menses. (*Ambra*). See also "Pruritus with burning urine part (2)". See "No. 9 Eczema general at different places."

Iching-on moustaches with ring worm—See "Ringworm, itching on moustaches."

Itching-intense—Intense itching but scratching is painful and the patient cannot bear to scratch very hard, as it hurts ; a mere rub suffices to allay itching ; stinging, smarting pain of the eruption. (*Croton-tiglium.*).

Itching of nose—Tingling sensation in the mucous membrane of the nose. The tingling and itching sensation must be so intense that the pain of bleeding is not felt. In itching of nose the *Arum-t.* patient will say that his nose is hot as it is on fire. Acid discharge from nose. The glands and neck and even the parotid (situated near the ear) may be inflamed and sore. (*Anm-t.*). See also "Eczema-on nose".

Itching-scratching causing burning—Voluptuous itching of the skin with or without eruptions causing burning after scratching. (*Sulf.*). See "Eczema", "Eruptions", "Scabies" under their different heads and "Burning sensation".

Itching -skin of old people—Itching on hands and feet also. (*Antimonium-sulph.*).

Itching without eruption—Old people have sensitive skin which itches intolerably without any eruptions. (*Baryta carb.*)

J

Jar—Slightest jar or even shaking the bed causes pain in the inflamed parts. In localised inflammation *Bell.* is the first remedy where there is great redness and swelling (*Bell*). See "Inflammation localised".

Jaundice—(1) Jaundice due to hepatic and gall bladder obstruction. Distension. The jaundiced skin and constant pain under angle of scapula. Liver enlarged. Gall stones. *Chelidonium* majus. This should follow Sulphur after one day. Begin treatment with *Sulphur.*

(2) Jaundice with enlargement of abdomen and constipation, stool clay coloured, soft, yellow and pasty. Tongue coated. Jaundice with arrest of menses. Enlarged spleen. A prominent liver remedy. (*Chionanthus.*) (Dewey).

(3) Of children from fright or anger. (*Cham.*).

(4) Eyes yellow. Sour eructations or vomiting. Flatulence and tongue yellow coated. (*Natr-phos.*).

(5) Alternating white and black stool. Bad taste in the mouth. Coated tongue, pain in right side and shoulder and jaundiced skin. Attack of bilious vomiting and diarrhoea. *Aurum-muriaticum-natronatum* followed by *Veronica officianalis* in high doses. (Dr. Nash).

(6) Jaundice with gall stones obstinate hepatic engorgement. Liver cancer. (*Choles-terinum.*). See "Infantile liver".

Jaundice chronic—Of chronic types of jaundice that attend bilious states, when the tongue is coated, the breath foul, sensation of heaviness and fullness in the hepatic region ; stitching pains in the whole abdominal cavity, flatus offensive (*Aloe*). See "Liver chronic enlarged".

J

Jaundice-liver hard and painful—(1) Liver hard and painful, yellow skin and eye, stool white or light coloured, urine dark yellow. Pain in the right side of abdomen near liver area. Flatulence of abdomen. Acute or chronic specially in children (*Chin.*).

(2) Nausea and vomiting. Tongue swollen showing marks of teeth with white or yellow coating (*Hydrastis.*). See "Liver inflamed with degeneration".

Jaundice-malignant—In last stages of malignant jaundice with fever and restlessness, and thirst for small quantity of water. (*Ars-s.* or *Cholesterinum.*)

Jaundice-liver painful—Liver region painful ; better rubbing part. Abdomen distressed. Can lie comfortably on stomach. (*Podo.*). See "Liver sore".

Jaundice-liver sore with growing hunger—Liver sore and painful ; relieved by lying on left side. Feeling of bearing down in abdomen. Sensation of gnawing hunger in stomach and patient must eat something. (*Sep.*).

Jaundice—As a result of anger, alcohol or purgation. Jaundice that have resulted from fits of anger also in hepatic (pertaining to liver), hyperamia (congestion of blood) when there are sticking pains and soreness in liver. There is frequent history of alcoholic excess or the use of drastic purgatives (*Nux-v.*). See also "Liver", "Infantile liver" under their different heads and "Prophylactic" Chapter V.

Note—*Natrum-sulph. 6x* plus *Natrum-phos. 6x* two tablets 3 times a day may be given in addition to above treatment. (Dr. Boericke).

Jaw-carious or cracking with growth of tumour and easy dislocation—(1) Caries or necrosis or decay of jaw. *Phos.*, if this fails then *Silicea*.

(2) Cracking in the joint or jaw. (*Rhus-tox.*).

(3) Pain in jaw joint as if sprained on swallowing. (*Arum-trip.*). See "Yawning".

(4) Easy dislocation of jaw. (*Petroleum.*).

(5) Growth on jaw. (*Thuj.*).

(6) Tumour of jaw. (*Helca., Plumbum.*). See "No. 2 of Caries" and "Tumour tongue".

Jaw-cyst—Cyst in the jaw with swelling inside cheek. It is painful and begins to enlarge more and more. (*Symphytum*). *Dr. Boericke.*

Jaw-swelling—Swelling of jaw after extraction of teeth with violent pains. (*Hecla.*). See "No. 15 of Teethaches".

Jealousy—(*a*) Bad effects of jealousy. With attempts to murder, with rage and distrust, with sexual mania. (*Hyos.*) The same jealous feelings women. (*Apis-m.*). See "Perverted affections" and "No. 2 of Insanity".

(*b*) (*i*) If the patient is peevish and malicious and talks much discontentedly to every person about his grievances. (*Lach.*). See" Peevish".

(*ii*) When the patient shows inclination to attempt to kill persons hence forward esteemed or loved or shows contempt to them. (*Platina.*). See "Perverted affections".

Joint cracking—(1) Cracking of joints on moving, (*Ginseng.*).

(2) In rheumatic subjects with fever, anxiety, restlessness and pain. (*Acon.*). See "Knee grating and weakness with swelling".

Joints-deposits—Joints become rigid on account of deposits, lumps and nodules. (*Tr. Ruta. 30*).

Joy—Effects of excessive joy. (*Coffea-cruda.*). See "Grief ailments due to".

K

Keratitis—Inflammation of cornea See."Blepharitis".

Kidney abscess—See "Liver abscess chronic".

Kidney affections—(1) Inflammation of kidneys with suppression of urine. Cutting pain in the lumbar region. Urine passed in drops and is mixed with blood. With much urging. (*Canth.*).

(2) *Terebinth.* is most reliable and most frequently indicated remedy in the early stages of renal disease, when congestion is prominent and when there is much pain in the back extending along the ureters. There is anasarca and the urine is bloody and albuminous,

(3) For albuminous nephritis of pregnancy. (*Merc-c.*).

(4) For acute Bright's disease. Oedematous swellings of the face and extermities, paleness, ascites, pains in the head, back and limbs. Urine heavily charged with albumin and contains blood corpuscles. Suppression of urine and eruption of skin like nettlerash. (*Apis-mellifica.*).

(5) Granular degeneration of kidneys with tendency to uraemic convulsions. (*Plumbum.*).

(6) For uraemic convulsions *Cuprum* is a valuable remedy.

(7) Swelling of the face very common in kidneys disorders. If the upper eyelids are swollen then *Kali-carb.* and in case lower eyelids are swollen then *Apis-mel.* See also "Bright's disease". "Nephiritis", "Uraemia", "Inflammation of kidney" and "Renal colic-severe pain caused by efforts to pass a stone locked up in ureter".

Kidney floating—For floating kidney the *Aur-m.* and *Calc-f.* are useful".

Kidney-function stopped in typhoid—See "Typhoid-kidney function stopped in typhoid".

Kidney-removal of stone and avoiding operation—Digging, sticking pain in one kidney region which radiates from one spot either sideways or up and down. The whole back is affected accompanied by stiffness and discomfort, the patient finds it difficult to get up. Burning in the bladder, violent sticking pain from the kidney down to the bladder. The urine is often pale with gelatinous sediment, there may be blood in it. With these indications it is quite possible for a kidney stone to pass after giving *Berberis*.

Kidney-stone in—A. (1) Violent sticking pains in the bladder extending from kidneys to urethra with urging to urinate. (*Berberis vulgaris*). This is head remedy for renal colic.

(2) Agonising pain, twists about, screams and groans, urine red with brick dust sediment. (*Ocimum-canum*.).

(3) Writhing with crampy pains, must move about. (*Dioscorea*.).

(4) Urine becomes turbid like clay water immediately after passing. Much pain at end of urinating. White sand, scanty, slimy, flaky urine. Tenesmus of bladder (*Sarsaparilla*.).

(5) When all remedies fail then *Pareira-brava* may be given in mother tincture in hot water in 5 drops doses every half hour.

(6) Prevention of gravelly urine, pain in back and loins. (*Berberls vulgaris* 6 hourly.) Tendency to store uric acid in the tissues. (*Urtica-urens*.).

B (1) Dr. Jahr says that *Puls., Cannabis, Sarsap*. and *Lyco*. have done wonders in his hands in alleviating renal colic and facilitating the passage of calculi through urethra.

(2) Dr. Jousset says that *Bell.* and *Cham.* are given in alternation when pains are violent, regardless of the disease which produced them in renal colic.

(3) Dr. Preston used *Arg-nit.* when there is dull aching across the small of the back and also over the region of the bladder. The urine burns while passing and the urethra feels as if swollen and the urine contains blood.

(4) *Ipomoea-nil.* has been used by Dr. Jacob James for the passage of stone from kidney to bladder. Dr. Hempel records many cases of renal colic cured with *Coccus-cacti.*

(5) *Eupatorium purpureum* has to be used when there is a considerable amount of gravel deposit in the urine, dull pains in the renal region and mixed with mucus and also urinary tenesmus.

(*a*) *Galium aparine* acts on the urinary organs ; is a diuretic to use in dropsies, gravel and calculi. See also "Calculi in kidney", "Stone in kidney", "Cystitis-inflammation of bladder" and "Renal colic severe pain caused by efforts to pass a stone locked up in ureter."

Kidney-cessation of its function—Polonged retention of urine or complete cessation of the function of the kidney with stinging, burning in orifice. (*Zingiber.*).

(*b*) For pain dependent upon the passage of gravel, uric acid etc. from the bladder, ureter or kidney, give *Hydrangea arbor.*

Kidney-floating or moving—Give *Calc. iod.* If this fails, then try *Sepia*.

Kidneys-both deranged—Continued urging for urine which sometimes escapes and is hot and burning. Urine brown or with brick dust sediment. Stool perfectly colourless. Jaundice sets in, slow, pulse alternating with quick pulse. Breathing difficulties, struggling for breath while talking. Heart weak ; great weakness and sinking of strength. Excessive nausea and enlarged liver (*Digitalis 200* at intervals).

Knee grating and weakness with swelling—(1) Sharp pain, weakness, grating sensation. (*Dioscorea.*).

(2) Stiffness, soreness, pain, swelling. (*Berb.*).

(3) For swelling of the knees, lumps, on the joints of hands and fingers give Sulf. and later *Calcarea*. See also "Gout" under its different heads.

(4) Abscess of knee. (*Taxus-baccata.*).

(5) Rheumatism of knee. (*Pulsatilla-nuttaliana.*).

(6) Weakness of knee.(*Cocculus-indica.*).

(7) White swelling of knee. (*Kali-carbonicum.*).

(8) Creaking of knee. (*Wild-bad.*). See "No. 11 of Rheumatism". Compare *Lathyrus sativa.*

Knife-cut—Sharp knife cut. (*Staphysagria.*). See "Wound-incised and clear cut" See "Cut sharp by knife".

Knife-homoeopathic—The use of *Myristica-sebifera* from 3*x* to onwards often does away with the use of knife It is almost specific for breaking open the carbuncles, fistulas and boils etc.

L

Labour pain causing blindness—The patient suddenly becomes blind during the process of labour, all light seems to her to disappear from the room, labour pain cease and convulsions come ; the urine is scanty and albuminous. Dr. Kent recommends *Cuprum-met.* See "Pregnancy-disorder No. 36".

Labour confinement made easy—*Caulophyllum* makes unexpectedly easy confinement if the pregnant woman takes it for a month before delivery.

Labour pains-distinction between true pains and false pains—

(a) True pains

(*i*) Come on and go off regularly, gradually increasing in frequency and severity.

(*ii*) Are situated in back and loins.

(*iii*) Are grinding or bearing down according to stage of labour.

(*iv*) Arise from contraction of uterus and the resistance made to its efforts and produce dilation of the mouth of the womb.

(*v*) Each pain is attended with a little watery discharge and tends to dilate the os.

(b) False pains

(*i*) Are irregular in their recurrence or in some instances are unremitting.

(*ii*) Are chiefly confined to the abdomen.

(*iii*) Are of colicky nature.

(*iv*) Are caused by cold, flatulence, indigestion, spasm, fatigue etc. and have no effect upon the mouth of the womb which is found closed.

(*v*) False pains are not attended with a little watery discharge and therefore they do not dilate the os.

If the character of pains point to true labour although the proper time has not arrived then *Puls.* will generally quite the abnormal. If after a few doses at intervals of 40 to 60 minutes the symptoms continue then *Cimcifuga* may be given in like manner. If still pains increase then the treatment prescribed under "Miscarriage-threatened" should be undertaken.

(*c*) If proper time for child birth has arrived and symptoms of labour have set in then the Practitioner is requested to take steps under "Labour-prophylactic for difficult labour".

(*i*) Besides, *Gelsimium* should be tried first for relaxation of a rigid and unyielding os uteri. It should be given from 1 to 5 drops in tincture every half hour.

(*ii*) For excessive painfulness in highly sensitive and irritable patients use *Cham.* in like manner.

(*iii*) For sharp and severe pains administer *Coffea*.

(*iv*) For pains recurring regularly for a time and then ceasing 2 or 3 doses of *China* are sufficient.

(*v*) *Bell.* is useful when pains are strong and normal but an apparent resistance in the womb itself impedes progress. The above medicines may be given every fifteen, twenty or thirty minutes according to the severity of case.

(*vi*) Normal secretion from vagina has dried up, passage hot and dry, tedious labour. Give *Jaborandi*.

(*vii*) If the pains cease suddenly and the face is red and there is stupor, snoring. *Op.* See "Pregnancy its affections" and "Pregnancy disorders".

(*viii*) Absence of pains may depend upon constitutional weakness, or upon transitory cause such as passion, opposition or annoyance. The small doses of *Puls.*, *Sec.* and *Op.* will prove useful.

Labour-prophylactic for difficult labour—(1) Dr. Dewey recommends *Gels.* for women who get habitual painful labour.

He also recommends *Cimic.* and *Caul.* as remedies that will facilitate labour if taken previously.

(2) Abdomen large after labour—(*Sepia, Colocynth*). See "Abdomen-pendulous after confinement", "Prophylactic of difficult labour" and "Delivery safe" for living birth, putting child in right position and avoiding false labour pains.

Labour-fever after labour—Muttering delirium, unconsciousness and foul adour from the mouth. Dr. Jahr says that a dose of *Sulphur* followed by a dose of *Nux-vomica* acts like a magic. *Opium* should be given when there is excitement and fetid discharge from uterus. *Kali-carb.* when the fever is attended with too great exhaustion and the patient is too weak to answer question. *Kali-carb.* is one of the best remedies following labour. See "Fever puerperal".

Labour-pains spasmodic in child birth—(1) The patient cries. 'OH' "I can not bear this", peevish and snappish. Labour pains unbearable. (*Cham.*).

(2) Dr. Jahr thinks that when pains are violent and painful *Coffea* helps most.

Labour-pains ineffectual—(1) Ineffectual labour pains. Worse in the morning. (*Nat-m.*).

(2) Pains come and go suddenly. (*Bell.*). See "False-labour pains".

Labour-pains ineffectual with desire to urinate—(1) Ineffectul labour pains, extending to rectum, with desire for stool or frequent urination are quickly relieved and become efficient after the administration of a dose of *Nux-v. 200* (*Nux-v.*).

(2) When due to tardy dilatation. (*Puls.* and *Secale.*).

Labour-pains irregular—Irregular labour pains. Labour pain changing to hip pain or some other pain suddenly. *Act-rac.* will regulate pains when the next pain comes, it will hold on to the end. Hysterical shivering in the first stage of labour. (*Act-rac.*).

Labour-retention of urine—(1) Paralytic weakness of the bladder after a woman has gone through strenuous labour causing retension of urine afterwards is miraculously removed by *Causticum*. See "Weakness of bladder after labour".

(2) For involuntary urine give *Sepia*.

(3) Constipation of later months of pregnancy. (*Collinsonia*.) See "Pregnancy its affections" also "Pregnancy-disorders of" under latters different heads, "Dribbling of urine", "Micturition" and "Retention of urine after labour".

Lacerated wound—*Hypericum*.

Lacerated wound in nerve area—In a lacerated wound involving parts full of small nerves, sentient (having sensation nerves) give *Hypericum* and do not start with *Ledum*. (*Hyper*.) See "Wound-infected and inflamed with pricks".

Lachrymation—(1) In open air and early in morning. (*Calc*.)

(2) Lachrymal fistula. Dr. Hempel recommends *Silicea*., *Puls*. See "Fistula lachrymal of the eyes".

Lactation—(1) Milk late appearing or afterwards diminishing in quantity. (*Asaf*.).

(2) To arrest the flow on weaning. (*Urtica-urens*). See "Fever-milk".

(3) Milk fever (*Acon*). See also "Weaning-engorgement of breast after weaning".

(4) When from sudden and powerful emotions, exposure to cold etc. the secretion of milk is suddenly checked and is followed by some internal or local congestion. (*Puls*. and *Calc-car*.). See "Milk suppression due to emotional disturbance".

(5) Milk fever—*Bell*., if this fails *Bry*. in repeated doses. See "Pregnancy-its affection" and "Pregnancy disorder of".

(6) Absence of milk. (*Mill*.).

(7) Abnormal. (*Rheum*.). See "Milk ceasing after starting".

Lactation-failure to menstruate—During nursing period when woman ceases to menstruate. A woman does not menstruate when she nurses the child. But when she fails to menstruate when the child ceases to be nursed and the woman begins feeling all sorts of mental and pelvic trouble, *Sepia* very often sets the menses in and cures her of other symptoms. (*Sep.*). See "Menstruation-failure after nursing-stopped".

Lameness after rest—Lameness and stiffness and pain on first moving after rest or getting up in the morning, relieved by continued motion. (*Rhus-tox.*).

Lameness and stiffness after re-union of fracture—See "Fracture union-stiffness and lameness".

Larynx—Itching, scraping and soreness in larynx and trachea. Tickling in throat and larynx. (*Ambra.*). See "Throat" under its different heads.

Larynx-in children who grasp larynx—Severe laryngeal cough compelling the child to grasp the larynx. Feels as if the cough would tear it. Hoarseness. (*All-c.*). See "Cough child grasping larynx".

Laryngeal diphtheria—False membrane in the throat. laryngeal. (*Act-rac.*). Dr. Hughes considers *Kali-bich.* as a specific for such a disease. See "Diphtheria" under its different heads.

Laryngitis-with hoarseness—Pain in the larynx along with hoarseness. The pain worse on talking and not swallowing. (*Phos.*). See "Hoarseness" under its different heads and "Pharyngitis".

Laughter—(1) Uncontrollable. Sings and laughs, then angry. Sudden changes from hilarity to melancholy. (*Croc-s*).

(2) Weeping interrupted by fits of laughter. (*Phos.*) See "Hysterical laughing".

(3) Involuntary laughter. (*Zincum oxydatum or Zincum sulphuricum*). Compare *Moschus* for uncontrollable laugher. See "Mocking".

Lean people—*Lyco.* is a remedy for lean people with feeble muscular development but with keen intellect. (*Lyco.*). See "Fat".

L

Left leg-feeling of shortness, contraction and lameness—(1) Left leg feels shorter than right leg. (*Cinnab.*).

(2) Pain in legs making lame. (*Dicsc.*).

(3) Painful contraction in calves when walking. (*Carb-ac.*).

(4) Pain from ankle half way up the leg causing lameness. (*Guaiac.*).

Legs-Cramps—Cramps in calves of legs, worse after midnight, only relieved by getting out of bed and standing. (*Cup. arsenitum*) (*Boericke*).

Leg-hanging down unbearable—See "No. 4 of Varicose left leg-hanging down unbearable". See also "Pain-shaking the part or hanging down gives relief."

Leucoderma—R. B. Bishamber Das begins the treatment with *Tuberculinum 200* and gives it every month with the following medicines. *Arsenic-sul-fl.* head remedy for leucoderma. It is to be given for a very long time in varying dilutions. At first give 3x trituration and after 2 months give 30 dilution provided there is no improvement from this lower dilution or when the improvement is arrested. If 30 dilution also fails or does not completely cure within 3 or 4 months try 200 dilution every week. *Hydrocotyle*: If *Ars-sulf. flav.* fails this remedy may be tried. It should be given in lower dilution 3x or 30 thrice daily. It should be tried for a long time.

Leucorrhoea-acrid—Acrid and watery, (*Nat-m.*).

Leucorrhoea-acrid, profuse and making parts raw—Acrid leucorrhoea making parts raw. (*Fluoric acid*). Leucorrhoea very profuse, dark, bloody. (*Agar.*). See "Menstruation-in its place leucorrhoea with pain" and "Acrid fluids".

Leucorrhoea-burning and pungent—The main characteristic of *Am-c.* is the acrid nature of all fluids that excoriate the surface they touch. Hence burning and pungent discharge. The genitals of the female become raw and sore from discharge. (*Am-c.*) See "Acrid fluids".

L

Leucorrhoea-copious white discharge—There is a copious white or an egg-like leucorrhoea. (*Agn.*). See "Prolapse of Vagina with discharge".

Leucorrhoea-fetid—Leucorrhoea a putrid, very fetid and exhausting. (*Kreosotum.*).

Leucorrhoea-instead of menses—Profuse, smarting corrosive instead of menses. (*Phos.*). See "Menstruation in its place painful leucorrhoea".

Leucorrhoea-of different types—(1) Like the white of an egg with a sensation as if warm water is flowing down the thigh and occurring between the periods. (*Borax*).

(2) Of fat women nearing menopause the discharge being watery with pain in back. (*Phos.*).

(3) Discharge of yellowish colour with offensive odour with itching in vaginal region. *Kreosotum 30* potency three times a day.

Leucorrhoea-of nursing mother—Yellow, mostly after menses with itching. It suits the woman who has been nursing her child a long time or nursing twins, prolonged nursing. (*Phos-a.*) See "Lactation-failure to menstruate".

Leucorrhoea-old with pains in hips—Old cases of leucorrhoea, discharge of a dark yellow colour, thick and sticky with lameness in the back across sacroiliac articulations. Pressing pains in the hips when walking. (*Aesc-h.*). See also "Menstruation" under its different heads.

Leukemia—A disease of the blood forming organs, characterised by uncontrolled proliferation of the leucocytes. Immature leucocytes usually are present in the blood, often in large numbers. According to Dr. Bellokossy the strongest remedy for this disease in his experience is *Natrum sulph.* The author has had no experience of treating such cases.

Liars—Worst liar in the world. Their morals are blunted. (*Opium.*).

L

Lice—(1) Carbolic acid is an excellent remedy for head lice.

(2) Lice in publc hair. (*Staphy.*).

(3) Specific for skin lice. (*Lyco.*).

(4) Lice in hair on head. (*Psorinum.*).

(5) Lilienthal recommends several medicines for lice two or three of them are *Oleander, Psor.* and *Sul.* For external use *Tincture Staphysagria M.T.* One dram and coconut oil one ounce be mixed together and rubbed externally on the affected parts. See "Head lice".

Limping—If due to trauma then *Arn*; if due to debility or constitutional fault then *Sulf. 30., Calc-c. 30.* See "Lameness and stiffness after reunion of fracture".

Lipoma—It is a kind of tumour which in the gross is obviously fatty, microscopically composed of fat cells usually of mature form but occasionally in part or wholly of embroynal type. Give *Bar-c.* alternately with *Uric acid* for outer application *Thuja M.T.* Compare *Lapis-alb.* and *Phyt.* See "Tumour". (*Dr. Boericke*).

Lips-cancer—*Conium, Hydrastis, Sep.* are some useful remedies according to Dr. Yudhvir Singh.

Lips-crack—Lip has got a deep crack in the middle of the lower and upper lips. (*Nat-m*). Lips-picking—Picking the lips until they bleed. (*Arum-triph.*). See "Face ulcers on lips."

Lips-tumour and swelling—(1) Hard tumour *Conium,* soft tumours. *Staphy.* See "Tumours".

(2) Swelling and soreness of upper lip. (*Rhus-venenata.*). See "Swelling of upper lips".

Liver abscess—Chronic hepatitis. Abscess of the liver and kidneys when there is vent for the pus but the toxic symptoms persist. (*Hepar sulph.*). See "Kidney Abscess"

Liver-its various troubles—(1) Torpid or chronically congested liver when diarrhoea is present. The liver is swollen and sensitive. The face and eyes are yellow with bad taste in the mouth. Tongue coated white. (*Podo.*).

(2) The liver is enlarged. Dull pain in the region of liver. The patient cannot lie on right side. Skin and conjunctiva are jaundiced. (*Mercurius*).

(3) Soreness and stitching pains in the region of liver. Swelling of liver, chilliness, fever, jaundice, and yellow coated tongue with bitter taste and craving for sour and acid things such as pickles and vinegar. (*Chelidonium*).

(4) Dull headache, worse in the morning, jaundice, the eyes have a dirty, yellowish hue, tongue coated yellow, aching in the limbs, dark urine. *Myrica cerifera* is an important liver remedy for above symptoms. (*Dr. Dewey*).

(5) Constipation, clay coloured stool. Hypertrophy and obstruction of liver. Chronic jaundice. (*Chionanthus*).

(6) Region of liver sensitive to touch, cirrhosis, pain in back and right side, sallow complexion. Dr. Alfred Pope claims that *Lycopodium* is more useful than any other remedy in old hepatic congestions as it acts powerfully on the liver.

(7) Enlargement of liver and spleen without fever (*Ferrum-cocl.*).

(8) Emaciation, insatiable thirst, ulcers mouth, diarrhoea with swelling of feet and legs. Slow fever with night sweats. (*Acetic acid.*).

(9) Intolerance of milk, thrown out as curdled as soon as milk is swallowed. Gastric disorders of disease. (*Aethu-c.*).

(10) Infantile liver with bronchial troubles. (*Antimonium tartaricum*).

(11) Dr. D.N. Ray applauds *Argent-nit.* for great emaciation and marasmus for liver affections ending in fatal dropsy.

(12) Dropsies of long standing depending on organic affections of liver ; jaundice with dull headache, bitter taste, lips and eyes red, nausea, stools pasty. Dr. D.C. Das Gupta has used *Carduus marianus* in tincture (M.T. 5 to 10 drops). per dose in various stages of disease with satisfactory results.

(13) Jaundice with soreness of liver yellow urine, hypertrophic stage. (*Chionanthus.*).

(14) Condition where there is cirrhosis with ascites. (*Lyco.*).

(15) Jaundic, hard and large liver, white stools. (*Chin.*). See "Infantile liver", "Jaundice" and "Cirrhosis of liver".

Liver-abscess chronic—Dr. Cooper speaks favourably of *Liquor Sodium chloroauratum* also known as *Aurum muriticum natronatum* in chronic, liver abscesses, gallstone lodgment of gallstone and its removal—Biliary concretions are removed by taking one grain of *Podophyllum* at bed time to be followed in the morning by 3 ounces of olive oil.

Liver-affection inherited—Where liver affections of any type are inherited by patient from their family. (*Lyco*).

Liver-children with hunger—Chronic trouble of children with hunger or intense hunger wanting to eat a little often with distension and wind trouble, undigested stool, desire for sweet things and aggravation between 4 and 8 p.m. function of liver seriously disturbed. (*Lyco.*). See "Hunger in children satiety soon".

Liver-bilious and deranged digestion—With chronic soreness of the liver, deranged digestion *i.e.* in bilious condition with numbness and tingling of tongue, lips and nose. (*Nat-m.*). See "Digestive troubles due to liver disturbance".

Liver-chronic enlarged—(1) Chronic liver enormously enlarged. Great soreness in the region of liver, fulness in head. Urine scanty. Dreadful taste in the mouth. Leucorrhoea before menses, walks always fast ; burning hands and feet. Menses flow offensive ; great flatulence. Eructations of wind and food. (*Natrum sulf.* followed by *Lyco.*). See "Cirrhosis of liver". "Jaundice chronic" and "Hepatitis inflammation".

(2) Enlargement of liver, biliousness, bad taste, coated tongue, constipation and severe pain in the back such as lumbago with violent shivering. Headache over the eye brows (*Euonymus europaes*) as recommended by Dr. M.G. Blackie.

Liver-infantile with spleen—Infantile enlarged liver and spleen ; use *Calcarea arsenica* 200. See "Spleen enlarged" and "Infantile liver".

Liver-inflamed with degeneration—Inflammation of liver. Degeneration of liver with anaemic condition. (*Phos*). Acute or chronic specially in children. Pain in the right side of abdomen near liver area. Liver enlarged, hard and painful to touch, jaundice with yellowness of skin and eyes. Urine dark yellow. Stool light coloured or white. Flatulence of abdomen. (*Chin. 200*). See "Jaundice-liver hard and painful".

Liver-sore—With chronic soreness of the liver, deranged digestion *i e.* in bilious condition with numbness and tingling of tongue, lips and nose. (*Nat-m.*). See "Bilious attack" under its different heads and "Jaundice-liver painful".

Liver-torpid sluggish and inactive with white stools—Torpidity of liver. Secretion of biles deficient. No appetite. Depression of spirits : Eyes yellow. Bowels constipated (*Merc. Sol.*) See "Hepatitis-liver enlarged".

Liver-spots i.e. fine branny desquamation of skin—*Nat-hyposulph* which is useful locally and internally for such spots. (1) Spots specially on abdomen (*Lyco.*).

(2) Spots of light-white colour in patches of the body. (*Apis-m.*).

(3) Spots of very dark colour on chest and arms (*Mezerium.*).

(4) Spots during climacteric period or in menorrhagia. (*Plumbum.*).

Liver-trouble in children with constipation—Patient goes without stool for days together. Liver hard with swelling of abdomen. (*Magnesia-muriatica.*). See "constipation-no desire for days together".

Liver-trouble with swelling—Oedema of the feet and legs ; could not lie comfortably on the left side ; breathing oppressed. *Ptelea 30th* which is a remarkable medicine in stomach and liver troubles as suggested by Dr. Boericke.

Lochia-discharge from uterus after labour—(1) When the discharge is too long, continued in too great quantity. (*Crocus.*).

(2) Sudden suppression of the lochia. (*Puls.*).

Lochia-the discharge from the uterus and vagina during the first few weeks after labour—Suppression of discharge due to anxiety or emotional disturbance (*Act-rac.*). See "Pregnancy-disorders of" and "Pregnancy its after effects".

Lock-jaw in tetanus—See "Tetanus part (6)."

Locomotor ataxia-degeneration of the posterior column of the spindal cord, leading to loss of power of co-ordination in the muscles of the legs—(1) The lower limbs appear heavy, the patient can scarcely drag them along, stagers when walking and feels tearing pains in the legs, calves and thighs. (*Alumina*).

(2) Ataxia gait, cannot walk in the dark without reeling, the legs, feel as if made of wood. (*Argentum nitric*).

(3) Paralysis of single muscles cannot rise or lift anything with the hand. Extention is difficult ; pains in muscles of thighs (*Plumbum met.*).

(4) Begin treatment by giving one dose of *Bacillinum 200* on empty stomach and wait for 3 days. As an inter-current medicines give *Strychnine-sulf. 1M* and *Atropine-sulf 1M* alternately each fortnight. No medicine 3 days before or 3 days after it.

Loneliness—Afraid of being alone. (*Sep.*). Compare *Phos.* See "Fear of remaining alone."

Loneliness-fear of darkness :—The patient fears to be left alone, is afraid of the dark, in a thunder storm etc. (*Phos*). See "Fear of darkness."

Loss-of appetite -Want of appetites for any kind of food with unquenchable thirst. Bitter taste, bloated abdomen after eating. (*Rhus tox*) See "Appetite absence".

Loss-of body weight—Losing weight gradually due to over-work. Disappointment, menses late and scanty. Gets angry when comforted (*Nat-m.* in various potencies.).

Loss-of control over motion—The patient loses control over his motion although he is not yet paralysed. Paralysis comes later if this condition is not remedied. (*Plumbum-met.*).

Lotion for eyes—Discharge of acrid matter, itching of eyes; inflammation of corneas, eyes red and painful; disturbance of accommodation, opacities. Ptosis : (1) Tincture *Euphrasia*. 20 drops.

(2) *Tr. Ruta* 20 drops.

(3) *Tr. Zincum sulph.* 20 drops.

(4) *Tr. Boracic acidum.* Mix these all in rose water or distilled water 1 ounce. Use 3 times a day with a dropper including once before going to bed.

Love disappointed—When disappointed love causes silent grief. (*Ignatia*).

(2) When disappointed love wants to break connection, (*Natrum-mur.*). See "Grief-ailments due to" and "Broodings".

Low-blood pressure—(1) Lowered blood pressure; rheumatic and gouty subjects; pulse small; feeling of suffocation while lying on left side; palpitation of heart; persistent vertigo. (*Vis*).

(2) Rumbling flatulence worse between 4 and 8 p.m. of early morning; low blood pressure of dyspeptics. great emaciation and debility; palpitation at night; pressing headache; wakeful at night. (*Lyco.*).

(3) With low vitality and flatulence in the upper part of abdomen; copious menses in females. (*Carb-v.*).

(4) *Tuberculinum* is to be thought of in persons who are wasting in health.

(5) Prostration; weak and tired on slightest exertion; anaemia; buzzing in ears; sleeplessness : headache; very yellow urine. (*Kali-p.*). See "Blood pressure high and low."

(6) *Ambra grisea 200* and *Viscum album 200* may be given alternately twice daily. *Cactus 200, Calc. phos,* and *Tincture Crataegus* 10 drops of each may be given. See "Hypotension".

Lumbago-backache or pain in loins—(1) Dull backache, walking almost impossible. Scarcely able to stoop, or rise after sitting specially with constipation and piles. Backache due to straining sacroiliac . Pain relieved by standing. (*Aesc-h.*).

(2) (*a*) *Gnaphalium* will sometimes cure a chronic back-ache, a tired aching in the lumbar region that saps ones strength and ambition. Worse from continued motion, better resting specially on the back. The more chronic the backache, better indicated the remedy.

(*b*) *Aconite* suits the acute forms and will often-time give prompt relief. Dr. Baehr prefers *Tartar emetic* even to *Rhus* and *Arnica*.

(*c*) For aching in nape and stiff neck, sore shoulder (*Guiacum.*). See "Stiff neck".

(3) Back-ache during pregnancy will often be suggestive of *Aesculus* when specially worse from walking or stooping.

(4) *Secale* has sudden catch or kink in the back. Compare *Macrotin*.

(5) Dr. Farrington says that *Rhus-t.* seems to be the best remedy for lumbago whether the pains are better from motion or not. After *Rhus-t.* Dr. Jahr often removed the remnants with *Bell., Nux-v., Plumb.* and *Puls.* In *Bell.* there is intense pain of sacral region and the patient can sit for only a short time, becomes quite stiff unable to rise again. In *Nux-v* the patients feel bruised and turning in bed particularly, painful and unable to turn in bed without first sitting up. He is extremely chilly and better after having hot drink and getting warm. See also "Backache" under its different heads.

(6) Pains in the back such as lumbago, biliousness, bad taste, coated tongue and costipation. Cutting pains in the cheek bones with violent shivering, with liver disorder and

gastric derangements. Drs. M. G. Blackie and Boericke recommended *Euonymum europea* as a successful remedy for such a condition.

Lumbago stiffness—(1) Stiffness in the back ; painful on motion ; a bruise or burning pain, from damp cold. Aching on attempting to rise, aggravation in commencing motion. Chronic lumbago, (*Rhus-tox.*).

(2) Back stiff specially in morning on rising and during damp weather. Weakness and dull pain in region of kidneys. Aching pains in lumbar region, pains streaking up and down spine into sacrum. (*Phytolacca.*). See "Backache stiff spine".

Lumps-pain—See "Chapter V for details".

Lumbar-abscess—*Staphy.* See "Abscess".

Lump-in abdomen—Lump near liver region. The following remedies may be tried according to symptoms :—

(1) *Conium 200.*

(2) *Kali carbonicum 200* ; feeling of lump in the pit of stomach. Take *Kali carbonicum 200* first thing in the morning. It is also one of the best remedies following labour.

(3) Watery excrescenes, spongy tumours. (*Thuja. 1000*).

(4) Powerful remedy for stony glands. (*Calcarea-fluorica. 1M.*).

(5) *Thuja 30.* After it *Graphites 1M* every sixth day.

(6) *Tuberculinum 1M.* After 3 weeks *Graphites 1M.*

Lumps-in the breast—(1) For lumps in the breast, either when nursing or even without it, *Hepar sulph.*, *Phytolacca* and *Conium* will dissolve most of those lumps and surgery will rarely be required. See "Breasts" under its different heads.

(2) Lumps in the breasts of suspicious appearance go away under the action of *Psorium.* See "No. 5 of Pregnancy-disorders of" and "No. 37 of the same".

Lungs-abscess--*Hepar sulph* has great power on all suppurative processes and should be given.

Lungs-breathing oppressed--*Arsenic* is particularly efficacious in many affections of the lungs, when breathing is much oppressed, respiration is wheezing with cough and frothy expectoration ; patient cannot lie down, must sit up to breathe. The air passages seem constricted, (*Ars-alb.*). See "Breathing-oppressed".

Lungs-congestion due to lying down--Congestion of lungs due to persistent lying down, great rattling in chest with great weakness. The main feature is great prostration (*Am-c.*). See "Congestion of lungs".

Lungs-congested in dropsy--Congestion of lungs in dropsy, congestion of lungs due to prolonged lying in the bed compelling the patient to sit up. This hypostatic condition gradually creeps upwards so that a large portion of the breathing space is destroyed. It has a rattling breathings also Difficult breathing. Gasping breath. Pulse is small and irregular. (*Apoc-can.*). See "Congestion of lungs in dropsy".

Lungs-lack of oxygen--The digtalis of lungs. Increases oxidation of the blood by stimulating respiratory centres and excretion of carbonic acid and increases the oxygen in blood. *Tincture* (*Aspidosperma.*). (*Dr. Boericke*).

Lupus--A chronic tubercular disease of the skin and mucous membranes characterised by formation of nodules and granulation tissue :--First given *Bacillinum* in 200 dilution and after a week give *Radium brom.* which is head remedy for lupus and if there is great debility, restless, better by hot application then give *Ars-alb.* All the above three medicines are to be tried for a long time to achieve success. According to Dr. Burnett if there is an eruption on nose and two cheeks, the skin peels off in little flakes, leaving the underlying skin red, then he gives *Bacill.* and if the patient has been vaccinated more than once then he gives *Thuja 30.*

According to Dr. Franklin *Hydrocotyle* is very benefical for this disease.

Lustful mania With desire to cut a... tear every thing specially clothes, with lewd, lustful talk, amorous or religious, (*Verat.*). Compare *Hyos.*, *Stramonium.* See "Mania-amorous or religious".

—: o :—

M

Mad animals-their bites—Bites by mad animals and in poisoned wound. *Cistus canadensis* See "Bites" under different-heads.

Malaria—(1) Intermittent fever or malaria. Chill between 9 and 11 a.m. ; heat ; violent thirst increases with fever. Dryness in the mouth with lot of thirst. Drinks good deal of water. A deep crack in the middle of the lower or upper lips. Small pearl like blisters near the corner of the mouth during the attack of fever. The tongue is mapped with red islands. The fever returns at intervals or on alternate days round about 10 a.m. with sleepiness during the heat and a lot of thirst. Symptoms relieved by sweating. Numbness and tingling in fingers and toes. Abuse of quinine. A dose of *Nat. m. 200* be given after the fever attack is over and another next morning 4 or 6 hours before the expected attack. (*Nam-m.*), should never be given during fever attack. (*Nam-m.*).

(2) Chill but without thirst during the first two stages of chill and heat. The thirst commences about the end of second stage when the fever starts declining. It is prominent during the stage of sweat. (*China*). In chronic cases to be given in higher dilutions of 200 or more.

(3) Fever returning at clock-wise perioditicity. (*Cedron.*).

(4) Fever with prolonged chill, hands and feet icy cold. Give *Menyanthes* in 200 or 1000 dilutions.

(5) Malaria fever with enlargement of liver and spleen. (*Ferrum-ars.*).

(6) Malaria fever with bilious vomiting constipation, burning in stomach, nausea, violent thirst with chill and dropsical sweating. (*Nyctanthes*)

(7) The paroxysm of fever comes at 10 or 11 A.M. or 3 and 10 P.M. Strong. chill with thirst. The heat stage is very violent and is frequently associated with yawning and sneezing. Thirst during sweat stage. The sweat is .exhausting and long lasting. (*Chinium-sulf.*).

(8) Bone pain as if broken. Nausea and chill as the chill passes off. Nausea increases at the close of the chill till the patient vomits a bitter watery substance. Heavily coated tongue with bitter laste. (*Eupatorium perfoliatum*).

(9) Dry hacking cough before the chill, burning in forehead and eyes ; moist mouth. Watery yellow stool. (*Rhus-tox*).

(10) Great prostration and restlessness. Intense, burning, thirst with irritability of stomach. Severe shaking chill with thirst for small quantity of water at short intervals. (*Ars-alb*).

(*a*) The persistent nausea in one or all stages. (*Ip.*).

(*b*) Irregularly developed paroxysm, thirst intense during heat, for small quantities. (*Ars-a.*).

(*c*) Bone pains, vomits bile at the end of chill, 7 to 9 A.M. (*Eupator-per.*).

(*d*) Chill, with red face better by external heat, frequent sighing. (*Ignatia*).

(*e*) Chill begins between shoulder blades and spreads. (*Caps.*).

(*f*) During heat cannot uncover without chill (*Nux-vomica.*).

(*g*) Chill 10 to 11 A.M. bursting headache during heat : sweats on every exertion. (*Nat-mur.*).

(*h*) Cough in chill, restless and dry tongue in heat tossing about. (*Rhus-tox.*).

(*i*) Great loquacity during chill and heat ; jaundice. (*Podo.*).

(*j*) Great sleepiness during heat and sweat, with pale face (*Ant-t.*). (Dr. Nash.). See "Ague" and "Fever-malaria" under different heads.

Grimmer starts treatment of malaria with *Nat-mur*. *Ars-alb*, 2nd. *Chin sulph*. 3rd for currbing Malaria and also affording protection against the disease. See 'Ague', 'Fever malaria' under different heads.

Malaria-nausea—Ip. is a well know remedy for malaria fever after quinine. There must be constant nausea, splitting headache and thirst during the period of heat. (*Ip.*). See "Nausea-persistent."

Malformation prevention of birth of off-spring with clubfoot, twisted hand, Spine curb and cleft palate—See chapter (*v*) for details.

Mammary-abscess—(1) Breast may get inflamed, very hot swollen and painful with throbbing until it breaks. *Bell.* and *Merce-vivus*. alternately every two hours. Should the patient shiver and breast break then *Bell.* and *Hepar.* for three or four days and *Hydrastis* three times a day.

(2) *Conium* has specific action on female breasts, and for tumours of suspicious nature and also to injuries of breasts from blow or pressure or exercise. See "Tumours".

(3) Breasts sensitive during nursing and excessive flow of milk. (*Phyt.*).

(4) Undeveloped breast. *Sabal-s.* (Dr. Dewey). See "Breast" and "Boils".

Mammary-glands undeveloped—*Sabal serrulata* is valueable for undeveloped mammary glands in women.

Mania-amorous or religious—(1) With desire to cut and tear everything, specially clothes, with lewd lustful talk amorous or religious. (*Verat.*). Compare *Hyos* . *Stram.*

(2) Any form of mania with increased sexual desire. (***Baryta-mur.***).

(3) Religious mania. (*Cal-carb.*).

(4) Comical, wants to be naked. (*Hyos.*). See also "Religious mania" and "Puerperal mania".

Mania-marked by extreme uncleanliness—Patient who defecates or urinates at any time or any place. (*Am-c.*). See "No. 4 of insanity".

Mania-of old people—*Hyoscyamus*; *Lach.* is patently adapted to mania consequency upon the infirmities of old age.

Marasmus (emaciation and wasting)—(1) A gradual wasting of tissues of the body from insufficient, imperfect food supply or from poor absorption of a good food supply. (Sukha Masan). *Abrot.* is very good remedy for marasmus of children The emaciation begins in the lower limbs and gradually spreads upward, so that the face is last affected ; that is the opposite of *Lycopodium, Natrum-mur.* and *Psorinum* (*Abrot.*). See "Rickets".

Marasmus-with hunger and fever—Extreme hunger, yet, in spite of this the patient emaciates rapidly. Acute cases with more or less febrile action. The face is yellow and shrunken. The action of glands is interfered with. (*Iodine*). See also "Hunger" and "Emaciation".

(2) Marasmus from defective nourishment. The neck is thin and the appetite is ravenous. Much thirst and the water is craved for all the time. Mouth and throat dry. Craving for salt may also be present. (*Nat-m.*).

(3) Sluggish children who are weak in memory, whose cervical glands are swollen, who are lazy, pot-bellied and who want to eat all the time. (*Bar-c.*).

(4) Emaciation of skin with a large abdomen ; skin falls down into folds. (*Cal-c*).

(5) Emaciation due to anemia. Deficiency of blood. (*Plumbum*). See also "Emaciation" under its different heads.

Mastitis-inflammation of breast—The gland is heavy, hard, and red ; the face is flushed. There is a throbbing head-ache and the eyes are sensitive to light. (*Bell.*). See "Weaning enlargement with flow of milk after weaning".

Masturbation and its eradication—(*a*) Weak feeling in the chest from talking. If the patient is a young man, married or single ; if again he seems weak in mind. Listless, apathetic reticent, if he is growing fast ; all, these things would indicate *Ph-a*. See also "Impotency due to masturbation".

(*b*) For eradicating the habit of masturbation in boys (*Staphy.*). See "No. 7 of Insanity".

(*c*) Worn-out constitution, headache, loss of confidence and a desire to be alone. Loss of sexual power and nervous dyspepsia (*Agn-c.*). See "Sexual weakness with morning erections only".

Mastoid-abscess—(*a*) Swelling, painful and caries of mastoid. *Capsicum, Aurum* and *Nitr-acid* are highly recommended by Dr. Farrington. (*b*) According to Dr. George Royal *Capsicum* can be given both externally and internally and by doing so, the medicine will give prompt relief in *Otolgia*. (*Earache*) also. See also "Ear mastoid" and "Otorrhoea".

Mastoid and its prevention from Surgery—*Capsicum* 10M will prevent the resort to surgery where there is a family history of throat trouble. Compare *Calc. sulf.* which will clear up in an amazingly by short time, the pus running out of both ear. Double mastoid.

Measles not coming out properly—(1) *Puls.* helps in bringing the measles out ; restlessness ; feeling of warmth ; desire for open air. Diarrhoea after measles. Compare Rhus-tox ; and Arsenic for measles if symptoms other than those of *Puls.* are present. According to Dr. Jahr, *Verat. a.* is the best remedy for retarded eruption.

(2) Eruptive fevers, rash not coming out *e.g.* scarlet fever, measles, small pox. The eruptions are usually of a bluish tinge instead of being bright red. The regular rash does not come out but in its place red spots, roseola-like, make their appearance; the usual uniform spread of the eruption has failed or has been suppressed. Bleeding from gums and nose. Great prostration and stupification. (*Ail.*). See Blood poisoning in infective fever".

(*i*) Diarrhoea after measles, which is very common. (*Puls.*). See "Diarrhoea-after measles".

(*a*) *Bry.* is an excellent remedy for measles. It aborts the disease and definitely cuts short its course. It prevents lung affection which is a common complication.

(*b*) *Morbillinum.* may be given firstly and all through, either alone or alternated with other medicines, as indicated. This medicine in 100 potency is very efficacious for various after-effects of measles. (Dr. D. Shephard).

(*c*) Catarrhal symptoms, chilly with restlessness, dry skin thirst at night. (*Acon.*).

(*ii*) Deafness after measles. (*Puls.*). See "Ear deafness after meales".

(*d*) Sore throat, swollen face, headache, dry cough. (*Bell.*)

(*e*) Inflammation of the mucous membrane of eyes and nose. Acrid tears and conjunctivitis. (*Euphr.*)

(*f*) The cough is dry at night. The child sits up to cough. There is much predisposition to earache and sometimes sickness in the stomach. (*Puls.*).

(*g*) Haemorrhagic measles, not running a favourable course. Great prostration and restlessness. Stools offensive and exhausting. (*Ars.*). See "Measles-German".

(*h*) Cough after measles. (*Silicea.*). (Drs. Dewey, Clarke and Rai Bahadur Bishamber Das.).

(*i*) Measles respond to *Belladonna* and a final touch with *Pulsatilla.*

(*iii*) Emaciation after measles. (*Hydrastis.*). See also "Eruptions in measles retarded" and "Retarded-eruptions in measles".

(*iv*) In measles with conjunctivitis and photophobia. (*Ferr-p.*)

Measles-complicated by respiratory symptom—Acute bronchitis or bronco-pneumonia. Conjunctivitis with purulent discharge from the eyes, profuse, yellow expectoration, coughing of stringy mucus. (*Kali-bich.*).

Measles German—(1) *Acon 3,* 1 hourly followed, if necessary, by *Bell. 3, 1* hourly. See "(*h*) of Measles not coming out properly".

(2) *Antipyrinum* is a useful remedy for this trouble. The complications and sequelae are the same as those of measles and must be treated in the same way according to indication.

Measles-prophylactics—*Acon , Ars , Puls.* Let measles not affect, take *Acon. 3* and *Puls. 3* each twice daily. (Clarke) or *Morbillinum 200,* two doses, at monthly intervals. See also "Prophylactic of measles".

Measles-restlessness—The patient is restless, wants to drink water in good quantity but requires a cover (*Rhust-t.*). Compare *Puls.* See "Restlessness" under its different heads.

Measles-skin disorder—Skin disorder with repeated attacks of boils or rash on the body and redness of mouth with blisters often take place after measles. For this *Sulphur, Merc-sol., Nat. mur.* and *Puls.* are suggested according to symptoms.

Melancholia :—The patient is the most melancholic and pessimistic man who takes dark side of all things. In his pessimistic condition he is always inclined to commit suicide. Self-condemnation and self-criticism are the key-notes. He imagines, he is neglected by others or he is neglecting other and his duty. (*Aur-met.*). See also "Broodings", "Grief ailments due to" "Depression-in mind". For prevention See "Chaper V"for details .

Memory-loss due to excesses :—Loss of memory in patients broken down with sexual excesses. Despair, suicidal thoughts and peevishness. (*Agn.*). See also "Brain-fag".

Memory-failing of old persons :—Failing of old persons, using words wrong to express themselves and mixing things up generally in writing, spelling and unable to do or during mental work on account of failing brain power. (*Lyco.*).

(*a*) Forgetful of things in his mind but a moment ago forgetful as if in dream. (*Anac.*). See also "forgetfulness" and "Absent mindedness".

(*b*) *Anacardium* Is also an excellent medicine for restoring impaired memory. It often cures the patient of all other troubles. There are few medicines to match with it in this respect.

(*c*) *Rosmarinus* is indicated when memory is deficient.

Memory-loss after small pox—*Anacardium orientale*. See "(f) of Small pox."

Memory-slow in learning—Children slow in learning in school and who make mistakes and cannot remember things. (*Agar.*). See "Children-late in learning to talk and walking".

Maninges-membrane of spinal cord injuries :—Meningial injuries of the back are sometimes very troublesome and may linger on very long There may be tearing burning, stinging pain along the nerves. *Hypericum* is the remedy. See "Spine-injuries".

Meningitis-inflammation of covering membrane of brain—Violent delirium, drowsiness, temperature high. Jahr thinks that *Bell.* is the first choice as it has a curative influence. Dr. Baehr says that if meningitis can be arrested in its course by any one remedy, it is *Acon*. *(i) Apis-mel* 6—30 a very effective remedy in cerebrospinal meningitis.

(2) In cerebral irritation, the child awakes with fear, rolls his head, cries out and startless in sleep, indicated in anaemic children. (*Zinc-met.*).

(3) General convulsions ; frightful distortions of limbs, with loss of consciousness. The head is spasmodically drawn back with stiff neck, dilated pupils, *Cicuta virosa* one of best remedies having a fine clinical record (Dewey).

(4*) Iodoform. 6*X. It is the most effective remedy in tubercular meningitis. It is also to be applied locally on the head after shaving the head of the child. See also "Hydrocephalus-increase of fluid in skull".

Meningitis-tubercular—(1) *Anac.* has been helpful in the tubercular meningitis when there is total loss of memory, mental dulness and confusion and incomplete paralysis of the voluntary muscles.

(2) For meningitis of convulsion type with coma. (*Aeth-c.*).

Meningitis-its prevention—See Chapter V for details.

Menopause—*Lach.* is useful in many complaints connected with menopause. There is feeling of pressure of vertex (crown) found mostly in women nearing menopause. (*Lach.*). Compare *Sulf.* which is to be used as an intercurrent medicine. See "Headache at climacteric".

Menopause bleeding—Unusual bleeding during climacteric or during pregnancy. She usually has warts on her neck and face which go brownish later on in life. (*Sep.*). See "Bleeding during pregnancy".

Menopause-earache —Give *Gels.* which will relieve pain and patient will pass urine.

Menopause-rheumatic arthritis—Small joints of hands and feet are involved. (*Caulophyllum.*). See "Climacteric cessation of menstrual function or menopause".

Menopause-rheumatism—*Lac. caninum* is an excellent medicine of rheumatism with neuralgia and pains coming during menopause. Legs feel numb and stiff with burning in palms and soles. (See "Rheumatism").

Menorrhagia-excessive menstruation—*Act-rac.* is one of our best remedies in menorrhagia where there is severe pain in the back down the thighs and through the hips with heavy pressing down. Severe pain all through the flow. The more the flow greater the pain. (*Act-rac.*). See "Haemorrhage utrine".

Menorrhagia-in dropsy— *Apoc can.* has amenorrohea with dropsy, it has also copious menstrual flow which may be frequent and lasting too long. From copious menstrual flow the patient becomes anaemic and then dropsical (*Apoc-can*). See "Haemorrhage-in dropsy".

Menses-short--Painful, late, scanty, lasting only for one hour. (*Euphr*).

Menstruation-absence—If the menses do not appear and vicarious bleeding takes place from the nose or lungs instead. (*Phos.*) This medicine may be useful in the cancer of womb or cancer of breast.

Menstruation-bleeding from nose or lungs—Menses too early and scanty. Weeps before menses. If the menses do not appear there is often vicarious bleeding from the nose or lungs instead or from uterus between periods. (*Phos.*). See "Nose bleeding instead of menses".

Menstruation-copious and early—Headache, colic, chilliness, leucorrhoea before menses, burning and itching of parts before and after menstruation. Menses too ealy, too profuse, too long with subsequent stoppage of menses and anaemia and vertigo. Suppressed menses of fat girls. (*Calc.*).

Menstruation-with colic and diarrhoea and vomiting—Premature, abundant, blackish, often in clots, preceded by gripping and colic. There is sensation of soreness in the whole pelvic viscera as if the inner parts were raw. The sensation of soreness which is deep-seated spreads throughout the menstruation. Exhaustion coming on every menstrual period with a copious diarrhoea during the first day of menses. An attack of cholera or which one might mistake for cholera coming the first day of menses (*Am-c.*). See "Diarrhoea in menses" and "Colic menstrual"

Menstruation difficult, parts sore—Too late, short scanty and difficult ; thick, black, acrid, making parts sore. (*Sulf.*).

Menstrual colic-pain—See "Chapter V" for details.

Menstrual disorder-in hysterical and rheumatic women—In the hysterical and rheumatic constitution. Irregularity of the menstrual flow. It may be copious, suppressed or scanty.

Severe pain all through the flow. The more the flow the greater the pain. Generally the most severe and most painful attack is at the beginning of the flow and with some women again just after the flow has ceased. "Each woman is law into herself". (*Act-rac.*).

Menstrual disorder-in hysterical and rheumatic and clots Flow lasting long :—Menses come much too soon and lasts 7 to 10 days. The flow dark and clotted 3 or 4 days. Severe pain at the beginning but relief after passing membrane or clots. Leucorrhoea white of an egg-like, before menses. Pains often labour-like, constricting, extending into the back, up the back. (*Gels.*). down the thighs. (*Cham.*). and sometimes to the stomach causing vomiting. (*Borax.*).

Menstruation — dysmenorrhoea difficult or painful menstruation with labour like pains—Difficult or painful menstruation since puberty. Menses a few days too soon and profuse lasting 5 days. Labour-like pains. (*Calc-phos.* in high potencies).

Menstruation dysmenorrhoea with difficult or painful menstruation with pains in legs—Difficult or painful menstruation. Suffers from great pain at every period from the every start. Menses every 3 weeks. Pain in the uterus and down the limbs. She cannot stand long on the feet, the pain aggravates. Cold feet. (*Calc-phos.*).

Menstruation-of girls too early and excessive—Too early, excessive and bright in girls. If late, blood is dark, sometimes first bright, then dark with violent headache. Complaints during puberty by wetting feet during menses. (*Calc-phos.*)

Menstruation-early and lasting longer—Menses are some what before time, rather too copious and last a few days longer than usual and all other complaints aggravate during this period. This aggravation may remain even after the menses are over. Blood black with faint spells. Nervousness and sensitiveness increases. (*Nux-v.*). Compare Puls. which has late menses and scanty flow lasting much shorter than usual and *Cal-c*.

Menstruation-early profuse with itching and swelling of labia—Menses too early and profuse. Menses appear seven days before time. Horrible itching of genitals with swell-of labia during menses. During menses left leg becomes quite blue from distended varices with pressure ; pain in leg. Discharge of blood between menstrual period is a common occurrence after every little accident. All uterus symptoms aggravate on lying down. (*Ambra.*) See "Uterus trouble during menses" and "Swelling of labia in menses with itching".

Menstruation-in its place painful leucorrhoea—Bloody leucorrhoea seems to take the place of usual menstrual discharge. (*China.*). See "Leucorrhoea-instead of menses".

Menstruation-irregular failure after nursing stopped—Flow scanty or profuse ; whether it is late or early ; whether it is painful or hot. Irregular menses of nearly every form, amenorrhoea (absence of menstruation) dysmenorrhoea (difficult and painful menstruation) of girls of delicate constitutions and sallow complexion. A woman does not menstruate when she nurses the child. But, when she fails to menstruate when the child ceases to be nursed and the women begins feeling all sorts of mental and pelvic troubles. *Sep.* very often sets the menses in and cures her of other symptoms. (*Sep.*). See "Lactation-failure to menstruate".

Menstrual flow-with pain in back—Difficult or painful menstruation when there is "severe pain" in the back down the thighs and through the hips (*Act-rac.*). See "Back pain in the back during menstruation".

Menstruation-in its place milk in the breast—Milk in the breast of non-pregnant women at the menstrual period. Milk in breast instead of menstrual flow. (*Merc-sol.*) as suggested by Dr. W. Boericke.

Menstruation-irregularities with bleeding from nose—Menstrual irregularities, with pain, with great abdominal and pelvic soreness and gastric symptoms. Bleeding from nose when menses should occur. (*Bry.*). See "Menstruation-bleeding from nose or lungs" and "Irregularity of menstrual flow".

Menstruation-lasting only for short time—Painful, late, scanty, lasting only for one hour. (*Euphr.*) See Mense-short.

Menstruation-scanty late and suppressed—*Puls.* is very useful in affections of uterus. But mental symptoms of ***Puls.*** namely, quite and of yielding disposition with a fearful mood etc. must be present. Amenorrhoea—absence of menstruation, menses usually late and very scanty and of short duration ; the flow stops and starts again, and so on. Suppression of menses. Menstrual trouble from wetting the foot just before menses. Menstruation may be painful with great restlessness, tossing in every direction. No thirst. Relief from walking slowly in open air. Pain in back. Nausea. Diarrhoea during or after menses. (*Puls.*). Compare *Nux-v.* which has opposite symptoms.

Menstruation pains relieved by flow scanty and short—(1) Though regular but too short, scanty, feeble, pains all relieved by the flow. Always better during menses. (*Lach.*).

(2) Menses too short, to scanty and insufficient. *Puls.* If it fails than *Sulph.* followed by *Puls.* again.

Menstruation-not starting at puberty with slow development—Menstruation not starting at puberty and development slow in girls. Dr. Kent has suggested *Lyco.* for such cases and had claimed that the medicine is wonderfully potent in such cases.

Menstruation-scanty with weeping tendency and vomiting—Menstruation is generally scanty with general depression of spirit and weeping tendency. Weeping is more irritated and disturbed by consolation. Menses irregular. Vagina dry. Pearl-like blisters near the corner of the mouth. Menstruation, pain (*Nat-m*). See "Derangements at pubetry '.

(2) Flow scanty. Spasms accompanied by vomiting. (*Curpum*). See also "Weeping tendency in girls".

Menstruation-severe colic pain before flow—(1) Severe pain before menstrual period. Severe pain 2 hours before the flow begins. The patient almost faints. Cramping, soreness through abdomen. Flow every 4 or 5 weeks, scanty and lasts 1½ to 2 days. Dark clots on first day. Pain between shoulder and sometimes headache. (*Lapis-albus.*).

(2) Pain during and before menses. The patient is restless. (*Act-rac.*).

(3) Excruciating pain with bending double before menses, colic pain in lower abdomen. (*Vib-o. 3 drops M. T.*)

Menstruation-suppressed—*Puls.* removes most of the symptoms in the sphere of female genital organ which come after the suppression of the menses. One has therefore, to think of *Puls.* when such symptoms occur after these suppressions. (*Puls.*).

Menstruation-with undeveloped breasts-suppressed for months together—A young girl having no menses going without periods for 9 months, one breast smaller than the other, valuable for undeveloped mammary glands. (*Sab.serrulata M.T.* three times a day at least for 3 months.).

Menstruation suppressed in plethoric girls—Suppression of menstruation or irregularity in plethoric girls. (*Acon.*).

Menstruation-Vicarious i.e. habitual discharge occurring in an abnormal situation—Vicarious habitual discharge occurring in an abnormal situation-menstruation :—*Eupionum.*

Mental-development slow and late in children—In *Agar.* it is mental defect a slowly developing mind. Children who cannot remember mistakes and are slow in learning. The patient is sluggish and stupid. Compare *Nat-m.* which has late learning to talk and *Calc-c.* which has late learning to walk. These two features are combined in *Agar.* See "Children late in learning to talk and walking".

Mental faculties dull-sleepy and dreading movement—*Gels.* patient is sluggish and sleepy and dreads movement. Mental faculties are dull. Cannot think clearly and does not want to answer questions. He desires to be quiet, does not want to speak or spoken to. He wants to be quietly alone and undisturbed. (*Gels.*) See "Weakness anaemic with mental prostration".

Mental shock-causing nervousness—A strong vigorous man becomes nervous, trembles, is easily excited. This happens very often after a big mental shock. (*Ambra.*). See "Depression-gloominess".

Mercury-inducing rheumatism and affecting heart—The patient has been taking mercury all his life and his liver is enlarged and his joints are enlarged. Mercury has super-induced rheumatic stage that has been rubbed away with linements until the heart is affected and with this comes hopelessness, insanity of the will. distrust of affections. *Aurum-met.* would come in as an antidote to both syphilis and mercury. (*Aur-met.*).

Metastasis—Changing of one so-called disease to another e.g. Mumps to orchitis. (*Abro.*). Compare, *Carbo-veg.* or *Puls.* See also "Changing disease".

Metastasis-gonorrhoea to testicles—Metastasis is the transfer of disease from a primary focus to a distant one by conveyance of causal agents or cells through the blood vessels or by lymph channels. Gonorrhoea pains transferred to testicles. Orchitis. *i.e.* inflammation of testicles. (*Puls.*).

Metastasis-mumps to testicles—*Puls.* See "Mumps changing to testicles".

Metritis-(Inflammation of uterus)—Indurated cervix, chronic inflammation of uterus and prolapsus. Ovaries indurated. Profuse menstruation and a tendency to habitual abortion. (*Aurum-mur-nat.*). See "Inflammation of bladder".

Metrorrhagia (uterine haemorrhage, specially between the menstrual period)—(1) Between the periods there is a profuse, brown, offensive discharge which may be stringy. Menses with pain in back and thigh. This may happen after abortion or confinement or from over-exertion. (*Acidum nitricum.*).

(2) Diarrhoea frequently precedes or accompanies the menstrual flow which is too early and too profuse, either in night or in morning. Between periods occasional flow of blood. *Bovista* which may be indicated in menorrhagia and leucorrhoea.

(3) The menses appear every two weeks and last from 7 to 8 days and in the interval bloody leucorrhoea rendering the patient anaemic. Gushing of bright blood on least movement. Useful at climacteric and such trouble. (*Trillium pendulum.*). See "Menorrhagia and leucorrhoea".

Micturition after marriage and labour—(1) Painful in young wives. (*Staphy.*).

(2) Constant dribbling after labour. (*Arnica*).

(3) Retention after labour, post operative. (*Caust.*). See "Labour-retention of urine" and "Wed-lock urine trouble after it".

Micturition-painful and uncontrollable :—Frequent micturition accompanying pains. Desire sudden and urgent but cannot be controlled. (*Thuj.*). See alse "Bladder-weakness of bladder with micturition".

Micturition sediment in offensive urine—Pressure on bladder and frequent micturition with tension in lower abdomen. Sediment in urine like clay : urine very offensive. (*Sep.*).

Micturition-in-young wives after marriage—Painful in young wives. Urinary trouble of young nervous women after marriage where urging to urinate becomes very troublesome to the young women. *Stphysagria* is the most comforting to the young wife under such circumstances. (*Staphy.*). See also "Urine trouble in young wives after marriage".

Migraine—(1) In nervous sick headaches which are caused by excitement and over-exertion with frequent scanty urination. *Scutellaria* in mother tincture to be given 5 drops a dose.

(2) Migraine and neuralgic affections. (*Tongo.*).

(3) Periodical nervous sick headache which comes on after the patient relaxes from a mental strain. The patient usually vomits a bitter bilious substance and the vomiting gives relief to the pains in the head. *Iris versicular.* If this fails then

Cyclamen may be tried if migraine is accompanied with sparking before eyes.

(4) *Damiana* is an excellent remedy for migraine. It should be given in M.T. in 15 to 20 drops doses every 2 hours. In severe cases it may be given every half hour and the patient will sleep after 2 doses. See "Headache, Migraine" and "Headaches" under different heads.

(5) Terrifically severe headache accompanied by high blood pressure. Headache which is throbbing and beating. Worst type of migraine. (*Nat-m.*).

(6) Migraine due to acidity and sluggishness of liver. (*Chionanthus.*).

(7) For migraine of children. (*Carb ac. 12*).

(8) For dimnishing the attacks of migraine. (*Cann-i*).

(9) For right sided migraine. :—*Prunus-spinosa.* 6 or *Sanguinaria* 200 ; for left sided migraine :—*Spigelia* 30 or *Thuja* 200.

(10) In migraine which is the result of fatigue, weariness and exhaustion. The headache is preceded by flashes of light before the eyes and is accompanied by vertigo. (*Coca.*).

(11) Headache starting at the back of neck and travelling up the head ending on the right temple causing sickness, sweating with offensive smelling, sweating feet. (*Silica*).

(12) Female patient walking in the morning with a severe headache two or three times a month, vision affected and headache always worst during menstruation Rising blood-pressure. (*Nat-mur.*).

(13) Sensation as though the temples were crushed together. Neuralgic pain about the zygoma (The bony yoke connecting the malar and temporal bone), and ear. These pains are aggravated by talking, sneezing or biting the teeth together. (*Verbascum thapus*).

(14) Headache in plethoric and healthy person. The cause of some disturbance of circulatory system. The headache is violent and throbbing. (*Belladonna.*).

(15) In hysterical patient when due to some grief. Women of sensitive and easily excited nature, inclines head forward (*Ignatia*). See "Headache Migraine" and "Headache under different heads".

Milk-ceasing after starting—Ceasing of milk after it has started or becomes scanty suddenly in women with previous history of secret vices and sexual excess. (*Agn*). See "Lactation".

Milk-not diminishing after weaning—Give *Belladonna*.

Milk-crusts on scalp wetting the pillow—Itching of the scalp. Much perspiration. Wets the pillow. (*Calc*.). See "Eczema-general part No. 12", "No. 5 of Itch" and "Eczema-scalp".

Milk-disagreeable—Always worst after taking milk (*Sepia*.). See "Cholera-infantum worst by milk".

Milk-not digested with diarrhoea—There is marked inability to digest milk in children with diarrhoea. It is vomited in large curds as soon as is taken. Then weakness causes drowsiness. (*Aeth*.). Compare *Mag-c*. and *Nat-c*. See "Crying of child, dentition, milk not digested", "Diarrhoea milk upsets" and "Indigestion of babies due to overfeeling".

Milk-fever—*Bell*. If this fails then Bryonia in repeated doses See "Fever-milk" and "No. (5) Pregnancy-its affection".

Mind-weeping tendency—The mental symptoms of *Sep*. are very characteristic and they must be present along with the bodily symptoms. She has an extremely weeping tendency, she is sad and cries on all occasions without always knowing the reason thereof. She is tearful when she narrates her trouble to anyone. She is indifferent. (*Sep*.) Compare *Puls*. See also "Weeping tendency".

Miscarriage-and its tendency—Threatened, fever restless-ness; thirst, anxiety and fear. (*Acon*. 1 hour). (a) Tendency to miscarry, sensitiveness of genital (*Zinc*.). (b) Tendency in the earlier half of pregnancy. (*Sabina*. 1 hour.) ; (c) Tendency in the later half. (*Secale cornutum*. 1 hour.). (d) In women who habitually miscarry at a certain period of pregnancy. *Viburnum-opulus*; should be given for some-time before. (*Vib-o*). (e) When due to syphilis give in mother tincture *Lueticum 30, Syphilinum* to be given twice a week throughout pregnancy (Dr Clarke). (f) Habitual abortion (*Helon.*). (g) *Cimcifuga* is a powerful restrainer of abortion. (h) *Viburnun opulus* will prevent miscarriage if given before the membranes are injured and when pains are spasmodic or threatening. See "Abortion threatened" "Haemorrhages during pregnancy if abortion apprehended".

Miscarriage-habitual—Miscarriage or abortion whether habitual or otherwise whether threatend or from accidental causes. It will also act as uterine tonic. Menstrual irregularties of sterile females with uterine displacements.

(*Virburnum prunifolium.*)

Miscarriage of-syphilitic-origin—Women with feeble. constitution are subject to uterine haemorrhages and miscarriages. (*Syph.*). Even there is no history of syphilis; give *Merc-sol.* in high potency. Next try *Sulph.* and *Calc-carb.*

Miscarriage-threatened—(1) Tendency to miscarriage specially at third month. Inflammation of ovaries and uterus after abortion. Promotes expulsion of mole. (retained foetal membrane and placenta) from uterus. (*Sabina.*).

(2) Threatened miscarriage from mechanical injury. (*Arnica.*) For continued haemorrhage with nausea and pain. (*Ipec.*). See "Abortion-tendency to miscarriage" and "Abortion threatened".

Mistakes commiting—(1) In calculating; in spelling and in writting. (*Lyco.*).

(2) Mistakes in measures and weights (*Nux-vom.*).

(3) Miss-spells common words; forgets names; cannot concentrate on study. (*Xerophyllum.*).

(4) Using wrong word or misplacing words (*China.*).

(5) Mistakes locality(*Glonoine, Nux mos, Petroleum.*). Try these three medicines in given order. See "Forgetfulness".

M

Mocking—Mocking at others and at relatives. (*Lachesis; Platinum.*). See "Laughter".

Morphia (opium)-habit—*Avena sativa* is a specific for removing morphine (*Opium.*) eating habit. Give 20 drops of M.T. in hot water 4 times a day. A prolonged use will be necessary to completely get rid of the habit. See "Opium-eating habit".

Morphia-vomiting after operation—Morphia effect on sensitive persons after operation are awful eructations with retching and vomiting and there is nothing to vomit. Give *Chamomilla* which will stop these within a few minutes and is practically the only remedy that stops vomiting from morphine. (*Cham.*) See "Vomiting due to morphine effect after operation". See also "Opium eating habit".

Mosquito-bite—*Ledum-pal.* will give immediate relief on mosquito bites (Led.). See "Bites also".

Mountain climbers—See "Physical acts requiring strength".

Mouth offensive after sleeping—Mouth covered with offensive mucus after sleeping. (*Rheum.*). See "Odour from nose and mouth".

Mouth open in sleep—Keeps mouth open during sleep (*Opium.*). See "(d) of adenoids growths" and "Catarrh of nose block".

Mouth-ulcerative—Ulcerative stomatitis with coated white tongue and a tough, stringy acid saliva. (*Kali-chloricum.*). See "Blisters in mouth", "Ulcers in mouth" and "stomatitis".

Mouth washed—Mouth wash in sore-throat and affections of the gums. Useful for consumptive cough also. 10 to 20 drops of tincture in a table spoonful of water. *Salv. off.* also known as *Sage*. Compare *Calendula* which can also be used as a mouth wash with drops in a tea-cup full of hot water. Tones up the gums after massaging them gently.

Mouth stomatitis—Mercurial stomatitis with gums ulcerated, tongue cracked and mouth exceedingly offensive.

(*Baptisia.*). (Dr. Dewey). See "Tongue-papilla bleeding and cracked" and "Stomatitis".

Mouth-bad taste—Bad taste in the mouth and nothing tastes well, not even water ; dryness in the mouth without thirst caused by rich greasy food, will be a good indicator of *Puls.* during digestive trouble. (*Puls.*). Compare *Merc-sol.* with similar bad taste in mouth but it has charcteristically moist mouth with somewhat more salivation and with intense thirst. See also "Taste" and "Taste-nothing, tastes well during digestive trouble".

Mouth-blisters near corner—Dry with lot of thirst. The lips and mouth ulcerated and cracked. Small pearl like blisters occurring near the corners of the mouth during an attack of fever or the menstrual period. (*Nat-m.*). Compare *Merc-sol.* and *Puls.* See "Ulcers-in mouth" and "Blisters in mouth extremely painful".

Mouth cracked—Cracked in corners. (*Graphites*). If it is ulcerated with cracks in a corner then *Nitric acid.*

Mouth-whole of it inflamed—The inflammation is intense and spreads all over the cavity of the mouth including whole of the throat, uvula and the gums become spongy and bloody (*Merc.*). See "Inflammation acute" and "Uvula-different complaints".

Mouth-offensive and raw—Raw feeling at roof and palate. Corners of mouth sore and cracked. Putrid odour from the mouth, excessive flow of acrid saliva. (*Aurum-t.*). See "Odour-mouth".

Mouth-offensive odour and swollen gums—The whole mouth is offensive in look and odour. Gums and teeth swollen. Intense thirst though the tongue and mouth are moist. This condition may happen in acute fever or any inflammation of any organ specially the glands or the instestine. (*Merc-sol.*). See "Thirst with offensive mouth", "No. 1 of gums" and "Tongue swollen with offensive mouth".

Mouth parched—Mouth and lips are parched and there is thirst for large quantity of water at longer intervals. Dryness of mucous membranes. (*Bry.*). See "Thirst-dry mouth".

Mouth ulcers in child's mouth—Mouth full of ulcers, very often with a foul smell. The child is usually prostrated and drowsy. (*Bapt.*). See "Ulcers in mouth".

Mouth-ulcers of adults—Ulcers of the gums, tongue, throat and inside of cheeks with profuse salivation. Fetid odour from the mouth. The edges of ulcers are irregular and undefined and have an unhealthy lardacious base and have surrounded with dark halo. Great thirst with moist mouth. (*Merc-sol.*).

Movements-increase in all complaints—All complaints increase on movement of any kind. All disinclination of movement generally by the patient or the particular part involved. Suffering of almost of any and every kind, whether whole body or of a part, is increased by movement. It makes no difference what the name of the disease is, if the patient feels greatly relieved lying still and suffers greatly on slightest motion and the more and longer he moves, the more he suffers. *Bry.* is the first remedy to be thought of (*Bry.*). (Dr. Dewey.). See "Fidgetiness part (b)".

Mucus-accumulation in air passages—(1) Great accumulation of mucus in air passages which cause rattling and inability to expectorate ; impending paralysis of lungs.

(2) Great accumulation of mucus ; violent degree of dyspnoea with wheezing cough, great nausea and anxiety. (*Ipec.*). The same medicine may be used when there is threatened suffocation due to accumulation of mucus.

(3) With discharge of tough, stringy, adherent mucus which cen be drawn into long thread (*Kali bichro.*). Compare *Hydrastis Lyssin,* when there is mucus from mouth and throat ; and also *Iris vers.*

Mucous colitis—(1) Membranous discharges, flatulence, and constipation and pain. (*Arg-n.*).

(2) Gelatinous stools, cutting pains in bowels and kidneys (*Codenium sulphuratum*.).

(3) Stools like scrapings of intestines, pains, thirst, nausea and vomiting (*Canth*.). See also "Colitis" and "Dysentery" under latters different heads.

Muco enteritis-pain—See "Chapter V" for details .

Mumps—(*a*) *Bell.* is an excellent remedy for mumps. It ma be alternated with *Merc-iod.* 30 every half hour. If these fa then *Phytolacca* may be tried when the tumour is harder and the skin paler. (b) When the ear is involved and the pain i very severe, *Puls. Parotidnum* which is a nosode to be given one dose 200 stopping all other medicines for that day. See "Ear pains of various types".

Mumps-changing to testes—Inflammation of mumps changin to testes or inflammation of the breasts. (*Abrot.*). See als "Changing disease" or "Metastasis-mumps to testicles".

Mumps-preventive—*Pilocarpinum* and *Parotidinum*. Th latter is a nosode. It should be given in 200 in a week for 2 c 3 weeks as preventive. It is used as curative when othe medicines fail in which case only one dose to be given stoppin all other medicines for that day. See "Preventives".

Mump-prophylactic—*Trifolium repens*. See "xiv of Prophyla ctic for other diseases".

Mumps-aborting and shortening the duration—If *Perot dinum* is given every two or three hours at the commencemen of mumps it may considerably shorten the period of diseas (*Dr. Clarke*.).

Mumps-trouble in testicles—Metastasis of mumps to testicle (*Puls*.). Compare *Abrot.* and *Carb-v.* See also "Metastasis".

Music-aggravating symptoms—Music intolerable. Hearir music very often aggravates many bodily symptoms, *e.g.* coug (*Ambra*.). Compare *Calc.*

Muscles-different troubles including atrophy—(1) Relaxe muscles, easily fatigued. Weakness of the legs. Loss of pow of extremities. (*Gels*.).

(2) Pain in the muscles from getting cold and wet. (*Dulc.*).

(3) Weakness of the whole muscular system, drawing pains and cramps in the limbs and the joints ; aching in the back. (*Verat-v.*) 2 hourly.

(4) Stiffness and weakness and pressure on shoulder, uneasyness in the limbs paralytic heaviness. (*Caust.*).

(5) Muscular atrophy ; *Plumbum* is the head remedy and covers symptoms from irritation to complete destruction of muscles. Complete loss of sensation, weakness, cutting, shooting in the neck ; shortening of muscles. Try *Kali-b.*, for muscular atrophy. The virus associated with this condition is destroyed by its use. (Clarke and R.B.B. Das.).

(6) Contraction of muscles. (*Cimex.*). See "Pain-of the tendon and muscles". See also "Atrophy of nipples in breasts" and "Strains of muscles, tendon."

(7) Weakness of cervical muscles—can hardly hold the head up. (*Cocculus ind.*). *Zincum, Ignatia* and *Agaricus* cover jerking and twitching of various muscles.

Muscles—Rigid, chiefly of neck and shoulder (*Senecio Jacobaea*).

Myelitis-inflammation of spinal cord—(*a*) (1) When the upper part of cord is involved shooting, stabbing pains in cord ; high fever. (*Bell*).

(2) Pain and inflammation of the spinal cord when due to an injury or blow on the spine. Pain from the least movement. (*Arn-m.* ; *Hyperi.*).

(3) Great rigidity of lower limbs pains, chilliness. (*Ox-ac.*).

(4) Chronic spinal paralysis. (*Plumbum.*). See "Spine inflammation".

(*b*) (1) Spinal cord thickened, cramps in calves, gums swollen. Gastralgia, constipation, stool hard, lumpy ; straining at stool or urination. Paralysis of lower extremities. Emission of urine drop. (*Plumb-iodat 30*).

(2) Involuntary stool ; no sensation of passing faeces, anus wide open ; burning pain in uterus ; insomnia with restlessness, anxious, dread ; paralysis of bladder ; craves acids ; trembling staggering gait ; varicose ulcers ; skin feels cold to touch ; covering not tolerated, wants part uncovered ; eructations of bad odour. (*Sec.*).

(3) Cramps relieved by pushing against the foot : numb and paralysed feeling of legs ; frequent urging to stool. Dry mouth, pain in lumbar region ; cramps in calves of legs ; renal insufficiency ; vertigo ; urine of high specific gravity ; pain in lumbar region and in lower shoulder blades. (*Cupr-ars.*).

(4) Must urinate when getting cold ; catarrh of bladder from taking cold, urine has thick mucus, purulent sediment ; suppression of menses ; cough ; stiff neck, pain in small of back as after long stooping ; perspiration on palms of hands. (*Dulc. 30.*).

(5) Pain and inflammation of spinal cord when due to injury or blow on the spine. Pain from least movement, extreme sensitiveness to touch, fear of attempting to stand. (*Arn-m 30* and *Hyper. 30*).

(6) All pervading debility, exhaustion and restlessness burning pains ; degenerative changes. Great anguish and restlessness ; cramps in calves ; must have head raised by pillows haemorrhoids burn like fire ; urine involuntary. Degenerative changes. (*Ars-a. 30*).

(7) Anaemia of spinal cord, burning, aching and weakness of spine, cold, clammy feet ; weakness and loss of power of cerebro-spinal system. (*Strychnia-phos.* 3rd trituration). See "Spine injuries" and "Poliomyelitis and its preventive", and "Spine inflammation".

Myopia-short sightedness – (*a*) *Physostigma* 3x, 4 hourly. See also "Eyes" under different heads.

(*b*) *Cyclamen* is useful for that kind. Patient who disinclined to work, and easily fatigued, and who complaints of flickering before the eyes.

Myositis—Progressive ossifying (converting) myositis (inflammation of muscles referring to voluntary muscles *i e.* general inflammation of muscles plus a progressive ossification of the same, for this disease.)

Calc-fluor. is an excellent medicine and should be tried for a long time. It is a powerful tissue remedy for hard, strong glands, varicosed enlarged veins and malnutrition of bones.

If the use of this medicine does not show any perceptible improvement then the following drugs may be tried in the given order according to R.B Bishamber Das :

(1) *Calc. Phos.*

(2) *Acid Fluor.*

(3) *Symphytum.*

Myxodema—It is a diseased condition due to deficiency of thyroid secretion or removal of thyroid glands or atrophy of the same characterised by loss of hair, increased thickness and dryness of skin, increase in weight, slowing of mental process and diminution of metabolism, with puffy face and hands, absence of sweating, brittleness of nails, apathy and lethargy. *Thyroidin* in 30 dilution should be given for at least 3 months. If no improvement within this time then try *Spongia* and later on *Iodine.* Dr. R.B. Bishamber Das further recommends *Lapis A, Oleum J.* and *Sulf.* for general affections of glands.

N

Naevus (birth-mark) (*a*) *Thuja. 30,* mother tincture of *Thuja* to be applied twice. *Radium bromidum* 30 to be given once a week along with *Thuja* which is not to be given that day. *Vaccininum 200* to be given once in a fortnight. (*b*) According to Dr. Aggarwal *Lyco.* and *Fluor acid* are best remedies for removing of the birth mark.

Nails blue, falling, pains and soft nails—Nails blue, *Oxalic acid* ; falling of nails, *Helleborus foetidus* ; pains under nails ; *Sep.* ; soft nails : *Wild-bad.* compare *Thuja* ; splitting nail : *Stannum.*

Nails-biting :—(1) Biting of finger nails till they bleed. (*Arum trip*).

(2) *Ambr.* works of nails biting.

(3) *Sanic.* is another most effective for nails-biting.

(4) Nail-biting due to nervous irritation. (*Ammon. bromat.*)

Nail-fingers mis-shapen—Both fingers and toe nails become thick, grow out of shape. (*Graphites*).

Nail of finger hurt—When never rich area, as finger ends or toe ends are injured or a nail has been torn off or nerve has been crushed between hammer above and bone below and nerve shows sign of inflammation and the pain can be traced upon the nerve. *Hyperium* is the remedy. (*Hyper*). See "Finger-end or toe-ends injured".

Nails growth deficient—Deficient growth of nails ; split nails (*Antim Crud.*).

Nail of iron in the foot or under finger—When a patient steps on a nail or a splinter sticks under the finger nail or into the foot or any other sensive part, give a dose of *Ledum.* This will always prevent tetanus. See "Splinter or nail into the feet".

Nail-fungus and abnormal outgrowth of finger and toe nails—A spongy, morbid excrescences of nails of toe and fingers. Painful cracks in the palms as well as in the soles. Itching of nail better by hot application. Application of cold water causes burning. Irritable before menses. Easily excitable : worries when alone, likes extra salt. Start treatment with *Sepia* 200 going gradually upto C.M. After this *Myristica* 30 may be given for a few days. Local application of *Calendula* ointment.

Nail in growing toe nail—*Magnetis polus australis 30-200* 4 hourly. Locally *Hydrasis* ointment.

Nail-miss-shapen, also due to tight shoes—(1) Brittle, distorted, crumbling, miss-shapen or soft. (*Thuja*).

(2) Nails grow rapidly : nails brittle and crumble, feeling as of a splinter under nail. (*Fl-ac.*),

(3) Finger nails thick, black and rough. Nails deformed and out of shape. Painful and sore.(*Graph.*).

(4) Inflammation at the seat of nails. (*Sil.*) local application of *Calendula M.T.*

(5) If the nail gets inflamed or suppurated and the soft structure around nails gets inflamed due to wearing tight or pointed toed shoes then Acid-*Nitric* or *Magnet australis 200* internally and externally application of *Hydrastis.* M.T. See "Onychia".

Nail-pain—Pain under finger nails with coldness of feet, swelling of finger joint. (*Berberis*).

Nail-psoriasis—Dr. A. Banerjee recommends *Chrysophatnic acid* 3X, 3 times a day. It can be used as a local application in ringworms, and other skin affections. Ointment of it be made with 4 grains to 8 grains with vaseline one ounce as recommended by Dr. Banerjee.

Nail-skin cracking—Skin around the nail dry and cracking (*Nat-m.*). See "Finger cracks."

N

Nail-white spots—Affections of finger nails specially if white spots on nails (*Sil.*).

Nails yellow—Finger nails become yellow. (*Am-c.*) See "Nails blue, falling, pains and soft nails.

Nape - muscles drawn—Head drawn back from contraction of muscle of neck. (*Act-rac*). See "Head-drawn back" and "Wry neck"

Narcolepsy—See "Sleepiness".

Nasal-Erythema—Hyperemia of the skin occurring in patches of variable size and shape :—Nose all red and swelled up, inflammatory action extending to the cheek, involving the eyes also. *Thuja 30th* for the erythema and if the nose stopped inside then *Kali-bichromicum 5*, five drops in water night and morning. As a local application a weak solution of *Kali bichromicum* (*1 to 2000*) be used according to Dr. Clarke.

Nasal polypus—(1) Dr. Jousset recommends *Calc-c. 2* doses per day per month and then rest for 10 days and then begin a new.

(2) For bleeding polypus. (*Sang.* and *Phos.*). See also "Polypus covering nostrils".

Nausea-heaviness in stomach, relief by pressure—Heaviness in stomach. Nausea characterised by (i) Aggravation by movement, (ii) Thirst for large quantities of water and (iii) Relief by pressure. (*Bry*). See "Vomiting with thirst".

Nausea-morning sickness in pregnancy—Vomiting many times each day, pain and retching, cramps, restlessness night and day. Dr. Hoyne cured within 24 hours by *Cupr acet. 30.* See also "Morning sickness" and "Pregnancy vomiting".

Nausea-persistent—Persistent not relieved by vomiting. Face usually pale with sleepiness after vomiting. Clean tongue ; *Ip.* relieves all kinds of nausea. (*Ip.*). Compare, *Puls.* See "Persistent nausea" and "Malaria-nausea".

Nausea-in pregnancy due to thought or smell of food—Nausea or vomiting in pregnancy at the very thought or smell of cooked food. The patient cannot even pass by the kitchen. *Colchicum* is a good medicine for this but *Sep.* is better in pregnancy. (*Sep.*). Compare Ars. See "Pregnancy vomiting".

Nausea-with retching without vomiting—Nausea and retching without vomiting. There is lot of rumbling in stomach (*Podo*). See "Retching".

Nausea-smell of food—The smell or sight of food causes nausea. (*Ars-alb.*). Compare *Sepia* and *Colch.* in pregnancy. See "Smell of food".

Navel bleeding and ulceration—(1) Bleeding from navel of infants. (*Abrot*).

(2) Ulceration of navel in newborn children (*Nux-mosch.*). See also "Bleeding from navel".

Neck-glands with discharge from nose—Along with excoriating discharge from nose, the glands of the neck and even the parotid (situated near the ear) may be inflamed and are sore. (*Arum-t.*). See "Glands swelling due to discharge from nose".

Neck gland-enlarged—Enlarged, suppurating, swelling ; also sore throat. History of tuberculosis in the family. Under *Bacillinum,* *Silicea* and *Baryta carb.* it spontaneously opened. Externally apply *Calendula M.T.* lotion. See "Glands or ulcer on neck tubercular" and "Glands enlarged of neck".

Neck-sprain—If due to wrong position in sleep neck is twisted thereby causing sprain of neck. In this condition *Rhus-tox.* 200 may be given 4 hourly which will relieve pain in a day. See "Head drawn back" and "Wry neck".

Neck-gland swelling—Glandular swelling in neck or any part of body. (*Merc-sol.*). See "Glands" under different heads and No. 13 of Eczema general at different places.

Neck-pain—See "Chapter V for details".

Neck-stiff—Due to draught or chill ; painful ; worse on moving the neck. (*Acon.* 1 hourly). See also "Stiff neck".

Necrosis of bone of lower jaw—Particularly of lower jaw but also of other parts as vertebra and caries of tibia. (*Phos*), *Calcarea fluor* and *Silicea* to be given alternately to cure and check necrosis of bone. See "Jaw carious and cracking" and "Caries of vertebra".

Necrosis of bone-of upper right jaw—Dr. Luther of Plymouth Michigan completely cured cases of maxillary—upper right jaw bone—necrosis by Silicea followed by Fluoric acid and then *Calcarea fluorica*.

Nephritis acute-pain—See ' Chapter V for details".

Nephritis-children (inflammation of kidney)—Nephritis acute in a child with enlarged neck glands. Teeth appearing slowly. 'Takes cold easily. Sluggish bowels. Enlarged abdomen. Grinds teeth. Fever, urine scanty. Aversion to being touched. (*Calc.*). See "Inflammation of kidney".

Nephritis-inflammation of kidney—The urine is dark. Casts are abundant and it contains much albumin, pale skin, watery diarrhoea and great thirst. Dr. Pope found Ars. 3x efficient in acute nephritis. *Acon.* is the first remedy and Arsenic may cure immediatey after it.

(2) Has high grade of inflammation, urine scanty, bloody, strangury, foul odour of breath. Dull pain in the back, *Terebinth.* is indicated in early stages of disease.

(3) Oedematous swelling of the face and extremities, paleness, pains in head, back and limbs, dull pains in the kidneys, scanty urine and frequent micturition, urine charged with albumin and contains blood corpuscles, patient apathetic. *Apis.* is most useful in last stages.

(4) Has pale, profuse urine with albumin casts and great reduction in urea, nausea, putrid eructations. 10 drops of *Aurum-chlor.* of 2x potency (freshly) prepared given before each meal and at bed time acts very well.

(5) For albuminuria of pregnancy. (*Helonis.*). See also "Kidney affections", "Brigt's disease". "Inflammation of kidney" and "Pregnancy nephritis."

Nerve injury—(1) Crushing—*Hyper.*

(2) Ascending neuritis after nerve injury—(*Hyper*).

(3) Tearing burning, stinging pain along nerve. (*Hyper*). See "Inflammation of nerve injury" and "Crushing of nerve".

Nerve sheath spine—Injuries to spine linger for years. But for the action of the nerve sheaths and meninges with tearing, burning and stinging pain along the nerves. *Hypericum* is the remedy. (*Hyper.*). See "Spine injuries".

Nervous-sudden blindness and colour blindness—Sudden dimness of sight. Dark ring about the eyes. Colour blindness. (*Sant*). See "Blindness", also "Night blindness" and "Sudden appearance of symptoms and blindness".

Nervous breakdown—Always brooding and listless in talks and action. Profound despondency with increased blood pressure. Disgust of life and thoughts. Peevish. (*Aur-met. 200*). See "Suicide-inclination to commit".

Nervous-deafness—The principal remedy is *Lach.* and should this fail give *Naja.* Dr. Jousset got great benefit from *Elaps corallinus.* See "Deafness".

Nervous-diarrhoea—Diarrhoea of nervous type from emotion excitement, fright and bad news. (*Gels.*). See "Diarrhoea nervous".

Nervous-dyspepsia from excitement—When digestion has absolutely ceased from brain trouble and from excitement. The characteristic symptoms relate mainly to the brain and nervous system connected with gastro-intestinal disturbances (*Aeth*). See "Indigestion from brain trouble or excitement". "Dyspepsia of adults from brain trouble and constant eating" and "Dyspepsia nervous".

Nervous-dyspepsia with pain in stomach—Dyspepsia of nervous type. The main symptom in the sphere of stomach is a pain, which is sometime removed by eating. (*Anac.*). See "Dyspepsia" under different heads.

N

Nervousnsss-exhaustion—In case of Ph-a. the exhaustion is primarily of nervous exhaustion and not due to loss of fluid in diarrhoea. (*Ph-a.*). See "Dyspepsia-nervous".

Nervous, irritability and prostration—The patient develops prostration of peculiar kind ; nervous prostration. The patient is emaciated. (*Nat-m.*).

Nervous-patient—*Tela-urane* calms such patients. It abates the excitement of circulation, promotes sleep, and induces, a sensation of quietade and comfort.

Nervous-prostration after infectious diseases—Great lassitude and prostration in all conditions. Specially at the end of serious infections diseased condition due to a fungus e.g. diphtheria, scarlet fever, pneumonia, and erysipelas etc. *Am-c.* competes well with *Ars.* for nervous prostration. (*Am-c.*). See "Prostration at the end of a serious infection disease".

Nervousness-no stamina to appear before public—The patient is weak-hearted, irritable and gives up hope. No stamina to appear before the public and say something. He is afraid to approach people in higher position. Excitable, anxious ; fixed ideas. *Sil.* will build up mental stamina, his spirits will rise and general weakness and depression of mind will vanish (*Sil.*). See "Mind-lack of stamina" and "Shyness-bashful".

Nervous-headache syphilitic—Old syphilitic bone pains in the head. These pains in the head are sometimes very distressing. These bone pains of the head usually called nervous headache are either syphilitic, hysterical or scrofulous. Pains extend from within out, aggravated at night. (*Asaf.*) See "Headache nervous" and "Headache syphilitic or hysterical".

Nervousness-due to sedentary life—The *Nux,* patient is nervous and irritable. He is rather thin, quick and active. He does a good deal of mental work and leads a sedentary life. (*Nux-v.*).

Nervous system-very sensitive to opposition—*China* is excessively sensitive in its nervous system. The menses are acute, mind is very sensitive to slight opposition or insult. It has an acute hearing. Sensitive to cold, draught, light, touch and sound. (*China*.). See also "Sensitiveness to opposition".

Nervous trouble-want of clarity or application—The patient losing all ambition to do anything ; either mental or physical labour. Great indifference ; cannot think with usual clearance ; cannot apply himself to study or mental operations ; ideas come slowly or not at all. (*Phos.*) See "Mental faculties dull".

Nettlerash (urticaria)—(1) Recent—*Apis*. If no improvement in a day or two then *Chloralum-hydratum*. 8 hourly..

(2) From chill and wetting, (*Dulc*.).

(3) When the irritation comes at night when warm in bed, (*Sulf*.).

(4) Stinging sensations, great irritation. (*Urt. urens* 6 hourly.).

(5) Lotion of *Urtica urens* M.T. or lotion of *Calendula M.T.* for external use

(6) When associated with liver affections. (*Astac-fluviatilis* 4 hourly.

(7) Inveterate cases with constipation. (*Nat-mur*. 8 hourly).

(8) Hives rashes of various kinds. (*Hydr*.). See "Urticaria" under its different heads.

Neuralgia-eye—Neuralgia of left eye with soreness of head. (*Kali-iod*.). See "Eyes" under different heads.

Neuralgia of face-pain in nerve due to exposure—Of face due to exposure to cold or draught, pain in joints. Face red and flushed but pale. (*Acon.*). See "Facial paralysis with neuralgia".

Neuralgia of face-pain crampy pressure relieves—Neuralgic pains are crampy in nature and must have the symptom of being relieved by hard pressure and warmth. If Coloc. does not help try Mag-phos. if relief is prompt from fomentation. (*Coloc*.).

Neuralgia of left side. (pain in nerve)—Neuralgia of the left side, left eye, left orbit, and in the left brachial plexus. Pains shooting, burning and tearing. Pains in neck and shoulder (*Spig.*). See "Paralysis-face of, left and right".

Neuralgia pain in nerves lightning like—*Mag-p* is wonderful pain remedy for neuralgia. Its main characteristic is lightning like character ; has a sharp cramping pain which flashes in and out and often changing places. It can be found along the nerves or muscles in the stomach or abdomen or in the pelvic region. Pain relieved by warmth or pressure. (*Mag-p.*). See "Pain lightning like".

Neuralgic pains-anywhere in the body ; relief by pressure (a) If relieved by lying on the painful side and also by hard pressure and warmth. (*Coloc.*). (b) For periodic headaches and occipital pains. (*Niccolum sulphuricum.*). See "Pressure relief" and "Headache periodical".

Neuralgia pains with numbness—Sensation of pain far in excess of actual pain. Numbness with pain. Peevish temper. For adults. (*Cham.*). See "Numbness of nerves".

Neuralgia-of right side—Symptoms like neuralgia on left. (*Sang.*). See "Neuralgia of left side pain in nerves".

Neuralgic-nerve pain with trembling of limbs—The prostration or trembling of limbs should be present. Mental faculties dull. Does not wish to speak or spoken to. *Gels.* centres its actions upon nervous system causing various diseases of motor paralysis. (*Gels.*). See "Trembling-of lower extremities in paralysis".

Neurasthenia-due to debility and different causes—(1) Due to debility or exhaustion of the nerve centres. Fatigability, lack of energy and disinclination to activity. (*Nat-m.*).

(2) *Kali-phos.* is an excellent remedy for nervous prostration, brain fag or exhaustion, shyness, nocturnal emissions and sexual powers diminished, are the main symptoms.

(3) *Mephitis* given in low potency tones up the nervous system.

(4) Nerves weak, brain tired and patient irritable. *Avena-sativa* in appreciable doses of tincture will calm and strengthen the nerve.

(5) Mental depression, disinclination to work and general debility. (*Coca.*).

(6) Debility arising from continued grief, over-exertion of mind, sexual excesses, nervous strain on body or mind characterised by indifference, apathy and torpidity of body and mind. Any attempt to study causes heaviness in the head and limbs (*Ph-a.*).

(7) Chronic worries, fears of misfortune and startled by slightest noise. (*Ig*). See "Depression mental" under different heads. and "Debility due to various causes".

Neurasthenia and general weakness—Especially associated with alcohol ; delirium, hallucination and migraine. Hysteria and insomnia alternate ; 3 or 4 doses per day of *Cannabis Indica*.

Neurasthenia-with depression—The *Anacardium.* patient is found mostly among the neurasthenics. Depression and impaired memory ; diminution of senses (smell, sight and hearing), syphilitics often suffer with these conditions. (*Anac.*). It is also useful in such cases due to weak digestion or nervous dyspepsia. See "Depression-low spirited and unsocial".

Neurasthenia-after sexual excess or nervous prostration, brain fag or exhaustion—After sexual excesses. Despair anxiety ; fear and peevishness from above cause. (*Agn.*). See "Sexual—neurasthenia. and always dwelling on sexual subjects".

Neurotic patient—These patients have no actual disease and are not really ill but they find it very difficult to live in normal life and are often afraid of tackling a job. They think they suffer from many symptoms of diseases. But there are often so many complaints that it is desirable to give a low potency of a remedy like *Coffea* or *Lycopodium* to help the sleeplessness or *Argentum nitricum*, to the patient who dares not go shopping alone ;

Aurum 6, can be given if the patient is depressed, and *Natrum muriaticum 6*, if the patient feels resentful that life has not treated him well. Compare *Coffea* for sleeplessness as suggested by Dr. M.A. Alient.

Neuritis in retro-bulbar area—Inflammation of nerve situated behind the eyeball. According to Dr. Norton *Arsenic* seems specially adapted to loss of vision.

Neuritis in stump (inflammation of nerve)—*All-c.* has marvellous power on such affection often met with in a stump after amputation or serious injury. The pains are almost unbearable, rapidly exhausting the strength of the patient. (*All-c.*) See "Stump neuritis" also "Amputation neuritis".

Night-aggravation—Aggravation at night is characteristic of Merc-sol. The pain increases at night. Perspiration without relief and profuse salivation. (*Merc-sol.*). See "Perspiration without any relief."

Night blindness—(1) *Bell*, 4 hourly.

(2) or *Hellebours* niger.

(3) *Lyco.* is the best remedy for night blindness. Sudden blindness with cutting pains. If it fails then *China-off.* should be tried.

(4) *Phys.* with or without glaucoma or myopia.

(5) If it is accompained by quivering or jerking then *Hyos.*

(6) Night blindness though the patient can see well during the day. (*Ran-b.*). See "Blindness" also "Night blindness" "Vision-different troubles".

Nightmares—Nightly raving. Nocturnal furious delirium. (*Acon.*). See "Delirium" and "Dreams".

Nightmares (dream characterised by great distress and sense of oppression and suffocation and sleeping with mouth open and eyes half closed)—(*a*) When due to indiscretion in diet (*Nux-v.*). (*b*) (*i*) When not traceable to obvious cause *Kali brom.* at bed-time (*ii*) *Paeonia* 1, 4 hour. (*c*) Fears to go to sleep lest she would die, sense of suffocation.

(*Ledum*). (*d*) In heart diseases. (*Am-c*). (*e*) In spermatorrhoea. (*Dig-s*). See also "Dreams" and "Insomnia". (*f*) Deep snoring, sleep with eyes half closed with mouth open. The respiration is nearly suspended. Cold perspiration. (*Op.*). (*g*) Cries and moans in sleep when there is derangement in the digestive functions by eating rich, fat food, cakes, nuts or meat. (*Puls.*). (*h*) Irritable and vindictive. Shocks in body and jerking in limbs during sleep. Sleep unrefreshing, many fantastical, anxious and frightful dreams, mouth putrid. (*Nit-ac*). (*i*) Difficult breathing. Breath foul. Wakes frightened at night, looks ghastly and shrieks. (*Ter.*) (*j*) People who are plagued with recurring dreams of throwing themselves from great height are relieved of their painful nightmares after taking *Thuja* as recommended by Dr. Banerjee. See "Sleeplessness-emotions disturbing" and "Mouth open in sleep".

Night-pollution—See "Emissions-nightly" and "Sleeplessness" under their different heads.

Night sweats—(*a*) With hectic fever of drenching night sweat with no thirst in fever. (*Abrot.*). Compare *Acetic acid*. See "Hectic fever". (*b*) In consumption with moist and coated tongue., *Baptis*. 2 hourly and with dry tongue *Ars*. 2 hourly. Compare *Pilocarpine*. See also "Sweat in fever" for Tubercular sweats, see "No. 16 of Tuberculosis" and "Chest-violent cough with might sweat".

Night walking—Gets up while asleep; walks about and lies down again. (*Sil.*). See also "Somnambulism".

Night-watching causing ill-effects—(1) If sitting up at night is always debilitating and produces greater weakness than usual. (*Phos-a.*).

(2) The mouth is dry, loathing of food, belching, nausea with faintness. The patient is sad and starts in sleep. (*Coc.*).

(3) When body and soul appear worn-out due to want of sleep and there is sensation of heat in the head and the patient is despondent. (*Cuprum.*)

Nipple-atrophy also cracked and ulcerated—(1) Nipples burn in mothers who have given newly birth to a child. (*Sulf.*).

(2) Nipples sore or cracked. Paint *Hamamelis M.T.*, rub gently *Graphites ointment*. Internally give *Ratanhia* 6th potency. It is also useful for ulcerated nipples. See also "Sore nipple inflammatory threating abscess" and "Atrophy of nipple and breast".

Nipples-retracted—Nipples are soft, they are retracted and can't be made to come out. Retraction of nipples is a suspicious sign, though there is no tumour.

Nodes (a hard swelling on bones and abnormal out-growth of bones)—(1) On bones of the skull. (*Kali-bic.*).

(2) Out-growth of bone. (*Cal-flour*). Compare *Rhus-tox*.

(3) Out-growth of long bones. (*Phos.*). See also "Bones-an abnormal out-growth".

Noise-frightening and disturbing—A little noise frightens and disturbs him. (*Nux-v.*). See "No. 2 of Fright".

Nose-abscess—*Aurum met. 200* is a good medicine. Dr. Kent recommends *Hep. sulph* 9x, thrice daily according to age.

Nose-adenoids—(1) The treatment should start with *Bacillinum 200* every fortnight. No other medicine to be given on the day of its administration for two days before and two days after it.

(2) For thin and weak children with tonsils. (*Calcarea-phos.*).

(3) For fat and pale children with perspiring head at night. (*Calc-carb.*).

(4) An excellent remedy for adenoids. (*Agraphisnutans* 3x potency).

(5) Another remedy is *Merc-iod.* for adenoids.

(6) In very obtinate cases when other medicines fail then the practice of giving *Sulph.*, *Calc-c.*, *Lyco.*, and *Sil.* one after

the other is most efficient course. See also "Catarrh of nose" under its different heads and also "Adenoid growth".

Nose-bleeding—(1) Bleeding of nose with red face. Nose red and swollen. (*Bell.*).

(2) Recurrent bleeding without appreciable cause. (*Ferrum-phos.*).

(3) *Millefolium* is another remedy without knowing the cause. Note :—In all such bleedings *Hamamelis M.T.* on cotton plug be kept in nostrils. See also "Epistaxis (nose bleed)".

Nose-bleeding while blowing—Bleeding from nose while blowing. Bleeding in children is very often cured with a dose of *Phos.* especially when there is small quantity of fresh blood wnenever the child blows his nose. Bleeding from nose instead of menses between periods. (*Phos.*). See "Catarrh of nose while blowing." and "No. 5 of Pharangitis due to silver nitrate and constant desire to blow nose".

Nose-bleeding-instead of menses—Bleeding from nose when menses should occur. Swelling of the tip of nose. Aggravation by movement. (*Bry.*). See "Menstruation-bleeding from nose or lungs".

Nose-bleeding in morning—Copious bleeding from nose and other orifices mostly in the morning. Dry blood gathers in nose. (*Ambra.*). See "Bleeding copious".

Nose-bleeding when washing—When washing face or hands. The blood does not easily coagulate and is dark in colour. Dried blood gathered in nose. (*Am-c.*). See "Bleeding-dark does not easily coagulate".

Nose-block on lying—(*a*) The nose blocks on lying specially in night. Feeling of dryness. Discharge scanty and excoriating. Crust and elastic plugs. Patient breathes through mouth. (*Lyco.*). (*b*) Nose of infant blocked. Cannot breathe, crying for expiring. *Sambucus* night and morning. See "Catarrh-of nose block" and "Infants nose blocked".

Nose-diseased bone of nose red tipped and pain—(1) Bones swollen. Hawks mucus from nostrils. Boggy mucous membrane of nose. (*Merc-b.-iodalus.*).

(2) Pain in nose. (*Rheum*).

(3) Redness of tip of nose. (*Silica*).

Nose-dripping while eating—Fluent discharge from nose. As soon as a man starts eating his nose begins to drip. (*Trombidium.*). See "Discharge offensive"

Nose-nasal dermatitis—Pimply, scaly nasal dermatitis ; extending upto cheek ; appearing as facial acne. The patient had obstinate constipation. The pimples of the nose and face used to get little white mattery beads and the patient was revaccinated. (*Thuja 30x* and later on *Thuja 100*).

Nose-picking—Picking at the nose constantly until it bleeds. *Arum. triph*.

Nose-perforation—*Kali Bich.*

Nose-polypi—(1) Polypi in nose with offensive odour (*Calc-c.*)

(2) *Lemna-minor* is head remedy for polypus.

(3) *Thuja* 30 internally and mother tincture locally.

(4) For stoppage of nose. (Teucrium.).

(5) When due to enlargement of nasal bone. (*Lemna minor.*). See "Polypi in nose with discharge" and "Polypus covering nostril".

Nose-red tipped—In drunkards. Red nose as if frost bitten. (*Agar.*). See also "Drunkenness".

Nose-septum ulcerated—Fetid smell discharge thick, violent sneezing, loss of smell, inflammation extending to frontal sinuses. (*Kali bich.*). See "Septum-ulcerated".

Nose - smell—(*a*) Fetid smell in nasal catarrh. (*Sil.*) (*b*) Fetid smell in cold of long standing (*Mer-sol.*). (*c*) Putrid smell with watery discharge. (*Kali-bi*). (*d*) Loss of smell on account of catarrh. (*Puls.* and *Nat-mur.*). (*e*) Impairment of smell with sore throat. (*Merc-cor.*). (*f*) Smell disminished in typhoid fever. (*Argentum-nit.*). (*g*) Loss of smell on account latent syphilis, chronic catarrh etc. (*Aurum-met.*). See also "Catarrh of nose" under different heads "Smell-sensitiveness" "Ozaena" and "Odour from nose and mouth".

Nose stopped when going out—The nose is stopped due to cold and cough. Every time the patient goes out in fresh or cold air the nose runs. Extremely sensitive to cold air. Cold air causes sneezing or running of nose. (*Hep.*). See also "Stoppage of nose of newborn", "Coryza-stopping of nose and sneezing" and "Cold after exposure"

Nose children scratching in acute diseases—Tingling sensation in mucous membrane of the mouth and nose. Children when they are suffering from acute diseases they scratch and pinch their lips and bore into the nose even when they are bleeding from scratching. This has been a guiding symptom in acute disaeses like typhoid, scarlet fever and other low type of continued fever conditions with delirium, excitement and maniacal manifestations. The tingling itching sensation must be so intense that the pain of bleeding is not felt. Acrid discharge from nose. Along with this excoriating discharge, the glands of the neck and even the parotid (situated near the ear), may be inflamed and are sore (*Arum-t.*). See "Itching of nose" and "Boring into the nose".

Nose-septum ulcerated Fetid smell. Discharge thick, ropy; Tough elastic plugs from nose, leave a raw surface (*Kali-bi. 30* attenuation and higher).

Nose-depression—When middle of nose becomes depressed, discharge is offensive, mixed with pus and blood. (*Kali-bichromicum*).

Nose-syphilitic—*Aurum-met.* is full of nasal troubles, with foetid discharge. The bones of the nose necrosed the nose flattens down. A few remedies have the power of curing these syphilitic nose-conditions. *Aurum-met.*, *Mercury* and *Hepar* are three of them. See "Syphilitic complications of nose throat and palate" and "Ozena".

Nose-watering with irritation in eyes—Watering both from nose and eyes but irritation in the eyes and not in the nose. (*Euphr.*). Compare *Allium cepa* if there is irritation in the nose but the eyes have no irritarion and simply water. See "Throat infection with running nose" and "Eyes watering with redness".

Nose watering-causing rawness—(*a*) Watering ; a watery discharge drips from the nose constantly, burns like fire and excoriates the upper lips and wings of nose until there are redness and rawness. (*All-c.*). (b) *Nux-v. 3* may prevent a cold if given early before the commencement of the running of nose Compare *Acon.* See "Watering from nose" and "Allergy catarrh".

Nose-child boring fingers in worms—The child very often bores the fingers in the nose and grinds teeth while asleep. He is very restless while sleeping. Jumps and jerks in sleep. Frequent swallowing as if something is coming up in the throat. This combination is very peculiar in *Cina* alone. *Cina* also itches nose but that is more nervous than congestive. It has no excoriating discharge from the nose. (*Cina*) Compare *Arum-t.* which has excoriating discharge. See "Worms" and "Finger boring during sleep".

Nosodes—Nosodes are remedies derived from morbid tissues and secretions containing the specific virus of diseases. The importance of these remedies is daily becoming more recognised. The nosodes should be used according to symptoms and not according to the disease. They have a particular influence in chronic and rebellious affections where there is a lack of reaction to curative measures. It is not possible in a book like this to specify all of them here. A few only, those which are frequently used besides others in my practice are mentioned.

(1) **Adrenalin**—It is most powerful and prompt astringent and haemostatic (to stop haemorrhage) an invaluable remedy in capillary haemorrhage from all parts of body *e.g.* nose, ear, mouth, throat, larynx, stomach, rectum, uterus, bladder ; in asthma and arteriosclerosis ; also in acute congestion of

lungs. Dr. Jousset reports success in treating angina, abdominal pain and heart failure during anaesthesia.

(2) **Ambra Grisea**—Adapted to hysterical subjects or those suffering from special irritation. Also for patients weakened by age or overwork, who are anaemiea and sleepless. Great remedy for the aged with impairment of all functions, weakness, coldness and numbness. One sided complaints call for it. Cramps in hands, fingers worse grasping anything.

(3) **Anthracinum**—Useful in septic inflammation, carbuncles and malignant ulcers. Glands swollen, cellular tissues oedamatous and indurated. Septicemia, ulceration, sloughing and intolerable burning, black and blue blisters.

(4) **Bacillinum**—Successful employed in the treatment of tuberculosis. It is specially indicated for lungs of old people with chronic catarrhal condition. Suffocative catarrh. Constant disposition to take cold.

(5) **Bacillus Coli**—(1) It is useful in coli infection.

(2) Puerperal-sepsis and chronic diarrhoea after delivery when fever is present. 30 to 200 potencies are useful.

(6) **Cantharis**—Attacks urinary and sexual organs. Intolerable constant urging to urinate is most characteristic. Gastric derangements of pregnancy. Acute mania of amorous type. Palpitation. Secondary eczema about scrotum and genitals following excessive perspiration.

(7) **Cholesterinum**—It is useful in obstinate hepatic engorgements (hyperaemia), and excessive amount of blood in a part usually with local oedema. According to Dr. Swan it is almost a specific for gall-stone colic : relieves the distress at once. Dr. Ameke claimed to heve to drived great advantage from its use in cases diagnosed as cancer of the liver, or in such obstinate engorgement that malignancy suspected. Burnett, claims to have twice cured cancer of the liver with it in condition when the diagonosis is in doubt, specially if the patient has been subjected to repeated attacks of biliary colic, *cholesterinum,*

Burnett claims, is very satisfactory and at times its action is very timely.

(8) **Diphtherinum**—Useful in diphtheria, post diphtheritic paralysis. Malignancy from the very start. Adapted to patients prone to catarrhal affections of respiratory organs.

(9) **Electricitas**—Every medical man knows the extreme susceptibility of some persons to the electric fluid, and the suffering they experienced on the approach of and during a thunder storm, or the contact of electric current. The medicine is useful in such cases like anaxiety, nervous tremors, restlessness, palpitation, headache, and approach of thunder storm.

The potencies are prepared from milk sugar which has been saturated with current.

Electricity should not be used nor electro-thermal baths taken when suffering from a cold if chest is involved as fatal results have followed. (*Dr. H.C. Allen.*).

(10) **Electricity**—It is useful for weeping, timid, fearful patient. It is indicated when a person dreads at the approach of thunder storm and suffers mental torture before and during electric-storm, also for involuntary hysterical laughter, dim-sightedness, blindness, incontinence of urine, asthma alongs. life, with palpitation of the heart and disposition to faint and for paralysis of arms.

(11) **Insulin** —This pancreatic harmone plays an important part in the process of sugar, metabolism.

(1) It is indicated in chronic intestinal disorder with loose bowels with enlarged liver.

(2) Ulcers, boils, bed-sores.

(3) Intractable eczema in patient with chronic liver trouble.

(4) Suppuration of the glands in the neck. 30th potency is preferable.

(5) In diabetes mellitus, the blood sugar is maintained while normal liver urine remains free of sugar.

(12) **Lac-caninum (dog's milk)**—It is of great value is sore throat, diphtheria and rheumatism when erratic pains alternating sides It has decided effect in drying up milk who can't nurse the baby. It is indicated in stiffness of neck and tongue. Menses too early, profuse, flow in gushes. Sciatica right sided. (Dr. W. Boericke).

(13) **Lac Felinum (Cat's milk)**—Great depression of spirits. Dr. Swan had a great success with it in eye cases where there is severe pain in back of orbit, indicating choroiditis (inflammation of choroid). It is also useful in ciliary (pertaining to eyelids) neuralgia, photophobia, asthenopia and dysmenorrhoea.

(14) **Lac vaccinum (Cow's milk)**—Headache, rheumatic pains, constipation ; and also for piercing pain in each hip joint.

(15) **Lac vaccinum coagulatum (Curds)**—Nausea of pregnancy.

(16) **Lac vaccinum floc (Cream)**—Diphtheria, leucorrhoea, menorrhagia, dysphagia.

(17) **Magnetis polus australis**—South pole of the magnet—Severe pain in inner side of nail of the big toe, ingrowing toenail, easy dislocation of joints of foot.

(18) **Malandrinum** (The grease of horses) – Great difficulty in remembering what was read. Gums swollen, ulcerated, receding from teeth : bleed easily when touched ; unable to brush at the teeth from sour and bleeding gums. Profuse foot sweat with carrion like odour. Probhylactic of small pox. A remedy for ill effects of vaccination causing eczema.

(19) **Malaria officinalis**.—Dizziness on rising from reading position. Frequent attacks of headache.

Eyes weak, blurring, reading difficult. Can't eat anything ; vomits everything. Intermittent : quotidian ; tertian fevers.

(20) **Morgan Co. (Bach)**—Is a bowel nosode and is found very useful in chronic gastritis, general congestion in the

pelric organs or defects of circulation—oedema and congestion of the feet and many of the skin complaints. (*Dr. M.G. Blackie*).

(21) **Medorrhinum**—Useful in ailments due to suppressed gonorrhoea. Children dwarfed and stunted. Oedema of limbs, chronic rheumatism. Violent pain in liver and spleen. Rests more comfortably lying on back. Weak memory. Impotence, sterility. Time passes too slowly with suicidal thought.

(22) **Naja**—Its action settles around heart : valvular troubles. Control of sphincter lost. Diseases primarily depending upon degeneration of cells. Irritating cough dependent on cardiac lesions. Threatened paralysis of heart, body cold, pulse slow, weak, irregular, tremulous. Damaged heart after infectious diseases.

(23) **Pituitary**—It is an extract of the posterior lobe of the pituitary gland. It is indicated in strangulated hernia, asthma, delayed puberty, and precordial pain. 30 potency would be suitable.

(24) **Sepsin**—Drs. Swan and Shedd introduced this by potentising it from septic pus and Proteus vulgaris. It is employed in typhoid, septic conditions in all froms *e.g.* septicaemia following abortions, ptomaine, gas poisoning, offensive diarrhoea and pulse abnormally rapid also post operative case with overwhelming sepsis.

(25) **Staphylococcin**—It is indicated in chronic cases of dysentery with discharge of blood and pus, and also in acne, abscess.

(26) **Streptococcin**—It is indicated with remarkable result in acute bacillary blood dysentery with temperature and toxemia. with septic symptoms in infections disease.

(27) **Sycotic Co**.—It is an important bowel nosode, it is indicated in recurring bladder infection. Very useful in chronic and recurring cystistis. (Inflammation of bladder).

(28) **Tuberculinum**—It is of undoubted value in the treatment of incipient (beginning) tuberculosis. Of great value also in epilepsy, neurasthenia and in nervous children. When

symptoms are constantly changing and well-selected remedies fail to improve and cold is taken from the slightest exposure. Chronic eczema, crops of small boils. To be used in all skin troubles along with *Syphilinum*.

(29) **Thyroidinum**—Goitre. Rheumatoid arthritis. Effective in undescended testicles in boys. Mammary tumour, uterine fibroid. Fibroid tumours of the breast. Has a powerful action in various types of oedema. Excessive obesity.

(30) **Ustilago Maydis (Corn-smut)**—Melancholia ; depression of spirits ; nervous headache from menstrual irregularities in nervous women ; falling of the hair and nails ; complete alopecia, not a hair on the head. Tendency to small boils.

(31) **Vaccininum**—Whooping cough. Inveterate skin eruptions, chilliness, indigestion with great flatulent distension. Frontal headache. Inflamed and red eyelids.

(32) **X-Ray**—Mental processes not clear, writes wrong words and letters. Sexual desire lost in man. Palpitation during evening causing cough. Sterility, anaemia and leukemia".

Nostrils—cracked—*Anthrok,* See "Finger cracks".

Numbness in feet staggering while walking—Numbness in fingers and soles of feet. Patient staggers while walking. Finger movements awkward. Cannot pick up small object. Pains coursing through limb and back. (*Alumina 200*). See "Sleeping-of limb pressure while lying down".

Numbness-of head with pain—Numbness is a great feature of *Asaf.* Numbness of the scalp or deep in the head, numbness here and there and numbness may be associated with pain. It has chronic movement. (*Asaf.*) See "Head".

Numbness or insensibility of nerves in different parts of body—(1) Sudden and complete loss of sensibility. (*Hydr-ac.*).

(2) Numbness of back and limbs. Numbness and sensation of swelling in ball of thumb. (*Ox-ac.*).

(3) Feeling as if ants crawling in the extremities deep in the muscles and the skin. Crawling in paralysed parts.(*Carb-s.*).

(4) Diminished sensibility of all parts, feeble circulation, soreness, music intolerable. (*Ambra.*).

(5) Limbs benumbed with paralysis. Numbness of whole body, coldness, of hands (*Cicuta-virosa.*). See "Paralysis" under its different heads.

(6) Parts cold and blue ; dead feeling as if frozen. (*Agar.*).

(7) Numbness of fingers and pricking of tips. Numbness insensibility and coldness, crawling sensation, worse by heat. Fingers and feet bluish or bent backwards and numb. (*Sec.*).

(8) Numbness of hands and fingers ; contraction of tendons on waking up in the morning in patients who are loquacious and worse during night or early morning and improved as the day went on. Worse by heat and after sleep. (*Lach.*).

(9) Numbness of hands and soles of feet. (*Raph.*).

(10) Numb feeling over whole of body. (*Con.*).

(11) Numbness in the forearms at night time. (*Arg-n.*).

(12) Numbness of left arm : Cactus, Aching, *Acon* .

(13) Numbness of tongue, lips and nose which come in connection which chronic soreness of liver, derangement of digestion such as biliousness : (*Nat-mur*). See "Nervous diseases" and "Rheumatic troubles with numbness crawling feeling."

Numbness, feeble circulation and sleeping of limbs—Numbness on different spots. Feeble circulation and numbness Limbs go to sleep on slightest pressure ; arms go to sleep when lying down. (*Ambra.*). See "Pressure-causes sleeping of limbs" and "Sleeping of limb pressure while lying down".

Numbness-with pain neuralgic and in rheumatism—There is numbness with pain. This holds good in cases of rheumatism and neuralgic pains. If therefore, there is numbness with over-sensitiveness for pain and peevish temper think of *Chammomilla*.

Nursing with falling of hair—Falling-off of the hair while nursing. *Sulf*, *Lyco.* or *Calcarea*. (Dr. C. Herring.). See "Hair" under different heads and "Falling out of hair".

Nymphomania (excessive sexual desire in women) with ovarian trouble and sexual delirium—(*a*) Excessive sexual desire specially in virgins, premature or excessive development of sexual instinct. Ovarian trouble and prolapsus with the profuse menses and excessive sensitiveness of the genitals, cannot bear to be touched. *Platina* is a head remedy for this trouble in women before and after delivery. (*b*) Almost uncontrollable sexual desire. (*Murex-purpurea.*). (*c*) Sexual delirium, talks about lewed subject, excessive menstrual flow. (*Stram.*) (*d*) Irritable condition of organs with congestion. (*Gratiola.*) (*e*) According to Dr. Nash the two other remedies namely, *Lilium* and *Platina* must be remembered in connection with Nymphomania. See "Excessive sexual desire".

—: o :—

O

Obesity—(*a*) Tendency to obesity specially in children and young people. Fat and flabby patient. Enlarged lymphatic glands specially in the neck (*Calc-c.*). If this fails then *Fucus—Vesiculos*us. (*b*) For peculiar tendency to obesity Dr. Nash recommends *Graphites*. See "Fat" and "Fat patient—tendency to obesity".

Obesity during menopause—*Graphites* which increases the menstrual flow if menopause is premature.

Obesity-general—(1) *Phyt.* If it fails to do good after a month's trial then *Am-bro.*

(2) Obesity in young people (*Ant-c*).

(3) Obesity—after abdominal operation—*Calc. carb*.

(4) Obesity in young people—*Antim crud.*

(5) Obesity—*Blatta orientalis* is most serviceable in stout and corpulent patient. See "Pet Animals".

Obstetric table—If the number of the day of the month on which the last menstruation occurred, is added to the date mentioned in the following table against the said month the expected date of labour is obtained :—

Month in which last menstruation occurred.	Expected date of labour-day of the month added to
January	October 7.
February	November 7.
March	December 5.
April	January 4.
May	February 4.
June	March 7.
July	April 6.
August	May 7.
September	June 7.
October	July 7.
November	August 7.
December	September 6.

Suppose last menstruation occurred on 20th January then the expected date of labour is 27th October.

Obstinate—(1) Obstinate children ; will not do things when asked to do. (*Cham.*).

(2) Obstinate children inclined to grow fat. (*Calc-carb.*).

(3) Resists wishes of others. (*Nux-vom.*).

(4) For excessively obstinate child give *Tuberculine* 30 or 200 potency. See "Child unmanageable" and "Weeping-child pretending".

Odour-flowers—Very sensitive to odour of flowers. (*All-c.*). See "Smell-sensitiveness" and "Odour strong things".

Odour-mouth—There is a bad odour from the mouth in *Lach.* and there may be abundant accumulation of tenacious mucus in the mouth. (*Lach.*). Compare *Merc-sol.* ; *Kali-carb.* See "Mouth offensive and raw".

Odour-from nose and mouth—(1) From mouth and the nose fetid odour comes. Face dark, great prostration. (*Ail.*).

(2) Bad odour from mouth after dinner, sour smelling breath. (*Nux-v.*).

(3) Like carion. (*Pyrogen.*). See "Mouth offensive odour and swollen gums" and "Nose smell".

Odour-offensive of body—(1) Offensive odour of body despite washing and bathing. (*Sulf.* or *Psor.*).

(2) Offensive with perspiration. (*Merc-sol.*).

(3) Like garlic. (*Phos*). See "Feet offensive" and "Perspiration offensive of body".

Odour-strong things—The patient cannot bear strong odour of any drug, petroleum, phenyle etc. Strong odours make him faint. (*Nux-v.*). See "Smell-sensitiveness" and "Odour flowers"

Oedema-face and lips—Pale and anaemic in look. Bloating of face. The bloating is all round the eyes or all over the face. (*Phos.*) Compare *Kali-carb.* and *Apis.* In the former bloating of upper lip and in the latter bloating of the lower lip. See also "Bloating".

Oedema-of different parts due to different causes—(1) In heart diseases due to hypertrophy of heart. (*Ars-alb.*).

(2) With diarrhoea in nephritis with anaemia. (*Phos.*).

(3) With debility and anaemia. (*China.*).

(4) From congestion of kidneys, with kidney affections, prostration. (*Tereb*).

(5) With albuminuria ; with intermittent fever ; from disease of liver or spleen. (*Aur-mur.*).

(6) Oedema of limbs and face without any apparent cause. (*Thyroidine.*).

(7) Acute dropsical swellings with suppression of urine. (*Scilla*).

(8) Oedema due to complete failure of kidney, which stops secreting urine. No urine passed on account of stopping of functioning of the kidney. Give *Vesicaria* in one drachm dose of mother tincture.

(9) Oedema of legs during pregnancy. The best remedy. (*Bry.* then *Sulph.*).

(10) Oedema of penis, vulva and about the mouth. (*Rhus-tox.*).

(11) Oedema of the lungs. Frothly expectoration is found in oedema of the lungs and may occur in Brights disease. The medicine cures the consumption also. (*Kali-hydroiodicum*).

(12) Oedema of left hand, foot and leg (*Cactus grandiflorus*).

(13) Oedema general or local ; face, ears, lower eyelids, genitals ; general anasarca, abdomen. (*Apis mellifica*). See "Penis" and "Vulva" and "Bloating's and swelling" under their respective different heads.

Oesophagus hysterical—Lump in the throat or suffocation is a sort of hysterical spasm of the aesophagus. (*Asaf.*). See also "Hysteria fainting".

O

Offensive foot sweat—*Calc-c.* Compare *Sil.* See also "Feet offensive" and "Smell foul of body".

Old age and its related symptoms—(*a*) A man of middle age looks and shows symptoms of old age. Also for patients weakned by age or over-work, who are anaemic and sleepless. *Ambra.* is a great remedy for the aged with the impairment of all functions, weakness, coldness and numbness usually of single parts : fingers, arms, etc. One sided complaints call for it. Feebleness and foregetfulness. (*Ambra.*). Compare *Baryta carb.*

(*b*) Dr. Hard suggests *Thiosinaminum-Rhodallin* for retarding old age with gastric, vesicle and rectal crises, arterio-sclerotic vertigo and deafness due to some fibrous change in the nerve. It will hold off senility, dose 2x attenuation B.D. (2) *Lycopodium* is another classic homoeopathic remedy for decrepitude common to old age. (3) Weakness of body and mind ; trembling and palpitation ; unable to sustain any mental work. Night cough and moroseness. (*Conium maculatum* 6th potency). (4) *Urtica urens* tincture will renew the strength in old age. See "Weakness—premature old age with impaired functions".

Old age-from excesses—Broken down constitution from sexual excesses and secret vices. Despair and anxiety. Pale and sickly. (*Ail*). Compare *Orchitinum* a testicular extract. See also "Senile decay" and "Sexual weakness".

One sided complaints—Complaints one sided very often. Perspiration on one side of body or on the affected side only. Pain in one side of head if hair is touched, or some spots, over-sensitive to touch on one side of body. (*Ambra*). See "Perspiration-one sided" and "Complaints one sided".

Onychia - inflammation of the nail matrix (mould)—(1) Affections of finger nails specially if white spots on nails. In growing toe nails. (*Sil.*).

(2) Eruption around finger nails. (*Psor.*). For open laceration and cut with much damaged skin apply *Calendula*

and aslo give *Calendula* internally. (*Calendula*). See also "Nails" under different heads.

Operation-collapse—(*a*) Collapse symptoms after a surgical operation, coldness of body, cold breath and profuse perspiration, will require *Strontium carb.* It relieves shock at once, and the patient gets warm and comfortable. (*Stront-c.*). (*b*) A single dose of high potency of *Phosphorus* given a day before abdominal operation will prevent nausea and other distress after operation. See also "Shock of operation-collapse" and "Chloroform".

Operation-after it urine retention—*Causticum* is to prevent the retention of urine after an operation. This is often quickly effective and will obviate the use of Catheter or when there is cramp in the rectum on trying to pass water after operation. Its use often prevents anti-biotics after surgery.

Opium-eating habit— ill-effects of opium eating habit. (*Verat.*). See "Morphia-habit".

Opium - ill - effects of tabacco and causing tobacco heart—Opium and its ill-effects ; bad effects of opium eating and tobacco-chewing. Tobacco heart from chewing tobacco. (*Verat.*). See "Tobacco habit" and "Morphia habit and how to get over it".

Optic-atrophy—(1) Atrophy of retina with intense pain on attempting to use the eyes, intolerance of light, wrose in the morning (*Nux-v.*).

(2) Atrophy of optic nerve with cataract. (*Phos.*).

(3) When due to paralysis of vision nerve. (*Bor.*).

(4) Dr. Blackwood says that *Santoninum* is highly serviceable in charoditis and atrophy of the optic nerve and Amblyopia (dimness of vision not due to refrative errors or organic disease of the eye, it may be congenital or acquired).

The following treatment is found benificial ;

(1) Give *Phos. 200* in first week for 3 days.

(2) *Nux-vom. 200* for first three days of second week.

(3) *Argentum nit 200* for first three days of 3rd week.

(4) *Carboneum sulphuratum 200* for first three days of 4th week. No medicine to be given in remaining 4 days of the week.

Optic-nerve sclerosis of the optic nerve—(1) *Phos. 3, 2* hours.

(2) *Strychnin, nitricum 3x,* 2 hours.

(3) *Carb.-sulf. 30,* 4 hours. (*b*) For atrophy of optic nerve, optic disc. pale arteries and veins congested. (*Carb-sulph.*) 1st attenuation. According to Dr. Blackwood *Santoninum* is reported to be highly serviceable in choroiditis (inflammation of choroid) and atrophy of the optic nerve and amblyopia (dimness of vision). See "Hemiopia"

Optic neuritis—(1) In the first stage—*Apis 3x* 2 hours.

(2) *Caraboneum sulphuratum 30.*

(3) Secondary inflammatory changes effusion, (*Arsen.*).

(4) To arrest atrophy. (*a*) *Phos.* 4 hourly. (*b*) *Nux-vom.* 2 hourly. See also "Eye-troubles" and "Vision"

Oral contraceptive—Three doses of *Nat-mur.* 200x taken by women on the first, second and third day after the cessation of monthly course, produces such reactions that fertilisation during the month becomes unlikely. These doses must be repeated after every menses till conception is not desired. See "Birth control".

Orchitis (inflammation of testicles)—(1) Gonorrhoeal orchitis, or that brought on from cold, where the testical is as hard as a stone and very painful. (*Clematis-erecta.*).

(2) Orchitis of right side with pain extending to abdomen and scrotum. (*Merc-c.*).

(3) Testicles hard and drawn up also inflammed. (*Bell.*).

(4) Swelling of spermatic cord and testicles with pain and tenderness. (*Spongia.*).

(5) As an intercurrent medicine give alternate fortnightly (*Phytolacca 200*) and *Aurum-met 200*. No medicine to be given 3 days before and 3 days after it. See "Hydrocele".

Orchitis (inflammation of testicle pain transferred)—(1) Inflammation of testicles. Gonorrhoea pains transferred to testicles. (*Puls.*).

(2) Testicles enlarged and very hard as a result of injuries (*Conium*). See also "Testicles and its different troubles".

Otalgia-pain—See "Chapter V for details".

Otitis (inflammation of ear)—(1) Inflammation of ear discharge putrid like putrid meat, from ear granulation : polpi creaking when swelling. (*Thuj.*).

(2) When external ear is swollen, red, violent pain and itching and sometimes closure of the whole external canal. Drs. Jousset and Farrington recommended *Puls.* and if *Puls.* does not help then *Merc-sol.* should be tried.

(3) The pus is thin, offensive, long lasting and the canal is sensitive to touch. *Tellurium* is an excellent remedy in otitis media (*Tell.*).

(4) *Kali-mur.* is one of the most useful remedies for inflammatory condition of the middle ear ; it seems to clear the eustachian tube which is closed in these cases. (*Kali-mur.*). See also "Ear inflammation" and "Ear" under latters different heads.

Otorrhoea offensive (discharge from the external auditory meatus)—Offensive. Mastoid disease with pain in temporal region with pushing out sensation. Burning in the ear with discharge of foetid pus and stitching in the ear from within out (of syphilitic origin). (*Asaf.*). See also "Mastoid", "Ear discharge syphilitic" and "Discharge offensive".

Otorrhoea (discharge from the external auditory meatus)—(*a*) Discharge from the external auditory meatus (opening). Both chronic and acute troubles particularly in children. Pus may be thick and greenish. Thirstlessness, heat feeling and restlessness relieved by slowly walking about in cold air. Hearing difficult as if the ears were stuffed. Discharge offensive. Diminishes acuteness of hearing. (*Puls.*).

(1) (*b*) *Chamomilla* is almost specific in infantile ear-ache.

(2) When discharge is caused by an abscess in the ear, perforation in the ear. (*Hep-s.*).

(3) In suppuration of middle ear with thin and acrid discharge specially in syphilitic ear condition. Hardness of hearing due to swollen tonsils. (*Mercurius.*).

(4) *Baryta carbonica* for deafness associated with swelling of tonsils. Also in noises in ears from arterio-sclerotic conditions.

(5) Deafness following purulent or inflammatory otitis media. Dr. Dewey recommends *Kali-mur.* as the most valuable remedy for this.

(6) Discharge with glandular swelling (*Merc-s.*, *Puls.*).

(7) *Silicea* says Dewey, is the most frequent indicated remedy in persistent chronic discharge from ear. Dr. Moffat advises changing to *Lapis albus* after use of *Sil.* for too long a time.

(8) When there is horribly offensive discharge the *Psorinum* though ordinarily for foul odour of discharge, *Merc-s.* should be given. See also "Ear-inflammation *i.e.* otitis and discharge" under its different heads and "Deafness".

Ovary-pain in right ovary—Pain in right ovary running down thigh of that side. (*Podo.*). When there is severe pain without swelling then give *Naja*.

Ovary-fibrous body—For fibrous bodies in ovary. *Calcarea, Platina, Staphysagria* and *Thuja*. See also "Fibroma or fibroid tumour".

Ovary-pain with sweating—Pain in right ovary and all over the body. Patient restless and thirsty. Sweating and coldness. Pains even worse in seating condition. (*Merc-sol.*).

Ovarian-colic (right sided)—Ovarian colic, gripping pains relieved by bending double; stitching pains deep in right ovarian region. (*Colocynth.*). See "Uterine colic".

Ovarian-neuralgia—*Lach.* is a good remedy for disease of female generative organs. It is of use in simple ovarian neuralgia and from that the actual tumours or even cancer of the left ovary and also in uterine displacement of various kinds. The pain in ovary travels from left to right. (*Lach.*). See "Tumours in ovary with neuralgia" and "Uterine pains darting to sides".

Over-feeding of children—(1) To check vomiting accompained by purging give *Ip.*, if no relief then give *Puls.*

(2) Purging with discharge of undigested food and child already debilitated by diarrhoea. (*China.*).

(3) Vomiting accompained by constipation. (*Nux-vom.*). See "Diarrhoea-of children with nausea in summer", "Wakeful and restless infants" and "Improperely fed babies"..

Overlifting, mis-step and strains—(*a*) (*i*) If lifting or carrying heavy loads or any sudden exertion of strength produces pain in muscles. (*Rhus-t.*).

(*ii*) When on account of overlifting violent piercing pains are felt in the small of back, which becomes worse on every motion then give *Bry.*, if it fails then Sulf.

(*iii*) If due to this exertion headache is caused then give *Cal-c.* or *Rhus-t.*

(*b*) Mis-step—(*i*) Pains in the limbs will be relieved by Bry. or *Rhus.* (*ii*) If stomach is affected then *Puls.* (*iii*) *Symph.* may be used when the pain seems to remain within bones, in all above cases *Colbch, Merc-s., Calc-c.* and *Sulf.* may help a good deal when troubles due to above causes become chronic.

(*c*) Strains : When a person while wrestling or while climbing a high fence or tree overstrains himself and feels sick at the stomach then give *Verat-a*. See "Strains of muscle, tendon".

Over-sensitiveness—The patient is sensitive to touch ; he is sensitive to pain ; he is sensitive to cold air. The patient is so sensitive to pain that she faints away during pain even when the pain is not very intense. If there is inflammation or painful swelling or eruption on the skin they are so sensitive that patient cannot bear to have cold air blown on the surface. (*Hep*). Compare *China-off.* See also "Hypersensitiveness".

Over-strain and over-work—(1) Over-strain both bodily or mental. (*Cocc-i.*).

(2) Over-work. (*Bell-p.*). See "Fatigue corporeal or mental".

Oxaluria and infantile colic (Calcium oxalates and phosphates in urine)—(1) Urine cloudy, burning in urethra, hungry feeling not relieved by eating, starvation, constipation. Ulcerated mouth—3 to 5 drops thrice of *Nitro-muriatic acid.* Specific for this trouble.

(2) Infantile colic ; child seems to be full of wind, greenish mucus with pain. Loss of appetite. (*Senna.*). See "Urine albuminous and other casts" and "Colic infants".

Ozena (fetid nasal ulceration caries and foetid discharge)—(1) Syphilitic ozena. Ozena is a chronic disease of the nose accompanied by a foetid discharge. It is due to atrophic rhinitis, syphilitic ulceration or caries. Putrid old catarrh of the nose. (*Asaf.*). Compare *Aurum, Aurum mur.* and *Cadmium-sulph*. See "Nose-syphilitic".

(2) Deep seated destruction of the tissues with caries of nasal bone. (*Aurum-met.*).

(3) Ulcers in the nose with a thick gluey discharge. (*Merc-cor.*).

(4) Formation of scabs and cracks in wings of nose. (*Petroleum.*).

(5) With thick purulent, fetid discharge swelling at the root of nose and ulceration. (*Calc-c.*). See "Caries of nasal bones".

Tuberculinum may be given as an intercurrent remedy as sometimes the disease may be based on tuberculosis of the nose. See also "Nose-smell". Locally use Tr. *Hydrastinum muriaticum M.T*.

—: o :—

P

Pain including bone pains—See "Chapter V for details".
Pain-in abdomen—See "Chapter V for details".
Pains-in abdomen aftar meals—See "Chapter V for details".
Pain-abdominal burning and pain in thigh with digestive trouble—See "Chapter V for details".
Pain in gastric ulcer—See "Chapter V for details".
Pain in arthritis—See "Chapter V for details".
Pain-in asthma—See "Chapter V for details".
Pain in bachache—See "Chapter V for details".
Pain-in brain—See "Chapter V for details".
Pain in breast—If there is pain in both the breast with scanty menses. (*Conium.*). If it is in the right breast then give (*Sang.*). If it is on the left breast then give (*Cimic.*).
Pain in bilious colic—See "Chapter V for details".
Pain-colic like and shifting rheumatic pain—See "Chapter V for details".
Pain-in coccyx—See "Chapter V for details".
Pain-in acute cystitis—See "Chapter V for details".
Pain-dull at the injured part—See "Chapter V for details".
Pain-Hernia—See "Hernia pain".
Pains-flying along nerve—See "Chapter V for details".
Pain-in gallstone—See "Chapter V for details".
Pain-in hands—See "Chapter V for details".
Pain-in headache congestive—See "Chapter V for details".
Pain-in hips—See "Chapter V for details".
Pain-in groin—See "Chapter V for details".
Pains-lightning like—See "Chapter V for details".
Pains in pelvis—See "Chapter V for details".
Pain-in lumbago—See "Chapter V for details".
Pain-in menstrual colic—See "Chapter V for details".

Pain-in muco enteritis—See "Chapter V for details".

Pain-in the neck—See "Chapter V for details".

Pain-in acute nephritis—See "Chapter V for details".

Pain-in otolgia—See "Chapter V for details".

Pain-in Injury—See "Chapter VII for details".

Pain-in proctalgia—See "Chapter VII for details".

Pains-in the punctured wound—See "Chapter V for details".

Pain-in renal colic—See "Chapter VII for details".

Pain-in rheumatic-pain—See "Chapter VII for details".

Pain-in sciatica-See "Chapter VII for details".

Pain-in shoulder spine—See "Chapter VII for details".

Pain-in small joints—See "Chapter V for details".

Pain-in skin bones—See "Chapter V for details".

Pains in sprained joints with black blue appearances—See "Chapter V for details".

Pain in stiffneck—See "Chapter V for details".

Pain after stretches and surgical operation—See "Chapter V for details".

Pain-in right arm—See "Chapter V for details".

Pain and weakness of the tendon and muscle—See "Chapter V for details".

Pain in tetanus—See "Chapter V for details".

Pain in decayed teeth—See "Chapter V for details".

Pain in suppression of urine—See "Chapter V for details".

Pain-shaking the part or hanging it down gives relief—See "Chapter V for details".

Pain-in stomach after eating—See "Chapter V for details".

Pain-with swelling of joints spreading over large surface See "Chapter V for details".

Pains-wandering locating in heart—See "Chapter V for details".

Pain immediately after taking food—*Abies-nigra*.

Palms and head sweating—Sweat of palms and head specially) in chidren. (*Sil.*). See also "Burning palms" and "Sweat on head and hands in sleep".

Palms and soles sweating—Sweating on palms and soles, (*Calc.*). See "Sweat offensive foot".

Palpitation after eating at night with oppression—(1) At night after eating, with feeling of coldness and with restless oppression of chest. (*Calc.*).

(2) Palpitation of heart, awakens from sleep. (*Cannabis-indica.*). See "Heart palpitation and pain".

Palpitation-increased by walking—See "Heart-palpitation increased by walking".

Palpitation from noise and heart failure of aged—(1) Shock felt in heart from sudden noise. From eructations on coughing when lying on left side. Nervous palpitation. Aggravation in evening. (*Agar.*).

(2) Cardiac pain, heart failure of the aged. (*Strophanthus hispidus*). See "Heart-noise disturbs" and "Heart-block" and Cardiac asthma dyspnoea'.

Palpitation-shaking the body in anaemia—In every case of anaemia of *Nat-m.* there is lot of palpitation and uneasiness in the heart. Violent pulsation of heart which shakes the body. (*Nat-m.*). See "Anaemia" under its different heads.

Palpitation of heart with sweating irregular pulse and breathlessness—(1) *Am-c.* is good heart remedy in which there is a severe palpitation which the slightest motion aggravates and which is associated with great prostration. The complaints of this medicine come on at 3 o'clock at the morning with palpitation, prostration, cold sweats, dyspnoea, weakness of heart, almost pulseless. Face pale and cold. A single dose given high usually suffices to stop the palpitation. (*Am-c.*).

(2) Palpitation with irregular and intermittent pulse. (*Dig.*). See "Heart" and "Heart weak".

Palpitation audible throbbing during sleep with anaemia –(1) *Aesc.* is useful in persons who suffer from palpitation when the pulsation extends to the extremities and throbbing of heart in sleep can be heard ; an audible palpitation. (*Aesc.*).

(2) Palpitation due to dilated heart and anaemia. (*Strophanthus.*). See also "Heart and audible respiration".

Pancreatic troubles after, eating with nausea—(1) Intestinal indigestion ; pain an hour or more after eating. Liver sore. Nausea. Deficient appetite. (*Iris-vers.* tincture in high potency).

(2) Catarrh of pancreas ; haemorrhagic pancreatis (*Bell.*). Violent vomiting of sour substance with diarrhoea of foamy stool which contains fat. Losing flesh while eating well. (*Iodine*). See "Dyspepsia".

Palpitation—Violent and with congestion—Violent with anxiety or congestion to the chest and visible beating carotids and temporal arteries. (*Aur. met.*). See "Angina pectoris palpitation".

Paralysis-affecting memory—Easily excited and angered. Memory impaired. (*Arg-n.*). See "Memory" under its different heads and "Anger complaints".

Paralysis-caused by electricity—Shock introduced by terror and caused by electricity.

Paralysis-eyes due to exposure—Paralysis of ocular muscles after exposure to cold. (*Caust.* also *Conium.*).

Paralysis-gradually affecting—For ascending paralysis, *Conium mac.* whereas for descending one *Zinc. met.* and *Baryta carb,* be given. See "Exposure to cold" and "Neuralgia of face pain in nerves due to exposure".

Paralysis-of intestines bladder—Partial or complete. Peristaltic action is entirely suspended. No desire even for movement. The faces tie there, which have to be removed by enemas ; the urine also retained from paralysis of fundus of the bladder ;

involuntary urination or stool from paralysis of sphincters. (*Opium.*).

Paralysis of upper eye-lid of right side—In rheumatic subjects where the paralysis of ocular muscles causes headache. Lids seem heavy and there is inclination to close eyes. (*Caust.*). See "Eye-lids drooping".

Paralysis of upper lid of left side—Associated with rectal inertia and consequent constipation. *Alumn.* which is very useful in cold dry cases of granulations. See also "Eyes troubles" and "Eye-lids drooping".

Paralysis-face (left and right)—(1) Paralysis of left side face. Heat in face. Burning vesicles in corners of mouth and lips. (*Seneg.*).

(2) Paralysis of right side of face. (*Caust.*). See also "Facial paralysis".

Paralysis-left arm and leg—(1) Paralysis of left arm and left leg of the child ; paralysed muscles jerk in the sleep waking the child. Puts feet out of bed. Tearful when cannot have her own way. (*Caust.*).

(2) The legs are so heavy that patient can scarcely drag them. Weariness while sitting. (*Alumina.*). See "Gout long bones".

Paralysis-lower limbs in infancy—Lower limbs paralysed in infancy. Repeated catarrh of nose, pharynx. Leucorrhoea instead of menses. Face flushed. Sensitive to cold. (*Phos.*).

Paralysis-lower limbs in pregnancy and of bladder in old age—(1) Trembling and weakness or paralysis of lower limbs only. Paralytic-weakness in the lower limbs soon after becoming pregnant. (*Agar.*).

(2) Paralysis of the lower extremities. Paralysis of bladder in old men. (*Nux-v.*).

Paralysis of one side of body with unintelligible speech—(1) Specially in old men, mental and bodily weakness. (*Bar-c.*).

(2) Speech unintelligible. (*Hyos-niger.*) 4 hrly.

(3) With great despondency and inclination to weep. (*Aur-met.*).

(4) Aching in occiput, numbness, tremor, speech difficult, *Gels.* 4 hourly.

(5) Speech slow. (*Lach.*). See "One sided complaints".

Paralysis-painful or painless—For painful condition *Cocculus* is helpful whereas for painless condition *Plumbum* be given.

Paralysis-single muscles and hand—Paralysis of single muscles. Cannot raise or lift anything with hand. Extension is difficult. Paralysis from over-exertion of the extensor muscles in piano players. (*Plumbum-metallicum.*). See "Muscles—different troubles including atrophy" and "Trembling of hands and feet".

Paralysis-retention-urine and stool—Paralysis causing retention of stool and urine. (*Opium.*). See also "Retention of urine".

Paralysis-of rheumatic origin—See "Rheumatic paralysis".

Paralysis-of sphincter—Stool involuntary, flow of urine intermittent. Partial paralysis of bladder. (*Gels.*).

Paralysis-tongue and face with indistinct speech, bladder paralysis—(1) (*a*) Paralysis of tongue with indistinct speech. (*Caust.*). (*b*) Facial paralysis of young people where tongue is implicated. (*Baryta carbonica.*). (*c*) Facial paralysis from exposure to cold dry winds. (*Acon.*).

(2) Local paralysis, vocal cords, muscles of deglutition (swallowing) of tongue, of eyelids. Bladder and extremities burning, rawness, soreness are characteristics. (*Caust.*).

(3) *Gels.* is useful in paralysis of tongue or any localised slight paralysis as may be observed in connection with the bladder in retaining the urine as well as in the paralysis of fundus (the base of an organ) so that it cannot be evacuated. Again there may be paresis (slight paralysis) when the flow is intermittent. See "Tongue paralysis", "Facial paralysis" and "Bladder with involuntary urine".

Paralysis of vocal cord—When child gets worse in sleep. Loss of voice. Larynx sensitive to least touch. It causes suffocation. (*Lach.*). See also "Voice loss of".

Paralytic condition-complete motor paralysis including eye muscle—(1) Complete relaxation of muscular system with apparent or real paralytic condition. *Gels.* centres its action upon nervous system causing various diseases of motor paralysis. (*Gels.*).

(2) Paralysis of eye muscles. Also for post-diphtheritic and infantile paralysis. (*Gels.*). See "Trembling of lower extremities in paralysis" and "Relaxation of muscles with prostration in walking".

Paralysis of rectum—See "Rectum prolapse and paralysis".

Paralytic condition of sphincter after labour—Constant dribbling of urine after labour which is due to the paralytic condition on the sphincter, bladder on account of the contusion is always removed by *Arnica.* See also "Labour-retention of urine" and "Urine retention after labour".

Paralytic weakness-of lower limbs—Heaviness and paralytic weakness of lower limbs. (*Ambra.*).

Paralytic weakness-in pregnancy of lower limbs—Paralytic weakness in the lower limbs soon after becoming pregnant. This comes with every pregnancy and she must go to bed. Weight in legs. Legs feel heavy. Trembling and jerking motion in the lower limbs. (*Agar.*). See also "Pregnancy" under its different heads and "Pregnancy-paralytic weakness in lower limbs".

Paralytic weakness of throat muscles after diphtheria—If after sore throat and specially after diphtheria inflammatory condition of the throat is followed by paralytic weakness of the throat muscle, making it impossible to swallow liquids or food and when food is forced into the nose instead of oesophagus. *Arum-t.* is particularly indicated. (*Arum-t.*). See also "Diphtheria followed by paralytic condition".

Parotid gland (near the ear) with shooting pain and swollen after measles—Dr. Farrington recommends *Kali bichromicum* for the ear symptoms, sharp pains shooting from the ears into the glands. See "Ear deafness after measles".

Peevish—(1) Peevish child. (*Cham.*).

(2) Peevishness, quarrelsome, intolerance of contradiction. (*Ferrum-met.*). See "Annoyance".

Pellagra-acutaneous (pertaining to skin) disease—Itching on getting warm. Eczema moist ; pimples cover the entire body. Urticaria on waking in the morning worst from bathing. (*Bovista.*).

Pelvic-infiltration—Inflammation of the tissues of pelvis. Dr. Blackwood suggests that *Mag-sulf.* is highly beneficial in reducing pelvic infiltration following acute inflammation. In such cases this medicine should be incorporated into a vaginal suppositary and inserted in the vagina. See "Inflammation acute" and "Vagina bleeding".

Pelvis-bearing down sensation—In women the most prominent symptom is a bearing down sensation in the pelvis as if all the organs specially the uterus would come out. Labour like pains in uterus. (*Sep.*).

Pelvis-lower back dragging pain in, and with leucorrhoeà—Dragging pain in pelvis with leucorrhoea and pressing pains in the hips when walking. Almost all the usefulness of *Aesc.* centres in its action in the lower back and pelvic region and ever prominent is the characteristic. (*Aesc.*). See "Back-ache low" and "Pains in pelvis".

Penis-different complaints—Cartilaginous swelling on penis : *Sabin.*

(2) Inflammation : *Hedysarum-idle-fansinidum.*

(3) For pains : *Geum rivale.*

(4) For sores : *Osm.*

See "Oedema dropsical swelling".

Penis—When there is itching on penis (1) when the penis is small and retracted then (*Ignatia.*).

(2) When the penis becomes small due to masturbation. (*Lyco.*).

(3) When there is burning during coition, and swelling. (*Kreosote*).

Peptic (pertaining to digestion) ulcer—(1) Intensely acrid eructations. The gastric symptoms with the most pronounced acidity are well authenticated and are the guiding symptoms of this remedy. It is useful in peptic ulcers. (*Robina*). See "Duodenal ulcer."

(2) Pencillin in homoeopathic potencies is very efficacious for peptic ulcer.

(3) Peptic ulcer of the bleeding type with tubercular bowels. (*Alumina phosphate*).

(4) For complete obstruction due to peptic ulcer. (*Podo, C.M.*).

(5) For perforated peptic ulcer *Kali bic.* is very effective according to Dr. Rexom. See "Duodenal ulcers", "Gastric ulcer" and "Ulcer of stomach".

Perception or recognition (the acquiring of impressions through senses)—(1) Perception diminished in typhoid. (*Colchicum.*).

(2) Perception diminished in constitutionally weak children. (*Baryta-carb.*).

Pericarditis (inflammation of the closed membranous sac covering the heart)—Fever ; semi-consciousness. Pains in the chest starting from the pit of stomach to the upper extremity of the lung behind the border of the first rib. (*Kali-hydro.* 30 and later on a few doses of the same of 200 potency).

Periodicity—Of affections or diseases *e.g.* fever, diarrhoea or pain. (*China*). Compare *Eupatorium purpur,* Ipecac, *Nat-m.,* Arsenic-alba. See "Fever-malaria periodical", "Calic periodical" and "Urticaria-annual".

Periostitis (inflammation of fibrous membrane investing the surface of bone)—Of tibia (the inner and larger bone of the leg) with purple skin in common feature of *Asaf.* Deep flat ulcers from bone and periosteal affections give out a watery bloody discharge which is very offensive. These ulcers bleed and are sensitive to touch. (*Asaf.*) See "Tibia pain" and "Discharge offensive".

Peritonitis (inflammation of serous membrane lining abdomen)—Stony heaviness, nausea, and vomiting (1) Aggravation by movement ; Thirst for large quantities of water. Relief by pressure. (*Bry*).

(2) Swollen abdomen which is tense like a drum ; retching and vomiting (*Bell.*).

(3) Fever with peritonial pain (*Aconite-n.*).

(4) (*a*) The abdomen is tympanitic with effusion ; riguor and sweats ; (*Merc-sol.*). (*b*) For further spread of suppurative process, give *Merc*. as suggested by Dr. Farrigton.

Persistent nausea—Patient is as sick before as after vomiting. This is called "persistent nausea". This condition is often found in connection with gastric trouble from dietetic errors. Constant neusea with almost all complaints with empty eructations, accumulation of much saliva in mouth and efforts to vomiting which does not relieve is in a nutshell the main symptom of *Ip.* Compare *Puls*. See "Vomiting-persistent".

Perspiration and its absence and also perspiration which attracts flies—(1) (*a*) Perspiration during sleep on being covered. (*China.*).

(*b*) Profuse perspiration arising from debility and profuse perspiration during sleep. (*Rhus-glabra.*).

(2) Absence of perspiration. (*Lach.*).

(3) Hysterical perspiration (*Nux-m.*).

(4) Profuse perspiration. (*Phos-ac.*).

(5) Exhausting and profuse sweat when asleep. (*Chin-a.*)

(6) Sweat on uncovered parts of the body. (*Thuja.*).

(7) Sweetish odour of perspiration which attracts flies. (*Calad.*).

(8) Offensive perspiration. (*Petr., Sil.* and *Staphy.*).

(9) Perspiration in flabby persons or children which wets the pillow. (*Calc-c.*). See "Sweat offensive foot" and "Wetting the bed".

Perspiration cold—(1) Cold perspiration in any disease whatsoever. There may be diarrhoea or may not be diarrhoea. There may be intense pain in joints or in abdomen or anywhere else. (*Verat.*).

(2) Profuse and exhausting sweat while asleep. (*Chininum-ars.*). See "Sweat-cold".

Perspiration offensive of body—(1) Offensive odour of body despite washing and bathing. (*Sulf.*).

(2) Perspiration offensive specially in axillae which fills the room when patient enters. (*Petroleum*). See "Odour-offensive of body" "(e) of Axilla...complaints" and "Urine offensive".

Perspiration-on foot offensive—Diseases from suppressed foot sweat, which if present is profuse and sometimes offensive. (*Sil.*) *Silicea* is also a head remedy for sweats on palms, hands and soles of feet. See "Sweat-offensive foot".

Perspiration-one sided—On one side of body. One sided complaints. (*Ambra.*). See "One-sided complaints".

Perspiration-on palms and head—Sweat of palms and head specially in children which wets the pillow. (*Calc-c.*). See also "Sweating on head" and "Sweat on head and hands in sleep".

Perspiration-profuse and its prevention—*Apomorphia* is not only a prophylactic for such a trouble but is indicated mostly in bad cases accompanied with profuse perspiration.

Perspiration-without any relief—Profuse perspiration without relieving any symptom *i.e.* feeling of fever or headache. This condition may be present in any disease *viz.* sorethroat, bronchitis, pleurisy, abscesses and rheumatism. (*Merc-sol.*).

Perverted affections—Most important point in 'the mental symptom of *Aur-met.* is that all its affections are perverted. The patient loathes life, longs to die, seeks method to commit suicide. Self-condemnation and self criticism is the key-note. An image of baffled life. (*Aur-met.*). See also "Suicide" and "Jealousy".

Perverted mind—*Anac., Hyoscyamus., Stramonium* and *Bell.* are the four pillars in homoeopathy which bring the perverted and illusioned mind to the sphere of intellegence and reasoning. (*Anac.*). See "Mind delusion and hallucination".

Pharyngitis-due to silver nitrate and constant desire to blow nose—(1) Where silver nitrate has been used as a local application. (*Nat-m.*).

(2) A fish bone sensation in the throat with hawking. (*Kali-bi.*).

(3) Acute tonsillitis. A congestion on either side of throat which is less bright red ; the pharynx highly glazed. Throat dry, smarting and burning. Also useful in syphilitic sore throat. (*Guaic. 3x.*)

(4) Chronic pharyngitis and laryngitis where there is a constant desire to clear throat for distinct utterance. An excellent remedy is *Wyethia 30* dilution.

(5) Constant desire to blow nose. Acute or chronic coryza with sensation of pressure and fulness at the root of nose. (*Sticta-pul.*) See " Laryngitis with hoarseness".

Phimosis (narrowing of the foreskin of the penis)—(1) *Mercurius. iod.* is an excellent remedy for phimosis.

(2) Discharge of pus, throbbing pain (*Hep-s.*).

(3) With swelling syphilitic. *Nitric-acid* is the head remedy.

(4) Phimosis with prepuce painful and swollen. (*Jacranda*). See "Urine retention in infants".

Phlebitis-Inflammation of a vein—Varicose veins and ulcers ; veinous congestion, passive veinous haemorrhage ; varicose, veins or haemorrhoids that bleed profusely. (*Hamamelis*). It can also be applied locally in form of wetdressing and giving enternally.

Phosphaturia—When the urine presents white sediment and also in the derangement of childhood when urine is milky (*Acidum phosphoricum*).

(2) When there is a history of prolonged lactation, leucorrhal discharges and general anaemia. (*Kali-hypophosorosum*).

Photophobia-(Intolerance or morbid fear of light)—"Showers of star like bodies". Great soreness about the eyes and into eye-balls. Sees firy objects. (*Aur-met.*). See "Eye troubles and troubles after operation on the eye".

Phthisis inherited—(1) Inherited phthisis. Emaciation, weakness and loss of appetite. *Acet-ac.* is very useful in complaints of pale, sickly people. (*Acet.-ac.*)

(2) Dr. Jousset recommends *Ars-iod.* alternately with *Calc.-phos.* in active stage with hectic fever. See "Tuberculosis", "Cough phthisis" and "Fever consumptive".

Phthisis incipient and galloping consumption—(1) Convulsive cough, with sweat twoards evening, with frequent pulse, expectoration of pus like mucus, worse in the morning and when lying on bed. Agar. fattens up emaciated T.B. patients. (*Agar.*).

(2) *Phos.* useful for galloping consumption alternately with *Ars-a.* See "Consumption-pulmonary" and "No. 12 of Tuberculosis".

Phthisis palliative— *Arum-t* . is palliative for phthisis. It has burning and raw feeling in the chest while coughing. The raw feeling may be along the trachea and in the chest. (*Arum-t.*)

(2) Dr. Jahr gives *Sulph, Calc-c* and *Lyco.* in the order given 2 or 3 doses of *Sulph.* first week, then 2 or 3 doses of

Calc-c. 2nd week and then 2 or 3 doses of *Lyco.* 3rd week and so on in confirmed cases with hectic fever and pus formation.

(3) In the increased manifestation of Phthisis Pulmonis *Ferrph.* has been found to be a great palliative with amazing recuperative power. See also "Consumption palliative".

Physical acts requiring strength—*Coca.* is of service in those witch are performing acts and feats requiring great strength also for mountain climbers where it relieves dyspnoea, palpitation of the heart and controls haemoptysis. (*Coca.*).

Pigeon chest i.e. narrow chest—Tall and slender persons with emaciation and debility with narrow chest will greatly be benefitted in getting their chest become normal if they use *Phosphorus* for long time at least for 3 months or so, as this is the only medicine which has special influence on the narrow chest.

Piles bleeding—external application—*Aesculas, Hamamelis* and *Phytolacca* 1 to 10 part to be applied in olive oil.

Piles—both blind and bleeding—(1) Both painful blind as well as bleeding piles. Bleeding piles due to highly seasoned food or sedentary habits combined with mental and physical strain and night watching and nursing. Temperamental symptoms must be present. As first aid, routine dose temporarily cures bleeding. (*Nux-v.* 200 at bed time followed by *Sulph.* next morning).

(2) *Mucuna M.T.* one drop a dose is specific for bleeding piles ; 2 or 3 doses a day will arrest the disease in 2 or 3 days. See also "Haemorrhoids—blind or bleeding".

Piles with distended veins in rectum—(*a*) Pile is purple. The rectum seems full of sticks with liver engorgement. The stool becomes jammed into the rectum against these distended viens and then ulceration takes place. Great piles remedy. (*Aesc.*). (*b*) Aches in anus, protrusion of piles. (*Ratanhia.*). See "Haemorrhoids of both types".

Piles-impeding the stool—Patient chilly. Burning and stringing piles worst from washing ; fissure present ; weak and irritated eyes which pour tears in the open air. (*Causticum.*).

Piles inflamed—*Plantango-m.* It is very useful as local application for inflamed piles. The M. T. of this medicine should be used, three times a day.

Piles-incessant bleeding also in pregnancy—(1) Dr. Burt says that no remedy can equal *Collinsonia* in obstinate haemorrhoids which bleed almost incessantly. Itching in the anus, obstinate constipation alternating with diarrhoea. It suits pregnant women who suffer from piles with pruritis.

(2) *Capsicum* for bleeding piles with pruritis.

(3) *Capsicum* for bleeding piles with great burning, itching stinging. See "Haemorrhoids bleeding" and "Haemorrhoids pregnancy".

Piles-itching—Itching and burning of anus ; redness around anus. (*Sulf.*). See "Haemorrhoids with itching".

Piles-after operation piles swollen—(1) Anus stretched for cutting piles. (*Staphy.*). Swollen pain worse sitting, with stitching and burning pains at the anus. (*Thuj*). See also "Stretches".

(2) "Blind piles very painful, pain in back and hips. (*Aesc.*)". See "Haemorrhoids of both types".

Piles-oozing of mucus—Continuous oozing of mucus staining the lilnen. Disagreeable to the patient. (*Antimonium crudum*).

Piles-prevention of recurrence—*Tuberculinum* 1000 acts well as an intercurrent medicine to avoid the tendency for recurrence.

Piles-throbbing pains in both types of piles—Bleeding or blind, the blood must be dark. Constricted feeling in anus and throbbing pains as if little hammers are striking on the painful piles. Warm usually aggravates these cases. (*Lach.*). See "Haemorrhoids blind or bleeding".

Piles with fissure—Piles bleed after every evacuation and spasm of the anus with splinter like pain and continued desire or stool. Patient, cold, thin and dark, being chilly. Melancholy and fat loving. (*Nitric acid*).

Piles-with pain and ulcerated pimples—(1) Haemorrhoids large, swollen, painful, itching. Ulcerated pimples around anus. Burning in rectum and anus. Large discharge of blood with natural stool. (*Kali-c*).

(2) Piles with ulceration, the anus, and surrounding parts are purple covered with crusts, ulcers within the anus very painful, the whole, mucous membrane studded with ulcers and cracks. (*Paeonia*). See "Haemorrhoids—with ulceration".

Piles-with weakness of sight, epilepsy and hysteria—According to Dr. Blackie *Ruta graveolen.* has a great reputation for such trouble when there are piles and inertia of bowels with difficult stool. It is often most useful when piles are starting and many patient have been clear completely from these symptom.

Pimples—Acne, simple in young persons. *Carb-v* , if plethoric, *Bell,* if pale, *Puls.* More chronic cases *Kali bromatum.* and *Radium bromidum 30* once a week. *Sulf.* may be given intercurrently with any of the above medicines. See "Acne", "Face-acne" and "Prickly heat".

Pimples : external application—Lotion of *Arnica* or *Ledum.*

Pimples-on face and ears—*Clematis* is a useful remedy for pimples on the face or about the ears and hair-line with small discharging crusts on scalp.

Plague also its prophylactic—(1) Dr. D.N. Roy is of opinion that *Buboninum* in 12-13 potency should be used as prophylatic and in lower potencies as curative agent as often as required. Dr. Mahendra Sirkar and Dr. Honingberger found *Ignatia* very useful both as a curative and prophvlactic agent.

(2) *Naja.* is said to be useful in India.

(3) *Hydro-ac.* during the stage of collapse. See "Bubo".

Plane of disorder and plane of cure—There is a strong tendency in the scientific world to depend on tests, which are gleaned by senses, but the realm of the immaterial must be recognised by the reason. Man is affected in the internals and in every cell by the disease. Crude drugs produce the opposite effects from the attenuated dose. Crude whisky produces a drunken condition, and attenuated dose of whisky will make a man who appears drunk feel better. In the attenuated forms. Primary and secondary effects, opposite effects are found. A class of man, belonging to the scientific schools thinks they discover the cause of bacteria to be grand parents who establish a family. If bacteria causes disease, we have many things to think about. Is it bacteria that causes the disease or is it the soil that is prepared for the bacteria to grow and cause the diseased symptoms ? On the north side of the house in the shadow where the ground is copiously watered the moss has crowded the grass. So the preparation of the soil preceded the development of any growth. There will be no growth in vegetation or bacteria if the soil is not prepared for it. Changes in the blood when the health is disturbed make a preparation of soil in the blood for the spontaneous development in the body of various forms to correspond to every change in bodily disorder. To assume that this spontaneous growth causes sickness is the reverse of the truth. There is no difference in bacterial growth and growth of any vegetation. Fluids that contain bacteria will act as agents of infections. You can kill the bacteria and inject the fluid and cause a condition in the blood similar to that in the body from which the blood was taken. So the fact is that the sepsis comes first then the germs grow. There is spontaneous development of sepsis in the blood. If the germs are left long enough they will kill off the poison. This is illustrated in the case of cadaver (dead-body). The scalpel that pricks the hand in the course of a post-mortem is more poisonous then the scalpel that pricks the hand after using it on the cadaver that has lain of six weeks and is mortified and green.

Pleurisy—Stitching pain in the chest. Lying on painful side relieves. Pain will increase by movements of parts. (*Bry*). See "Rheumatic-pleurisy".

Pleurodynia-pain over the intercostal muscles or pain in the chest—It is an affection of the muscles of the ribs. It causes pain and stitch in the side on moving, coughing, sneezing or on deep breathing. *Ranunculus bulb. 30* is the principal remedy.

Pleurisy-dry and wet—(1) Dry pleurisy during pneumonia and phthisis. First *Acon.* and then *Bry.*

(2) Purulent exudation complicated with bronchitis. (*Hepar*).

(3) When there is pus in pleura with great prostration and hectic fever. (*China.*).

(4) Profuse sero-fibrinous exudations indicated by dyspnoea, palpitation, profuse sweats, weakness, tendency to syncope with scanty and albuminous urine. (*Canth.*).

(5) *Ars-a.* is one of the best remedies for pleuritic effusion. (Dr. Nash.)

Pleurisy-pain—See "Chapter V for details".

Pneumonia—(1) *Ip.* 12 and *Bry.* 6 to be given alternately at least 2 doses of each daily gives good results.

(2) The temperature is high and respiration rapid with gastric irritability. Nausea. (*Verat-v.*).

(3) If pneumonia assumes a chronic form, sputa becomes foetid and badly coloured. (*Carb-v.*).

(4) Hectic fever and emaciation. Difficulty in breathing and warmth intolerable. Easily perspires. (*Hep*). first to be followed by (*Iodium.*).

Pneumonia-with blood discharge—In the first stage it aborts the disease, with a good deal of blood discharge, it is very valuable and often cures quickly. (*Ferr-p.*). See "Bleeding from lungs".

Pneumonia-with breathlessness—(1) Extreme breathlessness.

(2) The wings of the nose expand with a fan-like motion.

(3) Wrinkling of forehead. The characteristic aggravation time of 4 to 8 p.m. is also generally found in this condition. Neglected or maltreated. To hasten absorption or expectoration. (*Lyco.*).

Pneumonia-with burning and raw feeling—There is burning and a raw feeling in the chest while coughing. The raw feeling may be along trachea and in the chest. *Arum-t.* has cured pneumonia with these symptoms. The urine is scanty and sometimes suppressed. (*Arum-t.*).

Pneumonia-with cough and oppressed breathing—Of old people and pleuritic effusions. *Arsenic* is particularly efficacious in many affections of the lungs, when breathing is much oppressed. Respiration is wheezing with cough and frothy expectoration, patient cannot lie down, must sit up to breathe. The air passages seem constricted worse after 12 in night. (*Ars.*).

Pneumonia-exudation--The passage of various constituents of the blood through the walls of vessels into adjacent tissues or spaces in inflammation—Advanced stage of exudation with symptoms of mental anxiety and restlessness. Give *Sulf.* at once. Superficial symptoms to be treated with *Acon.* or *Ars.*

Pneumonia-maltreated consumption—*Lyco.* has often saved neglected, maltreated or imperfectly cured cases of pneumonia from running into consumption.

Pneumonia-of infants—Of infants similar to symptoms in bronchitis. Chest loaded with mucus, rapid and wheezing breathing. Face pale or bluish. Nausea. (*Ip*). See "Bronchitis infants".

Pneumonia in typhoid—*Lach.* is the best remedy in typhoid with lung complication. See also "Typhoid with pneumonia".

Poisoning-charcoal fumes—*Am-c.* is of use in poisoning by charcoal fumes. (*Am-c.*). See "Charcoal-fumes poisoning".

Poisoning by lead—Characteristic symptoms.

Poliomyelitis-inflammation of gray matter of spinal cord and its preventive—*Lathyrus*. See "Inflammation of cord". See "Myelitis inflammation, spinal cord".

Poliomyelitis-its preventive—*Lathyrus. 1 M,* works as preventive for this disease. Dr. Bond says that he had 100 percent recovery and many cases were aborted.

Polypi-with offensive odour—In nose with offensive odour. (*Calc.*). Compare *Thuj*. See "Odour from nose and mouth".

Polypi-in nose with discharge—Thick discharge from nose ; scabs are formed in it. Chronic catarrh, thick green mucus. (*Thuj*). See "Catarrh-of nose thick and large discharge".

Polypus—Soft tumour in the nose, uterus or vagina attached by a pedicle. If it is removed by operation, it reappears after sometimes. *Formica Ruf* 1x is very useful. When it bleeds then give *Phos.* 30 to 200 weekly and apply externally *Sanguinaria* 1x powder. (*Dr. Y. Singh*).

Polypus in ear and rectum—(*a*) In ear. (*Hydrastis.*). (*b*) In rectum with inflammation. (*Phos.*) See "Rectum prolapse".

Polypus-covering nostril—Polypus occupying entire nostril, stoppage of nose on the side he lies, greenish white discharge. *Teucrium* is head remedy for polypus. See "Nose polypi".

Polyuria—See "Urine-polyuria" which means passage of excessive quantity of urine.

Position-changing giving relief—Must change position constantly, with relief for a short time by the change. Cannot lie in one position for long. The patient constantly changes his position, turns sides, sits up, lies down or even walks about a little. But he cannot lie in one position for long. *Rhus-t.* patient cannot be quiet. This is just opposite of *Bry.* which is relieved by lying quietly. (*Rhus-t.*). See also "Restlessness changing position giving relief".

Post operative complicatious—*e.g.* Septicemia. (*Rhus-t*) See "Septicemia-post operative" and "Amputation neurites".

Post-operative gas pain—*China*.

Post-operative vomiting—After chloroform anaesthesia (*Phos.*). See also "Chloroform-vomiting".

Pot-bellied children—*Sanic.*

Potencies of medicines—(*a*) *Centesimal scale*-one drop of mother tincture and 99 drops of alcohol gives the 1st potency. One drops of the 1st potency and 99 drops of alcohol gives the 2nd potency. All the following potencies are prepared with one drop of the preceding potency to 99 drops of alcohol. They are called 1, 2, 3, 30 or 200 etc. (*b*) *Decimal scale*—As the tincture contains 1/10 of drug power, it corresponds to the 1st potency ; 1 drop of mother tincture and 9 drops of distilled water gives the 1x potency. One drop of 1x potency and 9 drops of alcohol gives the 2x potency. The next higher potencies are prepared with one drop of the preceding potency to 9 drops of alcohol. These are called 1x, 2x, 3x, etc.

Power of absorption-of fluid—Fluids anywhere in the body like the enlargement of the joints in rheumatism, exudations into serous sacs, pleura, meningeal membrane (inflammation of the membrane of brain or cord) peritonic membrane, after the acute symptoms are over but the swelling persists. A dose of *Sulph.* will very often help the absorption. (*Sulph.*). See also "Fluids-absorption".

Pregnancy-its affection—(1) Toothache of pregnant women. (*Mac-c.*). See also "Tooth-ache during pregnancy".

(2) Constipation of pregnancy. *Sepia 200* when *Sep.* fails then *Op.*

(3) (*a*) Milk egg. (*Ham.*). (*b*) For albuminous nephritis. (*Merc-c.*).

(4) After delivery when the breasts are swollen and painful with scanty, most suppressed flow of milk, (*Puls.*).

(5) Milk fever when the breasts are stony hard. Sensitive to touch and feel heavy. (*Bry.*). Compare *Bell.*

(6) When child moves so violently in womb, awakens the the mother causing cutting in bladder with great urging to urinate. (*Thuj.*).

(7) Threatened abortion more specially about the 3rd month, false labour pains with bloody discharge. (*Secale*.). Compare *Sabin*, *Corc-s*. and *Kreos*.

(8) Violent movement of the foetus. Threatened abortion due to fearful fright in the advanced stage of pregnancy. (*Op*.).

(9) Labour pains deficient, come and go suddenly. (*Bell*.). See "Labour" under its different heads.

(10) Child at birth pale, breathless, gasping although the cord still pulsates, inability of the newborn to respire. (*Ant-t*.).

(11) Syphilis : Child born with diseases and deformities due to syphilis. See "Syphilis in general".

(12) Inability of new born to respire : First give one globule of *Ant-t*. dry on the tongue. If it fails then *Opium* in the same manner. *Laurocer asus* is useful when there is gasping without breathing ; blueness of face and twitching of face muscles.

(13) Bleeding from navel of infant. (*Abrot*).

(14) Colic of pregnant women : Colic is as frequent in pregnancy as vomiting and anorexia (loss of appetite.). Generally the trouble consists of abdominal spasms that set during the first month of pregnancy and not confounded with labour pains. The best remedy is *Cham*. when there is wind in bowels, if this fails then *Nux-v*. or *Coloc*. If the pains are extreme not allowing the patient to rest.

(15) Desire of eating dirty things : For eating earth or lime *Nit-ac*. sand and ashes *Tarent-c*. ; for indigestible things chalk or charcoal *Alumina*. See "Desire for eating dirty things in pregnancy".

(16) Hiccough during pregnancy :—*Cyclamen* every two minutes.

(17) Dyspepsia of hysterical women during pregnancy *Nux-m*.

(18) Pregnant women falling :—First give *Arnica* ; if pains become violent then give *Cham*. after *Arnica*. See also "Labour" and "Lactation" under their different heads.

(19) The mother due to same metabolic defects gives birth to children who in infancy suffer from infantile liver then *Medorrhinum* will rectify if mother is administered this medicine during her pregnancy.

(20) If there is a fit after delivery immediatetly then remember *Hyocyamus 30* or *Strychninum 30* should be given at half hour or one hour in trouble.

Pregnancy-bleeding—Unusual bleeding during pregnancy or at a later stage *i.e.* 5th to 7th month is cured by *Sepia*. See also "Piles-incessant bleeding also in pregnancy" and "Bleeding-during pregnancy".

Pregnancy - complaints after delivery—Should the new mother run a temperature and generally feel very unwell. (*Lachesis.*).

Pregnancy - disorders of—(1) Albuminuria, *Apis-mel.* or *Euonymin 1x* trit.

(2) Aversion to food. (*Laur.*).

(3) (a) Backache with sense of weakness and dragging in the loins. *Kali-c.* 4-hourly or severe pain in the back before or during stool. (*Sars*). (b) *Kali-carb.* is one of the best remedies following labour.

(4) Bladder trouble, urine expelled by slightest exertion, coughing or sneezing. (*Caust.* 4 hourly.).

(5) Breasts painful. (*Con.*). (c) Fainting in child-bed or during lactation. (*Sep.*).

(6) Constant hacking cough. (*Kali-bi.*).

(7) Cramps. (*Verat-a.* 4 hourly.). (d) Discharge of lochia too great and too continuously long. (*Crocus.*).

(8) Desire of unusual articles of food. (*Chelidonium.*).

(9) Foetus displacement. *Puls.* is an excellent remedy for putting the foetus in the right place.

(10) Insanity during pregnancy. (*Stram. 200*). See also "Puerperal mania".

(11) Heart-burn with acidity. (*Calc.*).

(12) Heart-burn without acidity. (*Puls.*). (e) Gastric pains with eructation. (*Lyco.*).

(13) Morning sickness, *Symphoricarpus-racemosa 200* is a good all round medicine in desperate cases.

(14) Salivation. (*Merc-sol.*). Great falling of hair. (*Sep.* and *Nat-m.*).

(15) Swelling of feet and face. (*Apis.*).

(16) *Act-rac.* ensures in a woman a living birth who has previously delivered only a dead child.

(17) *Cal-fl.* is an excellent remedy in digestive troubles of pregnancy and given in later months facilitates delivery.

(18) Sleeplessness with anxious dreams. (*Anac.*). It is all useful for gastric nervous disorders. Compare *Coff.*

(19) Oedema of legs. The best remedy is *Bry.* then *Sulf.*

(20) Sleeplessness with delirium tremens. (*Act-rac.*). See also "Sleeplessness-during pregnancy".

(21) Frightful images at night. (*Kali-brom.*).

(22) The labour-like pains, the best remedy is *Caulo* ; it relieves in most cases.

(23) Constipation of pregnancy *Sepia 200th* potency. If it fails then *Opium* will often cure.

(24) Milk leg. *Hamamelis* is par excellence drug.

(25) *Nux-vom., Camphor* and *Puls.* may be given in the order given for retention of urine during pregnancy.

(26) Burning in anus during pregnancy. (*Capsicum.*).

(27) Frequent desire to urinate. Urine in few drops escapes before reaching vessel. (*Sepia* and *Caust.*).

(28) (a) Continued sick feeling day and night without vomiting. (*Tabac.*) (b) Hysterical shivering in the first stage of labour. (*Act-rac.*).

(29) Backache with sense of weakness and dragging in lions. *Kali-carb* ; with lameness and inability to walk. *Bellis. 30.* 4 hourly. *Kali-carb.* is one of the best medicines

following labour. Compare *Aesc-h.* for backache during pregnancy

(30) Diarrhoea, stools chiefly at night. (*Puls.* 4 hourly.). Compare *Nux-m.* and *Cham.*

(31) Diarrhoea with prostration and loss of flesh (*Phos-ac.* 2 drops 4 hourly.).

(32) In the interest of health of patient if medically advised then *Gossypium* in mother tincture in drop doses may be used for producing abortion though in homoeopathy there are no remedies which would create disease hence failure to produce abortion will be the general rule. (Dr. Clarke and R. B. Bishamber Dass).

(33) *Pituitrin* acts on uterus to check bleeding after delivery.

(34) After delivery fever and also for septic fever. (*Phyrogenium.*).

(35) Varicose veins during pregnancy—*Puls.* to be followed by *Lach.*, when attended with constipation, haemorrhoids and irritable temper then *Nux-v.*

(36) Blindness also night blindness :—during pregnancy. Night and day blindness in women. (*Ranunculus bulbosus.*). See "Labour pain—causing blindness."

(37.) Breast congestion after weaning :—*Puls.* most useful followed by *Calc-c.* (g) For constant flow of milk *Bell.*, *Calc-c.* and *Bry.* are the best remedies.

(38) Pendulous abdomen after confinement. (*Podo.*).

(39) Convulsions after child-birth or after loss of blood. (*Chin.*).

(40) Dyspnoea of pregnant females. Please See under "D" Dyspnoea of pregnant females.

(41) Haemorrhoids in pregnancy :—With prolapse during pregnancy or after child birth. (*Podo.*).

(42) During pregnancy inability to walk (*Bellis perennis.*). See "Delivery safe" also "Labour" under latter's different

heads, "Shivering-in labour and otherwise" and "Lumps in the breast".

Pregnancy of hysterical women changing symptoms—Cures all sorts of conditions and symptoms of women of hysteric, nervous, rheumatic and fidgety women with jerking, in the muscles. So markedly do her troubles alternate with each other, that alternation is in the nature of her case. She has nausea at one time ; she will come to you with one group of symp toms today and may come back to you with entirely different group in a couple of weeks. (*Act-rac.*).

Pregnancy-giving birth to dead babies—Women who habitually give birth to dead babies ; give *Act-rac. 1x* daily at least for 2 months before the actual time of delivery. See "Infancy-baby dying in infancy" and "Grown up dying in early age."

Pregnancy nephritis—*Apoc-can.* is an important remedy in this trouble with albuminuria, uraemia and convulsions. See "Nephritis—inflammation of kidney".

Pregnancy-paralytic weakness in lower limbs—Paralytic weakness in the lower limbs soon after becoming pregnant. This comes with every pregnancy and she must go to bed. Wieght in the legs. Legs feel heavy. Trembling and jerking motion in the lower limbs. (*Agar.*). See also "Weakness" under its different heads and "Paralytic weakness in pregnancy of lower limbs".

Pregnancy-swelling, including lochia, placenta troubles and baby's head hindering delivery—(i) Swelling of the lower extremities, of thighs, or even of external parts of sexual organs. Oedema with much prostration ; feeble, irregular pulse ; coldness of extremities ; *Arsenicum* ; extreme swelling with urinary difficulties : *Apis mellifica* ; affections of skin ; *Sulf.* (ii) If discharge of lochia continues beyond 3 weeks and for unduly long time then *Secale 3x* or *Sabina 3x* ; if *lochia* ceases suddenly then *Aconite 3x* ; if it smells foul then *Kreosote-3x* or *Carbo-veg. 3x*. (iii) If placenta not expelled nor detached within an hour of delivery then *Puls. 30* or *Secale 30* every

15 minutes. (iv) As regards excessive size of the head of child making delivery difficult use *Puls.* or *Secale.* Sometimes *Calc.*, *Sulf* or *Sil.* make the task easy. See "Lochia" under its two headings.

Pregnancy-vomiting—(a) Nausea or vomiting at the very thought of or smell of food. The patient cannot even pass by kitchen. *Colch.* is a good medicine for this but *Sep.* is better in pregnancy.

(b) According to Dr. Edson. *Amygadalus-perisca* will allay the vomiting of pregnancy than any remedy. Every case of retching and vomiting will yield under its use. See "Vomiting in pregnancy".

Premature-grey hair—The process is a lengthy one and requires patiece from the patient.

(a) Give *Thyrodinum 30* in dilution, 3 times a day, at least for one month.

(b) After this increase the potency of *Thyrodinum* to 200 dilution and give it every week for another month.

(c) If no improvement then give *Acid phos. 30,* 3 times a day in first week. In the second week give *Lycopodium 30* dilution T.D.S. per day.

In the 3rd week give *Wiesbaden 30* dilution T.D.S. This process is to be continued for at least six months.

Even after this if no improvement takes place then give *Pilocarpinum 1000* dilution every month for at least 3 to 4 months longer if necessary.

(d) Grey hair due to exhausting ailments. Give *Natrum-m* dilution 30 T.D S. for one month.

Phosphorus 30 dilution T.D.S. next month and soon. See "Hair" and "Greyness of hair and its prevention".

Premature old age due to excess—Broken down constitution from sexual excesses and secret vices. Despair and anxiety. Pale and sickly. (*Agn.*). See "Old age from excesses", "Debility and prostration due to loss of fluid".

Prematurely old-with impairment of all functions—A man of middle age looks and shows symptoms of old age. Also for patients weakened by age or over-work, who are anaemic and sleepless. Great remedy for the aged with impairment of all functions, weakness, coldness and numbness, usually of single parts, fingers, arms etc. One sided complaints call for it. Feebleness and forgetfulness. (*Ambra.*). Compare *Baryta carb.* See "Weakness-premature old age with impaired functions" and "Rejuvenator".

Prepuce-eruptions and warts—(1) Eruptions on it. (*Sil.*).

(2) Warts on it. (*Phos-ac*). See "Gonorrhoea-swollen prepuce".

Pressure-ameliorates—Amelioration from pressure. This is the reason why the patient always wants to lie on painful side or part. (*Bell.* the patient cannot lie on painful side.) Pain usually better by lying on painful side and patient reliev-ed by lying quietly and on painful side. (*Bry.*).

Pressure-causes sleeping of limbs—Limbs go to sleep on slightest pressure.

Arms go to sleep while lying down. (*Ambra.*). See also "Sleeping of limbs pressure while lying down".

Pressure-relief—Relief by hard pressure on painful parts is characteristic symptom of *China*. Compare *Bry.* also. See "Neuralgic pains anywhere in body relief by pressure".

Preventives—See ' Chapter V for details".

Prevention of cold—Hoarseness ; cough from tickling in throat. Narrow chested patient. (*Phosphorus*). See "Cold and its aborting".

Prevention of inflammation—After injury *Ledum* ; *Hypericum*.

Prevention of bronchitis.—See "Bronchitis and prevention of its attack in different weather".

Prevention of Cold—In the beginning stage, when there is sensation of cold in the body, yawning and bruised feeling all over, two or three drops of M.T. *Spirit Camphor* should be taken in sugar or sugar of milk every one or two hour. Often the attack is thus cut short.

Preventive for punctured wound—*Ledum.* See "Prophylactic for other diseases".

Preventive for snake poison—*Euphorbia prostata.*

Prickly heat—(1) Prickly heat simple. (*Sulf. Apis.*).

(2) Red pimples on face and neck ; scalp red ; itches violently at night, itching and eruptions of small red pustules. (*Juglans-regia.*). See "Face-acne" and "Pimples".

Principles of cure—Two-thirds of all homoeopathic cures are accomplished by the following two methods :—(1) By finding a peculiar symptom and giving a dose of medicine exactly adopted to the symptom.

(2) By removing the 'block' and then if necessary giving the indicated remedy in cases where clearly the antecedent can be found. The other chronic cases which will not be more than one third of the total are cured by trial for finding the exactly selected right remedy.

Process of digestion—The process of digestion starts in the mouth and is carried on in the stomach and small intestines. When digestion is complete certain substances pass through the walls of the blood vessels in the lining of small intestines and are then carried in the blood stream to the other parts of the body. The residue which is left behind in the bowels consists water and various kinds of debris. The water is required by the body and is also absorbed into the blood from large intestine. What remains, contains an important element of our food known as roughage which consists of rough fibres from stalks, leaves, fruits and grains, which act as a broom to sweep all the debris out of the bowel. Some of the substances which are absorbed into the blood from the small intestine are also waste materials. These are eliminated by the kidneys and are disposed of in the urine. There is a constant process of breaking down and building up of tissues going on in the body. The breaking down process is known as *Katabolism* and the building up as *Anabolism*. The balance of the two is what we call *Metabolism*. During the years of growth the metabolism of the body has a bias towards *Anabolism*. During old age and in wasting diseases *Katabolism* is in excess. Throughout the majority of life the two are balanced but metabolism is never static, old parts are constantly being thrown out and new ones are supplied.

Proctalgia-pain neuralgic pain, in anus or rectum—See "Chapter V for details".

Progressive muscular atrophy—(1) This is a fatal disease and its prognosis most dismal. No system either Ayurvedic, Unani or even modern system of medicine have been, to my knowledge unable to find a sure cure for it. However Homoeopathy gives a slight ray of hope for this disease. According to veteran Homoeopath R.B. Bishamber Dass *Plumbum met.* is the head remedy and covers symptoms from simple irritation to complete destruction of muscles. It not only covers the muscles of brain but also of lungs, extremities and muscles of other organs. Complete loss of sensation, weakness, cutting, gripping twisting trembling, shooting in the neck, contraction and atrophy of deltoid, oedema, unsteady gait, shortening of muscles ; worse at night and from motion. Hypertension and artereosclerosis. Drs. N. Boericke and Blackwood also testify that this medicine is beneficial for progressive muscular atrophy, infantile paralysis and low motion ataxia. *Plumbum met.* 200 and 1000 dilution.

(2) For sensitiveness of spine, great pain in spine which is worse at night. General trembling and weakness of extremities rigidity of calves, also debility, walks and stands unsteadily, worse at night from cold and better from fresh air.

Symptoms of incoordination, loss of control and want of balance everywhere, mentally and physically. Withered and dried constitution. If female then leucorrhoea foul and uterine haemorrhage. fearful and nervous. (*Argentum-nitric.*).

(3) If there is hypertrophy (morbid enlargement of an organ) and atrophy in others, the make up of the patient should be kept in view—a tall hollow chested individual with tubercular or syphilitic diathesis (a constitutional tendency to certain diseases scrofula,rheumatism etc.)

Burning with trembling, numbness and weakness are the ranking symptom. Arms and hands become numb. Ascending sensory and motor paralysis from ends of fingers and toes. (*Phosphorus.*).

(4) For muscular atrophy destroying the virus associated with this disease, wandering pains along the bones ; worse cold, can't walk, kidney, heart and liver are also affected. Symptoms are worse in the morning ; pains migrate quickly, rheumatic and gastric symptoms alternate. (*Kali bich.*).

(5) *Arnica. Cupr met.* and *Baryta iod.* may be tried in the given order if the above remedies fail. See "Muscles—different troubles including atrophy."

Prolapse of rectum (falling down of a part)—A feeling of foreign substance as of a ball or weight in the rectum. (*Sep.*). See "Rectum prolapse".

Prolapse of rectum in child or after child-birth—Either with or without diarrhoea in children or in women after child-birth (*Podo.*). Compare *Rhus-tox.* and *Nux-vom.* For children *Ferr. phos.* is also useful. See also "Rectum-prolapse with or without diarrhoea".

Prolapse of uteri after delivery—Specially after child-birth from over-lifting or straining. (*Podo*). Compare *Rhus-tox.* and *Nux-vom.* See "Uterus-prolapse after child-birth or straining".

Prolapse of uterus (falling down of a part)—Acute ; with a pressure feeling as if something would come out. (*Sep.*). See "Uterus prolapse".

Prolapse of uterus with diarrhoea—*Aloe* has cured prolapse of uterus of long standing when it is associated with fulness, heat of the surface of body, tendency to morning diarrhoea, and dropping down to uterus. (*Aloe.*). See also "Uterine" under its different heads.

Prolapse of vagina with discharge—The vagina is much relaxed. There is copious white of an egg like leucorrhoea. (*Agn.*). See "Leucorrhoea-copious white discharge".

Prolapse of vagina with pain—Vagina, painful specially on coition. (*Sep.*). See also "Vagina-bleeding".

Prostate-discharge—Discharge at the time of stool. (*Agn.*). See "No. 8 of Spermatorrhoea." also "Emissions".

Prostate-enlarged of the aged person—Difficult urination. Aching pain in the back, suppression of the urine dependent upon the passage of gravel or uric acid. *Hydrangea-arborescens* works as sedative for the pain in the bladder, ureter or kindneys. (Potency 200 or 10M).

Prostate gland and its affections—(1) Acute cases of enlarged and inflamed prostate. Difficulty in passing urine. Burning while urination. The gland is hard swollen and painful. (*Sabal serrulata*).

(2) Prostate enlaigement in the aged. (*Ferr pic.*).

(3) Frequent pressing to urinate with small discharge, patient strains much ; cases from syphilis or badly managed gonorrhoea. (*Thuj.*).

(4) Chronic hypertrophy of prostate with difficulty in voiding urine ; it stops and starts. (*Con.*).

(5) Tenesmus, frequent urination, and great discharge due to prostate hypertrophy. *Chimaphila umbellata*.

(6) Prostate hypertophied, frequent micturition after urinating, renewed straining with dribbling of urine. Enlargement in old age. (*Bar-c.*),

(7) Enlarged prostate with pus and mucus in urine. (*Nat-s.*).

(8) Retention of urine in very old people from enlarged prostate when there is a great deal of trouble in urinating, (*Triticum repens.*).

(9) Intolerable urging and tenesmus constant desire to urinate. Urine drop by drop. (*Nux-v.* and *Cantharis* half hourly alternately).

(10) (*a*) According to Dr. Nash *Chimaphila* and *Cannabis indica* are very useful remedies in prostatic trouble of serious nature. When there is sensation of swelling in the perinaeum or near the anus with mucus in the urine.

(*b*) In cases of enlarged prostate glands with swelling of genitals. (*Dig.*). See "Urine-prostatic hypertrophy".

Prostate-irritation—Prostate disorders ; irritable bladder with vesical catarrh or gravel. (*Barosma crenata.*).

Prostate—after stricture—Acute affection of prostate after mal-treated stricture. (*Merc-c.*). See also "Gonorrhoea" and "Stricture".

Prostate—urine retention—Prostate hypertrophied. Retention of urine. (*Bell.*). See also "Retention of urine" under its different heads.

Prostration-extreme with depression—Gastric symptoms important, vertigo, pain in stomach with vomiting. If fever, the patient is as cold as ice, urine mixed with pus and blood. Give *Cal. sulf. 200,* twelve hourly in one week. *Staphi*-1M may be given as an intercurrent medicine each fortnight.

Prostration-with burning pain at midnight with hands and feet cold and sinking of vital power—With hands and feet cold and sinking of vital powers. Wants to toss about if still strong enough to do so. Intense burning and burning pains. *Arsenic* symptoms occur usually at midnight between 12 and 2 and sometimes between 1 and 3 P.M. (*Ars.*). See "Weakness—at midnight sinking sensation"

Prostration—of, child drowsy—The child is usually prostrated and drowsy and confused and inclined to fall asleep even when answering questions. Mouth full of ulcers, very offensive stools. (*Bapt.*). See "Drowsiness".

Prostration—relaxation of muscular system hands and feet tremble, lying drowsy and general fatigue—In acute cases. The patient desires to lie quietly with closed eyes. Trembling of hands and feet on attempt to move. Desires for lying still. Somewhat drowsy, complete relaxation of the muscular system with apparent or real paralytic condition. There is a feeling of lassitude or general fatigue. (*Gels.*). See also ' Relaxation of muscles with prostration of walking".

Prostration—at the end of a serious infectious disease— Great lassitude and prostration in all conditions specially at the end of serious infectious disease due to a fungus *e.g.* diphtheria, scarlet fever, pneumonia and erysiplas etc. *Am-c.* competes well with *Ars.* for nervous prostration. (*Am-c.*) See also "Diphtheria—when patient progressing" "Convalescence after lingering disease" and "Nervous prostration after infec-tious diseases".

Pruritus—*Sepia, Tarentula hispania* is another good medicine. See 'Itching female organ'.

Pruritus of whole body—Intolerable itching of whole body specially when getting warm and in bed, scratches till the skin bleeds which is painful. Brittle skin on fingers. (*Alumina.*).

Pruritus vulvae—When there is itching and soreness of genitals that disturb sleep. See Itching female organ. (*Ambr-gr.*).

Pruritus with burning urine—(1) Specially from warmth; itching and burning urine (*Sulf.*).

(2) For pruritus of ani, *Radium bromide* 30 once a week. This is also useful for pruritus of vulva. See also "Itching-anus", "Itching-female organ" "Urethra-itching" and "Genitals-females".

Psoric-antidote—*Sulphur*

Puerperal fever—See "Chapter V for details".

Pulmonary Tuberculosis its prevention—See "Chapter V for details".

Purgative—Persons who are used to cathertics and of sedentary habit, easily tired with great debility, constipation with dull head-ache. (*Tr. hydr.* 30.) ; for chronic constipation give one drop of *M. T. Hydr.* in water before going to stool first thing in morning while for obstinate constipation the patient should frequently take *Hydr. 3x* in drop doses in water in the morning to get rid of this trouble.

Psoriasis—(a) First start with *Sulf.* and then give *Ars-br.* (b) Itching of back of finger joint, unhealthy skin ; slight injuries suppurate. Ends of hair become trangled. (*Borax.*) (c) Psoriasis itching—*Thyroidin*. in low potency is useful is distressing itching of psoriasis.

Ptomaine poisoning—After decayed food or animal matter or alcoholic drinks and chewing tobacco. But it should have :

(1) burning pain,

(2) restlessness and

(3) *Ars.* thirst for little quantity and often ; warm drinks are preferred. (*Ars.*) First of all give *Acon.* in repeated doses and it acts admirably. Next try *Verta-a.* and then *Ars-a* ; for collapse stage think of *Camphor* and *Carb-v.* See also "Food-poisoning".

Ptosis drooping of upper eyelids—(1) Upperlids specially left, hangdown as, if paralyzed, burning dryness in eye ; useful in cases of granulation. (*Alumina*).

(2) Drooping of eyelids of rheumatic origin ; sensation of heaviness in upper lids as if he could not raise easily. (*Causticum*).

(3) Sensation of stiffness in eyelids and in muscles of eye of rheumatic origin. (*Kalmia.*). See "Eyelids drooping".

Puberty-derangements—The girl often weeps while stating her symptoms. She is submissive and usually good natured. Menses usually late, scanty in flow and slightly blackish in colour. Flows sometimes, stops then and flows again and so on. Menstrual trouble from wetting the feet just before menses. She feels too much hot, intermittent flow with evening chilliness, with intense pain and great restlessness and tossing about. First menstruation delayed. Pain in back. Nausea. Diarrhoea during or after menses. *Puls.* mental symptoms of quiet and of yielding disposition with a tearful mood must be present. *Puls.* patient may be irritable. (*Puls.*). See also "Derangements at puberty".

Puerperal-fever—If there are stretching pains in puerperal fever then *Kali carbonicum.*

Puerperal mania (following child-birth)—Aimless wandering from home. Delusions of impending misfortunes. Melancholy, with stupor and mania. Sullen indifference. Frenzy excitement, shrieks, curses. (*Verat.*). See also "Mania-amorous or religious "Fever puerperal", Part. (2) of "Insanity" and No. 10 of "Pregnancy disorder of".

Pulse—Pulse of *Gels.* has the characteristic that it is slow when the patient is at rest and is greatly and suddenly accelerated if the patient tries to move. Like *Bell.* it has the congestion of brain but neither the fever nor the congestion is so intense as in *Bell* Pulse more rapid in the morning than in the evening. Abnormal pulse is regular in rhythm, moderately full in volume, swelling under the examining fingers.

(1) Thready tremulous pulse. (*Colchicum*).
(2) Pulse small, quick, intermittent, compressible. (*Secale*).
(3) Slow pulse. (*Laurocerasus*).
(4) Pulse quick, irregular and intermittent. (*Crataegus*).
(5) Every fourth beat of pulse omits itself with great regularity. (*Calu-ars.*).
(6) Slow pulse with palpitation of heart. (*Ars-iod.*). Dr. Norton recommends this medicine in all heart diseases.

There is relationship between pulse, respiration and temperature. Normally for every degree of temerature above normal, there occur 10 extra beats of the pulse and 2 extra respiration as the following will show :—

Temperature	*Pulse*	*Respiration*	
94 F.	80	18	
100 F.	100	22	per minute
105 F.	150	34	

See "Respiration".

Pulse-normal—The normal pulse in full, strong and regular and the variation from the above must be due to radical disease or injury. (*Gel.*).

Pulling of penis by children—Child continually pulls at the penis. *Merc-sol.* and *Cantharis* to be tried in the order given. See "Penis".

Punctured wound inflammatory—Punctured injury to a nerve which later on takes inflammatory condition. (*Ledum.*). For external application *Ledum. M.T.* lotion. See also "Wound punctured".

Pus-formation—*Hep.* comes into use only when the pus is formed or about to form. Sometimes when pus has not been formed the very formation may be stopped and the inflammation may subside. If the pus has been formed it will hasten the pointing and bursting of the abscesses with rapid healing thereafter. In cases where suppuration seems inevitable *Hepar* may open the abscess and hasten the cure. Compare *Metc-sol.* which is indicated much before there is indication of formation and *Hepar* follows it if pus threatens to form or has already formed. (*Hep.*). See also "Inflammation-tending to form pus" and "Suppuration".

Pus-in axilla-armpit full of pus—The whole armpit covered into a bag of pus. (*Hepar-sulph. 6. T.D.S.*).

Pus-infection prophylactic—*Arnica.*

Pus-prevents formation—Prevents formation of pus ; to be given after *Hepar-sulf.* for healing, discharge of ulcer which has burst open after use of *Hepar.* ; *Silicea* ranks among the first of remedies for inflammation ending in suppuration. (Dr. Nash). See "Boils-pus averted" and "Inflammation tending to pus".

Pyelitis (inflammation of pelvis of a kidney)—Dr. Hughes thinks *Uva-ursi M.T.* to be most effective remedy. See also "Inflammation of kidney".

Pyorrhoea—(1) Gums separate from teeth ; pus oozes out ; all teeth loose ; bad smell from teeth. (*Kali-c.*).

(2) With spongy gum, bad odour from mouth. (*Merc-c.*).

(3) A lotion of mother tincture of *Symphytum* 1 gram in 4 ounces of water is a good application to the gums in pyorrhoea.

(4) Equally efficacious is *Eucalyptus g.* oil for local application on the gums after cleaning the teeth. It controls the development of bacteria and stimulates local cells. See "Gums and Teeth".

Pyorrhoea-alveolaris—Teeth decay next to gums, very sensitive, gums retract. (*Thuj.*). See "Tartar".

Pyorrhoea-crumbling teeth and bleeding gums with gum boil—(1) Teeth black and crumbling. Salivation, spongy gums bleed easily. (*Staphy.*).

(2) Painful inflammation worse by cold or hot things, gum boil. *Sil.* 4 hourly. See also "Teeth" under its different heads.

—: o :—

Q

Quinine-its antidote—The best antidote is *Ipecac*, then comes *Ars-a*. and *China*. The other useful antidotes are *Natrum-m*. and *Verat-a*.

Quinsy-acute inflammation of the tonsils—(1) Initial chill and fever, anxiety and restlessness with pain and soreness. (*Acon*. 3 hours.).

(2) Severe tonsillitis with pricking pains. (*Sil*.).

(3) Septic tonsillitis : Gunpowder to be alternated with *Bar-c*.

(4) Shooting pain principally during swallowing extending to the ears. Sometimes complete inability to drink. The fluid returning by the nostrils. Swelling of the palate, uvula and tonsils with headache. *Bell*. in alternation with *Mercurius* two hours between each dose. (J. Laurie.).

(5) With eruption of vesicles on mucous membrane. (*Phytolacca*). (Dr. Clarke.). See also "Tonsils" under their different heads.

Quinsy-(acute inflammation of the tonsil with fever and peritonsillar tissues usually tending to suppuration and its prophylactic—Prophylactic. (*Bar-c. 30*).

Quinsy—See "Tendency to Quinsy".

Quinsy-its prevention—See "Chapter V" for details.

Quotidian-intermittent fever—The stages of fever appear around the clock *e.g.* chill at 10 A.M., vomiting at 12.30 p.m., headache at 4.30 p.m. and so no. For complaints that appear in the same months every year. Dr. V. Krishnamurty of Madras suggests ***Urtica urens***. See "Periodicity" "Fever malaria periodical" and "Colic periodical".

R

Rabies—(*a*) *Hydroph. 30* shoud be taken 3 times a day for a week and then *Bell.* night and morning for 6 months at least. (*b*) To prevent convulsions after bites of mad dogs give this medicine evening and morning every week till it produces fever and diarrhoea. (*c*) *Stramonium* is nearest similimum to hydrophobia. (*d*) Jones suggests that by keeping up free perspiration by the use of *Jaborandi* the poison of rabies might be eliminated from the system. See also "Dog bite".

Rachitis-its prevention—See "Chapter V" for details.

Rage-fits of—For fits of rage. (*Mosch.*). See "Anger complaints".

Ranula-under the tongue—(*a*) A retention cyst of the tongue in front. (*Thuj.*). (*b*) Hard and large in size, *Merc-sol.* to be alternated with *Thuja*. Compare *Fluor-ac*. See also "Tongue cyst".

Rash-on child's body—*Acon.* if there is fever and frequent pulse ; *Ip.* if diarrhoea is present. *Bry.*, if constipation and distension of bowels. See "Eruption with blisters spreading redness".

Rash-papular—A very disagreeable rash on the body. The eruption occupied the skin over the chest, stomach, and duodenum and itched a good deal on going to bed. The patient is costive and anaemic. (*Thuja* 30 infrequent doses). Compare *Sulphur-iodatum* which is good for papular eruption on the face.

Rat-bites—Made safe by use of *Ledum* from its subsequent complication of tetanus or any other form of septic condition. *Ledum* will not only prevent inflammatory complication but will also prevent shooting pain. (*Led.*). See "Bites".

Rat-bite external application—Bites by rats or scorpions, apply *Ledum-pal*. mother tincture externally. See also "Bites" under their different heads. See "Internal Homoeopathic medicines".

Rational use of curative agents—In considering the curative agents you have to consider the 3 kingdoms—the man, mineral world and the vegetable world. There are no changes possible in a man that cannot be produced, caused or aggravated by drugs. Man's diseases have their likenesses in the substances that make up three kingdoms. Man himself is *Microcosm* of the elements of the earth. This earthly elements (minerals) strive to rise through the vegetable kingdom into man. Every element and creature below man in the created universe seeks to degrade man exercising such an influence as will elevate itself at man's expense, as if through jealousy. The study of man as to his nature, as to his life, as to his affections underlies the true study of Homoeopathy. A rational doctrine of therapeutics begins with the change wrought in a man. We may never ascertain causes but we may observe changes. Hahnemann emphasised the symptoms of the mind, hence we see how clearly the master comprehended the importance of the direction of the symptoms, the more interior first the mind, the exterior last-the physical or bodily symptoms.

SUMMARISE

Man :

Diseases in general.
Diseases in particular.
Remedies in general.
Remedies in particular.

The examination of an epidemic is in all nothing but a consideration of a similar number of provers. When a given epidemic comes upon a land and if as many cases as possible are most carefully written out, then the prevailing disease may be viewed collectively as a unit as if one man has suffered from all the symptoms observed. It is similar to a course applied to a large group of provers in order to bring out the totality of symptoms of a drug. Every epidemic or every man, sick, must be fully wrought with, first the generals and then the particulars ; remember that the particulars are always within the generals. Great mistakes may come from going too deeply into the particulars before the generals are settled. An army of soldiers without the line of officers could not but be a mob. Hence consideration of all particulars without first considering the generals would be like a confused mob in our materia medica. We must avoid confusion of mind that often comes from thinking in the old way, not knowing what to call a disease and what to consider as only the results of a disease. A practical illustration comes to us at once when we think of Hahnemann's prevision, in as much as he was able to say that Cholera resembles *Cuprum, Camphor* and *Veratrum.*

Ravenous hunger—See "Appetite increased and ravenous".

Reaction - creating reaction—When carefully selected remedies fail to produce a favourable effect specially in acute diseases due to depression of vital force or psora. *Sulf.* frequently serves to rouse the reactive powers of the system and clear up the case. It has power to meet and overcome certain obstacles to the usual action of drug. Give a dose of *Sulf.* and wait for a few hours in an acute case and wait for a few days in a chronic case and then administer the indicated medicine. See also "Blocks" and "Creating reaction".

Reaction-lack of—When well chosen remedies do not act.

(*i*) Lack of reaction in persons of lax fibre. *Capsicum.*

(*ii*) In patients where there is no pain, drowsiness. *Opium.*

(*iii*) In nervous affections when well chosen remedies fail. *Valerian or Ambra.*

(*iv*) Collapse, coldness of knees, breath, perfect indifference. (*Carbo-veg.*) Each one of the above medicines may be called for when there is defective reaction.

(*v*) *Psorinum* may succeed in Psoric obstruction, vital reactions when *Sulphur* fails.

(*vi*) *Laurocerasus* may be used in case of excessively low vitality.

R

Reappearance of skin trouble—Many a time an internal disease which has been cured after suppression of any skin trouble will be cured with *Sulf.* after the original skin trouble reappears on the skin. (*Sulf.*). See "Suppressed skin trouble". See "Eczema; itching and recurring".

Rectum-aches—Aches as if full of broken glasses. Anus burns after stool. Protrusion of haemorrhoids. (*Ratanhia.*). See "Anus fissures".

Rectum-haemorrhage,dark blood and also from anus—(1) When the blood is of dark colour and is passed with stool painlessly. (*Ham.*).

(2) *Nitric acid* and *Muriatic acid* are head remedies for bleeding from anus without reference to any cause. See Bleeding from mucous membrane, and Part 'b' "Haemorrhage of" "Haemorrhage continuous of" "Haemorrhage" during pregnancy if abortion apprehended.

Rectum-haemorrhoids—The rectum seems full of sticks due to blind haemorrhoids with liver engorgement. (*Aesc.*). See "Haemorrhoids of both types".

Rectum-prolapse and paralysis--(*a*) A feeling of foreign substance as of a ball or weight in the rectum. (*Sep.*).

(b) Paralysis of rectum. (*Tab.*). See "Prolapse rectum".

Rectum-prolapse with or without diarrhoea—Prolapse of rectum either with or without diarrhoea in children or in women after child birth. (*Podo.*). See "Prolapse of rectum in child or after child birth".

Rejuvenator—For old men who suffers from different painful ailments due to old age, specially suited to tired, languid and exhausted subjects. Indisposition for mental exertion ; sleepless on account of indigestion. General muscular weakness-persons who look older than they actually are. (*Mag-p.* to be given in highest potencies in hot water). See "Prematurely old-with impairment of all functions"

Relapse-of typhoid fever—*Ant-c.* is best, then comes *Ip.* See "Fever typhoid relapse" "Hands and feet tremble, lying drowsy and general fatigue".

Relaxation-of muscles with prostration on walking—Relaxation and prostration in acute diseases. The patient desires to lie quietly preferably with closed eyes. Trembling hands and lower extremities on attempt to move. If he attempts to move hands tremble, if he attempts to walk the legs tremble. All these tremblings from weakness of the nervous system specially in acute febrile cases should attract the notice to *Gels.* The eyelids droop in acute condition. The patient is drowsy. The pulse is weak. Complete relaxation of muscular system with apparent of renal paralytic condition. (*Gels.*). See also "Prostration-relaxation or muscular system hands and feet tremble, lying drowsy and general fatigue".

Relationship of remedies-complementary and antidoting When a remedy has done its best in relieving a case it is important to know the remedies that can follow well and cure a case partly affected by the former. A drug is said to be complementary to another when the former completes a cure which the latter begins but is unable to effectuate it. In other words when the relationship between the remedy and one of the remedies that follow well is very close, the latter is said to be complementary to the former. Sometimes a complementary medicine may precede the principal medicine. Some remedies are listed both as a complementary and as an antidote to the same remedy. This anamoly is explained by the fact that such drugs, show often, the power of antidoting or neutralising the unwanted effects of and yet not interfering with the curative action initiated by the previously administered drugs. It may be noted that a second prescription should be one of those medicines that follow well. The term 'compatible is a generic term which includes complementary and those followed well by'. (b) (i) Incompatible or inimical remedies :—The use of any of these after the principal remedy has been administered is harmful ; such a procedure renders the disease complicated and more difficult. (ii) Antidotal relation—An accidental over dose of any remedy may harm the system. A prescriber who can not antidote a drug effect is like the driver of a motor who cannot put the brake. Some drugs are found to neutralise the effects of drugs previously given. The knowledge of this relation between remedies is clinically very useful as sometimes we have to counteract the dangerous medicinal aggravations or trouble-some accessory symptoms when they appear after the administration of a partly similar remedy in a case. So in case of each remedy it is necessary to know the remedies it antidotes or is antidoted by. At the end I have with great pains prepared a chart comprising 6 columns which gives at a glance a true picture mostly of those remedies suggested in this prescriber on the basis of standard authorities.

Religious mania—(*a*) When there is conflict between two wills. The external and internal. (*Anac.*). (*b*) Mania of religious or amorous, lascivious (*lust-ful.*) type. (*Verat.*). Compare *Hyos.*, *Stram.* See also "Mania amorous or religious" and "Will".

Renal colic-pain—See "Chapter V" for details.

Renal (pertaining to kidney) colic-severe pain caused by efforts to pass a stone locked up in ureter and suppression of urine—(1) For colic due to indigestion. *Nux-v.* is the head remedy to be given in hot water. Pain may be in any part.

(2) Abdomen hard, violent spasms of colic. Aggravated by cold drinks. (*Cupr-met.*).

(3) Colic in women and children. Colic from anger, digestion is at standstill, abdomen distended like drum. (*Cham.*). See "Anger complaints".

(4) Abdominal pains radiating in all directions, cramp in legs and obstinate constipation. Stony hardness of abdomen. (*Plumbum.*).

(5) Violent stitching pains in bladder extending from

kidneys into urethra with urging to urinate drawing of testicles, urine pale with mucus (*Berb.*).

(6) Dr. Jahr says that *Puls. Cann-i., Sarsap.* and *Lyco.* have done wonders in his hands in alleviating renal colic and facilitating the passage of stone through urethra.

(7) Dr. Jousset says that *Bell.* and *Cham.* are given in alternation when pain is violent, regardless of the disease which produced them. They act like morphine.

(8) *Nitric-a.* should be thought of when the urine contains oxalic acid.

(9) Dr. Jacob uses *Ipomea-nit.* for passage of stone from kidney to bladder when there is severe pain in either renal region extending down the ureter on the corresponding side. The distinctive feature is that these pains excite nausea.

(10) *Ocimum* is useful when the urine contains considerable blood.

(11) Dr. Hempel records many cases of renal colic cured with *Cocus-cacti.* extending to bladder accompanied by frequent emmision of dark scanty urine.

(12) *Cantharis* is one of the best remedies during the paroxysm of renal colic. Ferrington says that it relieves local irritation permitting nature to get rid of stone with less suffering to the patient.

(13) Tendency to stone, uric acid in the tissue, gouty subjects. *Urt-ur. M.T.* 5 to 8 drops in water.

(14) *Pareira brava M T.* a few drops in warm distilled water every half hour when all other remedies fail.

(15) Colic when the griping pains forcing the patient to bend double, colic caused by flatus, undigested food. There may be present diarrhoea ; also useful in menstrual colic. (*Coloc.*). See also "Colic-renal (pertaining to kidney) stone in kidney."

(b) suppression or retention of urine, difficult or painful urine ; blood and sand in urine, tenesmus after urinating *Stigmata maydis M T*. 20 drops and *Magnesia phos* 12x trituration may be given in alternation in hot water.

(2) Renal and vesical irritation. Frequent, urine heavy, phosphatic. Brick dust sediment, violent colic. (Give *Thalspi Bursa Pastoris M.T.* 10 to 15 drops in hot water.).

(3) Red adhesive sand in urine which is very offensive. (*Sepia*).

(4) Colic with gout. Urine highly coloured and very offensive, changeable colour brown ; acid. Excess of uric acid. *Benzoicum acidum*.

(5) Renal colic ; violent pain along ureter, left side. Incessant nausea. (*Tabac.*).

(6) Gall-stone colic ; urine fetid with white sediment Expels renal stones when formation of stones is due to uric acid. Constipation. *Calc-c. 30*. Give *Tuberculinum 1 M*, as an intercurrent medicine.

(7) Urine looks like lime water. Prevents, the accumulation of gravel and renal calculi. Has to be used for a long time. (*Calc. renalis*).

(8) 15 drops of Tincture Ether may be put in half a glass of warm water and a dose may be given every 10 to 15 minutes during attack.

(9) Tightness and pressure across the lower limbs ; accumulation of wind in bowels expelled with much difficulty and relief after it ; stiching pains in the spleen ; the colic occurs or is worse at night. (*Ignatia* every hour).

(10) Colic with nausea and profuse saliva ; severe and pinching pain with hardness of abdomen particularly about the navel, prostration, chills and shuddering. Sometimes diarrhoea. (*Merc.* every half hour.)

(11) According to Dr. Bhanja *Citrated Borate* of *Magnesia* has been used with great success in alleviating renal colic and expelling renal calculus and gravel. During pain as much of the medicine as can stand on the point of knife is to be taken after one hour or so. It is reported that the medicine very promptly

diminishes the pain and the passage of calculus is not attended with any pain. For prevention of renal colic with gravely urine, pain in back and loins, give 5 drops, of *Tr. Berb-vulg* See "Urine albuminous and other casts".

Respiration-breathing oppressed and puffing of cheeks—(a) *Arsenicum* has proved useful in diseases of respiratory organs. *Arsenic* is also particularly efficacious in many affections of the lungs when breathing is much oppressed. Respiration is wheezing with cough and frothy expectoration, patient cannot lie down, must sit up to breathe. The air passages seem constricted. Worse after 12 in night (*Ars-alb.*). See also "Dyspnoea" under its different heads. (*b*) Sonorous breathing and puffing out of cheeks. (*China*. 2 hour.). See "Breathing oppressed", "Heart-respiration", and "Pulse".

Restlessness-changing position giving relief—Must change position constantly, with relief for a short time by the change. Cannot lie in one position for long. The patient constantly changes his position : turns side, sits up, lies down or even walks about a little. But he cannot lie on one position for long. *Rhus-tox.* is famous remedy for restlessness. Thus *Rhus-tox.* patient cannot be quiet. Quieter he tries to be the more restless he becomes. This is just opposite of *Bry.* which is relieved by lying quietly. There is not much of mental factor in *Rhus-tox.* restlessness. It is relieved temporarily by changing position. (*Rhus-tox*). Compare *Ars.* and *Acon.* which are also restless medicines. Thus great trio of restless remedies are *Ars.*, *Acon.*, and *Rhus-tox.* See also "Position changing giving relief at midnight" and "Changing position giving relief".

Restlessness at midnight, more mental—With prostration and sinking of bodily strength. Anxiety of mind with thirst. He is more disturbed in mind by application of heat. *Arsenic* symptoms occur usually at midnight between 12 and 2, sometimes between 1 and 3 in the after-noon. (*Ars-alb.*). Compare other restless remedies. *Acon.* and *Rhus-tox.* which are more bodily restless. See also "Prostration with burning pain at midnight" and "Weakness at midnight with sinking sensation".

Restlessness-moving his body with fidgetiness—Though *Phos.* is not as anxious and restless as *Arsenic* it has a peculiar fidgetiness all over the body. He cannot sit or stand still for a moment. The child must be moving or doing something. *Phos.* has less anxiety though he may be always moving this or that part of his body. (*Phos.*). See also "Fidgetiness".

Restlessness-tossing in bed throwing covering—Restlessness with anxiety and thirst to a certain extent. Tossing about in bed. Throws off covering. Anxious looks along with restlessness. (*Acon.*) *Ars.* and *Rhus-tox.* and other restless medicines may be compared.

Retarded eruption of measles—According to Dr. Jahr *Verat-a.* and according to Dr. Herring *Camph.* are the best medicines to bring out suppressed measles. See also "Measles-restlessness" and "Eruptions in measles retarded".

Retarded eruption-of small-pox—If the eruptions are not well out in spite of *Variolinum* try *Sulph.* ; if the result is not satisfactory *Bry.* should be given in repeated doses. After *Bry.* a dose of *Sulph.,* may help to bring out the eruptions. See also "Small-pox no regular rash and its stages".

Retching (unsuccessful attempt at vomiting)—(1) Dry retching without vomiting. Diarrhoea. Hardly any thirst. (*Podo.*).

(2) Vomiting of milk. (*Aethus-c.*).

(3) Sudden vomiting of milk in infants (*Merc-s.*).

(4) Acid or bilious vomiting. (*Iris-v.*).

(5) Violent retching or continuous vomiting and having nausea. (*Symphoricarpus-racemosa*). See also "Vomiting" and "Milk not digested with diarrhoea".

Retention of urine in dropsy—Scanty urine accompanies many complaints amongst the early symptoms of dropsy. Painful micturition ; urging to pass urine constantly. The kidneys are not acting and scarcely any urine passes. The bladder is sometimes only partially full but the patient cannot pass urine (*Apoc-can.*). See also "Prostate-urine retention" and "Urine in dropsy".

Retention-of urine after strenuous labour and of infants with bloated face—(1) Paralytic weakness of the bladder after a woman has gone through strenuous labour causing retention of urine afterwards is miraculously removed by *Caust.*

(2) Retention of urine of infants will be removed by *Acon.* If this fails then *Puls.*

(3) Child very drowsy and sleepy, face bloated, urine retained. (*Op.*). See also "Paralysis-retention urine" and "Labour retention of urine".

Retina detachment, haemorrhage and its reabsorption and apoplexy of retina—(1) Detachment of retina due to injury. (*Arnica-m.*).

(2) The retina is inflamed and there are opacities. Detachment of retina. (*Aurum-met.*).

(3) Haemorrhage in the retina. Inflammation of retina. Retinal vessels large. Pain in the upper part of eyeball. (*Dub.*).

(4) Stinging pains in the eyes with swollen lids. Detachment of retina. (*Apis-mel*). "See also "Eyes" under its different heads.

(5) Apoplexy of the retina especially when arising from and accompanied by congestive headache. Aching pains in the eyes and retina. (*Bell.*).

(6) *Gels* is an excellent remedy for haemorrhage in the eyes resulting in blindness. Give *Gels. 200* twice daily morning and evening. If *Gels.* fails then *Phos.*

(7) For reabsorption of effused bloods. (*Lach.*). See "Eyelids drooping".

Retina-Hyperaesthesia (exaggerated sensibility of nerve-filaments)—Pain extending back into head ; lachrymation and impaired vision. Useful in restoring power to the weakened ciliary muscle. (*Lilium tig.*).

R

Retinal Haemorrhage—*Hamamelis virginica* hastens absorption of intra-ocular haemorrhage.

Rheumatic pain with stiffness and soreness—Rheumatic pains in joints with soreness and stiffness in the buttocks, knees and wrist. The joints feel stiff as if they wanted oil. Headache over eyes ; urine violet smelling. (*Salol.*). (Dr. Boericke).

Rheumatism in different parts of body and its line of treatment—(a) (1) Pain in soles of feet and heels. (*Tart-ac.*). The pure acid 10-30 grains dissolved in water.

(2) Pain in wrists and ankles with fever, it diminishes the amount of urates. (*Trimethly*).

(3) *Gultheria* oil in 10-20 drops never fails to arrest the pains.

(4) *Colchicum* is a head remedy for gout and rheumatism. Albuminous urine and scanty.

(5) Rheumatic finger joints with flatulence. (*Lyco.*).

(6) When the pain attacks the back, back of the neck and back of the head with restlessness and pain in the eyes. (*Act-rac* 1 hourly.) See also "Head-drawn back".

(7) Small joints of the hands and feet the joints ache and swell while the patient is walking. (*Act-sp.*).

(8) Rheumatism of the finger joints with tendency to heart complications. (*Lith-c.*).

(9) Rheumatism of the wrist. (*Viol-o.* and *Ruta.*).

(10) Rheumatism of the right shoulder. (*Mag-c.*).

(11) The knee is swollen, has a doughy feet and the pain is worse at night, usually the trouble is of syphilitic origin. (*Kali-hy.*).

(b) The line of treatment of father Muller's dispensary is as follows :—Give *Acon.* for fever. *Bry.* when the muscles are chiefly affected, when the pains are steady and always in the same place, increased by motion, touch or cough. *Rhus.* for steady pains increased by damp and cold weather, worse by rest better by motion. *Merc-viv.* when the joints and bones are affected, pain worse by heat and cold, worse at night with abundant oily perspiration. *Puls.* when the knees, ankles and small joints are affected, when the pains shift about, are worse at night, in warm room and by rest, better by motion and in the fresh air. Dulc. sub-acute cases due to getting wet ; *Cimicifuga* when the pains are in the waist and back, back of the neck and in the head. *Sulph.*, in all cases to be given intercurrently. See also "Arthritis, hyper-sensitivation with rheumatic constitution" and "Gout".

(*c*) (1) Rheumatism of neck. Stiff neck, head drawn back. (*Lachnanthes*). (2) Severe drawing erratic pains (which change place every minute) and stiffness in small joints, fingers toes and ankles etc. Aching wrists ; pains on closing hands. Rheumatism of women. Habitual abortion from uterine debility. (*Caul.*). (3) Rheumatism of left shoulder and deltoid (muscle of the left shoulder) ; shooting, tearing, stinging, swelling. Better from continued movement of the parts or slow movements. (*Ferr-met.*). (4) Rheumatism of syphilitic or gonerrhoeal origin. Left side affected ; chilly patient. Tearing in muscles and joints, worse at rest, better in dry weather, worse damp and humid atmosphere ; lameness (*Thuj* in 'M' potency.). (5) Migratory rheumatism with alternation of sides *i.e.* it may attack one ankle first and then other and then comes back again to the original locality. It may attack knees, hips and shoulders in this way. The key-note symptom is erratic pain alternating sides. (*Lac-can.*).

Rheumatism-in the feet—Rheumatism begins in the feet and travels upwards. This is opposite of Kalmia, which goes the other ways. *Ledum* may be indicated in both acute and chronic forms of this complaint. In the acute form the joints are swollen and hot. (*Ledum.*).

Rheumatism in lower extremities with breathlessness—In lower extermities. Difficult breathing, clothing all removed from neck and breast, choking and gasping for breath. (*Lach.* followed by *Abrot.*). See "Dyspnoea".

Rheumatism in joints aggravated in damp weather—Pain aggravated in damp weather which drives the patient out of bed and makes him walk about. Pain in joints maddening and send the patient to delirium (*Verat.*). See "Wet weather-cold air".

Rheumatism with bad teeth—Bad and unhealthy teeth specially pyorrhoea. (*Phyorrhin* nosode in high dilution.).

Rheumatism-bad weather excites attacks—(*a*) *Calcarea, Dulcamara, Rhus-tox, Lycopodium* and *Hepar-sulph*.

(*b*) When change of weather causes a relapse—*Calcarea, Silicea, Sulphur, Dulcamara. Rhus-tox* and *Lachesis*.

Rheumatism due to checked diarrhoea or constipation—Due to checked diarrhoea or constipation. Relief from diarrhoea. (*Abrot.*). Compare *Nat-s.* and *Zinc*. See "Constipation causing rheumatism".

Rheumatism with diabetes—(1) *Lac-ac.* (2) *Phaseal* is an important remedy for gout accompanied with diabetes.

Rheumatic-deafness—The best remedy is *Sulph.* Sometimes *Dulc., Bry.* and *Caust.* may be useful. See "Deafness due to different causes Part 15".

Rheumatism - deformed and swollen joints—Deformed and swollen joints after attack of rheumatism. (*Iodum.*). Compare *Pituitary gland,* a nosode which is often used in deforming rheumatism by Dr. Barishac. See (ix) of "Arthritis hyper sensitivation".

Rheumatism - of any type without taking the totality of symptom—*Colchicum* which has a specific power of relieving chronic gouty attacks.

Rheumatism - in dropsy with inflammation of all joints—Inflammatory in dropsy. Inflammation of the ankle, joints of the toes, of the fingers, inflammation of the joints all over the body. Joints pit on pressure with dropsy. But with the scanty urine, want of sweat, with the febrile condition he is all the time chilly and wants the parts well wrapped where *Apis.* wants them uncovered. He may be chilly with fever or without fever. (*Apoc-can.*). See also "Dropsy swelling of feet".

Rheumatism in lower limbs and also in upper limbs—*Ledum p.* is used for lower limbs while *Kalmia* is used for rheumatism of upper limbs. It has very sudden excruciating pains.

Rheumatism-nervous patients—*Asaf.* is the remedy which is full of rheumatism and gouty symptoms ; gouty affections in general in nervous constitutions. When such a nervous constitution finally produces gouty formations, then nervousness often disappears, for it has been relieved by deposit in joints ; a transformation has since taken place. (*Asaf.*). See "Gout-nervous".

Rheumatism-soreness and aching of muscles and joints—Rheumatism aching and soreness in muscles and joints, compelling patient to change sides. Bed feels too hard. *Arnica* followed by *Sulf.* See "Changing position".

Rheumatism-pains spreading at neck and extremities—Pains spread over a large surface, at nape of nack, loins and extremities, better by motion, hot painful swelling of joints. Pain along ulnar nerve. (*Rhus-t.*). See also "Pain-wandering".

Rheumatism-pain and swelling in all joints—Pains in joints and muscles, knees stiff and painful. Hot swelling of feet, joints swollen with stitches and tearing. Every spot is painful on pressure and worse on least movement. Joints red, swollen and stiff with pain, will be worse at the slightest motion or movement. (*Bry.*). See also "Pain colic like and shifting rheumatism pains".

Rheumatism-pains wandering with swelling of different parts of body—Pains wander from joint to joint or from place to place throughout the body with swelling aud redness of joints. Such a changeableness should be present in her disposition *e.g.* obstinate, yielding, tearful, irritable, mild and pleasant. She is immediately soothed by consolation. Feet inflamed ; legs and feet are heavy and weary. Hip joints painful. Knees swollen. Tensive pains in thighs. Sleeplessness and chilliness. No thirst. Relief from walking slowly in open air. (*Puls.*). Compare *Aur-met.* and *Kali bichromicum* if digestive trouble. See also "Wandering-joints pains".

Rheumatism with gastric troubles—Chronic gout with gastric and urinary deposits. Compare *Nux-v.*, *Antim-cru.*, *Natrum-muri.*

Rheumatic pains-in back and neck and head drawn back—In muscles of back and neck. Violent aching down the back. Head drawn back from contraction of the muscles of the back. Mental state following disappearance of rheumatic condition. (*Act-rac.*). See also "Head-drawn back" 'Lumbago-stiffness" and "Back-ache".

Rheumatic pains-with cold extremities—Shifting, cold extremities. (*Bell.*). See "Chapter V for details".

Rheumatic dysmenorrhoea—In the rheumatic and hysterical constitution. Irregularity of the menstrual flow. It may be copious, suppressed, or scanty. Severe pain all through the flow. The more the flow the greater the pain. Generally the most severe and most painful attack is at the beginning of the flow and sometimes after the flow has ceased. Each woman "is a law unto herself". (*Act-rac.*). See also "Dysmenorrhoea or difficult or painful menstruation in hysterics".

Rheumatic fever with various complaints—(i) High fever, thirst and redness of cheeks, shooting extremely violent pains at night ; excessive irritability of temper. *Acon.* a dose every 2 hours at night. It may prove of great service as an intermediate remedy during the course of treatment. (ii) Paralytic weakness, soreness and stiffness of limbs ; chilliness, pain over the whole body ; puffy swelling of face ; bitter taste in mouth. (*Gels.*). (iii) Intense aching pains specially in the back and shoulders, headache, nausea, sometimes vomiting, flushed face ; cold, clammy perspiration. (*Verat-v.* a dose every 2 hours.) (iv) Tearing pains with numbness of paralysed parts, feverishness ; tossing ; perspiration confined to head. Aggravation at night, temporary relief from sitting up in bed. (*Cham.* a dose every 3 hours.) Dr. Laurie further recommends *Bry., Merc., Cimic., Puls., Nux-v., Rhus-t.,* and *Cact.* for fevers after rheumatism to be given according to symptoms. See "Heart weakness due to rheumatism".

Rheumatic-heart—Chronic rheumatic pain in the ankle and knee. Murmurs in the heart. Can sit while propped up on pillows, small pulse. Pain in the heart. (*Abrot.*). See also "Endocarditis-rheumatic heart" and "Heart weakness due to rheumatism".

Rheumatic heart due to suppression of disease—Cardiac weakness or inflammation of the lining membrane of the heart or its valves or enlargement of the heart. The condition of heart may be a sequence of rheumatic state which has been removed by suppressed methods. (*Aur-met.*). See also "Heart-weakness due to rheumatism".

Rheumatism-hereditary—*Silicea* is useful in such cases when pains are worse at night, worse from uncovering, better from warmth.

Rheumatic pain-in influenza—(1) Aching all through as if in bone. (*Eupato-perf.*).

(2) Violent pains in the joints. (*Mer-s.*).

(3) Dr. Dewey highly recommends *Phos.* as the great post-influenzal tonic. See also "No. 3 and No. 4 of fever influenza".

Rheumatic pain - in knee—A great rheumatic remedy particularly for a single joint like a knee is *Pulsatilla* according to Dr. Blackie.

Rheumatic ophthalmia (inflammation of conjunctiva)—Dr. D.C. Das Gupta recommends *Acon., Bry., Euphr, Merc-s., Puls., Rhus-t., Spig., Sulf.,* and *Verat-a.,* according to symptoms. See "Eyes" "Vision" under different heads and "Inflammation of eye-lids, loss of lashes and eczema".

R

Rheumatic pleurisy—It yields in most cases to *Arn-m.* but when it cannot do any thing try *Bry.* and *Rhus-t.* Dr. Jahr recommends the use of *Nux-v.*, *Lyco.* and *Cimic.* Try also *Ars.*, *Senega* and *Bacill.*, according to symptoms. See "Pleurisy".

Rheumatic pains-in thigh—*Ferrum-magneticum.*

Rheumatic pains-oversensitiveness to pain and peevishness—Hyper sensitiveness to the pain ; the patient must be peevish and snappish which is the peculiar mental condition of *Cham.* Violent pains are usually at night and compel the patient to leave the bed and walk about. Numbness with pain. (*Cham.*). Compare *Ferr-met.*, *Rhus-tox.*, *Verat-a.* But over sensitiveness to pain and peevish temper will decide for *Cham.* See also "Hyper sensitiveness" and "Bones pains due to injury or fracture".

Rheumatic paralysis—*Rhus-t.* is specially adapted to all forms of paralysis which are rheumatic in origin or brought on by getting wet or exposure to dampness in any form or for paralysis caused by nervous fevers and typhus.

Rheumatic troubles-with numbness and crawling feeling—stiffness and pain with cold, numb and crawling feeling, buttocks, back and limbs asleep. Specially for rheumatic troubles of children starting in cold damp and after winter rains. (*Calc-p.*). See also "Numbness of main parts (2) and (3)".

Rheumatic tooth-ache—The first remedies to be tried according to symptoms are *Merc-s.*, and *Puls.*, then try *Bry.*, and after that *Cham.*, the other possible remedies are *Nux-v.*, *Rhus-t.*, and *Spig.* See "Teeth-aches".

Rheumatic symptoms in spine due to injury—In spine due to injury caused by a fall or due to inflammatory changes may need *Rhus-tox.* and finally *Calcarea.* See also "Spine injuries" under its different heads.

Rheumatoid arthritis-chronic of knee—Osteoarthritis of the knee. Swelling, stiffness, and pain of rheumatic arthritis are removed in very short time by *Berberis-vulgaris* given in 3x potency. (*Dr. Jugal Kishore*).

Rheumatoid-arthritis (arthritic pain in fingers)—Pain in heels, weakness and shaking of hand in writing. (*Antimonium-crudum.*). (Dr. Anshuez).

Rhinitis—Inflammation of nasal-mucous-membrane :—Nose swollen involving tonsils and cervical glands. Discharge purulent and even bloody and slight exposure to draft on exposure of any kind causes one attack after another. *Lemna Minor*. (Dr. Blackwood).

Rickets including curvature and malformation of bone—(1) Rickety children, thin, perspiring head and feet. (*Silicea.*).

(2) Curvature specially of spine or long bones ; extremities crooked and growing imperfectly. (*Calc-c.*).

(3) Malformation of bones with loss in weight. (*Calc-c.*).

(4) Drs. Dewey and Jousset recommend *Phos-a.* as principal remedy for rickets.

(5) *Tuberculinum* to be administered every forthnight as intercurrent remedy.

(6) When there is tendency to rickets ; the limbs are tender and motion is painful. (*Ferr-p.*).

(7) Give *Psorinum* for stopping the sweating head of rickety children, if *Silica* is unable to do so. See also "Bones-rickets" "Curvature of bones" and "Emaciation".

Riding-causing inability to walk—Bruised and sprained by riding, the legs and buttocks becoming sore and permanent contraction of the tendency of lower limbs. (*Cimex-lec.*).

Right sided complaints—*Anac.* has a special affinity for right side of body and so is *Am-c.*

Right sided hernia—*Lyco.* and for left sided hernia *Lachesis.* If there is pain around neval *Belladonna.* See "Hernia".

Ringworm itching and on moustaches—(*a*) (*i*) Itching not relieved by scratching. (*Sep.*). (*ii*) *Bacillinum* is head remedy and should be given once a week 200 for adults. (*iii*) Father Muller gives *Sepia 30.* and *Sulf. 30* intercurrently. (*iv*) Externally ointment of *Phytolacca* to be applied in all cases. See "Eruptions-itching".

(*b*) Ringworm on moustaches and other parts : *Ant-c, Graph., Lyco., Merc-iod.,* and *Sulf.* according to symptoms. (*ii*) For violent itching and the eruptions are moist and offensive *Staphy.* to be followed by *Rhus-t.* (*iii*) Dry ring worm on face not relieved by itching. Eruptions like ringworm every spring on different parts of body. *Sep.* (*iv*) Itching of hands and feet. Ringworm on any part of body. *Tell.* is a head remedy for such a trouble. *Tellurium* is also an excellent remedy for curing ringworm specially on the face. Dr. Burnett's special remedy for ringworm trouble is *Bacillinum* in high potency.

Ringworm-in the hair and in other places—Vesicular eruption. Red spots, eruption on face, genitals and hands, (*Dulcamara,*). See "Eruptions on genitals" and "Eruptions-in hair of forehead".

Ringworm-on face and chest—On chest and face of the child. The child keeps up a chewing motion during sleep and rolls its head. (*Hell.*). *Calc-c.* should be thought of in plethoric persons. For ringworm specially on face and body of adult. (*Tellurium.*). See "Eczema-on face".

Ringworm on the scalp of children extending to face, neck and eyes—(1) Begin with *Rhus.* and follow it with *Sulf.*

(2) When moist and offensive with violent itching. *Staphy.* to be followed by *Rhus.* again.

(3) When the disease extends to the forehead, face and neck or when the eyes or eyelids become red and inflamed. (*Hepar.*). See also "Eczema-scalp" and "Milk crusts on the scalp".

Ripe cold—(1) The mucus assumes thicker consistency instead of watery discharge and the nose may be alternately stopped or running. *Puls . Bry.* will be useful to remove the remaining symptoms.

(2) *Merc. sol.* may be given when the cold is ripe and discharge is yellowish green. See "Cold-ripe".

Rolling relief from it—Rolling from side to side relieves the distress. Extreme restlessness ; must keep in constant motion. (*Tarentula.-h.*) (Dr. Kent).

Rubbing eyes—When the patient rubs eyes frequently and black spots appear before the eyes then give *Caust.* See "Eyes".

Rubella German measles-its prevention—See "Chapter V for details".

—: o :—

S

Sacrum (the lower bone of pelvis on which spine rests) pain extending to hips—Pain through the sacrum into the hips while walking specially in haemorrhoidal patients (*Aesc.*). See "Walking" and "Gout-long bones."

Sadness—(1) Sadness worse during music. (*Graph.*).

(2) Sadness after grief. (*Ig.*).

(3) Weakness caused by sadness. (*Acid-phos.*). See "Grief-ailment due to" and "Melancholia".

Saliva-producing rawness, headache and constant spitting—(a) (1) Whenever the discharge of saliva flowing over the lips produces rawness, smarting and burning of the lips starts bleeding (*Arum-t.*).

(2) Accompanying nervous headache. (*Iris-v.*).

(3) Saliva runs out during sleep. (*Bar-c.*).

(4) Copious salivation after eating. (*Allium-sat.*).

(5) During pregnancy. (*Kreos.*). See "Acrid fluids". (b) Constant spitting ; accumulation of much saliva in mouth. Taste sour. (*Am-c.*).

(1) Bloody saliva. Gums spongy profuse flow of saliva which has foul odour. (*Nit-ac.*).

(3) Tongue white, swelling of lower lip. Saline salvia, involuntary urination during first sleep. Fetid breath and urine. (*Sep.*).

(4) Mouth and tongue scalded. Profuse flow of saliva ; ropy ; drops from mouth when talking. (*Iris-v.*). (c) Constantly wants to spit saliva viscid in connection with headache. (*Epiphegus.*) which will cure the headache also.

Saliva-from mouth hanging—Profuse secretion of ropy saliva ; glairy mucus ropy, hanging in string from mouth to receptical. (*Iris.*).

Salt-craving—Abnormal craving for salt. Patient salts every thing he eats. (*Nat-m.*). Compare *Caust.* See also "Craving-for acids and refreshing things" and "Craving for salt".

Salt-counteracting its bad effects—Craving for salt. *Phos.* often counteracts the bad effects of desire for salt. (*Phos.*). Compare *Nat-m.*

Scar injured with pain—If there is old scar which is injured or bruised by coming into contact with something hard and starts burning and stinging with the pain running along the course of nerve use, *Hyper.* See also "Cicatrix" and "Nerve injury".

Scar-syphilitic—Old of syphilitic origin. They turn purple, threaten to suppurate, become painful or even turn black. (*Asaf.*). See also "Syphilis".

Scabies on different parts of body—(a) (1) *Mercurius* and after a few days *Sulf.* alternately.

(2) If the vesicles are small and dry *Carbo-v.* or *Hepar.* once night and morning.

(3) If the pustules are large and become yellow. (*Lach.*).

(4) Scabies,cracks and ulceration of nostrils. (*Anthrako-kali.*).

(5) Itching without eruptions worse by scratching at night. (*Dol.*).

(6) Violent itching of scalp. (*Olnd.*).

(b) (1) When itches spread all over the body and are attended with maddening scratching. The hairy portion of the body itches more, sore red blotches, better by bathing in cold water. (*Fragopyrum.*).

(2) Itching without eruption. Dr. Dewey has verified this symptom. *Dolichos* will sometimes control diabetic

itching and is specially useful in senile pruritus. Worse at night. Worse across shoulders.

(3) Itching all over, worse at night when warm in bed. Itch in bends of elbows when some of the vesicles become pustular. (*Merc-s.*). Dr. Herring recommends *Merc-s.* first, then after a few days *Sulf.* and so on alternately. Occasionally it is well to start with *Rhus-t.* in repeated doses. This should be followed by *Sulf.* and this again by *Rhus-t.,Sulf. 200* once a week.

(4) Prof. Dr. Bhanja cured a case of most exasperating type of itches all over fingers, wrists and thighs swelling, inflammation and burning pain of worst type. He at first gave 3 doses of *Anthracinum 30* to be taken every half hour. After gap of one day *Croton 30* was given and later on *Anthracinum 200* potency was prescribed. Complete cure was effected within very short time.

(5) Skin dirty, dingy look. Body with a filthy odour. Warmth of bed excites violent itching. Wants warm clothing in summer. Extreme sensitiveness to cold. Inveterate case with symptoms of tuberculosis. (*Psor*). See "Eczema", "Eruptions" and "Itch" under their different heads.

Scalds-injury by hot liquids and ulceration of bowels— (1) *Cantharis* is an excellent remedy for all stages of burns and scalds. It prevents blisters. The injured part should be immersed in a few drops of mother tincture. (*Canth.*).

(2) If the burns are deep, destroying skin. (*Kali-bi.*).

(3) Suppuration after burns. (*Hep.*).

(4) Internally *Cantharis* and *Capsicum* are the best remedies to relieve burning. Dr. Herring says that *Cantharis M.T.* 5 to 8 drops in a half tumbler of water for external use is most efficacious.

(5) In burns when there is ulceration of bowels and in nervous patients. (*Stram.*).

(6) For shocks when there is inflammation of lungs, ulceration of bowels and hurried, difficult breathing. Dr. Laurie

recommends *Phosphorus* given alternately with *Aconite.* See also "Burns".

Scarlet fever—Prophylactic : *Bell. 30* ; *Eucal-glo.*

Sciatica-chronic—Chronic sciatica, arthiritis, gout, rheumatism and the disease of the spinal cord. (*Medorrhinum.*). See "Specific".

Sciatica left and right sided—(1) Left sided sciatica ; better motion. Darting pains in left thigh relieved by motion. (*Kali-b*).

(2) Right sided sciatica, sharp shooting pain extending to knee, worse by motion. (*Colch*).

(3) The pains are darting and tearing, aggravated by motion. (*Phyt.*). Compare "Viscum".

(4) Lightning like pains with twitching of parts ; has to change position. Pains shoot down into the foot. (*Nux-v.*).

(5) Intractable cases either side, chronic or acute. (*Carb-s*).

(6) Intense neuralgic pains, whole trunk affected. Worse from motion. Better while sitting in chair. *Gnaphalium* (Dr. Dewey).

(7) Aching in back and thighs, in all joints. Legs and arms feel heavy. (*Cotyledon-tinctora.*).

(8) Violent jerks in the limb and the patient suffers from obstinate constipation, chronic cases with weakness and stiffness of affected parts. (*Lyco.*).

(9) Pain in sacrum, passing into right thigh down ; sciatic nerve worse when pressing at stool, coughing, laughing also while lying on affected side. (*Tell.*).

(10) *Hypericum M.T.* may be applied locally for sciatic neuralgic pain of leg.

(11) When patient feels sore all over from head to feet, muscles sore and stiff can hardly move without groaning. (*Phyto.*). has given most brilliant victories of such cases of sciatica.

(12) Sciatica with stiffness in neck and shoulders and pain

in left arm give *Iodum* which will cure such cases as recommended by Dr. Benerjee. See "Lumbago" and "Backache".

Sciatic-pain—The combination of following 4 Biochemic drugs have proved very successful in removing the sciatic pain. The patient cannot erect and has to stoop down while walking : (1) *Calc-flour. 6x.*

(2) *Calc.-phos. 6x.*

(3) *Ferrum-phos. 6x.* and

(4) *Kali-muri.6x.* All the above medicines mixed together in a tumbler of tepid water and may be divided in 4 doses—one dose may be taken at interval of 3 hrs. Thus 4 doses per day may be taken until relief is obtained. See "Chapter V for details".

Sciatica-oedema—Sciatica with oedema of the extremity following inflammation of vien. (*Apoc-c.*).

Sciatica-left sided with pains and cramps and numbness in calf or feet—(a) Worse cold damp weather at nignt. Left sided. (*Rhus-tox.*). (b) Some authors consider *Gnaphalium* to be specific for sciatica. Pains accompanied by cramps alternating with numbness. It is also useful for pains in calf and feet.

Sciatica and lumbago relieved by pressure and by pulling the legs up—(1) Relieved by hard pressure and warmth, or by pulling the legs up. The pains being crampy in nature. But *Mag-phos,* will relieve these pains earlier if warmth has a more marked relieving action than pressure. (*Coloc.*). See "Pressure ameliorates".

(2) *Acid-sulph.* for cases of sciatica and lumbago when well selected medicines fail.

(3) *Viscumalbum* has the credit of curing a number of severe and long standing cases according to Dr. Dewey.

(4) Painful affection and persistent. *Bry.* 3 times a day with *Merc.* night and morning, if worse at night *Cimicifuga* 3 times a day and *Gels.* at bed time 2 hourly, if sleepless, *Nux-v.* 3 times a day for removing stiffness.

Sciatica-right sided pains while moving—(1) Right sided *Lyco.*

(2) For pains in legs while moving or sitting use ***Dioscorea.***

(3) *Kali-phosphoricum* and *Magnesia-phosphoria* tissue remedies are also useful in every sciatica.

Scorpion-bite—*Ledum.* See also "Insects bites or stings" and "Bites".

Scratching-of skin—Scratching after putting of the clothes. *Nat. sulph. 12x,* 3 grains 3 times a day.

Screaming of children also while urinating—Piteous moaning and crying. (*Cham.,* 2 hourly.).

(2) Crying before passing urine. (*Bor.* 2 hrly.).

(3) Night screaming. (*Kali brom.* 8 hourly.).

(4) During sleep cries, starts, anxiety continues after waking. *Calc. 30,* 8 hrly.

(5) Piteous crying, continual crying and whining, gets only short sleeps. (*Ant-t.* 2 hourly).

(6) Weeping moaning, howling. (*Cicuta-v.*). See also "Crying of child teething trouble" under "C".

Sea-sickness and also when riding in carriage—(1) ***Tabacum*** to be given high.

(2) *Petroleum* is specific for sea-sickness, nausea, vomiting. Also for nausea from riding in a carriage.

(3) When riding in a carriage caused by swinging. (*Cocculu.*) See "Car sickness".

Sedative causing calmness of mind—Very irritable, sensitive to all impressions. Even the least ailment affects the mind. Anxiety, nervous dread. Great despondency, Hysteria. Slightest labour seems a heavy task. (*Tr. Nux-v. 1M+Kali-phos. 12x*). Prepare a mixture afresh each time with one minim (m)of *Nux-v.* in a small cup of water in which 4 globles of *Kali-phos.* be dissolved and administer a tea spoonful of mixture when required at short intervals.

(b) Sedative for promoting sleep, quietness in cardiac affections and similar irritative condition. (*Aranea-diadema*) as recommended by Dr. Lilienthal.

Sedative-for pain in the bladder ureturs or kidneys—(*Hydrange-arbar.*) for the pains dependent upon the passage of the gravel and uric acid, etc.

Sedative - general—According to Dr. Guy, *Bellis-perennis, Cimicifuga* and *Hyper.* all in M.T. 2 to 5 drops of each taken as a unit dose will certainly relax a patient who, has headache, cannot get sleep, when once awakened, with great depression, who has mania and is hysterical. It requires no repetition.

Senile decay due to degenerative changes—Diseases of old man when degenerative changes begin *e.g* cardiac vascular and central hypertrophied prostate. Grief over trifles. (*Baryta carb.*). Compare *Orchitinum*. See "Old age from excesses" and "Weakness-premature old age with impaired functions".

Sensation - peculiar over the body—Peculiar sensation over the body. Sensation of coldness and warmth, pins and needles and other peculiar sensations. Aggravation after sexual intercourse. (*Agar.*). See "Coldness of body" and "Numbness and insensibility of nerves in different parts of body".

Sensitiveness disturbed by noise, offended on triflings—The patient is over-sensitive *i.e.* even a harmless joke or a word is taken seriously by him and he is offended beyond measure. He is inclined to get excited and angry over small things. He has very often of a very malicious disposition sometimes even revengeful. He is disturbed by the slightest noise. A little noise frightens him. (*Nux-v.*). See "Hyper sensitiveness" and "Anger complaint".

Sensitiveness to opposition and sensitive to cold and light—Excessively sensitive in nervous system. Mind is very sensitive to slight opposition or insult ; patient is very sensitive to cold, drought and a slight touch to the painful part increases the pain. Over-sensitive to light and sound etc. (*Chin.*).

See "Annoyance", "Peevish" and "Nervous system very sensitive to opposition".

Sensitiveness-sudden emotions with nervous diarrhoea—There is sensitiveness of the nerves and the patient is susceptible to mental disturbances such as sudden emotion, all things of fright or anticipation of an unusual task to be performed *e.g.* nervous diarrhoea. (*Gels.*). See "Nervous diarrhoea and also for surgical case".

Septic infections and its prophylactic diphtheria and typhoid—(1) *Ars-alb.*

(2) Sepsis due to injuries. (*Echi.*).

(3) *Rhus-tox.* is best prophylactic for cases of surgery to be given for 48 hours, in 30 dilution every 3 hours.

(4) For complaints of septic condition in diphtheria, typhoid and gangrenous affections. (*Baptisia*). See "Surgical shocks", "Operation collapse", "Fever septic", Prophylactic for other disease. "Surgical Antibiotic" after it and "Wound on scalp".

Septicemia-blood poisoning ; for relieving septic fever after delivery fever—*Pyrogen* is an excellent remedy for septic fever. It is specific for after delivery fever. See "Fever-septic" and "Blood-poisining".

Septic-throat—See "Throat septic".

Septicemia due to post-operative complications—Post operative complications (*Rhus-t.*). See "Operation collapse".

Septicemia - wound caused while conducting post-mortem—Wound incurred during postmortem examination. Both local and general symptoms severe.(*Lachesis 12th* 3 times a day).

Septicemia caused by prickcut or other injury causing swelling—Small cut or injury, or by pricks or scratches by any sharp infected instrument and such injuries become much swollen and inflamed or discoloured. (*Pyrog.*). See "Cut-sharp with knife".

Septic states in different diseases—In ulcers, gangrene, diphtheria, carbuncle and plague, etc. (*Lach.*).

Septicemia - wound caused while conducting post-mortem—Wound incurred during postmortem. Both local and general symptoms severe. (*Lach.*).

Septum-ulcerated—Round ulcer, distress at root of nose, chronic inflammation of frontal sinus. (*Kali-bich.*). See "Nose, septum ulcerated".

Serious conditions with cold sweats collapse—*Carb-v.* is the medicine which is usually used in very serious conditions. Complete collapse. Hands, feet and surface of the body cold and blue. Paleness of the surface of the body. Perspiration over the whole body. Patient lies motionless as if dying. Pulse thready and quick. Cold sweats on the limbs. (*Carb-v.*). Compare *Verat-a.* See "Collapse" under its different heads and "Perspiration cold".

Serpent or other venous insects Bite—(a) Serpent bites or of other venomous insects. *Cedron* Tincture of pure bean scraped on wound. (b) *Golondrina* is an antidote to snake poison. It renders the body immune to the influence of snake poison. See "Bites" under its different heads.

Sexual - desire irresistible leading to mania—*Phos.* excites the sexual appetite in both sexes. It is almost irresistible and leads the patient into a mania in which he will expose himself. This is succeeded by the opposite extreme of impotence though the desire remains after the ability to perform is gone. (*Phos.*). See also "Impotency desire but inability" under its different heads and "Excessive sexual desire".

Sexual desire too strong—(*Iod*). Sexual desire diminished ; testicle, atrophict (*Kali iod*), sexual ejeculation, ejaculation does not follow coition in spite of every effort ; absence of erection in the morning, emission of semen involuntary with erection.

Sexual dribbling of semen—Dribbling of seamen while frolicking with women. (*Con.*).

Sexual excitement ineffective with orgasm wanting in nervous persons—Violent sexual excitement before and during but at the time of ejaculation the orgasm is wanting, it is passive and pleasureless ejaculation. This occurs in man with spinal weakness, nervous men who have tingling and crawling all over. Burning in the prostate during ejaculations. (*Agar.*). See "Emissions".

Sexual irritation-emission—*China officinalis* is useful in involuntary emission of semen from the slightest irritation and the patient feels exhausted and debilitated. (*China-o.*). See "Sexual weakness with morning erections only".

Sexual-neurasthenia always dwelling on sexual subjects—Especially after self-abuse. Persistent dwelling on sexual subjects. Spermatorrhoea, emissions with backache. Weakness (*staphy.*). See also "Neurasthenia after excess" and "Impotence sexual excess".

Sexual weakness with morning erections only—With preversion. The patient has lived in excesses and now suffers from relaxed and cold genital emissions, prostatic discharge at stool. Has morning erections but no more. History of repeated gonorrhoea. (*Agn.*). *Agnus-castus* followed by *China.* and *Lyco.* makes this victim a different. See "Debility due to excess".

Shivering-due to uncovering, no liking for draught—(1) Chilliness ; least uncovering of bed-clothes brings no shivering. He is worse in the cold air. He does not like a draught, and wants a good cover. The moment the cover is removed he feels extremely chilly. (*Nux-v.*).

(2) Continued shivering, rigour beginning in limbs. (*Acon.* $\frac{1}{2}$ hourly).

(3) Immediately after a chill has been taken. (*Camphor* $\frac{1}{4}$ hourly). See "Chilliness must cover head".

Shingles—See "Herpes Zoster."

Shivering with blueness of extremities and collapse in labour and otherwise—(1) Hysterical shivering in the first stage of labour. (*Act-rac.*). See "Hysterical shivering".

(2) Shivering with blueness of extremities and signs of collapse. (*Carb-v.* ¼ hourly).

(3) *Chill* ; effects of wet cold or cold drinks. (*Bellis.*).

(4) Shivering in the evening without thirst. (*Phos.* ¼ hourly). See "Pregnancy-disorder of".

Shock due to injury or operation—(1) Post-traumatic (*Arnica.*).

(2) Post-operative. *Strontia-carb.* (*Carbo-veg.* is the physicians' remedy for shock). See "Collapse-after operation".

Shock-in injury—(1) *Arnica* is an excellent remedy for the first hours for bruised condition after an injury and shock of injury. (*Arnica*).

(2) *Arnica* is very suitable for sore bruised condition of the body. Therefore it is an important remedy in injuries, bruises and shock from injuries. See "Injury" under its different heads and See "Accidents".

Shock-of insuline and aspirin—*Carbo-veg., Ant-t.* and *Lyco.* have proved good results in shock of Insuline injection.

Shock-of family tragedy—*Opium* is great remedy for patient in shock, specially these who have a history of having never, felt the same after some family shock. (*Opium.*).

Shock-of operation collapse and resulting various trouble—(1) Collapse symptoms after a surgical operation with great prostration, coldness of body, slow oozing of the blood. Cold breath and profuse perspiration will require *Strontium carb.* It relieves a shock at once and the patient gets warm and comfortable. (*Stront-c.*).

(2) *Verat-v.* is very good for surgical shock.

(3) If the temperature is subnormal immediately after the operation and the blood pressure is low *Camphora* is highly recommended by Dr. Dewey. It precedes *Verat-a.*

(4) A single dose of high potency of *Phosphorus* given a day before abdominal operation will prevent nausea and other distress after operation.

(5) Vomiting after operation due to morphine—Morphine effects of sensitive person after operation, awful eructations with retching and vomiting and there is nothing to vomit. Give *Cham.* which will stop these within a few minutes and is practically the only medicine that stops vomiting from morphine.

(6) *Nux-v.* relieves vomiting after operation with much irritability and retching.

(7) Neuralgic pains in the stump of amputated limbs relieved by *Allium-cepa* and for sharp pains due to amputation of fingers give *Hypericum.* See "Septic infection and its prophylactics". "Amputation neuritis" also "Operation collapse" and "Morphia vomiting after operation".

Shooting pain from wound—If the pain shoots from the wound up the nerve, then it is *Hypericum.* See "Pain-dull at the injured part" and "Wounds on palm and sentient parts".

Short stature—R. B. Bishamber Dass suggests that *Tuberculinum, Baryta-carb., Thuja* should be given alternately every week in 200 dilution for 6 months or more. Stature can only be expected to be increased between the ages of 10 to 17 ; earlier the age the better the results. See "Dwarfishness".

Shoulder-pain—See "Chapter V for details".

Shyness-bashful due to excitment and lack of confidence—(1) Shy of appearing in public, bashful, cowardice, vacant feeling of mind. (*Gels.*).

(2) Bashfulness with great mental excitment. (*Coca.*).

(3) Shyness due to lack of confidence, fear and cowardice. (*Bar-c.* and *Kali-phos.*). See "Fear" under its different heads and "Mind-lack of stamina".

Sickness-in air travel—*Bell.* is preventive in aviation (*Bell.*) If the sickness arises out of downward motion in aviator then give *Borax*. If *Petroleum 30x*, 2 doses for a few days before taking the journey are given, then this will prevent sickness.

Sickness in car—While in the car, in the hills, *Tabacum* to be given high. Compare *Cocculus* and *Peteroleum*. See "Sea sickness" and also while riding in carriage and car sickness.

Sickness-while riding in train or carriage or in sea voyage—*Tabacum* to be given high. Compare *Cocculus* and *Petroleum*. *Petroleum* is specific for sea-sickness, also for nausea from riding in carriage. When riding in a carriage caused by swinging. (*Cocculus-ind.*). See "Car-sickness". For sea voyage sickness Dr. Kent recommends *Antim-crud*. or *Hyoscyamus 200*

Sinus—Headache, sore throat, eyes burn. Stuffed up nose. Nose does not stop running ; chronic catarrhal, purulent discharge ; slow digestion. Ethmoid (Bone at the base of skull forming the upper bony nose) and front sinus. According to Dr. W. Boericke *Eucalyptus-globulus* is an effective remedy. Dr. A. Dalzell recommends it for bronchial asthma also. See "Catarrh of nose block and Catarrh-nasal".

Sinus shooting pain in eye-brows, head jaw and ears—(1) Any organ which is hollow is called sinus. Pain in sinus is called sinusitis. Such a pain mostly occurs on eyebrows after having cold. If the pain is on right eye-brow or is right sided sinusitis then give *Sang-n, 30* ; but if the pain is left sided and on left eye-brow then give *Sep. 200* ; but if the pain is on both sides then give *Sticta-pulmonaria 3x*.

(2) Sinuses left after breast abscess. *Silic 6, 3* hourly.

(3) Shooting and hammering pain in head, jaw, ear and face during attack of catarrh. (*Iodum*).

(4) Give *Silicea 200* every fortnight and no medicine two days before and after that. During the interval give *Kali-bi., 30* four times daily every four hours. It may be given in inflammation of sinuses. Deep down in the nasal track : *Ferrum phos.* and *Silicea* (*Biochemic*).

(5) The patient has a corrosive nasal discharge with burning sensation in the nose and eyes, feverish, with headache and cannot sleep. (*Ars-alb.*).

(6) Face is hot but patient feels chilly ; has a fluent coryza with lachrymation, which is acrid. (*Euphrasia.*).

(7) Thick yellow discharge from posterior part of the nose. Mucus drops down in the throat. Constipated with coated tongue. (*Hydrastis.*).

(8) Has chills up to the back and fullness of headache and face, sneezing and fluent coryza, fever remits and recures again (*Gels.*).

(9) Intense headache above eyes and facial bone with catarrhal trouble. (*Merc-iod. rub.*).

Skin-body red with ulcers and eczema in bends—Whole body red as if covered with scarlet eruptions. Putrid flat ulcers with pungent burning sensation. (*Am-carb.*). It is also useful for eczema in the bends of lower extremities, between legs about anus and genitals. See also "Ulcers-multiple brown and dark coloured" and "Eczema general". Skin dry : sensitive to cold bathing scaly pustular eruption with burning and itching, worse at night. *Antimonium-crudum* which is also useful for horny excrescenes any where on that skin. (*Antim-crud.*).

Skin-discolouration—See "Discolouration of skin".

Skin - chapped—Apply externally *Calendula M.T.* See "Chapped-hand and cracks in finger tips".

Skin - eruptions suppressed—*Sulf.* is the leading remedy for many skin eruptions. Burning and itching with or without eruptions are the characteristic sensation of skin in *Sulf. Sulf.* will bring the eruptions out mostly and then cure them. Many time an internal disease which has been cured after suppression of any skin trouble will be cured with *Sulf.* after the original skin trouble reappears on the skin. (*Sulf.*). Compare *Psorinum* which is an invaluable remedy for all skin troubles. See "Suppressed—skin trouble".

Skin - sensitive to cold—Itching, redness and a burning sensation in the hands and feet. (*Agaricus-m.*).

Skin - scratching—In case of desire for scratching after putting off the clothes, remember, *Nat-sulf. 12x* 3 gr. 3 times a day.

Skin - sensitive to pressure—The skin may be so sensitive to light pressure that the patient cannot bear the weight of the clothes or of the bed sheet even. He wants them to be lifted from the skin. On the contrary, again, *Lach.* patient may stand a little deep pressure but cannot bear the slightest touch either with fingers or with clothes on the painful portions. This is because the surface nerves of the skin become very sensitive where as deeper nerves are not so. (*Lach.*). See "Pressure" under its different heads.

Skin lichen—An eruption of red pimples generally ending in scurf—Much worse in the warmth of the bed. (*Syphli*). Compare *Anti-c.* and *Kali Ars.*

Skin-scratching—See "Scratching of skin".

Skin-shrivelled of old people—Shrivelled. Women of very lax muscular fibre ; everything seems loose. Open ; no action Vessels flabby, *Secale-cornutum* is useful remedy for old people with shrivelled skin and thin.

Skin-slight injuries fester—(1) *Sep.* widely indicated in skin trouble as *Sulf.,—Sep.* and *Sulf.* follow each other in skin troubles. What *Sep.* cannot cure *Sulf.* very often finishes. (*Sep.*).

(2) When slight injuries fester. (*Petr.*). See "Injury-children tending to form pus", "Contusion-skin ruptured" and "Bruise, skin".

Skin-tendency to suppurate by injury—(1) Unhealthy skin which whenever there is wound or injury tends to suppurate. The skin is pale and muscles are lax. *Sil., Calc-carb.* See "Inflammation—tending to pus" and "Suppuration". "Skin", "Suppressed eruption". See "Itching distressing extremely".

Skin-wheal—An elevation of the skin seen in some forms of nettle rash like that produced by the strokes of a whip stick—Such wheal are very common in young children causing great distress to the patient when they get warm and wet and is often almost maddening. *Chloralhydrate* (*Chloralum*) and *Urtica urens* and also *Persicaria. urens* are very useful in such cases when red blotches caused suffering to the patient. *Bacillinum* is also useful.

Skin troubles—Dr. Purse says that if 5 or 6 drops of *Spongia M.T.* are given daily than any skin disease can be cured in a short period.

Skull-fracture—Terrible pain. *Glonoinum* for terrible pain of badly fractured skull as suggested by Dr. John.

Sleep - aggravation after—Aggravation from sleep is a very characteristic symptom of *Lach*. Patient sleeps into aggravation so if a symptom becomes worse after sleep and is, in addition to it, if it is left-sided symptom *Lach.* is almost a sure cure. It does not matter whether the patient sleeps during the night or during the day. He wakes up with aggravation of symptoms. In all these cases one must think of *Lach*. See "Child frightended" and "Delirium".

Sleep cat nap type—When the patient lies awake from 3 a.m. and then sleeps when he ought to be awake. (*Nux-v*) ; when the patient awakes precisely at the same hour. (*Sel.*). See "Unrefreshing sleep" and "Insomnia".

Sleep child and gnashing teeth—The patient imagines to see ghosts and dreadful animals. Child starts up from very often and gnashes his teeth. If the child feels suddenly ill with red face and redness of eyes with semi stupor ; starts up in sleep, goes into spasms. *Bell* will act as oil in troubled waters. (*Bell.*). See also "Teeth gnashing by a child".

Sleep too much before examination or before meal—Give 10 drops of *Scrophularia-nodosa* twice daily. It is very useful for students before examination.

Sleepiness—Irresistible sleepiness. (*Cimex.*). With lassitude and no desire for work. (*Indol.*). See "Drowsiness".

Sleepiness, sudden short spells of sleep after reading, eating and after stool—(1) Irresistible sleepiness. (*Cimex.*).

(2) Sleepiness, morosness, lassitude, stupor, disinclination to work, great dejection and melancholy. (*Cyclamen.*).

(3) Sleepiness with lassitude, wants to lie down all the time. No desire to work ; continuous dreaming. (*Indol.*).

(4) While reading. (*Nat-s.*).

(5) After eating. (*Mag-c.*).

(6) While eating. (*Puls.*).

(7) After stool or after vomiting. (*Aeth-c.*).

Sleeplessness-emotions disturbing including cardiac sleeplessness—(1) From depressing news, recent grief. (*Ig.*).

(2) (a) From good news. (*Coffea.*). (b) Entire inability to sleep caused by aching of bones. (*Daphne-indica.*).

(3) Where business care of the day keeps him awake. (*Bry.*). *Ambra-grisea* is another medicine for worry of mind.

(4) From worry and business trouble. (*Ambra-g.*).

(5) Obstinate and intractable form of insomnia. (*Cannabis indica. M.T.* 10 drops.). Sleeplessness of children during dentition. (*Cimicifuga-rac.*).

(6) Due to nervous breakdown. (*Tabacum.*).

(7) *Avena sativa* 10 to 15 drops will induce sleep in nervous and exhausted persons.

(8) Dr. Dewey says that *Passiflora inc.* in massive doses of 10 to 30 drops of mother tincture in repeated doses will induce sleep when mental irritation or pain is the cause of wakefulness.

(9) Cardiac sleeplessness to excitement and nervousness, with dry asthma and harrasing cough. (*Tela-aranearum.*). See also "Dreams" and "Insomnia".

Sleeplessness due to pain, nervousness and with excessive yawning—(1) Over-sensitiveness for pain and peevish temper. *Cham.* will often put the patient to sleep if along with this sleeplessness other symptoms of over-sensitiveness to pain, peevish temper and for children the desire to be carried about are present. (*Cham.*).

(2) For excessive frequent yawning. (*Ig.*). See "Over-sensitiveness", "Yawning" and "Fracture-sleepless patient".

Sleeplessness-during pregnancy—(1) A dose of *Coffea* or *Bell.* will often bring back sleep. See "Pregnancy-disorders of No. 18".

(2) Also for sleeplessness during pregnancy Dr. Curtis recommends *Anac. 200.*

(3) *Opium* given a little dose can make a sleepless patient sleeps a natural sleep.

Sleep-unrefreshing and child awakes at night playing—Unrefreshing sleep during later part of night ; flatulence. Perspiration during sleep on being covered. (*Chin.*) For little babies who wake up and play the whole night. (*Cyripedium.*). See "Unrefreshing sleep" and "Wakeful and restless infants".

Sleeping of limbs, pressure while lying down—Limbs go to sleep on slightest pressure. Arms go to sleep while lying down. (*Ambra.*). See "Pressure-causes sleeping of limbs" and "Numbness and sleeping of limbs".

Sleeping-with half open eyes—*Lycopod.*

Sloughing with oedema and ulceration—*Ammonium-causticum.* See "Wounds sloughing".

Slow development-with sweating head—Slow growth, slow closing of fontanelles in emaciated children with sweating head (*Calc.p.*). See "Emaciation with sweating in head in children.

Small-pox with eruption on face and to prevent pitting—(1) Of great value in this disease provided the characteristic dark blue colour is present. *Lach.*, *Antimonium-tartaricum* to be given in the 2nd stage when pustules have formed. Externally *Calendula M.T.* or *Thuja M.T.* in olive oil to be painted frequently to prevent itching and pitting in all cases of small-pox.

(2) Eruptions more prominent on the neck and face, suppurative conditions of confluent type of small-pox. Prostration. To dry up sore, *Insulin* is wonderfully useful. See "Fever-eruptive with irregular rash".

Small-pox-preventive and for disfigurement—*Variolionum, Vaccinium, Variolinum 200* to be given once a week as preventive and as curative of disfigurement of the face by small-pox to be given every week 200. According to Dr. M.G. Blackie *Thuja* is both preventive and curative in an edidemic of small-pox. It aborted the process and preventing pitting. See "Prophylactic-of small-pox" and "Disfigurement face".

Small-pox also haemorrhagic small-pox, with no regular rash and its stages—(a) The eruptions are usually of bluish tinge instead of bright red. The regular rash does not come out. The usual uniform spread of the eruption has failed or suppressed. Continued dreamy state while awake. Great prostration and stupefaction. *Sarracenia* is another excellent remedy both curative and preventive. (b) (1) *Initial stage*—Dr. Jahr prescribes *Variolinum 30* at the commencement and he thinks that it aborts the disease more than any other remedy ; 4 or 5 doses of it should be given in 24 hours, then given a dose of *Sulph. 200* after 6 or 7 hours, again give *Variolinum 30.* If the temperature is very high, then *Bell. 3x, Gels. 3x* may be used after *Variolinum* to reduce the temperature. When the case takes unfavourable course from the start-the extremities are cold, face puffy, feeble pulse, then Dr. Jousset recommends *Ars-a.* For intense back-ache and rheuamatic pains, headache Drs. Hughes and Dewey recommend *Gels.* and *Bry.* specially *Cimicifuga* ; intense back-ache and rheumatic pains more, then *Verat-v., Ant-t.,* are recommended by Dr. Jousset.

(2) *Stage of eruption*—Dr. Jahr extols *Variolinum* in this stage too. Both Drs. Jousset and Hughes are in favour of giving *Ant-t.* when it has great skin and throat irritation, pain, pain in back, vomiting and drowsiness. *Thuja* according to Boeninghausen is the best remedy in the stage of eruption.

(3) *Stage of suppuration*—Dr. Jahr proposes to give *Variolinum* in this stage. Drs. Jousset and Dewey recommend *Rhus-t.* during the suppurative stage when the face becomes swollen and there is a fever, prostration with alternate chill and fever and very troublesome itching. Boeninghausen gives *Thuja* and says that it causes early drying of pocks and causes recovery without pitting.

(4) *Stage of desquamation*—Dr. Jahr thinks that *Variolinum* with *Sulph.* intercurrent will cure case speedily and less pitted. Dr. Lilienthal thinks that *Verat-v.* alternate with *Cimicifuga* rapidly dries and peels off the scab. (c) Eruptions retarted : *Bryonia* to be given in repeated doses. After *Bryonia* a dose of Sulph. may help to bring out eruptions. (d) Haemorrhagic small-pox : The best remedy is *Ars-a.* then *Phos.* and *Lach.* The other useful remedies are *Crotalus* and *Rhus-t.* (e) Catarrhal condition : The most useful remedies are *Ant-a.* then try *Phos, Rhus-t, Ars-a.* (f) Loss of memory after small-pox. Try *Anacard.* See "Memory loss-after small-pox". (g) 'Diarrhoea : *Ant-t., Ars, Merc-s. Rhus-t.* Compare *Thuja.* (h) Head-ache : Dr. Jahr recommends *Bell. Bry.* ; and *Rhus-t.* Deafness after small-pox. (*Sulf.*). See "Eruptions in measles retarded" and "Deafness (7)".

Small-pox-back-ache—Back-ache of worst type. (*Variolinum*). (*Dr. Burnett*).

Small-pox-external application—For itching in small poxes *Calendula M.T.* in olive oil one to 10 parts. See "Eruptions in measles retarded".

Smell of food causing nausea—Cannot bear the smell of food or sight of food. It causes nausea. (*Ars-alb.*). Compare *Colchicum* and *Sep.* See "Nausea-smell of food".

Smell-foul of body—Putrid condition of the whole body. Foetid perspiration of the feet, foetid discharges from the ear, foetid urine, smelling like horses, urine. (*Nitricum acidum*).

Smell-sensitiveness and its loss—(1) Great sensitiveness, faintest odours unbearable. (*Bell.*).

(2) All odours too strong, (*Carbol-ac.*).

(3) Every thing smells bad, (*Aur-met*).

(b) Smell fetid (1) Putrid smell with watery discharge. (*Kali-Bichr*). (2) Putrid smell when blowing nose. (*Aur-met.*). (3) Foetid smell in nasal .catarrh. (*Silicea.*). (c) (1) Smell : Loss of smell with cough and stoppage of nose. (*Am-mur.*). (2) Loss of taste and smell after catarrh of influenza. (*Mag-m.*) (3) During catarrh with loss of taste. (*Sang.*).

(4) Impairment of smell with sore throat. (*Merc-cor*).

(5) Inflammation of nasal cavities with bad smelling, greenish discharge from the nose. Loss of smell and allergic cold. (*Thuja*). See "Cold loss of smell and taste", "Nose-smell" and "Odour under different heads."

Smog-smoky for—To check its ill-effects such as headache, choking cough, difficult breathing etc. use *Sulph-acidum. 200* or 30 potencies. 2 or 3 doses per day either dry or in solution for problems of smog.

Snake bite oozing black blood—Oozing of black blood after bite. This tendency of bleeding black blood which does not coagulate runs through all the snake poisons. (*Am-c*). See "Bite", under different heads.

(b) *Panama* and *Cendron* are considered to be specifics for bites of venomous snakes. Tincture of pure bean scraped also on wound. See "Serpent bite" and See "No 5. of Bites".

Snake poisoning prophylactic—An antidote to snake poisoning Its use renders the body immune to the influence of the snake poison. (*Golond.*). See "Prophylactics for other diseases".

Sneezing with cold—Common cold with much sneezing ; influenza. (*Acon.*). Compare *Hep*. See "Cold-cold air causing sneezing".

Sneezing-with cold and its immediate relief—See "Cold-sneezing and immediate relief from it".

Sneezing-morning coryza—Morning coryza with violent sneezing. Earlier symptoms will be the sneezing which comes with increasing frequency. (*All-c.*). See "Coryza-stopping of nose and sneezing".

Sneezing-susceptible to cold—Every time the patient goes out in fresh or cold air he sneezes and his nose runs. Nose stopped. Extremely sensitive to cold air. (*Hepar.*). See also "Cold-cold air causing sneezing".

Sneezing-violent and excessive—(1) Violent sneezing. (*Agar.*).

(2) *Cyclamen* should be thought of when excessive sneezing is prominent symptom. See "Cold sensitiveness" and "catarrh of chest".

Snoring—(1) When due to obstruction in the nose. Enlargement of nasal bones. (*Lamna-minor.*).

(2) Caries or enlargement of nasal bone. Snoring with swelling and redness of nose, with obstinate catarrth ; noisy breathing. (*Hippoz.*). See "Nose polypi".

Snuffle-stuffing nose of infants cannot breath—Nose blocked. Child awakes suddenly, nearly suffocating, turns blue. Choking cough at night. Cannot breathe. Give *Sumbucus* night and morning (Dr. Laurie). See "Nos. 10 and 12 of pregnancy-its affections" and "Infants-nose blocked".

Soles—(1) Pains in ; pains on stepping ; Pain in heals. (*Achilles*).

(2) Violent spasmodic pains in the soles and heels, preventing, stepping, burning in feet and soles, heels and balls of toes ; painful as if on stepping toes sore as if ulcerated (*Phos. acid.*)

(3) Burning in soles and heels when walking. (*Graph*).

(4) Cramps in legs and feet ; asleep ; and shift. (*Secale*).

(5) Neuralgic pain in instep and ball of toes, pain as if stepping on something hard in middle of ball of toes. (*Brom.*).

Soles burning with feet out—Burning of soles. The patient puts his feet out of cover. (*Sulf.*) Compare *Cham.* See "Burning-palms", "Feet burning" and "Feet out with burning sole".

S

Somnambulism-sleep walking and sitting in room—(1) Walking or doing any other action while in sleep. (*Artemisia-vulg.*).

(2) Rising and sitting about in the room while sleeping. (*Nat-m.*).

(3) With night terrors drowsiness and imbecility. (*Kali-br.*). See also "Night walking".

Sore-cold—(1) *Calc-f.*

(2) Cold sore on lips. (*Sulphur iodatum*). See "Abscess No. 16".

Sore painful covered by a scab—Sore dry and covered by a scab hard as a horn. Painful. *Merc., proto-iod.* also known as *Mercurius-iodatus-flavus*.

Sore-mouth—In consumption cases, in syphilitic, in throat troubles. Bad odour in the mouth. (*Lach.*). See "Mouth under its different heads".

Sore nipple inflammatory threating abscess—(1) If the inflammatory swelling well-developed. (*Bell.*).

(2) If abscess threatened. (*Mercurius.*). See "Nipple atrophy also cracked and ulcerated".

Sore throat extending to wind pipe—Sore throat extending down to trachea (wind pipe) or even to bronchi. Hoarseness. (*Carb-v*). See "Hoarseness damp air".

Sore throat its prevention—See Chapter V for details.

Sore throat left sided—Chronic with much hawking, mucus sticks and cannot be forced up or down. Left sided. Pain in the throat usually runs up to the ears. Warm water makes the pain worse. (*Lach.*). See "Tonsillitis with something left sided causing paralysis of vocal cord.

Sore throat-with pain in mouth and fever—(a) Throbbing pain as if pus is going to form. Pain in the throat as if a splinter or stick sticking in the throat. The patient is sensitive to cold. (*Hepar.*). Compare *Bell., Merc-sol., Lyco.,* and *Lac-can.* (b) (1) *Bell* must have high fever, intense redness of throat, fever.

(2) *Merc-sol* : —Moist thick and indented tongue. Moderate fever and good amount of sweating without relief.

(3) *Lach.* Tonsillitis starts in the left side and may go out to the right. Very sensitive to touch and aggravation of symptoms after sleep.

(4) *Lyco.* Tonsillitis starts in the right side may extend to the left, with stopping up of the nose.

(5) *Lac-can.* (dog's milk). If in any case the pain in the tonsils starts on one side and goes back to the original side *i.e.* alternately one day worse on one side and next day worse on the other side.

(6) *Hepar* : There is much throbbing pain as pus is going to form The patient is sensitive to cold. There is pain like splinter sticking into throat. Think of *Hepar.* See "Throat sore with pain and fever","Tonsils to be prevented from surgery".

Sore throat - with raw mouth and swollen glands—Inflammation of throat ; inflammation is intense and spreads all over the cavity of the mouth including whole of throat ; uvula and the gums become spongy. All glands about throat swollen with sharp pains to ears. (*Merc-s.*). See "Throat-inflammation spreading and glands swollen" and "Tonsillitis-ulcerated and swollen glands".

Sore throat - recurring—The patient has painful and offensive mouth ; swallowing difficult. He is very chilly and keeps covered up. In such cases *Hepar-sulph.* is very effective in preventing recurrence of sore throat

Sore throat - redness and throbbing pain—*Bell.* is the first remedy if redness and throbbing pain persist and it comes suddenly. A sense of constriction as if throat is narrowing. Burning and dryness. (*Bell.*). "Tonsils-red with throbbing pain".

Sore throat - tendency to it—(*Baryta carb.*).

Sour - everything—Everything from mouth to anus sour. Sour vomiting and sour stool. (*Calc.*). See "Vomiting sour" and "Diarrhoea-of children sour smelling".

Spasms of child during sleep—Startling from sleep during fever of children and jerking of muscles of finger and toes. Red face and redness of eyes with semi stupor. (*Bell*). See also "Startling of child in fever", "Child frightened" and "Convulsions during fever of children".

Specific for appendicitis—If *Bapt. C.M.* in acute appendicitis is given as a unit dose then it will often abort the need for surgery. If one dose is not sufficient then it may be repeated fortnightly to avert the surgery.

Specific - for the stings—*Urtica urens* . See "Stings".

Specific of cholera—Spirit *Camphor* 8-10 drops on ordinary sugar without water every half an hour upto 3 or 4 doses acts like magic. Repeat it every time after vomiting or purging even if the interval is a minute.

Specific for epilepsy—Dr. Hughes recommends *Hydrocyn-ac.* to be specific.

Specific for haemoptysis—*Hamamellis.*

Specifics-different diseases—(1) For Angina pectoris. (*Latrodectus-m.*).

(2) For influenza 3x for the attack and 30th potency for resulting debility. (*Carbolic acid.*).

(3) For sick head-ache ; *Chionanthus virginica* 5 drops of 2x dilution 3 times a day for a week, then twice a day for a week, then once a day for a week and later on whenever the attack comes on.

(4) For chronic nose-pharyngeal catarrh with greenish crusts and when the patient himself smells foul odour from the discharge of nose : (*Elaps.* 6.).

(5) For nose-bleed of long standing. (*Ferr pic.* or *Vipera.*).

(6) For sciatica and lumbago when patient has frequent desire to urinate. (*Gins.*).

(7) Inflammatory rheumatism. (*Gaultheria.*).

(8) Bleeding piles :—Give *Hyper 1x* internally and apply the same externally on piles.

(9) Barbers' itch and obstinate skin diseases. (*Sul-i.*).

(10) Ulceration of cornea particularly of children. (*Tuber.*).

(11) *Nitric acid* is almost specific for diarrhoea after antibiotics specially the Mycines according to Dr. Hubbard.

(12) Specific for after delivery (*Pyrogen*).

(13) For bites of venomous snakes—*Panama* and *Cedron Tincture* to be scraped on wound.

(14) For small pox *Variolinum* to be pushed from start to finish.

(15) Specific for cholera : See "Specific for cholera".

(16) For sterility : See "Specific for sterility".

(17) For styes of every description. *Puls.*

(18) Specific for hoemorrhoids— *Mucuna* one drop of dose of mother tincture is a specific for bleeding haemorrhoids, two or three doses a day will arrest the disease in a couple of days. *Fiscus religiosa* may be tried if *Mucuna* fails.

(19) Specific for vomiting of blood for gastric ulcer. (*Geranium-Macul-atum.*)

(20) Specific against syphilis and intolerable bone pains specially at night. (*Kali-iodicum.*).

Specific—According to Dr. Y. Singh *Nat-sulf.* 6X and *Nat-phos* 6X. are specific remedies for diabetes. One should be taken in morning and the other in the night continuously for some days.

Specific appendicitis—If *Bap.* C. M. in acute cases is given as a unity dose then it will often abort the need for surgery. If one dose is not sufficient then it may be repeated fortnightly to abort the surgery.

Specific for masturbation and nymphomania in female—*Gratiola*.

Specific for epilepsy—Dr. Hughes recommends, Hydrogcyaenic acid to be specific.

Specific for ex-ophthalmic goitre—*Fucus vesiculosus*.

Specific for haemoptysis—*Hamamellis*.

Specific for hysteria—See "No. 2 of Hysteria consolation aggravates."

Specific for small-pox—*Variolinum* is specific for small-pox. Push it from start to finish. It is the best remedy in all stages and the most reliable remedy. An occasional dose of *Sulp. 30* may be required as an intercurrent remedy. (Dr. D. C. Das Gupta).

Specific for sore throat—Tendency to sore throat, which is recurring. The patient ; has painful and offensive mouth ; swallowing difficult. He is very chilly and keeps covered up. In such cases *Hepar-sulf.* is very effective in preventing recurrence of sore throat.

Specific for sterility—*Aurum-mur-nat.* See "Sterility barrenness in females".

Specific for stings—*Urtica urens.* See "Stings".

Specific-for tetanus—*Mag-phos.* is a specific against tetanus and has cured many severe and advanced cases in the convulsive stage as suggested by Dr. Grimmer. See "Tetanus".

Sphincter stretched, dilated and piles operated—(1) Stretched. (*Staphy.*).

(2) Stretched urethra by catheter or bougie (*Staphy.*).

(3) After dilation of cervix. (*Staphy.*).

(4) Anal sphincter in pile operation. (*Staphy*). See also "Stretches".

Sphincter stretched surgically causing tearing pains—Stretched surgically. Where coldness, congestion of head and receding tearing pains occur from stretching sphincter or tearing of sensitive part takes place *Staphysagira* is the remedy ; 'Stretching' and 'tearing' are the key-words here. (*Staphy.*). See "Stretches".

Spermatorrhoea (involuntary discharge of semen due to various causes)—(1) For bad effects of masturbation where there is great emaciation with dark rings in the eyes. Peevishness and shyness. The boy becomes gloomy. (*Staphy.*).

(2) The nocturnal emissions about three in the morning or later. The erections are weak and excitable. Great weakness follows all indulgence (*Calc.*).

(3) System weakened, erections improper, semen escapes too soon during coitus, patient distressed. (*Pho-a.*).

(4) Emissions occur with or without dreams. Indicated in advanced stages. (*Calad.*).

(5) Suitable to old men physically impotent. (*Agn.*).

(6) Bad effects of masturbation, headache, weak digestion, frequent emissions. (*Nux-v.*).

(7) Passive loss during sleep vertigo on rising in the morning. (*Selenium 30,* 8 hourly.).

(8) Loss of prostatic fluid when the stool is large and difficult. (*Sil.* 30.). "Impotency" under their different heads.

(9) *Conium* is specially the remedy where nocturnal emissions are brought on by suppression of the natural desire and there are pains in the testicles ; emissions on the slightest provocation.

(10) Dr. Mahendra Sarkar cured a case of noctural emission of 6-7 years standing with *Puls.* 30 when a patient is highly depressed with dry tongue, langour, distaste for water but good appetite and head light.

Spinal-sclerosis—Thickening and induration of connective tissue of spine, backache, week joints, hips, legs, and sensation of numbness. (*Oxalic acid.*).

Spinal headache-due to debility—Debility due to nervousness and excessive sensibility of the patient causing headache.

Give *Silicea* which will work as a tonic as suggested by Dr. Hughes.

Spine-inflammation when urine escapes with paralysis of lower extremity—Inflammation in inflammatory condition of the lower parts of the cord which feels sore after an injury to the spine causing aches etc. *Carbo-animalis, Silicea* and *Thuja* have cured them even after years.

(2) *Lathyrus-sativus* is useful for indurated and rigid paralysis and for motor paralysis of lower extremities; must hurry or urine is voided involunarily. Polio. See "Myelitis inflammation of spinal cord".

Spine-injuries—(1) Injuries. (*Hyper.*).

(2) Pain shooting up. (*Hyper.*).

(3) Local soreness. (*Hyper.*).

(4) Inflammatory condition of lower parts. (*Carbo-animalis, Sil., Thuj*).

(5) Injuries to spine higher up. (*Hyper.*).

(6) To prevent inflammatory change after injury. (*Calc.*).

(7) Pain on rising from seat; in old injury. (*Rhus-t.*). See "Rheumatic symptoms in spine due to injury" and "No. 5 of Concussion of brain or spine" and "Myelitis—inflammation of spinal cord".

Spine-stiffness with numbness—(1) Stiffness of whole spine. Tingling inside spine. Chilliness over the back. Crawling, creeping, formication. Bearing down pain in female with symptoms of spinal irritation. (*Agar.*).

(2) Numbness of feet and hands, muscles of the back rigid: spinal irritation. (*Phys.*). "Backache stiffness".

Spitting-constant—See "(b) of saliva producing rawness" and "constant spitting".

Spleen enlarged—(1) Deep seated pain in the splenic region. Enlargement of spleen. Pains on left side with shortness of breath. It is remedy par-excellence for this disease. (*Ceanothus M.T.* in drops.). Compare *Chelidonium, Berberis* and *Conium.*

(2) Enlarged spleen after malarial poisoning. (*Aranea-diadema*.).

(3) Sensitive, swollen and enlarged spleen usually after intermittent fever. (*Cap*.).

(4) Spleen enlarged and along with it the liver specially after malaria. General anaemia and dropsy. (*Cedron*.).

(5) Dr. Burnett highly speaks of Spirtus *Glandium quercus* (*Acron*.) as a splenic remedy either in the acute or in the chronic stage even when ascites and dropsical swelling of the legs are present with hypertrophy of the organ. It will increase greatly the quantity of urine. See "Liver" and "Jaundice".

(6) Pain in the left side, relieved by lying on the right side. (*Scil*.).

(7) For congestion, inflammation and enlargement of spleen. (*Chin-s*.).

(8) Cutting pain in the region of spleen extending to hips, enlargement and tenderness in the region. (*Grindelia*.).

(9) Enlarged liver and spleen with fever. (*Ferr-ars*.) ; without fever. (*Ferr-met*.). See "Liver-infantile with spleen".

Splinter or nail-into the feet—When a patient steps on a nail or splinter sticks under the finger nail or into the foot or any other sensitive part give a dose of *Ledum*. This will always prevent tetanus. (*Led*.). See "Nail in the foot".

Spondylitis-inflammation of vertebrae—*Lachnanthes 200*, one dose is to be taken in the morning and evening. From next day *Mag-phos. 30x, Kali-mur. 30x, Calc.-fluor. 30x*, four tablets of each should be taken alternately for some time.

Spots-brown yellow saddle on face, on cheeks, face and nose—(1) Brown spots on face, chest, abdomen. A yellow saddle across upper parts of the cheek and nose or roundish yellow spots on the face may be cured with *Sep*. These will be found in a woman along with menstrual and other uterine trouble. (*Sep*.).

(2) For naevus, the external use of *Bellis-perennis* is very useful.

(3) Brown spots on hands and arms (*Thuja-occ.*). See "Freckles" and "Liver spots".

Sprain-in joints—*Arnica.* Weakness, tenderness to be removed by *Rhus-tox,* and subsequently by *Calc.* They all go together. See also "Weakness in-sprained joints".

Sprained-joints sore, soles and ankles weak and legs give out on rising—(a) Swollen joints, easy spraining and difficult to rise from chair. *Arnica* will very often take the soreness out of the sprained joints. Black and blue appearances of the sprained parts will go away in a surprisingly short time. Externally *Bellis M.T.* in hot water to be applied in compressed form. See also "Pain-in sprained joints" and "Ankles-swollen".

(b) (1) When the swelling about the joint is so soft that a pit is left when pressed by fingers. (*Samb.*).

(2) Over-strained or over-exercised. Legs give out on rising from chair, hip and things so weak (*Ruta.*).

(3) Ankles swollen. Easy spraining of ankles. Soles painful, can hardly step on them. (*Led*).

Squints—(1) As a sequel to convulsions. (*Bell.*).

(2) Of either eye due to loss of power of internal muscle. (*Alumina.*).

(3) With worm symptoms. (*Cina.*)

(4) Internal squint of either eye. (*Gels.*).

(5) If squint is due to after-effects of anti-toxin drugs. (*Diphth. 1M.*).

Stammering with embarrassing speech, heavy tongue and certain letters not pronounced—(a) *Stram.* 6 hourly (b) (1) *Bovista* adapted to stammering of children.

(2) *Hyos.* 6 hourly, if *Stram.* fails. Both to be tried for long time.

(3) When he swallows words, speech embarrassed. (*Cic-v.*).

(4) Stammering from childhood or caused by or aggravated by excitement or from vexation. Distortion of mouth tongue when speaking. (*Caust.*).

(5) When due to heaviness of tongue (*Nat-c.*).

(6) Difficulty and stammering in pronouncing certain letters or words. Letters like 'S' or X,V,T,P. (*Lach.*).

Startling of child in fever—Child in acute fever condition startles, grasps the nurse and screams as if he is afraid of falling. (*Gels.*) See "Spasms of child during sleep" and "Child-frightened".

Stealing habit and tendency—(1) Habit of stealing in mania. (*Stram.*).

(2) General tendency. (*Staphy.*). See "Deceiving".

Sterility-barrenness in females and sterility in males—(a) (1) When not traceable to any organic defect with depression, menses scanty late or absent. *Aur-met.* Compare *Agn.*

(2) When due to weakness of uterus *Aletris-f.* Compare *Seuecio-aureus.*

(3) Irregularity of menses with leucorrhoea and constipation. (*Sep.*). Compare *Borax* when menses too soon, nausea and pain in stomach. Favours easy conception.

(4) When from excessive and premature menses. *Calc-c.*

(5) With dwindling of breasts and overies. (*Iod*).

(6) Sterility in women with excessive sexual desire. (*Platina.*).

(7) According to R. B. Bishamber Dass *Sepia.* is head remedy for sterility. There is irregularity of menses with leucorrhoea and constipation.

(8) R.B. Bishamber Dass recommends *Aurm-m-nat.* as specific for sterility. It cures ulceration, swelling of the ovary. also covers habital abortion and prolapses of the uterus. To be given in 2x trituration. (b) (1) Sterility in males : impotence of long-standing. Loss of sexual powers with lascivious

fancies. Semen thin and odourless. Sexual neurasthenia (exhaustion of nerve force). On attempting coition penis relaxes. (*Sel.* 4 hourly).

(2) Impotence, involuntary emissions discharge too quick, spasms during coition, effects of masturbation, disposition to handle organs. *Bufo. 30-200* night and morning. See "Impotence" and "Impotency".

(c) (1) When there is a fault in the ovaries, menses are scanty and there is pain in the breasts. (*Con.*).

(2) When much leucorrhoea is present. (*Bor.*).

(3) In obstinate cases of sterility think *Natrum-carb.* (Dr. Moor).

(4) Dr. Rummel recommends *Phosphorus* which has exact relation to the male and female organs for sterility.

(5) Dr. Boericke suggests *Agnus* and *Nat-m.* given according to symptoms.

(6) Impotency in the male and sterility and uterine atony in the female (*Eup-per*).

Still-birth-its prevention—See "Chapter V" for details .

Stiff neck-spraining on moving and rheumatic pains—(1) From damp and cold, pain in the nape after lying with the head in an uncomfortable position. (*Dulc.* 1 hourly.).

(2) Stiff neck spraining on moving it, head twisted to one side. (*Lachn.*).

(3) Head and neck retracted, rheumatic pain and stiffness in muscles of neck and back. (*Acet-r.*).

(4) From a draught or chill, tearing in the nape, painful stiff neck, worse on moving, pain extending from neck to shoulder. *Acon* or *Bell.* will suffice. See "Neck stiff", "Chapter V" for details .

Stings-their bad effects—Bad effects from sting and bites (*Acets ac.*). See "Bites animals" and "Bite sting".

Stings of bees scorpions and wasps—They may be treated by external application of *Apis-tincture* in watery solution and internal administration of *Apis 30* (Dr. Iyer). *Ledum 200* for scorpion itch. Give 6 pills every 5 minutes till the stingings pain comes down and then stop it.

Stings of venomous insects—*Ars. alb.* See also "Insect bites of stings".

Stomach-dilatation enlargement—In dilatation of stomach and chronic digestive disorders in *Hydrastinum-muriaticum*. It may be used locally in aphthos, sore mouth, ulcers, ulcerated sore throat, ozaena etc. See "External Homoeopathic medicines".

Stomach-eructations (belching) with burning and white tongue—(1) Pulsation in the pit of stomach which is perceptible both with sight and touch, loud eructation of wind from stomach. Spasmodic contraction of stomach. Pressure and burning behind the stomach and sudden violent single stitches of pain at short intervals coming from within outwards. (*Asaf*).

(2) Eructation of wind and fluid, tasting of food taken with heart burning. Tongue white. (*Ant-curdum*). See also "Eructations the act of belching with distension".

Stomach-fainting feeling at night to eat—(1) Fainting feeling in stomach and must eat then. Gets up at night to eat. (*Phos.*). See "Hnuger gets up at night".

(2) For gastric and intestinal trouble.. (*Petroselinum.*). See "Hunger gets up at night".

Stomach gnawing hunger and forcing patient to eat while milk causing diarrhoea—(1) The important symptom regarding the stomach is a peculiarly empty feeling or sensation of gnawing hunger and the patient wants to eat something immediately the gnawing starts. It is known as "all gone sensation in the stomach". (*Sep.*).

(2) Diarrhoea from milk stomach relieved by eating, drives him out of bed for eating. (*Natrum-carb*). See "Hunger gnawing-relief by eating". See "Pain in stomach after eating".

Stomach pain-relief by eating—(a) Which is sometimes relieved by eating. (*Anac.*) (b) For pain in stomach give *Bell. 200* in water every 5 minutes. See 'b' of abdomen pains".

Stomach sinking sensation with vomiting pain and flatulence—(1) Weak, empty, sinking sensation in the stomach with hunger at 11 A.M. (*Sulf.*).

(2) Vomiting pain in pit of stomach, flatulence. (*Carb-ac.* 3, 2 hourly). See "Hunger sinking sensation eating every 3 or 4 hours".

Stone-its prevention and expulsion in bladder and derangements or inflammation with partial paralysis—(*a*) (1) Irritability at the neck of bladder, dribbling of urine or retention, red brick dust sediment or bloody, (*Nux-v.*). Compare *Cantharis* during attacks.

(2) *Vesicaria* is recommended to favour expulsion of gravel and sand in urine. Dr. Laurie recommends *Dulcamara*, *Hydrastis, Sulphur* and *Calcarea* as indicated medicines.

(3) *Chionanthus* is powerful to prevent the formation of gall stones and promotes the discharge of those already formed. See "Cystitis inflammation of bladder".

(b) Derangements or inflammation of bladder due to cold, stimulants, and mechanical injury—(1) If fever, dry, hot skin. *Acon.*

(2) Very scanty urination. *Canth.* or *Puls.*

(3) Spasm. *Dig., Hyos.*

(4) Mucous deposit. *Puls., Dulc.*

(5) Chronic case. *Dulc. , Hyder.*

(6) For dissolving concretion give *Lith.* 3x (trit.) to 30, four times a day.

(7) For partial paralysis of bladder with spasmodic condition of sphincter. *Op.* See "Bladder" under its different heads.

Stomatitis-inflammation of soft tissues of mouth—(1) For most violent ulcerative stomatitis. (*Nitc-ac.*).

(2) Very sore feeling in the mouth, redness of tongue, elevated papillae, lips and corners of mouth cracked, nose sore. (*Arum-t*).

(3) When due to mercury : (i) *Nit-ac. 6,* 2 hourly ; (ii) *Hep. 6,* 2 hourly. See "Mouth stomatitis" and "Mouth ulcerative".

Stone in kidney with agonising pain—(a) (1) Violent sticking pains in the bladder extending from kidney to urethra with urging to urinate. (*Berb-vul.*). It is a head remedy for renal colic.

(2) Agonising pain, twists about, screams and groans, urine red with brick dust and sediment. (*Ocimum-Canum*).

(3) Writhing with crampy pains must move about. (*Dioscorea*).

(4) Urine becomes turbid like clay water immediately after passing ; much pain at the end of urinating, white sandy, scanty, slimy, flaky urine. Tenesumus of bladder. (*Sars.*). (b) *Carduus marianus* has the reputation of preventing further formation of stones. See "Gall-stone colic".

(5) When all remedies fail then *Pareira brava* may be given in mother tincture in hot water in 5 drops doses every half hour.

(6) Prevention ; gravelly urine, pain in back loins. (*Berb-vulg.* 6 hourly.).

(7) Tendency to store uric acid in tissues. (*Urt-u.*). (c) (1) Dr. Farrington recommends *Cantharis* as one of the best remedies during the paroxysm of renal colic as it relieves the local irritation while Dr. Jousset thinks that it is indicated in the quantity of blood voided in urine and in the inflammation of genito urinary organs. When *Cantharis* failed then Dr. Preston used *Arg-nit.*, when there is dull aching across the small of back and over the region of bladder. The urine burns and urethra swollen.

(2) Dr. Jacob James recommends *Ipomoea* for passage of stone from kidney to bladder.

(3) Dr. Hempel cured many cases of renal colic with *Coccus-cacti*.

(4) *Ocimum* is also useful when urine contains considerable blood. See also "Calculus in kidney" under its different heads "Kidney-stone in" and "Colic-renal stone in kidney".

Stone-its passing causing pain—When there is pain attending the passage of biliary or renal calculi then repeated doses of *Calc-c.* in 30 dilutions will go a long way in relieving such a pain.

Stool-involuntary in children and craving to swallow it—(1) Involuntary stool even solid in little children who may drop the stool over the carpet without knowing that they have done so. (*Aloe.*). See also "Involuntary stool of children."

(2) A craving to swallow his own stool or urine or dung lying in street. This sometimes happens with chronic patients with loss of memory. (*Vera-a.*). See "Involuntary stool of children".

Stoppage-of nose of new born—(1) *Nux-v.* is the best remedy. If the complaint still continues then give *Sambucus*.

(2) If the nose is stuffed up and the child is keeping its mouth open to breathe and cannot sleep, long continued coryza (*Am-c.*). See also "Nose stopped when going out" and "Infant's nose blocked".

Strains and weakness of muscle, tendon—*Rhus-tox.* follows *Arnica* well in removing the pain and weakness of the tendons and muscles. See "Weakness of the tendons and muscles" and "Pain of tendon and muscles".

Strangulated - Hernia—Slipping of one part of intestine to another. Passage of pure bright red blood, mucus with tensemus. Give *Aconite* for relieving pain. (Dr. Shepherd).

Strangury-painful urination, the urine, being vioded drop by drop and urine retained due to paralysis of bladder—(1) Violent pains in bladder, with frequent urging to urinate, cutting pains, urine passed drop by drop, with great pain. (*Canth.*).

(2) Burning and smarting on passing urine ; urine red, brown, blacky or smoky in appearance. Has much pain in the back in kidney and bladder troubles (*Ter.*).

(3) In woman specially. (*Copaiva* ½ hourly.).

(4) For violent pain, constant desire to urinate, urine dark red, offensive. (*Merc-sol*).

(5) When urine is retained owing to some sort of paralysis (*Helleborus, Nux-v* and *Ars-a.*). See also "Urine-frequent and painful".

Streaks red and blue—(1) Stripes (A discoloured mark) red lines, and streaks extending upto the arms and legs (*Hypericum.*).

(2) Bluish red streaks extending to arms and axilla and also up and down the legs. (*Myristica seb.*).

Stretches and remover of catheter pains—(1) When the urethra has been stretched for removing a stone or by use of bogies and catheter, dilation of cervix has been done or anal sphincter for treatment of piles etc. *Staphysagria* will remove the subsequent difficulties. These stretches after surgical operation may cause great distress with painfulness and symptoms of collapse causing cold sweat etc. These are also removable by *Staphy*.

(2) A dose of *Aconite* given shortly before passing a catheter will prevent pain if there is any difficulty. (Dr. Clarke). See "Pain after stretches" and "Catheter fever".

Stricture-inability to pass sound and removal of this inability—Dr. Bokowitz claims that in case where one is unable to pass the sound,the injection of *Lobelia-tincture* into the urethra and held there for a short time will obviate all the difficulties.

Stricture of urethra—The flow of urine is by fits and starts or the patient has to wait a long time before being able to pass water. The urine is turbid and milky or dark and secretion is diminished. It is very difficult to empty the bladder completely. (*Clematis.*). See "Dribbling of urine".

Strokes—Semi-consciousness, dullness and inability to concentrate. Patient nervous and irritable. *Opium* first and later on *Cicuta*.

Stricture-prevention—*Clematis-erecta* is a good remedy for gonorrhoea. On account of slow or intermittent flow of urine indication of formation of stricture and this medicine if given early and high will prevent it.

Stumps neuritis—It is a wonderful remedy for traumatic neuritis often met in a stump after amputation or serious injury. Pains almost unbearable. (*All-c.*) See "Amputation neuritis".

Stupor of child with red face—If the child feels suddenly ill with red face and redness of eyes with semi-stupor, starts up in sleep, goes into spasm. *Bell.* will act as oil in troubled waters. (*Bell*). See "Child-frightened" and "Startling of child".

Stupor-sudden in eruptive fevers—Continued dreamy state while awake, child whines or cries all the time. Pupils dilated. Fetid odour comes from the mouth and nose. Great prostration. The course of disease is usually sudden and goes into serious condition suddenly in diphtheria, measles, smallpox etc. (*Ail.*). See "Eruptive fevers-rash failing" and "Prostration of child drowsy".

Styes-margins aggulinated eyes—In eyes-lids ; aggulinated at night, dry scabs on edges forming nodules on lids. (*Thuj.*).

Styes-on lower-lid—Styes chronic particularly of children, leaving little nodules specially on lower lids but also on both lids. *Staphy* very effective.

Styes-margins and their prophylactic—(a) For chronic cases and for tendency for recurrence. (*Heper.*) (b) *Staphisagria* is a prophylactic against styes. See "Tumours recurrent".

Styes-margins itching—Recurrent styes. Margin of lids itch. (*Staphy* ; *Sil*).

Styes-upper lids—Specially on upper lid ; from eating fat, greasy rich food. *Puls.* It is specific for styes of every descriptions in every stage of disease.

Sudden appearance of symptoms and blindness—(1) *Mer-c.* has more intense symptoms which appear suddenly and vehemently. (*Merc-c.*).

(2) Sudden blindness. (*Acon.*). See "Blindness-also night blindness".

Suddenness-of disease in children—If the disease starts suddenly and with great intensity, redness and swelling and painfulness. *Bell.* is the remedy. So if the child feels suddenly ill with red face and redness of eyes with semi-stupor, starts up in sleep, goes into spasms. *Bell.* will act as oil upon troubled waters. It is one of the best remedies for diseases of children. (*Bell.*). See "Convulsions" and "Cholera-infantum-sudden and extreme prostration".

Sudden-loss of memory—Forgetful of things in his mind but a moment ago,forgetful as if in dream. Everything seems to be in a dream : patient is greatly troubled about his forgetfulness ; confused. (*Anac.*). See also "Memory" under its different heads and also "Forgetfulness".

Summer complaints-of children during dentition—Trembles during dentition. Anguish, crying and expression of uneasiness and discontent *Aethusa-cynapium* most frequently indicated in diseases of chidren during dentition, summer complaints when with diarrhoea there is marked inability to digest milk and poor circulation. Milk causes diarrhoea (*Aeth-c*). See "Dentition" under its different heads.

Summer diarrhoea-due to over eating—Worse in the morning on first moment, on rising and often occurs as an effect of over-eating in the summer. Constipation is its general character. It often occurs as a result of dietetic errors specially when warm wheather sets in after cold. (*Bry.*). Compare with *Nux-vomica* diarrhoea which is also worse in the morning is mostly caused by over-eating and is apt to put in the dysenteric type It is caused from continued over-eating and inactivity, the abuse of drugs, coffee, tobacco or alcohol. The *Puls.* diarrhoea is more apt to occur in the night from over-eating and is attended with great rumbling of bowels. It is caused from too rich foods, pastries, fat foods and ice cream in excess. See "Diarrhoea due to over eating in summer" and "Overfeeding of children".

Sucking of thumb—Child sucks her thumb and bites her nails, afraid of worms, birds and small animals. Give *Nat-m.* in 1 M. dilution every week.

Sucking-disinclination—(1) When the child refused to take the breast, although applied within few hours after delivery. One dose of *Cina 200* in dilution need be given if this fails then *Merc-sol.* 6th dilution should be tried.

(2) When the child takes the breast readily but immediatley therafter returns the milk. (*Silicea*). See "Lactation".

Suicide—In his pessimistic condition of the patient he is always inclined to commit suicide. He meditates always upon death, upon suicide, has no love for life which he thinks worthless. (*Aur-met*). See also "Mania", "Melancholia" and "Perverted affections".

Suicidal thought with broken down constitution—Despair, anxiety, fear, peevishness and suicidal thought of persons with broken down constitution from sexual excesses and secret vices and sex-weakness with perversion. (*Agn.*). See also "Broodings" and "Depression suicidal".

Sun-burn—When exposed parts to sun's rays become painful bathe them with *succus-calendula*. It may be mixed with a little water if so desired.

Sun-headache—Sun headache due to exposure to sun-heat. The patient is distressed with a headache every time he is exposed to the sun's heat for sometime. (*Lach*). See also "Headache—due to exposure to sun".

Sun-stroke-with laboured respiration and its prevention—
(a) Pale face, fixed eyes ; white tongue, laboured respiration.

The temperature is high and often times there is unconsciousness. Severe headache, jaws clenched. Involuntary eructations *Glonine* every five minutes later larger intervals. (b) (1) For sun-stroke *Nat-m.* is an excellent medicine.

(2) Much flushing of heat ; tremor of limbs ; surging of blood to head and face throbbing throughout whole body. (*Amyl-n.*).

(3) Face flushed, blood-shot eyes. Throbbing headache with high fever (*Bell.*).

(4) For prevention of sun-stroke *Gelsemium* is an excellent medicine.

Sun-stroke with pain, mental sluggishness—(1) Gnawing pain in the back of head extending to spine. Mental sluggishness. Throbbing in the back of neck. Bowels constipated. (*Nat-sulf.*).

(2) Breathing difficult or obstructed, face bloated. (*Opium*).

(3) For collapse. (*Camphor*).

(4) For nausea and vomiting. (*Silicea* and *Theridion.*).

Suppression of milk-due to emotional disturbances—(a) Little anxiety of emotional disturbance, causing suppression of milk. (*Act-rac.*). (1) If suppressed from fit of anger then *Cham.*

(2) When no cause discernible for non-appearance of milk. (*Caust.*).

(b) For non-appearance of milk and for increasing the flow of milk in nursing women, *Ricinus—communis* is an excellent remedy according to Dr. Dewey. (c) The breasts are swollen, painful and the flow of milk is absent or scanty. (*Puls.*). See "Milk suppression due to emotional disturbance" and "Lactation".

Suppressed-skin trouble—Many a time an internal disease which has been cured after suppression of skin trouble with ointment etc. will be cured with *Sulf.* after the original skin trouble reappears on the skin. (*Sulf.*). For suppressed small-pox see under proper head "Retarded eruptions of small-pox" and "Skin eruptions suppressed".

Suppuration—In diseases where suppuration seems inevitable *Heper.* may open the abscess and hasten the cure. (*Hep.*). See also "Pus formation" and "Injury-children tending to form pus".

Surgical shock—Post-operative shock with cold sweat on fore-head, pale face ; rapid feeble pulse. Cold perspiration on the forehead ; vomiting and cramps in extremities. (*Verat.*).

(2) For temperature sub-normal, blood pressure low and respiration slow give *Camphora*. Compare *Carb-v.*, *Opium* and *Digitalis* for shock. See also "Shock of operation", "Collapse" "Operation-collapse" and "Septic infections and its prophylactics".

Swallowing and boring finger in nose by a child—Frequent swallowing as if something is coming in the throat. The child bores fingers in the nose and grinds teeth. (*Cina.*). See "Finger boring during sleep" and "Nose children scratching in acute diseases".

Sweat-cold with sinking forces—On forehead ; complete prostration with cold, cold breath, blue skin and pinched nose. Rapid sinking forces. The whole body icy cold. (*Verat*). See "Perspiration cold".

Sweat-cold due to surgical stretches causing great distress—The stretches after surgical operation may cause great distress with painfulness and symptoms of collapse causing cold sweat. Where coldness, congestion of the head, the receding tearing pain occur from stretching sphincter or tearing of a sensitive part takes place. *Staphysagria* is the remedy. "Stretching" and "Tearing" are the key-words here. See also "Stretches".

Sweat in fever—With hectic fever or drenching night sweat with no thirst in fever (*Acet-ac.*). Compare *Abrot.* See also "Night sweats" and "Hectic fever".

Sweat on head and hands in sleep—Sweats in general or sweats on exertion, sweating on hand and palms. In children sweating on head and forehead during sleep. (*Bry.*). See

"Perspiration on palms and head" and "Emaciation with sweating head in children".

Sweat offensive foot—Offensive foot-sweat and of axilla intolerable *Rhus.* at bed time for a week, then *Sulf.* for a week. If both fail then *Silicea*. Dr. Laurie recommends that a dose first *Silicea* night and morning every third day, until six doses have been given, then pause a week, proceed with *Rhus.* in like manner returning again to *Silicea* if necessary. Either intermediately or in long course a dose of *Sulphur* night and morning for a week then pause. See also "Perspiration on foot offensive" and "Axilla-different complaints".

Sweating-on head—The sweat on head is a prominent symptom in *Calc-p.* See "Perspiration on palms and head".

Sweating-in infectious disease—Of weak and anaemic persons at night after infectious disease like influenza, *Ferr-p.* will be useful.

Swimmer-trembling—Swimmers trembling violently when coming out of water in spite of warm towels and standing in the sun. (*Gels.*).

Sweat things-liking by a patient—*Lyco.* patient desires sweet things. Aggravation between 4, 7 and 8 p.m. (*Lyco*).

Swelling-of abdomen with pain extending to lower limbs—With pain in lower abdomen extending to genitals, rectum and coccyx ; better sitting (*Parafine*). See "Abdomen pains".

Swelling-persisting and absorption of fluids—*Sulf.* has an unique power of absorption of fluid anywhere in the body. It may be in joints or serous sacks. After the acute symptoms are over, but the swelling persists a dose of *Sulf.* will very often help at the absorption of the fluids and finish the cure. (*Sulf.*). See also "Fluids absorption".

Swelling-compresses hot for it—See "Inflammation—compresses hot".

Swelling of feet in dropsy—Swelling of feet and leg (*Merc-s.*). See "Dropsy-swelling of feet"

Swelling-in glands—In glands which are inclined to form pus or swelling in any part of the body. The pain increases at night, perspiration gives no relief. (*Merc-c.*). See "Glands swollen and inflamed".

Swelling-with inflamed glands—Acute swelling with inflammation of glands *e.g.* neck etc., the patient should be thirsty, restless and chilly. (*Rhus-t.*). Compare *Merc-sol.* where the patient is somewhat restless, will not usually keep cover and will perspire profusely without much relief. See "Pains with swelling" and "Glands swollen and inflamed".

Swelling-of labia in menses with itching—Horrible itching of genitals with swelling of labia during menses. Menses too early and too profuse. Discharge of blood between menstrual period is a common occurrence after every little accident. All uterine symptoms aggravate on lying down. (*Ambra.*). See "Menstruation-early profuse with itching and swelling labia".

Swelling-of upper lips—*Silicea* and *Nitric-ac.* See "No. 2 of lips tumour and swelling".

Swelling-localised—In localised inflammation *Bell.* is the first remedy when there is great redness and swelling. Shaking of bed causes pain in inflamed parts. (*Bell.*). See "Inflammation localised".

Swelling-of nose with loss of smell and sneezing—Swelling of nose with fetid discharge. Loss of smell. Violent sneezing. (*Kali-bichromicum.*). See "Nose smell", "Glands swelling-due to discharge from nose" and "Nose-septum ulcerated".

Swelling-pus formation—Painful swelling or eruption on the skin. The patient cannot bear to be touched when pus has formed or is about to form. *Hepar.* follows *Merc-sol.* very often well specially in cases of boils and inflammatory swellings. (*Hepar.*). See also "Pus formation".

Swelling-on right side—Starts on right side and may go over the left. (*Lyco.*). See also "Inflammation" under different heads also "Tonsillitis with swelling causing suppuration and Eruption right sided".

Sycosis—An inflammatory disease affecting the hair follicles particularly. The skin is unhealthy and presents the various forms of eruptions. There is a tendency to ulceration with sticking pain. There is a foul perspiration of the feet, foetid discharges from the ears, foetid urine.

Sychotic antidote—*Thuja*.

Synovitis-inflammation of the knee joints—(1) Violent pain in the knee joint more outside and to the front. Shooting pain in the knee with white swelling and burning.

(2) Acute traumatic synovitis with effusion in the joints; the pains are aching and tearing (*Ledum*.).

Syphilis—*Asaf.* is a medicine for syphilis at times with induration and inflammation of periosteum (membrane covering the surface of bone) and glands, old scars turn purple threaten to suppurate and become painful or even turn black (*Asaf.*). See "Scar syphilitc".

Syphilis in general complicated with gonorrhoea and congenital during pregnancy—(*a*) (1) *Merc-sol.* is the head remedy for all stages of syphilis. Chancres are red which spread inwards with yellowish fetid discharge. To be given in low potencies in acute cases and in very high potencies in chronic cases.

(2) *Cinnabaris* is useful in syphilis complicated with gonorrhoea. Discharge of pus through urinary passage.

(3) *Merc-dulc.* is useful in syphilis of the females where there are many condylomatous growths in and around the external genitals. See "Condylomata".

(4) *Merc-c.* Chancres with expansive ulceration in mouth, gums and throat. Fetid breath and enlarged tonsils.

(5) *Carbo animalis* has copper coloured blotches on the skin, specially on the face, induration in general and of axillary glands hard as stone. See "Axilla-different complaints".

(6) Congenital during pregnancy and nursing, the mother should take *Merc-s.* 6 night and morning and *Leut. 30,* once a week. If in spite of this child shows signs of syphilis it should have *Merc-sol.* night and morning. (b) (1) According to Father Mullers dispensary *Merc-sol.* and *Acid-nitric* in the first stage ; *Merc-cor* and *Kali-iod.* in the 2nd stage. *Mezer.* for nightly pains in bones. In the tertiary stage, give *Kali-iod. Aurum-mur.* Use lower potencies 2x or 3x. (2) Dr. Berjeau considers that *Merc-cor.* and *Merc.* are most prominent remedies for bubo. The former for acute and the latter for indolent type while for stony hard and indurated glands *Badiga* is recommended.

Syphilis pain in bones—*Aur-met.* is useful in old syphilitics when the bones are breaking down in any part of the body ; the shin bones, nose bones, ear bones, any of the small bones. The complaints are aggravated at night. The pains are violent. The bones ache, as if they would break. Pains in the joints rendering them immovable. Inflammation of the bones with caries (*Aur-met.*). See also "Bones-ache" and "Head-ache syphilite".

Syphilitic antidote—*Mercury.* See "Anti-psoric" and "Anti-psychotic".

Syphilitic iritis eyes with ulcers, discharge and inflammation—Syphilitic eye complaints with ulcers on the eye-balls. Ulcers on the cornea, which are ameliorated in the air, with a sensation of numbness in the eye. Inflammation of eyes with severe sharp stitching pains that come from within out are met by *Asafoetida.* The discharge from the eye is acrid, bloody and offensive. (*Asaf.*). See "Eyes syphilitic".

Syphilitic complications of nose, throat and palate—In old cases when the syphilitic miasm attacks the bone of the nose, affections of the throat, palate and uvula with offensive smell from the roof of the mouth. The medicines that are specially related or specially useful in this form of ulceration in old syphilitic will be *Kali-bi., Lach., Merc-cor., Merc.* and *Hepar.* but in those syphilitic cases that have been mercularised *Hepar.* and *Nitric-acid* should be thought of. See "Nose syphilitic". "No. 4 of caries" and "Bones pains".

T

Tachycardia—abnormal rapidity of cardiac action— Sharp cutting pain in heart ; heart's action heavy and slow, lungs feel compressed, cannot be fully expanded. Choking sensation of throat. (*Abies-nigra*.). Compare *Agnus.*

Taking the case and questioning the patient—(1) The most difficult problem in homoeopathy is taking the case. A good taking of case means a good and effective prescription. No prescription can be made out of a case taking badly and not according to Hahnemann's principle of Homoeopathy. There is saying that "Where the practitioners of other systems stop, the homoeopathy begins". This means that practitioners of other systems stop at the diagnosis. The treatment portion then follows almost automatically but in Homoeopathy one has got to diagnose a disease, to know its pros and cons, its future development, its chances of cure etc. But real homoeopathic diagnosis *i.e.* the diagnosis of the medicine then starts after the pathological diagnosis has been fixed. For the latter purpose *i.e.* for the purpose of fixing the medicine-diagnosis we have to take the case in a way quite different from followers of other systems. In a well taken case where the case is accurately taken, almost, any novice, could prescribe on them. It is an interesting fact that a case taken cautiously and in minute details usually leads the physician easily to the pathological diagnosis also, thereby dispensing away with the pathological tests. Symptoms due to mechanical causes such as fractures, dislocation, stone in the bladder, etc. require mechanical intervention and should ordinarily be got set right by mechanical means. Of course complications arising afterwards can be treated with great benefit homoeopathically. Homoeopathic way is the medical way following the right indications given by the disease and that way is always open weather we treat the case successfully or not.

(2) The answers to the following questions put to the patient particularly in a chronic case will usually help the Prescriber generally to find out a correct remedy.

(1) Name, age and occupation of the patient.

(2) Let the patient describe his or her main complaint.

(3) What does the patient think about its cause.

(4) How did it start and since how long.

(5) What time of day and night the patient's complaint is better or worse.

(6) What will the patient do that will give relief in the complaint or make it worse. For example, is it better with rest, movements, heat cold or pressure or worst.

(7) Which season agrees with the patient, summer, winter or wet weather.

(8) How is patient's appetite, what food is liked most. Any particular food upsets the patient. Any special dislike for food.

(9) How much water does the patient drink daily. State rough amount. Does the patient like cold or warm drinks.

(10) Does the patient has a regular stool or is constipated.

(11) How often does the patient pass urine by day and night. Does the urine escapes a little if it is held for long.

(12) Does the patient has normal sleep. Any fearful or funny dreams in sleep.

(13) Past history : From which disease the patient suffered in the past. For example, fevers like malaria, influenza, typhoid, diarrhoea, dysentery, skin diseases like ring worms, eczema, itch, boils etc. Any accident, operation or injury.

(14) How often the patient has been vaccinated for small-pox.

(15) Family history : Any common disease in the family *i.e.* parents as skin disease, allergic conditions, arthritis, T.B. pleurisy or cancer etc.

(16) Has the patient any sexual mal-adjustment in life.

(17) Enquire about patient's temperament. Is it mild, gentle weeping, nervous, sad or irritable.

(18) Does the patient like company or prefer to be alone.

(19) Any other information that patient would like to give.

(20) For female patients only: Whether she has menses regular. Whether she has menses every 28 or 30 days. Any pain before, during or after menses ? Is the flow normal or does she bleed freely ? How many days the pain lasts ? Any abortion ? Does she has sensation that her internal parts feel like coming out when she squats for stools or lift heavy weight ?

Talkativeness-monopolising the talk—Patient is famous for his talkativeness. He will monopolise all the talks to him-self in a company with a rapid change of subjects and jumping abruptly from one idea to another. (*Lach.*).

Talkativeness-during fever—The *Podo.* patient becomes very talkative during high fever. The higher the fever more is the talkativeness. The chills are very violent and are followed by intense fever. (*Podo*). See "Fever patient talkative with intermittent fever".

Tallness-unusual—Try *Sulf. 30. Calc-carb. 6, Bell. 3* and *Silicea* 6 according to symptoms.

Tartar-its prevention and removal—*Calc-renalsis* prevents formation of tartar while *Fragaria,* removes tartar from teeth. See "Pyorrhoea" under its different heads.

Taste and its loss—(*a*) Food tastes bitter. (1) *Nat-m.*

(2) *China.*

(3) *Puls.* (*b*) Milk tastes digusting. *Nux-v.* 4 hourly. (*c*) Every thing tastes salty. (*Bell.* 4 hourly). (*d*) Food seems tasteless, milky coated tongue (*Ant-t.*). (*e*) Taste lost with loss of smell after cold. (*Mag-m.*). (*f*) Loss of taste with tongue thickly coated white. (*Ant-c.*). (*g*) Complete loss of taste. (*Nat-m., Mag-c.*). (*h*) Bad taste in the mouth in the morning, food and drink tastes sour : Bad odour from the mouth. Sour bitter taste. (*Nux-v.* 4 hourly.). (*i*) Bad taste after sleeping. (*Rheum* 4 hourly.). (*j*) Sour taste to all food. (*Lyco.* 4 hourly.). See also "Cold loss of smell and taste", "Mouth bad taste" and "Nose smell".

Taste nothing tastes well during digestive trouble—Bad taste in the mouth and nothing tastes well, not even water. Dryness in the mouth without thirst caused by rich greasy food, will be good indicator for *Puls.* during digestive trouble. (*Puls*). Compare *Merc sol.* which has similar bad taste in mouth, salivation and thirst. See "Dyspepsia with bad taste with rich food and vomiting" and "Indigestion with bad taste in mouth".

Taste-sour—After eating sour taste in the mouth. Pressure in the stomach for 1 or 2 hours. Tightness about the waist. Must loosen the clothings (*Nux-v.*). See "Sour every thing". "Acidity-with wind" and "Diarrhoea of children sour swelling"

Taste-sour eructations—In mouth sour eructations, vomiting and diarrhoea, every thing sour. (*Calc*). See also "Eructations the act of belching with distension".

Tears or watering from eyes with swollen lids—Constant flow of tears, or water from the eyes where there is no mucus or gumming. Burning in eyes. Lids swollen. Eyes appear wet with tears. (*Nat-m.* 30. one dose at least per day until improvement takes place.) See "Eyes burning". "Watering from eyes" and "Eyes watering with redness".

Tearing and starches after operations The starches after surgical operation may cause great distress with painfulness and symptoms of collapse causing cold sweat. Where coldness, congestion of the head and receding tearing pain occurs from stretching sphincter or tearing of a sensitive part takes place, *Staphy* is the remedy. Stretching and tearing are the key words here. (*Staphy.*). See "Stretches and remove of catheter pain".

Terrible disease of cancer—Dr. Yudvir Singh has suggested medicines for cancer in the different part of the body.

(1) *Carcinosin* potency 200 or 1000 should be given in all cases of cancer. This medicine should be given as an inter-current medicine either weekly or monthly along with other indicated medicine.

(2) Cancer of the breast or other places where there are thick muscles. (*Conium 200 or 1000*).

(3) Cancer of the tongue. Specially in cases where the patient has neuralgia of face. (*Kali-cyanatum 30, 200*).

(4) Cancer of uterus. *Hydrastis, M.T.* should be given internally and its lotion of 200 potency should be used for douching the part.

(5) Cancer of mouth, throat or cheek. In such cases the patient craves ice-cold water as it relieves pain. (*Phos. 30, 200*).

(6) Cancer of stomach when the patient vomits water or as soon as it gets warm in the stomach. (*Phos.*)

(7) Cancer of oesophagus. Painful cracks in the corner of the mouth. (*Condurango*).

(8) Cancer of the bone (*Hekla-lava 3x Trit*).

(9) For pains in cancer give *Aconite-radix.* One or two drops in an ounce of water every one or two hours until the pain is relieved.

(10) In all such cases *Radium-brom.* 30 and *Selenium* should be given once a week.

Teeth—See "Denture causing ulcer".

Teeth-aches of various types and also due to false teeth—(1) Pulsation toothache due to inflamed dentine or sockets. Painful ulceration at the roots of the teeth and pain in hollow teeth. Gums are swollen (*Mercurius.*).

(2) Pain and swelling from wearing false teeth. (*Arnica.*).

(3) Tearing pains in carious teeth extending to molar bone of the affected side. (*Spig.*).

(4) Teeth sensitive to touch with swollen cheeks. Pains periodic. Worse by lying on affected side. These pains are boring and stabbing and sometimes become very severe. Drs. Hughes and Hale think that no remedy can be compared to *Plantago major*.

(5) Abscesses about the roots of the teeth and dental fistula. Worse when cold air gets into the mouth (*Silicea.*) See "Fistula at the root of teeth".

(6) Gums unhealthy and tendency to decay of the teeth. They turn black and crumble in children. (*Staphy.*). See "Gums".

(7) When due to cold. (*Acon.*).

(8) Throbbing shooting pain extending to the head. (*Bell.*).

(9) When the pain is intolerable and maddening to head. (*Cham.*).

(10) When the pain extends to the ears and neck, when the teeth loose, when the gums and face are swollen, when pain increased by cold and contact and extends to the bones or several teeth at the same time. (*Merc.*).

(11) When the pain is of intermittent type and of a burning character worse at night, increases at night. (*Ars.*).

(12) When pain is on one side only affecting several teeth. (*Puls.*).

(13) When due to severe pain the patient is tossing about in anguish and the pain makes him frantic and if pain is temporarily relieved by holding cold water in mouth then *Coffea* will remove such a pain.

(14) In a hollow tooth which is paining put a swab steeped in *Tr. Aconite* and give a dose of it internally and it will remove the pain.

(15) Toothache with swelling about jaws. Abscess of gum magical relief can be had from *Hecla lava*.

(16) Toothache worse at night. (*Aranea-d.*).

(17) When teeth are decayed with spongy, bleeding gums. (*Kreos.*).

(18) *Magnesia Carbonica* is specially useful in toothache of pregnancy and Dr. Levitt mentions *Sepia* as almost specific in this condition. See "Jaw swelling" and "No. 7 of bites".

Teethache rheumatic—See "Rheumatic tooth ache".

Teeth-bleeding after extraction and nervousness—(1) Bleeding after extraction for hours, blood is very red and fluid. (*Phos.*). Also wash mouth repeatidly with cold water in which a few drops of *Tr. Hamemelis* have been added.

(2) Pain and nervousness after extraction of teeth. (*Staphy.*).

(3) Dr. Holcombe recommends *Hecla lava 30* dilution for neuralgic pain remaining after extraction.

(4) Extraction of tooth causing swelling of gum. (*Pencillin 200*). See "Pyorrhoea alveolaris" under its different heads and "Wounds bleeding extracted teeth", and See "Teeth extraction-fragnments of bone and splinter left".

Teeth decaying in children—Decay of teeth specially in children. Teeth begin to decay at roots, crowns remain sound ; rumble, turn yellow. Gums retract. (*Thuj.*). See "Decay of teeth in children".

Teeth extracted causing offensive discharge—Extracted teeth had dead bone under it, offensive discharge from the gum of lower jaw. (*Silica* and *Phos.*), give in alternate doses will throw out the bone itself. Dr. G.M. Deshpande recommends *Ledum* will expel such pieces easily.

Teeth-decayed pain—See "Chapter V" for details .

Teeth-gnashing by a child—The child gnashes his teeth and tries to bite or strike. Signs are sometimes as violent as in *Stramonium* but the congestion of the face and eyes is the main distinguishing feature. (*Bell.*). See "Sleep-child and gnashing teeth".

T

Teeth-grinding by child—Grinding of teeth by child while asleep. The child bores fingers in the nose. Jumps and jerks during sleep. Restless at night. (*Cina.*). See also "Grinding of teeth".

Teeth-grinding hysterical—Grinding of teeth at night in hysteria. (*Asaf.*). See "Hysteria and Hysterical" under different headings.

Teeth-gums swollen—Gums and teeth swollen ; offensive breath ; flabby tongue, tongue with imprints of teeth on the sides. Secretion of too much salvia. (*Merc-sol.*). See "Gums".

Teething-children distress—Distress of teething children. Green stool, foul odour and colicky pain. Abdomen bloated ; stool green watery corroding the anus, like stirred egg ; stool feels hot and smells like a rotten egg. Consoled when carried about. (*Cham.*). See "Dentition diarrhcea" under different heads.

Teething children-spasms—(1) Ailments of teething children. Spasm during dentition. No fever. (*Mag-p.*). See "Dentition difficulty".

(2) The child drowsy, has a pale face and brain symptoms occur during dentition. (*Zincum.*).

(3) *Acon.* and *Bell.* for fever ; swollen gums ; *Cham.* for diarrhoea. See "Convulsions child grinding teeth".

Teething trouble-its prevention—See "Chapter V" for details .

Teething troubles incidental to dentition—(1) Teeth develop slowly. rapid decay of teeth. Troubles incidental to dentition. Sweating on head. Remedies the whole constitutional defect. (*Cal-p.*). Compare *Cham.* which is good for acute trouble of this period.

(2) Dentition is very painful and difficult, child tosses all night, constipation or undigested diarrhoea, teeth when erupted show marks of decay, teeth become yellow end then decay. (*Kreos.*). See "Dentition-difficulty" under its different heads.

Tendency-to catch cold and aborting its attack—Every time the patient goes out in fresh and cold air, he gets cold he sneezes and nose runs. Extremely sensitive to cold air, wants to close all the doors and windows. Cough and cold aggravated when exposed to least cold air. The cough is loose and rattles but no mucus comes out though it appears as if lot would come up. Nose stopped. Suffocating cough of a child. (*Hep.*). (b) *Amon carb.* will often abort a recent cold while *Nux-v.* 3, may prevent a cold if given early before running of nose. See "Sneezing susceptible to cold", "Cold drought sensitive".

Tendency-to Quinsy—To eradicate the tendency to quinsy : (*Psorinum.*).

Tendons and muscles-their weakness with pain—*Rhus-t.* follows Arn. well in removing the pain and weakness of tendons and muscles. When weakness persists then use *Calc-c.* See "Weakness of the tendons and muscles with pain".

Tenesmus of rectum and bladder in dysentery—In dysentery the tenesmus or urging of the bladder and rectum at the same time and urine passing drops with much pain along with the stool. *i.e.* the tenesmus of the rectum must extend to bladder area also in order that *Merc-c.* may act or *vice versa i.e.* along with the symptoms of the bladder the constant urging for urination there shonld be urging to stool in dysentery. (*Merc-c.*). See "Dysentery with tenesmus".

Tennis-elbo—*Ruta-g.* See "Wrist, its affections".

Testes-atrophic and enlarged—Atrophy of testicles in boys. The testes and ovaries are involved and undergo a state of hardness. infiltration. *Aurum-met.* cures chronic enlargement of the testes. (*Aurum-met.*). See "Hydrocele" and "Glands-chronic enlarged".

Testicles-and its different troubles—Atrophy, infammation and enlargement. (1) If there is fever and restlessness. (*Acon.* 1 hourly.).

(2) Due to gonorrhoea. (*Clematis erecta.*)

(3) Syphilitic. (*Merc-bin.* 4 hourly.).

(4) When due to a blow or other injury with pain and red swelling. (*Arn.*). See "Hydrocele indurated testes."

(5) When born with hydrocele. (*Bry.*).

(6) Stony hardness of testicles with burning and cutting pains. (*Conium.*).

(7) Chronic enlargement with pain in cord and testicles: (*Aur met.* 30. 4 hourly).

(8) When syphilis is the cause then Dr. Baehr recommends *Nit-ac.*

(9) When arising from metastasis of mumps then *Rhus-t. Bell.* and *Bry.*

(10) *Clematis-e.* will also be useful if the testicle is drawn up spasmodically with aching pains.

(11) Induration of : *Agn.*

(12) Inflammation of : *Cham.*

(13) Retraction of : *Oleum animale.*

(14) Undeveloped. *Aurum-met.*

(15) Swelling of : *Agn. Calc-p., 'Variol.*

(16) Undescended testicle. *Aurum-met* Compare *Aur. mur. nat.* and *Aur. mur.* which are also very useful for this trouble. (*Aur-met.* 200-10 H.S.) See "Orchitis Hydrocele indurated teses".

Tetanus—In Homoeopathy *Hypericum* works like anti -tetanus Serum. See "Specific for Tetanus".

Tetanus and lock Jaw—*Ledum* is the preventive of tetanus whereas *Hypericum* is the remedy for tetanus after the initial symptoms have started. But if wound is not a punctured wound but it is a lacerated wound involving parts full of small nerves, sentient nerves, give *Hypericum* at once and do not start with *Ledum.* Do not waste your time with *Arnica* either. Hence the golden rule is in a punctured wound give *Ledum.* and in a lacerated wound in a nerve-rich area give *Hypericum* both for preventive as well as for cure of tetanic or inflammatory consequences. (b) Tetanic convulsions, distortion of eyes and face with dyspnoea. *Nux-vomica* is the leading remedy. (c) *Passiflora-inc*. is specific for tatanus 10 drops doses of M.T.

(2) Tetanus of infants. Stiffness of jaws. (*Bell.*).

(3) In persistent tonic spasms specially of the muscles of face jaws and back, embarrassed respiration with frothing of mouth. Drs. Hempel and Hughes cured several cases with *Hydrocyanic acid* and strongly recommend this remedy.

(4) Convulsions sudden, rigidity with perspiration, oppressed breathing. In suppurating wounds or when the discharge of pus stopped. (*Cicuta-virosa*). See also "Convulsions" under their different heads.

(5) According to Dr. Phares the best remedy in the world for tetanus is *Viburnum-prunifolium.*

(6) Lock-jaw in tetanus : side to side movement of jaw. *Gels.* every hour. It relaxes muscular system. Dress the umbilical cord with *Calendula lotion.*

Tetanus due to-ill-effects of injection of virus—*Ledum pal.* 200.

Tetanus-injury—After injury to avoid risk of tetanus give *Ledum. 200* continuously for 3 days.

Tetanus-pain—See "Chapter V" for details :

Tetanus-preventive and curative—*Ledum* ; curative, *Hyper.*

Tetanus-preventing its after affects—*Mag-phos.* acts quickly in preventing the after effects of tetanus.

Tetanus threatening—When tetanus is threatening with coldness of parts give *Ledum 200* daily for 3 days.

Thinking-including student not minding his studies—(1) Thinking of past troubles. *Nit-ac.*

(2) Inability to think or fix attention. An excellent remedy for students who have no mind to study. (*Aeth-c.*). See "Broodings", "Melancholia" and "Memory-slow in learning".

Thirst-absence in fever with cold feet—No thirst in high feverish state with feet icy cold. Delirious condition. Very often face red. (*Bell.*). See "Fever-without thirst and bad taste".

Thirst-cold water vomited when warmed and patient taking warm things—Thirst for large quantities of water which must be ice cold. Cravings for cold, cold iced drinks or ice-creams. Cold water is tolerated but as soon as it gets warm in the stomach it is vomited. *Phos.* patient cannot touch anything warm whether it is drink or food. (*Phos.*) See "Vomiting with thirst for cold water and bleeding tendency".

Thirst-complete absence—Complete absence of thirst. (*Aeth.*). See "Fever-without thirst and bad taste" and "Dyspepsia with taste with bad rich food".

Thirst-drinking largely or sipping—For large quantity of water. A thirst of *Rhus-t.* patient wants to drinks quite a good quantity of water at a time whereas *Arsenic* patient sips only little water at a time but very often.

Thirst-dry mouth—There is dryness of mouth but no thirst. Thirstlessness and feeling of heat and aggravation by warmth : (*Puls.*). See "Mouth parched"

Thirst-eyes and nose running with parched mouth—For large quantities at longer intervals, dryness of mucous membrane. Mouth and lips parched. Aggravated from motion. (*Bry.*). See "Nose watering with irritation in eyes".

Thirst-in chill—*Ignatia* has the thirst during the chilly fever and at no other stage.

Thirst-intense for small quantity of water—(1) Intense thirst. Drinks often and in little quantities preferably warm drinks. *Ars-alb.*

(2) Violent thirst but immediately vomited *Dulc. 2* hourly.

Thirst-intense with mouth offensive—Intense thirst though the tongue and mouth are moist. Tongue is flabby and swollen with imprints of teeth all around it. The whole mouth is offensive in look and odour. *Merc-sol.*

(2) Must drink large quantities of water during fever. *Bry*. See "Mouth offensive odour and swollen gums".

Thirst-large quantities of water—Thirst for large quantities of water during fever and restlessness. (*Acon*). See "Fever with thirst".

Thirst-light in acute fever—When there is light thirst in acute feverish condition along with tremblings from weakness of nervous system then *Gels*. It is most probably the remedy.

Thirst-unquenchable—Unquenchable thirst during chill. (*Nat-m. 2* hourly).

Thirst-water disagrees—*Apocynum* has thirst and wants cold drinks but water disagrees. Though he desires cold drinks it causes distress in stomach. He is better with hot drinks but still he wants cold drinks. He drinks and vomits. (*Apoc-can.*) Compare *Apis* for dropsical symptoms, which is hot while *Apoc*. is chilly. Compare *Phos*. for cold drinks. See "Vomiting in dropsy and hysterical vomiting".

Throat-complications after diphtheria—Throat purple, swollen, ulcerated accompained by great exhaustion, with enlarged tonsils and glands when patient is getting along very nicely but dies of heart failure, in great many cases if *Ammonium-carb*. were given in time it would save life. (*Am-c.*). See "Diphtheria-when patient progressing".

Throat hysterical lump—Lump in the throat of suffocation is a sort of hysterical spasms of oesophagus. (*Asaf.*) See "Hysteria-fainting and also for "Cerebro spinal meningitis"

Throat-infection with running nose—Acute infection of throat with irritating eyes and running nose. (*Euphr.*) See "Nose watering with irritation in eyes" and also "Coryza-with irritating eyes".

Throat-inflammation spreading and glands swollen—Inflammation of throat ; inflammation is intense and spreads all over the cavity of the mouth including whole of throat, uvula and the gums which become spongy ; all glands about throat swollen with sharp pains to ears. (*Merc-c.*). See also "Syphilitic complications nose, throat and palate" and "Sore throat with raw mouth and swelling glands".

Throat-paralytic and swallowing difficult—If after sore-throat and specially after diphtheria inflammatory conditions of the throat is followed by paralytic weakness of the throat muscle, making it impossible to swallow liquids or food and when food is forced into the nose instead of oesophagus. *Arum-t.* is particularly indicated. (*Arum-t.*) See also "Paralytic weakness of throat muscle after diphtheria".

Throat-septic—Raw, smarting, excoriating sensation. *Hydras.* use as a gargle in a septic state of the throat with fever arrests destructive process at once, according to Dr. Hill.

Throat-sore with pain and fever—(1) *Bell.* must have high fever, intense redness of throat.

(2) *Merc-sol.* Moist, thick and indented tongue. Moderate fever and good amount of sweating without relief.

(3) *Lach.* Tonsillitis starts in the left side and may go over to the right. Very sensitive to touch and aggravation of symptoms after sleep.

(4) *Lyco.* Tonsillitis starts in the right side and may extend to the left, with stuffing of the nose.

(5) *Lac-c.* (Dog's milk). If in any case the pain in the tonsils starts on one side goes back to the other side and again goes back to the original side *i.e.* alternately one day worse on one side and next day worse on the other.

(6) *Hepar.* There is much throbbing pain as if pus is going to form. The patient is sensitive to cold. There is pain like splinter sticking into throat. Think of *Hepar.* See "Sore throat with pain in mouth", "Tonsils" and "Fever with throat trouble"

Throat-ulcerated during menses with leucorrhoea—A small lump will come and then enlarge until it reaches the tonsil and then ulcers will come and fill both sides. The roof becomes very red and there is dryness and choking. Dry choking compels coughing and difficult swallowing. The sore-throat usually comes before menses. It commences on one side and goes over the other ; swelling outside the neck with the ulceration in the throat. The ulcers do not disappear until after the flow eases and then also it subsides slowly. White leucorrhoea ; discharge before menses. *Mag-carb*. See also "Menstruation" under its different heads.

Thrombosis (a blood clot in the heart) including hemiplegia and cardiac asthma—(1) Bothrops lanceolatus (yellow-viper). It is a head remedy for thrombosis. It is also useful in thrombotic pneumonia (manifestion of an unusual character) as hemiplegia (paralysis of one side of body) slowing of heart and inability to articulate.

(2) *Lach*. for thrombosis with high blood pressure.

(3) *Sumbul* is said to be very useful in thrombosis. Also useful in cardiac asthma. Pain sharp and stitching in the left chest and shooting into the arm and neck frequent attacks of palpitation, breathlessness ; must lie on right side with head high. (*Spigelia anthelmia*.) to be given in 1M potency. See also "Heart" under its different heads.

Tibia-pain—The inner and larger bone of leg. Breaking pain in tibia. (*Agar*.). See "Periostitis" and "Pain in shin bones".

Ticklishness—To affect with light touch on uncomfortable feeling producing laughter (*Solanium*.).

Timidity i.e. wanting courage and inclined to fear and faint hearted—*Ammonium-causticum, Datura-arborea*.

Timings of occurring chill—Chill often takes place in some of fevers. Chill in malaria fever is an indicator of the particular medicine when it occurs in particular time :—

1 P.M.—*Ferr-phos*.
2 P.M.—*Cal-carb., Lachesis*.
3 P.M.—*Apis Chin-s*.
3—4 P.M.—*Lyco., Thuja*.
4—8 P.M.—*Lyco*.

5 P.M.—*China.*
Forenoon—*N.V., China*
Seventh day—*China.*
Midday—*Gels.*
Midnight—*Ars., Nux-v.*
1—2 A.M.—*Ars.*
3 A.M.—*Thuja.*
4 A.M.—*Ferrum-met.*
5 A.M.—*China.*
6—7 A.M.—*Podophyllum.*
7—9 A.M.—*Eup. perf.*
9—11 A.M.—*Nat-m.*
11 A.M.—11 P.M.—*Cactus.*
Periodic—*Arnica, Cedron, China-s., Ipecac.*
Every spring—*Lachesis* (Dr. Yudhvir Singh)

Thunder-storm—One affected by thunder-storm should take *Bry.* during storm and later *Silicea.* See "Fear of loneliness and thunder storm".

Tobacco-craving—*Daphne-indica.* See "No. 2 of cravings".

Tobacco-habit and how to get over it—*Nux-v.* 3-4 hourly. When craving comes a *Camphor pilule* should be chewed. See "Opium-ill effects and of tobacco causing tobacco heart".

Tobacco-heart—Tobacco heart from chewing tobacco. (*Verat.*). See "No. 13 of Heart".

Tobacco-heavy smokers—Necotin poisoning causing damage to heart, lungs and blood vessels. (*Tabacum.*).

Tongue-biting—Biting of tongue in sleep. (*Phos-a.*).
The tongue in normal health is light red, moist and clean.

Tongue-its effections :—

(*i*) Biting of : *Sec., Thuja.*
(*ii*) Blistered : *Nat-m.*
(*iii*) Blue : *Gymnocladus-canandensis.*
(*iv*) Burning in : *Podo., Sanic.*
(*v*) Cramp in : *Lyco., Ruta.*
(*vi*) Coated white : *Nat-m.*

(*vii*) Cramp in : *Piper-nigrum*.

(*viii*) Heavy : *Nat-m., Piper-nigrum*.

(*ix*) Inflammation : *Canth., Crot-h.*

(*x*) Nodules on : *Aur-met.*

(*xi*) Numbness of : *Lithium muriaticum*.

(*xii*) Oedema of : *Apis.*

(*xiii*) Parched : *Olnd.*

(*xiv*) Peeling of : *Ranunculus-scleratus*.

(*xv*) Ring worm of : *Sanic.*

(*xvi*) Sensibility of lost : *Colch*.

(*xvii*) Stiffness of : *Chimaphila maculata, Niccolum,* including *N. metallicum* and *N-carbonicum.*

Tongue-cancer and hard nodules—(1) Ulcer of tongue with indurated edges. Power of speech lost but intelligence in tact. (*Kali-cyanatum*).

(2) Stony hard nodules. (*Aurum-met*).

Tongue-coated—*Ip.* has a clean tongue or a tongue with a slight coating with vomiting or nausea, whereas *Puls.* has a heavily coated tongue. See "Fever malaria with nausea".

Tongue-cyst (a tumour beneath tongue)—Ranula under the tongue. A retention-cyst of the tongue in front, *Thuja., Merc-sol.* may be given in alternation ; with *Thuj.* tumour is hard and large in size. See also "Ranula".

Tongue inflamed—See "Glossitis"

Tongue maped and cracked—(1) The tongue is mapped with red islands. (*Nat-m.*).

(2) Cracked, painful, bleeding. (*Art-t.*).

(3) Cracked in centre. (*Rhus-v.*).

Tongue-pappilla (conic eminence) bleeding and cracked—The tongue is red, the papilla elevated, it is raw and bleeding. Tongue cracked, bleeding, burning and painful. Putrid odour from the mouth. Excessive flow of saliva which is acrid. (*Arum.*). See "Mouth stomatitis".

Tongue paralysis including paralysis of bladder and fundus—(1) The head remedy is *Caust*. Another important remedy is *Plumbum*. which should not be forgotten if other remedies fail to act. See also "Paralysis-tongue".

(2) Another excellent medicine for paralysis of tongue when the tongue feels heavy, difficult to move is *Guaco*.

(3) *Gels*. is useful in paralysis of the tongue of any localised paresis (slight paralysis) or may be observed in connection with bladder in retaining the urine as well as in paralysis of the fundus (the base of the organ so that it cannot be evacuated). Again there may be a paresis when the flow is intermittent. See "Paralysis-tongue and face".

Tongue-swollen with offensive mouth—Tongue is flabby and swollen with imprints of teeth all around it. The whole mouth is offensive in look and odour. Gums and teeth swollen. This condition may happen in acute fever or any inflammation of any organ specially the glands or the intestines. Intense thirst though the tongue and mouth are moist. (*Merc-sol*.). See also "Mouth offensive odour and swollen gums" and "Fever with throat trouble".

Tongue-swollen with triangular tip—(1) *Rhus-t* tongue has a triangular tip with the rest of the tongue coated.

(2) Tongue swollen, sore. (*Oxal acid*).

Tongue-ulcer and also due to syphilis- Ulcers under the tongue, *Lyco*. due to syphilis. *Mercurius*. See "Ulcers in mouth".

Tongue-white with coating and blisters White coated tongue with red tip and border. Bright red colour of lips (*Sulf*.).

(2) Blisters with burning. (*Nat-m*.). See "Blisters in mouth".

Tonic for different troubles (1) Nervous headache and fatigue. Numbness of the limbs as if paralysed. (*Avena-s* M.T. 10 to 15 drops in half a wine glass of water).

(2) Enfeebled patients after chronic diseases. The remedy acts as a tonic increasing appetite, exerts an action on the

organs of nutrition and assimilation and stimulates excretory organs. (*Gentianalutea.*).

(3) Dr. Baker suggests a mixture of dilution of (*Hydrochloricum acid, Alfalfa Q.* and *Ignatia* an another tonic and appetiser. See "Appetiser".

Tonsillitis-hearing affected—Chronic tonsillitis when accompanied by hardness of hearing. (*Hep-s.*). See "No. 12 of deafness".

Tonsils-with inflammation of middle ear—(1) Soft palate and parotid. (parotid gland situated near ear.) (*Bapt.*).

(2) *Baryta-carb.* not only prevents tonsillitis but also the inflammation of middle ear which frequently results from it. It is the biggest tonsil medicine. But if tonsils are enlarged from vaccination then give *Thuja.* If due to tuberculosis then give *Bacill* and then *Baryta-carb.* See "Ear inflammation *i.e.* otitis".

Tonsils-red with throbbing pain—Enlarged and red. Redness and throbbing, *Bell.* is the first remedy if redness and throbbing pain presents and it cures suddenly. A sense of constriction as if throat narrowing. Burning and dryness. (*Bell.*). See also "Sore throat-redness and throbbing pain".

Tonsils-suppurating—Suppurating tonsils from every cold. Tonsils inflamed, with swollen veins. (*Baryta-carb.*).

Tonsils and adenoids-surgically removed—*Bromium 3x* is an excellent remedy for the sequelae of surgical removal of tonsils and adenoids. (Dr. Sukeskar). See "Adenoid growths" breathing with open mouth.

Tonsils due to silver nitrate—Where Silver-nitrate has often been used. (*Nat-m.*).

Tonsils-to be prevented from surgery—(1) Chronically enlarged, neck glands : rawness in the throat, with shooting pain on attempting to swallow. Chronic enlargement of the surgical glands—bad taste. Patient chilly with eruption around the ear, with accumulation of mucus in the nose and throat. *Baryta-carbonica* will clear it up and considerably reduce the tonsils in size and thereby minimizing the chances of the operation, See "Sore-throat with pain in mouth and fever".

(2) Red throat with swollen or oedematous uvula. Pain on putting out his tongue and this pain-shoots up to the ear. The mouth is offensive and the tongue raw and has a yellow coating. The throat has got infection accompanied by pains in bones and joints and also acute backache. *Phytolacca* clears the throat completely and it looks normal and the inflammation does not recur. (Dr. M.G. Blackie).

Tonsillitis-with cold, cough with hydrocele—(1) Child with high fever, loss of weight, restless during sleep, snoring and grinding of teeth in sleep. Right sided hydrocele also. History of T.B. in family. (One dose of *Thuja 200* and later on *Thuja 1M, 10M*, at intervals. Ultimately *Bacillinum* in successive potencies of 200, 1M and 10M, with excellent result according to Dr. Wadia).

(2) Sore throats with frequent tonsillitis and enlarged tonsils. (*Tuber.*).

Tonsils-gargle—*Tr. Sulph. Acidum.* may be used in the strength of one to six in a little warm water as a gargle. It may as will be used as a spray for tonsils.

Tonsillitis-its prevention—See "Chapter V for details".

Tonsillitis-fever with offensive mouth and inflammation of intestines—Secretion of too much saliva ; spongy and swollen gums. The whole mouth is offensive in look and odour. Saliva fetid. Sore raw and burning throat. Putrid sore throat. Aggravation at night. No relief after perspiration. Fever with creeping chilliness and bronchitis. This condition may happen in acute fever or any inflammation of any organ specially in the glands of the intestines. Intense thirst though the tongue and mouth are moist (*Merc-sol.*). See "Quinsy" and "Fever with throat trouble".

Tonsillitis with swelling left-sided causing paralysis of vocal cord—Left sided pain usually running to the ears. Swelling and pain. The colour of the throat is bluish red and not purple. Throat and neck sensitive to touch. Bad odour. Aggravation of symptoms after sleep. Paralysis of vocal cords. causing loss of voice, larynx sensitive to least touch, it causes suffocation when the child gets worse in sleep. (*Lach*). See "Sore throat left sided".

Tonsillitis-recurring—See "Sore-throat recurring".

Tonsillitis with swelling-right sided causing suppuration—Right-sided. Swelling and suppuration of tonsils. Ulceration of tonsils. Better warm drinks. Swelling may go over to the left. (*Lyco.*) Compare *Lach*. See "Swelling on right side".

Tonsils-septic—*Pyrogen 200* or *Kali Phos. 6* respectively.

Tonsillitis-sore throat with pain—Throbbing pain as if pus is going to form. Pain in the throat as if a splinter or stick sticking in the throat. The patient is sensitive to cold (*Hep.*). Compare *Bell, Merc-sol., Lach., Lyco.*, and *Lac-caninum* for sore throat. See also "Sore-throat with pain in mouth and fever".

Tonsillitis-swelling spreading to glands and mouth cavity—Inflammation of throat ; inflammation is intense and spreads all over the cavity of the mouth including whole of throat, uvula and the gums which become spongy, All glands about throat swollen with sharper pains to ears. (*Merc-c.*). See "Swelling with inflamed glands".

Tonsillitis-ulcerated and swollen glands gangrenous—In throat there is an appearance like that of diphtheria. Purple, swollen, ulcerated and bleeding and gangrenous accompanied by great exhaustion with enlarged tonsils and glands. The glands outside the throat and neck are enlarged and felt as lumps. (*Am-c.*). See "Diphtheria-swollen", Fever glandular due to swollen enlarged tonsils", and "Sore throat with raw mouth and swollen glands".

Tooth-ache during pregnancy—(1) The best remedy for it is *Sepia*-globules dry on tongue.

(2) If the pain proceeds from a single carious tooth. (*Cham.*).

(3) If the pain is violent and patient cries with pain. (*Coff.*).

(4) If the whole side of jaw is affected and the pain shifts. (*Puls.*).

(5) If the pain proceeds from decayed tooth to facial bone. (*Nux-v.*).

See "Pregnancy-its affections" and "No. 19 of Teethaches".

Tooth-ache-with changing temperature and bleeding—The tooth-ache violently from every change of weather or from change of temperature in the mouth. Gums settle away from the tooth and bleed. The jaws-ache or the roots of the teeth-ache. The teeth become loose, a general scurvy condition (*Am-c.*). See "Teeth-ache of various types also due to false teeth".

Tooth-ache-relief by cold water—(1) Relieved by holding cold water in the mouth ; worse from warm things and heat. (*Puls.*).

(2) *Hyoscyamus* and *Mercurius* are frequenty indicated in most of such troubles. See "Teeth-aches of various types also due to false teeth".

Tooth-ache with swelling, of glands, shifting and swelling of face—(1) At night ; rapidly shifting. Better by heat and hot drinks and worse by eating and drinking cold things. Ulceration of teeth with swelling of glands of face, throat and neck. (*Mag-p.*).

(2) *Kreosotum* cures a large number of tooth-ache cases, 1 hourly.

(3) Externally in all cases of tooth-ache apply *Plantago.* M.T. See "Teeth aches of various types also due to false teeth" and "Gum pain".

Tooth-ache-external application—Apply with a swab M.T. of *Plantago* which will relieve pain quickly.

T

Tooth-ache-warm water increases pain—(1) If warm water increases pain for adults. (*Cham.*).

(2) *Plantago* major be given every 10 minutes and applied in tincture for immediate relief. See "Teeth-aches of various types also due to false teeth".

Toxemia-intestinal of children—Chronic intestinal toxemias of children with fetid stools, eructations. (*Bapt.*). See "Fever of children with foul smelling stool".

Toxin-elimination—*Veratrine* relaxes vascular (pertaining to blood vessels), tension and stimulates the elimination of toxin by skin, kidneys and liver.

Tracheoma-wind pipe—Raw feeling along the trachea and in the chest. (*Arum-t.*).

Tracheoma—*Chimaphila-maculata, Cuprum-sulphuricum* and *Mercurialis-perennis* according to symptoms. See "Eyes" and "Vision".

Tranquiliser-for neuratic patients—On account of nervousness or neurosis patients approach a physician for various ailments for which they have been examined and found normal. But the patient still complains of chronic headache, a ball sansation in the abdomen, his inability to walk or to go to his office. The patient is most unhappy. His unhappiness due to various causes such as disappointed love, severe jolt in office, failure in the examination or in business. The greatest tranquiliser for him will be *Ignatia* to be followed by *Nat-mur.* which will make the patient normal.

Traumatic (pertaining to wounds) neuritis amputation and fever—(1) *All-c.* has a marvellous power on such affections often met with in a stump after amputation or serious injury. The pains are almost unbearable, rapidly exhausting the strength of the patient. .(*All-c.*). See also "Neuritis in stump".

(2) For fever produced by wounds including catheterism give *Acon.* 1 hourly. and when of typhoid character give *Ars.* and when hectic, give *China.* See "Catheter fever avoiding its pain".

Travellers-friend—Those who have to travel by train, by air, by buses and have to cover long distances for sufficient long time generally develop muscular soreness and railway spine. Statsis and swelling by constant sitting at one position. *Bellis*. perennis will give them a great relief.

Trembling of hands and feet—Cann't write ; cann't hold a glass of water, trembling of hand in paralysis. (*Lalium temulentum*). See "Paralysis-single muscle and hand".

Trembling with forgetfulness in old age—Trembling and tottering, feebleness of mind, forgetfulness, which is common in old age appear earlier ; weakness, coldness and numbness, usually of single parts, fingers, arms, etc. (*Ambra*). See "Old age" under its different heads and "Forgetfulness with absent mindedness and loss of memory", Senile decay due to degenerative changes" and "Numbness of nerves".

Trembling of lower extremities in paralysis—Trembling of hands and lower extremities on attempt to move. If he attempts to move hands tremble, if he attempts to walk then legs tremble. All these tremblings from the weakness of the nervous system specially in acute febrile cases should attract the notice to *Gels*. The eyelids droop in acute condition. The patient is drowsy. The pulse is weak. Complete relaxation of muscular system with apparent or real paralytic condition. (*Gels*.). See "Paralytic complete-motor paralysis including eye muscle" and "Eyelids drooping, swollen itching and ulcer along sides".

Trembling tongue—*Lach*. has trembling both in the acute disease like typhoid etc. and in chronic cases. Most important is the trembling of the tongue when protruded and it is difficult to protrude the tongue on account of trembling. (*Lach*.) Compare *Gels*. See "Paralysis-tongue and face with indistinct speech" and "Tongue paralysis".

Trismus-Tense spasm of the muscles of mastication—Lock jaw and paralysis of the tongue (*Linum*.).

Tuberculosis causing different troubles with galloping consumption and with indistinct speech—(1) *Phos*.

indicated in the incipient and later stages with the symptoms of cough, oppression and general weakness. To be given in a very high and in single dose and not repeated. If given too low and repeated it will fearfully aggravate. (*Phos.*).

(2) To subdue the hectic fever of the disease : (*Dig*).

(3) Dry racking coughs of consumption. (*Sticta.*).

(4) Dry teasing coughs at night, the expectoration has little specks of blood in it. (*Laur.*). See "Cough phthisic".

(5) For lessening cough, the expectoration, sweats and hectic fever. *Kali-hydroiodicum* and *Cannabis-sativa* to be given in alternation.

(6) The patient too weak to talk. Hetic fever ; chills at 10 A.M. profuse sweat at night, worse about 4 or 5 in the morning, hoarseness, expectoration yellowish, or yellowish, green sweetish mucus. (*Stann. met.*). See "Hectic fever" and "Night sweats".

(7) Large cavities in the lungs, profuse night sweats, hectic or suppurative fever. (*Silicea.*).

(8) Glands being large and nodular, stool frequent of varying colour with much flatus. (*Calc-i.*). See "Glands on neck tubercular".

(9) Suffocative hoarseness, cough that shakes the brain, offensive sputa ; sweat fetid, and breathlessness. For the last stage of tuberculosis of lungs. (*Carb-a.*). See "Cough-respiration oppressed".

(10) Diarrhoea in last stages of consumption. (*Saccharum lactis*). See "Diarrhoea in tuberculosis".

(11) When accompanied with haemoptysis, continuous hoarseness, dry cough, preventing the sleep at night. Breathlessness while ascending. (*Helix-tosta C.M*).

(12) Galloping consumption. Drs. Jousset and Hughes use *Cal-c.* in alternation with *Phos*, in galloping consumption. See "Consumption" under its different head.

(13) In threatening tuberculosis with acid dyspepsia and intolerance of milk *Cal-c.* is recommended for fat subjects and *Cal-p.* for thin subjects. Both these remedies follow *Tuberculinum* well and will cure the remnants of disease left by them.

(14) Diarrhoea in tuberculosis. *Phos-ac*. and *China-ars*. are the favourite remedies of Dr. Carter for this trouble. See "Diarrhoea-in tuberculosis".

(15) Thuberculosis haemoptysis spitting of blood Dr. F. Cartier recommends the following for abundant blood. *Germanium maculatum* (M.T.), *Acalypha* (M.T.). *Millifolium* M.T. and *Ferrum acet*. See "Haemoptysis-blood-spitting from lungs".

(16) Tubercular sweats. Dr. F. Cartier recommends *Acid-phos, Agaricin, Pilocarpine,* and *Sambucus*.

(17) Tuberculosis heart troubles. Dr. Jousset recommends *Cal-fl.* and Digitalis. See "Heart failure after infectious disease" See also "Phthisis" under its different heads. Tuberculosis of intestines. (*Phos*). (2) Great emaciation, abdomen enormously distended, stools frequent with flatus, nothing but skin and bone. (*Calc-i.*). (c) *Agar.* fattens up T.B. patients. (d) Tuberculosis pulmonary chronic and in the last stages dry or mucopurulent expectoration. High fever with chill and anorexia (*Baptisia*). See "Consumption palliative" and "Consumption pulmonary".

Tuberculosis-lack of digestive power—*Vanadium* acts as a tonic digestive functions and in early tuberculosis.

Tumours at different places—(1) Fatty tumour specially about the neck. (*Baryt-c.* 4 hourly).

(2) Tumour of the breast, nipple retracted. (*Hydr.*). See "Nipple-atrophy".

(3) Strong hard tumours on the breast. (*Conium.*). See "Breast-pain in menses" and "Mammary-abscess".

(4) Large uterine fibroid tumour covering the entire womb, frequently repeated haemorrhages as if the patient would bleed

to death, discharges horribly offensive. (*Lapis-albus.*). See "Uterine tumour or fibroid with consequential haemorrhage".

(5) Lumps and enlarged glands in breasts, milk coagulates and becomes stingy, bloody milk in nursing women. (*Phyt.*).

(6) For fibroid tumours with painful menses give *Fraxinus-ame.* 10 drops of mother tincture at bed time and *Veratrum alb. 30* dilution every morning (*Fraxinus Americana* and *Veratrum album*). See "Fibroma or fibroid" and "Uterine tumour or fibroid with consequential haemorrhage".

Tumour-in abdomen—Lump in liver region :—The following medicines may be tried according to symptoms :—

(1) *Conium 200.*

(2) *Kali-carbonicum 200.* First thing in the morning. Feeling of lump in the pit of stomach. It is also one of the best remedies following labour.

(3) *Thuja-1000* wart-like excrescenses, spongy tumours.

(4) *Calcarea-fluorica. 1 M.* Powerful remedy for hard stony glands.

(5) *Thuja. 30.* After it, *Graphites 1 M.* Every six day.

(6) *Tuberculinum. 1 M.* After three weeks *Graphites 1 M.* See "Abdomen-lump".

Tumour-brain—See "Brain tumour".

Tumour-in brain—It is rather a serious trouble which may cause the diminuation of vision, headache, vomiting and other trouble also. Under modern system of medicine generally the removal of such tumours is done by brain operation which is not without risks. R.B. Bishamber Das an old and eminent Homoeopath suggests the following treatment :

(1) Begin the treatment by administering a dose of *Tuberculinum 200,* which will arrest the disease and cure headache also. *Tuberculinum* is also useful in benign mammory tumour.

(2) Headache with vertigo on turning the head. Heaviness and painful pressure extending to the nose. Confusion as if

head were too full. Stitching pain in skull. Worse from cold and wet weather, icy coldness in and on the head. (*Calc-carb*).

(3) In case *Calc-carb.* fails then *Calc-fluor.* and *Calc-Phos.* may be tried in alternate doses.

(4) For arresting and absorbing bony brain tumour. (*Merc. Iod.*).

(5) Lightning like pains through the sides of head over the eyes and nose, worse from the back of pillow. Syphillic history. Lancinating pain in upper jaw. Profuse, acrid, hot, watery, thin discharge from nose. Much thirst, flatulence. Inflammatory conditions of the nose in young married women with leucorrhoea (*Kali-iod*).

(6) Slow developing tumours, activated by traumatism (The state of system induced by a severe wound). Throbbing in vertex (top of head). Pains in eyes and ears. (*Hypericum*).

Tumours-fatty on lips and breasts also—(1) Fatty tumours appearing here and there over the body. (*Bar-c*). (b) Hard tumour on lip. (*Conium*) ; soft tumour on lip. (*Staphy.*).

(2) Inflamed indurated masses in the female breast slowly developing. (*Plumb-iodat.*). See "Lips-tumour and swelling".

Tumour-in ovary—Ovarian tumours have disappeared under the action of Podo. See "Ovary-fibrous body".

Tumours-in ovary with neuralgia—*Lach.* is a good remedy for diseases of female generative organs. It is of use in simple ovarian neuralgia and from that to actual tumours even cancer of the left ovary and also in uterine displacements of various kinds. The pain in ovary travels from left to right (*Lach.*). See also "Ovarian-neuralgia" and "Ovary-fibrous body".

Tumours-recurrent including those surgically removed—Recurrent. The tumour removed twice by knife and it recurred every time. Big as hens' egg. The patient better by wrapping up the head. He lacked confidence in his ability. Timid in going into a new enterprise though able to perform the task if entrusted. (*Sil.*). See "Cicatrix" and "Styes recurring and their prophylactic".

Tumour-tongue—Tumour just at the root of tongue. The growth bluish and painful. Fast increasing in size of suspicious nature. Patient unable to chew food. (*Anthrac.* 200 in the morning and *Carb-a. 200* in the evening.). See "Jaw carious and Ranula under the tongue".

Tumours of urinary passage—*Analinum.*

Tumour of womb—Involving the whole body of the womb, horrible discharge and with intense burning : *Lapis alb.*

Tympanitis and dyspepsia in typhoid including digestion weak after typhoid—Tympanitic condition marked in typhoid ; low type of typhoid : trembling and jerking of muscles ; emaciation ; mental symptoms. (*Agar.*) See 'Tympanitis' No. 9 in "Fever typhoid"

(2) *Carbo-v.* the main remedy then *Lyco* ; *Asaf., 'Terebinth.* (b) Dyspepsia after typhoid :—Digestion weak after typhoid, flatulence, eructations give temporary relief. The simplest food disagrees specially fatty food. Excessive wind in the upper portion of abdomen pressing upwards in the chest and causing distress in the heart. Relieved by belching wind or passing flatus. (*Carb-v.*). Compare *Puls., Lyco* and *China*. See "Dyspepsia after typhoid".

Typhoid-of children—Fever of children. Child is half dozing and half confused, mouth ulcerated, at times foul smelling : loose motions with foul smelling stools : great prostration. The tongue is dry. Great typhoid remedy in its first stage. (*Bapt.*). See "Fever of children with foul smelling stool".

Typhoid-debility—For great debility after typhoid or other exhaustive disease *Sel.* has proved very efficacious. Strength failing the patient suddenly in hot weather. When the patient begins to walk and feels great general weakness in legs, weakness in spine a dose of *Selenium 200* animates and invigorates the patient speedily and to an extent that cannot be believed by a sceptic. (Prof. Dr. Bhanja.). See "Debility due to excess" and "Weak digestion after typhoid".

Typhoid-delirium with involuntary stool and urine—Delirium ; low muttering speech, involuntary stools and urine. Stupor. Restlessness ; picking at bed clothes and nose. (*Hyos*). See "Delirium in Typhoid".

Typhoid-diarrhoea with offensive stool and urine—*Arum-t.* has a diarrhoea which is associated with typhoid fever, it is like the yellow corn meal and musky. The faeces are also acrid and make the anus and adjoining parts raw and burning. The typhoid patient picking the nose and the lips until they bleed. The urine is scanty and sometimes suppressed. (*Arum-t*).

(2) Yellow, brown, cadaverous stool. (*Rhus-t.*).

(3) Offensive involuntary stool and urine, paralysis of bladder. (*Ars-a.*).

(4) Greenish mucous stool while emanating (*Nitr-ac.*). See "Diarrhoea in typhoid watery and acrid" and "Diarrhoea—in typhoid".

Typhoid-falling of hair—*Fluoric acid* is recommended by Dr. Boger for terrible falling of hair after Typhoid. See "Hair".

Typhoid fever—*Arsenic* is one of the best medicines for fever of typhoid character. It should not be given too early and should be given after *Rhus-t.* (*Ars-alb.*). See "Fever typhoid" under its different heads.

(2) According to Dr. Burnett *Pyrogenium 6* will rapidly cure nearly every case of typhoid. See "Fever typhoid".

Typhoid fever and its treatment—(1) The typhoid patient picking the nose and the lips until they bleed. Diarrhoea associated with typhoid stool like the yellow corn meal and musky. Urine scanty and sometimes suppressed. The faeces are also acrid and make the anus and adjoining parts raw and burning. (*Arum-t.*). See "Fever typhoid with delirium and diarrhoea".

(2) R.B. Bishamber Das begins the treatment by giving *Ars-alb. 3* drops doses every 2 hours *i.e. 6* doses daily If no improvement is seen then *Sulphur 200* to be given on empty

stomach and no other medicine that day. Starts again *Ars-alb.* 30 from the following day. If no improvement is seen during next 4 days then *Psorinum 200* on empty stomach next day and no other medicine that day and starts again with *Ars-alb.* from the following day. If this a'so fails during the next 4 days then *Tuberculinum* 200 or 1000 is given next morning on empty stomach. Waits for two days and then again start with *Ars.* The normal symptoms for *Ars.* are restlessness, thirst for small quantities of water at short intervals and prostration.

(3) When typhoid is accompanied with diarrhoea, with foul stools, stupor and prostration then *Baptisia* is indicated which cuts short the period if given in early stages.

(4) *Acid-muriatic* is indicated in haemorrhages from intestines. The eructations are constant with unconsciousness and extreme prostration. The jaw hangs down and the patient is on the very brink of grave.

(5) For sleeplessness in typhoid give *Absinthium.*

(6) Digestion weak after typhoid. See "Dyspepsia after typhoid" and "Digestion weak after typhoid".

Typhoid-haemorrhage intestinal—*Secale* in very bad cases when the patient is on the verge of death. *Mellitolium* ; *Ham.*, *China*, *Terebinth* and *Kreosote* are useful remedies according to symptoms. See also "Haemorrhage in typhoid" and "Haemorrhages in typhoid from bowels".

Typhoid-kidney function stopped—(1) Complete cessation of the function of kidney after typhoid. After urinating continues to ooze in drops, (*Zingiber.*). See "Uraemia".

Typhoid-with pneumonia—(1) With pneumonia, cough and bronchitis. Stupor and low muttering delirium. Thirst for large quantities of water which must be icy cold. Bleeding tendency. Arterial bleeding. Burning in palms. (*Phos.*).

(2) *Lachesis* is best remedy in such cases with lung complications. It is the most useful remedy in typhoid fever in 2nd and 3rd week.

(3) *Hyoscyamous* is a leading remedy in the typhoid form of pneumonia and has performed wonders. See "Pneumonia in typhoid" and "Fever typhoid with ear and lung complication".

Typhoid-relapse—*Ant-c.* is the best ; then comes *Ip.* See "Fever-typhoid relapse" and "Relapse of typhoid-fever". Typhoid vaccine in higher potency is a preventive remedy for typhoid.

—: o :—

U

Ulcers of different types—(1) Ulcers with sensitive edges and fetid discharges (*Asterias-rubens* 6 hourly),

(2) Pus has tendency to form an adherent scab under which more pus collects. (*Mez.*).

(3) Ulceration between toes. (*Sanic.*).

(4) Ulcers with violent scratching. (*Sulf.*) See "Itching causing burning".

(5) Skin readily ulcerates in rachitic children (*Staphy.*).

(6) Ulcers in folds of skin. (*Carbo-veg.*).

(7) Malignant gangrenous ulcers also for carbuncles, boils. (*Tarentula.*). See "Carbuncles".

(8) The ulcer is deep and secretes a thin and offensive discharge. *Mcrcurius* a dose night and morning. See "Discharge-offensive".

(9) For varicose ulcers and the condition of veins from which they arise. (*Ham.* every 12 hours.).

(10) Externally lotion and ointment of *Plantago* M.T. to be used in all cases. See "Varicose leg". (b) Ulcer bleeds easily, has burning sensation, is painful and its margins are hard. (*Ars-a.* 30). (2) Ulcer about joints of fingers. (*Bor.*). (3) The ulcer is deep and secretes a thin and offensive discharge. (*Merc.*). *Verat-v.* may be given as an intercurrent remedy in relieving the pricking and burning and generally subsiding the congestion. (4) Ulcer on heels from friction. (*All-c.*). (5) For irritable, painful, easily bleeding ulcers and the indolent callous and the appetite faulty. (*Hydr.*). Apply *Hydr.* also externally in double stregth. (6) Septum ulcerated. Tongue dry and feeling of hair on tongue. Ulceration of uvula and tonsils. Ulcers on previously inflamed feet. No tendency to heal. (*Kali-b.*). See "3oils" under different heads.

U

Ulcer-corneal with lacrhymation and pain in eyebrow—
(1) Corneal ulcers in new born infants. (*Arg-nit.*).

(2) Intense sensitiveness to light, much lachrymation. Little redness. (*Conium.*).

(3) Marked pain in the region of eyebrow at night ; granular lids ; pus pustules, of cornea (*Croton Tiglium*). See "Eye—troubles part (2)".

Ulcer-delayed healing—(a) Not healing quickly. Inflammation tendency to form pus. (*Sil.*). (b) *Galium* aparine favours healthy granulations on ulcerated surfaces. See "Wounds unhealthy no tendency to heal".

Ulcers-excoriating—Putrid flat ulcers with a pungent burning sensation. An ulcer excoriates the parts around it. (*Am-c*). See also "Boils-throbbing".

Ulceration-in lungs not healing—Of lungs, intestinal tract, and mammae ; prevents suppuration. Ulcers not healing quickly. (*Sili.*). See "Bleeding from lungs".

Ulcers-in mouth—(1) Mouth full of ulcers, very often with foul smell. The child is usually prostrated and drowsy. The tongue is dry. (*Bapt.*). See "Mouth—blisters near corner".

(2) *Merc-sol.* is the first and best remedy. If it does not help then a dose of *Sulph.* should be given. See also "Digestion mouth ulcerated", "Mouth-ulcerative" and "Blisters in mouth extremely painful".

Ulcers-local application—According to Dr. Boericke *Mag-sulf.* is used to a considerable extent-externally in saturated solution as an agent for reducing inflammation and also anti-pruritic cellulitis and other local inflammation and septic condition. Use compresses saturated with solution in 1x4. The 3rd potency of pure salt. See "Wound infested and inflamed with pricks".

Ulcers-multiple brown and dark coloured—Ulcers on leg. Brown crust on the ulcers, surrounded by very dark copper coloured skin. No syphilis. Drops what he holds in her hands if spoken to suddenly. Dry cough. Very nervous. Sensation of a closely fitted cap on head. (*Kali-sulf.*). See also "Skin—body red with ulcer" and "Boils in crops".

Ulcers-painful covered by scab—See "Sore painful covered by scab".

Ulcer-of stomach—Gastric ulcer is much more common in males. Usually gnawing or burning pain at a fixed time after food confined to a small spot at the pit of stomach with a corresponding pain at the back ; vomiting ; the vomited matter frequently contains blood coagulated by the ulceration of gastric juice. *Arsenic, Hydrastis, Baptisia, Mercurius-cor. Acid sulphuric, Phosphorus,* according to symptoms. Dr. Jahr says that *Phos.* afforded him the most essential aid for vomiting of food mixed with bile and blood. (b) (1) Ulceration of stomach, sour eructation, vomiting of all food taken, pain and distension of stomach. Loss of appetite. (*Acetic-acid*). (2) *Uranium-nitr.* is said to arrest the tendency of formation of ulcers. See "Gastric ulcer", "Duodenal ulcer" and "Peptic ulcer".

Ulcers-syphilitic and offensive—Deep flat ulcers from bone and periosteal affections give out a watery, bloody discharge which is offensive with a pain shooting outwards from the ulcers. These ulcers bleed and have a tendency to burrow. The ulcers are also very sensitive to touch. Of syphilitic origin. (*Asaf.*). Compare *Hepar* and *Nit-ac.* See "Syphilis" "Periostitis" and "Discharge offensive".

Unconsciousness due to injury and convulsions—(1) When alternating with delirium. (*Phos.*).

(2) In shock from injury (*Arn-mont*).

(3) Unconscious during convulsions. (*Cic-virosa.*). See "Fainting" under its different heads and "Coma".

Under-development in children—*Calc.* has under development of body tissues with enlargement of lymphatic glands in the neck. (*Calc.*). See "Delayed—mental development" and "Children late in learning to talking and walking".

U

Union of bones—*Calc-p.* is an excellent remedy when broken bones do not unite quickly. (*Calc-p.*). See "Fracture" under its different heads and "Bones-fracture and its non union".

Unsocial—Low spirited, disheartened, depressed, unsocial, almost imbecile. (*Anac.*). See "Company-aversion".

Unwanted hair—Sometimes the hair grow on the face and lips of women due to overactivity of some glands. According to Dr. Yudhvir Singh *Thuja, Lyco, Nat-mur, Phos* and *Thyrodinum* may be tried according to symptoms of the patient.

Uraemia (the retention in the blood of urinary constituents due to failure of kidneys to excrete them also including surgical operation—(1) Headache, vertigo, and coma. (*Cupr-ars.*).

(2) Slow and difficult urination. Uraemia acute and chronic. (*Morph.*).

(3) Acute form of uraemia with diarrhoea. The patient may be suffering from diabetes in which case urine becomes scanty, darkened. (*Cupr-ars.*).

(4) For suppressed urine in cholera. (*Verat-a.*).

(5) With unconsciousness, pupils dilated, convulsion strong urinous odour from body. (*Hellebours.*).

(6) Uraemic symptoms following operations on the genito-urinary organs. (*Cupr-ars.*).

(7) Uraemic convulsions *Hydrocyanicum acidum,* (Pilocarpinium.). See also "Inflammation of kidney", "Diabetic Coma" and "Kidney-affection".

Unrefreshing sleep—Unrefreshing sleep, wakes tired, and fed-up in the morning. Sleepy in the evening, lies awake towards the end of the night and mostly sleeps again in the morning hours. He sleeps as soon as he takes a book in hand. He is sleeply after eating early in the evening (*Nux-vomica.*). See "Sleeplessness" under its different heads "Sleep-unrefreshing and child awakes at night playing" and "Sleep-cat-nap types".

Urethra-bleeding from urethra—The blood is fresh and red. (*Phos.*). Compare *Hamamelis* where blood is blakish and thick. See "Bleeding under its different heads".

Urethra-itching—Smarting, itching in urethra. Sour smelling urine which is copious with burning (*Ambra.*). See "Itching female organ" and "Pruritus with burning urine" and "No. 7 of Itching in different parts of body".

Urethra-stretching for stone—When the urethra has been stretched for removing stone or by use of bougies and catheter, dilation of cervix has been done. *Staphy.* will remove the subsequent difficulties. These stretches after surgical operation may cause great distress with painfulness and symptoms of collapse causing cold sweat etc. These are also removable by *Staphy.* See "Stretches and remover of catheter pain".

Urethritis with swelling and split urine—In psychotic patients which, *Cannabis-sat.* does not relieve ; urine stream split, cutting after urination ; discharge thick ; urethra swollen and inflamed. (*Thuj.*). See "Gonorrhea-swollen prepuce".

Urging to stool—(1) Urging to stool but only little of flatus follow relieving the urging only for sometimes. There may be absolute constipation with the stool but the urging with flatus continues throughout the day in a chronic patient. ***Nat-sulf.*** helps here also.

(2) Lumpy stool mixed with water, very often jelly like mucus with the stool and sometimes without it. May expel good quantity of thick jelly like mucus before the stool (*Aloe.*) See "Constipation-no urging".

Urine-albuminous and other casts—(1) Albuminous *Apis-mel.* is head remedy for albumin in urine. During pregnancy also.

(2) Urine scanty with albumin and swelling. (*Hell*).

(3) Albumin in urine during or after typhoid. (*Acid Phos.*).

(4) Alkaline. In typhus. (*Baptisia.*). In catarrh of bladder (*Cantharis*).

(5) Urine black in inflammation of kidneys. (*Colch.*).

(6) Fatty or waxy casts. (*Phos.*). Urine contains fatty globules. (*Merc-cor.*).

(7) Head remedy for oxalates in urine. (*Ox-ac*).

(8) Phosphates : *Ammonium, Magnesium-p., Raph.*

(9) When urine is red. (*Bov.*).

(10) Scant urine in diabetes. (*Ratanhia*).

(11) Scanty with albumin and swelling. (*Hell.*)

(12) Specific gravity high. (*Arnica-m.*).

(13) Uric acid in urine with gastric and rheumatic troubles. (*Nat-s.*).

(14) Diseases resulting from urates in urine. (*Thlasp-b-p.*).

(15) Turbid urine rendered clear and non-irritating. Phosphatic deposits dissolved and growth of pus producing bacteria arrested. Prevents the decomposition of urine in ureters, bladder and kidneys. *Ammonium formald* commercially known as *Cystogen*. Dose 5 to 7 grains two to four times daily dissolved in hot water after meals. Compare *Urotropin*. (Wm. Boericke.). See "Albuminaria and Oxaluria".

Urine-constant desire for urination—There is a constant desire to urinate, only a small amount can be passed then give 5 drops of Tr. *Camphor* in wine glass of warm water every hour.

Urine-child crying Child afraid to urinate, screams before urinating. (*Borax.*). See "Crying of child-before urinating".

Urine-dribbling after labour and ordinarily—(a) Constant dribbling of urine after labour which is due to .the paralytic condition of sphincter bladder on account of the contusion is always removed by *Arnica*. and (b) Constant dribbling ordinarily. (*Verb.*). See "Dribbling of urine" and "Labour-rentention of urine"

Urine in dropsy—Scanty urine is one of the early symptoms of dropsy. Urine can suddenly becomes copious, removing the dropsy and suddenly it becomes very scanty and dropsy returns, the patient may drink plentiful but it all becomes dropsical. Dribbling and the urine being voided drop by drop. He takes lesser water but lets out more. (*Apoc-can.*). See "Retention of urine in dropsy".

Urine-escape involuntary also if not attended—(a) Increased secretion Involuntary escape. During first sleep at night, also from slightest excitement. (*Caust*). (b) Urgent desire to urinate. It may escape if not attended to quickly. (*Petroselinum.*). See "Incontinence involuntary evacuation of urine" and "Dysuria' either in diabetes or dyspepsia.

Urine-polyuria-excessive secretion of urine—(1) Profuse urination during menses. (*Phytolacca*).

(2) Urine passed in quantity larger than the fluid taken within 24 hours (*Acid-phos.*).

(3) Frequent urination with or without diabetes (*Argn-nit.*).

(4) Profuse urination in dyspepsia. (*Uranium-nit.*).

(5) Urine is passed several times during night, which may be due to indigestion. (*Nux-vomica 200.*).

Urine-frequent and painful and wetting bed and its suppression—(1) Micturition abnormal. Burning or scalding, painful emission drop by drop. (*Canth.*). See also "Strangury-painful urination".

(2) Constant ineffectual desire, emission in drops. (*Cop.*).

(3) Frequent desire, passes only a few drops. (*Apis.*). (ii) Frequent urging after drinking water. (*Carls-bad.*).

(4) Frequent urination in old people at night, (*Caust.*). (ii) Frequent and profuse urination with or without diabetes. (*Arg-n.*). See also "Bladder polyuria". (b) Suppression and retention. (*Camph.*). If no effect within one or two hours then *Terebinthina* every 15 minutes. (c) Involuntary evacuation at night. (1) In first sleep. (*Sep.*). (2) In children with phthisical tendencies. (*Bacilinum testium.*). (d) In children when difficult to awake. (*Kreos.*), (3) From too profound

sleep. (*Kali brom*). (4) Specific for wetting the bed by sickly girls involuntarily during first sleep. (*Sepia*). (5) Urination involuntary in sleep, the bed that has been wetted several times becomes uncleanble. (*Benz-a.*). (6) Wetting the bed at night. Passing urine at night in dream which awakes patient at night. (*Lac-c*). See also "Wetting the bed" "Micturition" "Bladder polyuria" and "Uraemia".

Urine-headache due to not attending it—Urine feels cold ; phosphate, milky urine. Headache from not attending to urinate. Scanty urine in rheumatic, gouty hysterical subjects. (*Agar.*). See "Headache-due to not urinating".

Urine-involuntary escape when walking or coughing—Involuntary escape of urine when walking or coughing, pain just after urinating. Has to wait a long time for it to pass if others are present. (*Nat-m.*).

Urine-involuntary and passing with difficulty—Involuntary urination when walking, coughing or sneezing. (*Zinc-met.*). Compare *Caust., Caps* ; *Ferr-met.* See "Incontinence involuntary evacuation of urine".

Urine-large-quantities and also suppressed—(a) Large quantities of pale urine with thirst. Weakness, pallor, loss of flesh. With sugar in the urine or without it. (*Acet-ac.*). (b) Urine suppressed : Urine scanty and sometimes suppressed Action of *Arum-t.*, is to start urine flow immediately (*Arum-t*). See "Diabetes".

Urine-milky—*Cina* urine becomes milky on standing or leaves a white stain on the ground. (*Cina.*). See "Urine albuminous and other casts."

Urine-milky in children—Milky urine which settles into whitish sediments. This characteristic is very often present in children. (*Ph-a.*).

Urine- offensive—(1) Urine is very dark with very intense urinous odour. (*Benzoic acid*).

(2) Urine dark, smelling like horse urine. (*Nitric-Acid*).

(3) Urine offensive and sourish (*Sepia*). See "Offensive foot sweat" and "Perspiration offensive of body"

Urine pus in—Pus in urine with great pain in the region of kidneys. (*Calc-sulph.*). See No. 15 of urine-albuminous and other Casts".

Urine-with painful micturition—See "Dysuria".

Urine-prostatic hypertrophy—(1) Retention ; prostates hypertrophied. (*Bell.*).

(2) In affections of prostate, dances with agony. (*Apis-m.*).

(3) Prostatic trouble, constant desire to pass urine at night, cystitis. Difficult urination. (*Sabal Serrullata*). See also "Prostate glands-and its affections".

Urine-retention in infants—Give *Aconite*. If this fails then *Puls.* but Dr. Herring recommends *Sulph.* See "Retention of urine after labour".

Urine-retention due to irritation and inflammation of kidney and bladder—*Cann-i.* and *Canth.* are useful when attended with inflammatory irritation of kidneys and bladder See "Inflammation of kidney", "Cystitis-inflammation of bladder" and "Kidney affections".

Urine-retention after labour—(a) Paralytic weakness of bladder after a woman has gone through strenuous labour causing retention of urine is miraculousy removed by *Causticum.* (*Caust.*). (b) *Nux-v.* and *Ars-a.* are also useful when the urine is retained owing to some sort of paralysis. See "Labour retention of urine" and "Paralytic condition of sphincter after labour."

Urine-smelling sour—Sour smelling urine which is copious with burning, smarting, itching in urethra (*Ambra.*). See "Sour every thing" and "Vomiting Sour."

Urine-suppressed—(a) Urine scanty and sometimes suppressed. *Arum-t.* is to start urine flow immediately. See "(b) urine frequent and painful and wetting bed and its suppression" "Urine large quantities and also suppressed", Kidney cessation of its function.

U

Urine suppressed pain—See "Chapter V for details".

Urine-troubles-sediment, other kinds of deposits in urine (1) Red deposite in urine. Child cries before urinating (*Lyco.*).

(2) White deposit of oxalates with pain in back. (*ox-ac.*).

(3) With deposit of phosphates. (*Ph-a.*). See also "Oxaluria" "Urine albuminous and other casts" and "Urine milky".

Urine-trouble after wedlock—Urinary trouble of young nervous women after marriage where urging to urinate becomes very troublesome. (*Staphy.*). See also "Micturition-in young wifes after marriage".

Urticaria-annual—Paroxsym sudden appearance of symptoms of urticaria appearing annually with burning and itching of skin ; hot as if on fire. (*Rhus-radicans. 200.*). See "Periodicity."

Urticaria better in cold air—Nettle rash ; better in cold air. (*Calc.*). See "Cold air causing sneezing."

Urticaria with burning—With burning and restlessness. (*Ars-alb.*). See "Burning-sensation" and "Restlessness" under latter's different heads.

Urticaria in different conditions—(a) *Urticaria* disappears in summer and reappears in winter. (*Psor.*). (b) Urticaria chronic with nettle rash on the whole body with itching (*Astac-fl.*). (c) Urticaria brought on by eating meat. (*Ruta.*). (d) When due to gastric disorder, with loaded tongue. (*Ant-crud.*). (ii) For swelling of whole body due to urticaria : (*Fragaria*). (e) If there are febrile symptoms. (*Acon.* every 2 hours.). (f) When rash is attended by severe headache with redness of the face. (*Bell.*—every 3 hours.). (g) Intense, intolerable fiery itching of the skin ; face becomes blotched, swollen and disfigured. The patient finds it impossible not to scratch or rub the affected area (*Urt-u.*). (Dr. Fisher). (h) Lotion of *Urtica-urens* M.T. to be applied externally in all above cases. See Nettle-rash. (i) A drop of *Tr. Camphor* on sugar taken removes the trouble of urticaria when it comes on after taking sour fruit or vinegar. (j) In chronic cases during or before intermittent fever there is much itching. (*Hep-s.*) (k) *Thyroidinum* is almost a specific for urticaria. The more oedematous the urticarial rashes and the more extensively they appear over larger area of the body the better will be the indications for the use of this remedy. (l) No remedy is so successful in relieving the distressing itching and formication of the skin due to chronic urticaria as *Sul-ac.* (m) *Urticaria* brought on by exposure on sour stomach. *Dulc.* 3. It is an excellent medicine for urticaria (n) When urticaria and other skin affections resist treatment then try *Skookum chuck*. See "Itching, distressing extremely" and "Fever and Cough and urticaria".

Urticaria-after exertion—Urticaria after every exertion. (*Psor.*).

Urticaria-external application—Apply lotion of *Urtica uren M.T.*

Urticaria-while going out—On going in open air ; better in warm room. (*Sep.*).

Urticaria itchings—Itching and burning (*Nat-m.*). See "Itch".

Urticaria with palpitation, diarrhoea on waking—Urticaria on excitement with rheumatic lameness, palpitation and diarrhoea. Urticaria on waking in the morning, worse from bathing. *Bovista* which has a marked effect on the skin producing eruption like eczema.

Urticaria itching-red and swollen—Intense itching red, swollen (*Rhus-t.*). See also "Nettle-rashs".

Uterine-colic—Must draw up double with great restlessness (*Coloc*). See "Ovarian Colic".

Uterine-haemorrhage—*Agn.* cures uterine discharge. The vagina is much relaxed (*Agn.*). See "Haemorrhage-uterine".

Uterine-haemorrhage-in dropsy—Haemorrhage from uterus in dropsy. Though it has amenorrhoea with dropsy, it has also copious menstrual flows, which may be frequent and lasting too long. From copious menstrual flow, the patient becomes anaemic and then dropsical (*Apoc-can.*). See "Haemorrhage-in dropsy".

Utrine-pains darting to sides—Pains of uterus darting from side to side. (*Act-rac.*). See "Pains in pelvis" and "Ovarian neuralgia".

Uterine-tumour or fibroid with consequential haemorrhage—(a) *Fraxinus Americana* 10 to 15 drops tincture to be given at bed time in mother tincture in alternation with *veratrum-alb. 30* dilution in morning.

(2) Womb packed with fibroid tumours, hot, burning feet though some times shivering all over (*Kali-iod.*).

(3) Fibroid with profuse debilitating bleeding (*Lapis-albus.*).

(4) Profuse haemorrhages due to fibroid. *Epihysterinum 30,* once or twice a week.

(5) Intractable bleeding from uterus due to fibroid tumour. (i) *Ficus religiosa.* (M.T.) 4 hourly. (ii) *Thlaspi bursa pastoris* (M.T.) 5 drops 4 hourly. (iii) *Hydrastinum-muriaticum.* (Dr. Clarke). (iv) *Aurum - muriaticum-natronatum* have more power over uterine tumours than any other remedy. (Burnett) See also "Fibroma or fibroid tumour" and "(d) of tumours at different places".

Uterus-trouble during too early menses with itching—All uterus symptoms aggravate on lying down. Menses too early and too profuse. Horrible itching of genitals with swelling of labia during menses. (*Ambra.*). See "Menstruation—early, profuse with itching".

Uterus-bleeding from—(*a*) Bleeding from uterus. The blood is fresh and red. *Phos.* has bleeding tendency and not oozing. The patient is pale and anaemic in look (*Phos.*). See "Haemorrhage uterine". (b) Uterine haemorrhage. (*Geraninum-maculatum* in 5 to 10 drops dose of tincture). See "Haemorrhage uterine".

Uterus enlargement—Enlargement and subinvolution of the uterus, when attended with prolapses and a bearing down sensation ; subinvolution means imperfect return to normal size of uterus after functional enlargement or after delivery. (*Fraxinus-americana*).

Uterus-pains before flow and displacement—(*a*) The pain in the uterus is usually more before the flow starts and is relieved by flow of blood. Uterine displacements of various kinds. (*Lach*). See "Pain in pelvis." (*b*) *Lilium-tig.* is very efficacious for uterine displacement.

Uterus-Prolapse after child birth or straining—Specially after child birth ; from over-lifting or straining. (*Podo.*). Compare *Rhus-t.* and *Nux-v.* See "Prolapse of uteri after delivery."

Uterus-prolapse—Prolapse of uterus. *Aloe.* has cured prolapse of uterus of long standing when it is associated with fulness, heat of the body, tendency to morning diarrhoea and dragging to uterus. (*Aloe*). See "Prolapse of uterus."

Uterus ulcerated—Ulceration and congestion of the mouth and neck of uterus. Actual prolapse of uterus (*Sep.*).

Uvula-different complaints--(1) Swollen, inflamed or ulcerated. (*Merc-c*). Compare *Hamamelis* 2 hrly.

(2) Uvula elongated, relaxed and scraping in throat. (*Alumen.*). Compare *Apis-m.* which is specific and head remedy for elongation of uvula.

(3) Elongation of uvula with throat badly swollen. (*Mancinella*).

(4) Elongation with cough, worse lying down. (*Hyos.*).

(5) Burning in uvula : *Tussilago-petasites.*

(6) Pain in uvula : (*Trifolium pratense.*).

(7) Uvula relaxed : (*Alumen*).

(8) Uvula ulcerated : (*Iodium.*).

(9) For local application on elongated uvula apply *Merc-cor.* in low *trituration* and it will give relief immediately and permanently. See "Sore throat" and "Throat inflammation spreading and glands swollen".

V

Vaccination—ill-effects of vaccination. (*Sil.*). See also "Diarrhoea small-pox" and "Diarrhoea-after vaccination and chronic".

Vaccination-child unwell since—ill-effects of vaccination. Child has never been well since last vaccination. Diarrhoea after vaccination or skin trouble. (*Thuj.*).

Vaccination - discomfort from pustules—It does not neutralise the effect of vaccination but simply relieves the pain and dicomfort arising from pustules without interfering from its course. (*Arn.*).

Vaccination-fever—Begin with *Merc-sol.* 30 two doses, follow it with two doses of *Hepar-sulf.* and lastly two doses of *Thuja* 30. (Dr. Guha). See "Fever due to vaccination."

Vagina-bleeding and with inflammation—(1) Discharge of blood from vagina after pressing at a hard stool. (*Ambra.*).

(2) Inflammation of vagina and vulva : *Ig.* 4 hourly. See "Prolapse of vagina with discharge" and "Fistula of vagina".

Varicose-leg with pain—(1) Varicose legs with purple areola. Venous congested part is purple or blue. (*Aesc.*).

(2) If there is much pain in the veins. (*Puls.* 2 hourly).

Varicose with ulceration-left leg hanging down unbearable—(1) The left leg becomes blue with distended varices. (*Ambra.*).

(2) In old-standing cases (*Fluor-ac.*).

(3) Varicose ulcers. Ulcerated legs which discharge freely and are extremely painful. (*Pyrog.*).

(4) Scarcely able to move about due to pain in legs. (*Ham.*).

(5) Veins in legs tending to ulceration. (*Fl-ac.*).

(6) The patient keeps the legs elevated. When they are allowed to hang down it seems as if they would burst and the pain is unbearable. Bursting feeling is the key-note of *Vipera.*

(7) Varicose vein in plethoric persons. Throbbing pains in legs. (*Bell; Glon.*). Lotion of *Ham.* may be applied locally in all cases of varicose veins.

Varicose with piles during pregnancy—*Puls.* to be followed by *Lach.* When attended with constipation, haemorrhoids and irritable temper then *Nux.* See "Pregnancy-disorders".

Variola-small-pox prophylactic—Prophylactics are ; *Ant-t., Hydr., Kali-cyanatum., Malandrinum., Thuja., Vaccinum., Variol.,* See "Small-pox preventive and for disfigurement."

Veins and arteries difference between them—Veins are blood vessels through which the blood from all parts of the body returns to the heart while arteries carry blood from the heart to all parts of the body and this flow is actually propelled by the heart with some force. Thus bleeding from arteries, rush out in jets and the blood is of clear scarlet colour. Bleeding from veins has a darker colour and the flow is continuous, not in jerks.

Venous-bleeding from any organ with blackish blood—Venous bleeding from any organ *e.g.* lungs, stomach, bowels, uterus, nose etc. Blackish blood and not the red arterial blood. (*Carb-v.*). See "Haemorrhage venous from any organ with blackish blood".

Venous stasis with ulcers and inflammation (stagnation of blood current)—(1) General and local venous stasis is the general rule with *Asaf.* Varicose veins surround the ulcers. (*Asaf.*).

(2) Acute inflammation of veins. The useful medicine, Dr. Jousset says is *Ham.* See "Varicose leg with pain"

Vertigo of the aged from motion—Of the aged after rising. (*Phos.*). See "Vertigo due to senility".

Vertigo-while closing eyes and rising from bed—(1) When closing the eyes. (*Thuj.*).

(2) On rising from bed with vomiting and faintness after eating. (*Sel.*).

(3) Dr. Boericke says that *Phosphorus* displays great curative powers in every imaginable case of vertigo.

Vertigo on rising or turning—(1) On rising. (*Acon.*).

(2) On turning the head side-wise or turning in bed or looking around side-wise *Conium*. (Dr. Nash.).

Vertigo-due to senility in different postures—(1) In old men. Vertigo comes on any time. Vertigo with weight in vertex-crown. Worse after sleep also eating. Lies down on account of vertigo with a feeling of weakness in stomach. It is the dizziness belonging to senility and to premature old age. (*Ambra.*). See "Weakness—premature old age with impaired functions" and "Prostration with burning pain at mid-night with hands and feet cold".

(2) Vertigo on looking up (*Calc.*).

(3) Vetigo due to anaemia, of loss of blood, flushes bright during attack. (*Ferr-p.*).

(4) Vertigo from looking down, *Phos.*, *Spig.*, *Sulf.*

(5) From odour of flowers, *Nux-v.*, *Phos.*

(6) During and after meals, *Grat.*

(7) From motion in carriage, *Cocc.*

(8) When stooping, *Nux.*, *Bell.*

(9) When ascending, *Calc.-Os.*

(10) When descending, *Bor.*

(11) When moving head from pillow, *Lac vacc.*

(12) Tendency to fall forward due to vertigo. *Spig.*, 30 ; tendency to fall backwards, *Nux-v.* 3x-200 ; tendency to fall on one side, *Sulf.* 30. See also "Giddiness".

Vesicles-yellow—Yellow vesicles are common in *Anacardium* with intense itching of the eruptions. (*Anac.*). Compare *Rhus-tox* See "Eczema of vesicular type".

Virus including haemorrhage—During epidemic of Virus conjunctivities according to a news published in Evening News of Hindustan Times *Platina 200* acts rapidly. It should be given at the intervals of half an hour. Three such doses will be sufficient and soon after the first dose the patient starts feeling comfortable and within 24 hours the patient shows no signs of eye flue.

(2) Putrid condition of the whole body. According to Dr. Nash *Nitric acid* is useful for pricking ulcers, excrescences condylomata haemorrhage from all outlets or the body, blood being bright red. See "Hoemorrhage-bright blood" and "Condylomata".

Vision-different troubles—(1) Colour blindness. (*Phos.*) See also "Colour blindness".

(2) Deception of colours or figures before the eyes. (*Agar-m*).

(3) Red spots before the eyes (*Hyos.*).

(4) Black spots before the eyes. (*Sulf.*).

(5) Flashes before the eyes. (*Bell.*).

(6) Blindness when due to paralysis of optic nerve. (*Bovista.*). See "Optic neuritis".

(7) Temporary attacks of blindness. (*Acon., Merc.*)

(8) Night blindness when the patient can see nothing after twilight. (*Acon.*). See "Night blindness"

(9) Night blindness when black spots float before the eyes. (*Lyco.*). If sparks appear before the eyes then *Veratrum.* If this fails then give *Hyos.*

(10) Day blindness when the patient can only see in the evening. (*Sulf.*). See "Day-blindness".

(11) For dread of the light with headache (*Euphr.*).

(12) Cataract. In incipient stages with myopia give *Caust.* 1M. every month. *Phos.* is also good remedy for a cataract. See "Cataract".

(13) For glaucoma (*i*) *Spigelia.,* (*ii*) *Prunus-spinosa* may be tried in the order given. See "Glaucoma".

(14) For granular lids. (*i*) *Hep-s.* (*ii*) *Graph.* to be tried in the order given.

(15) Granular lids when lashes turn inward towards the eyes and inflammation. Lower lids entirely inverted. (*Borax.*).

(16) In-growing eye lashes when *Borax* fails then try *Puls.*

(17) When due to blocking of lachrymal duct ; tears flow. (*Rhus-tox.*).

(18) Nodules on the eyelids. (*Conium*). (*ii*) *Staphy.*

(19) Polypus under eyelids (*Kali-bi*). ;

(20) Tumour on upper or lower lids. (*Zinc-met.*).

(21) Vision right half not visible. (*Lithium-carb.*).

(22) Vision lower or upper not visible. *Aurum-met.* See "Eyes" under their different heads also, "Eye troubles" and "Blindness also Night blindness".

(23) Pallor of optic-discs, contracted visual field and shrinking retinal vessel. (*Acetanillidum*).

(24) Atrophy of optic nerve ; retinal congestion ; optic disc pale ; vision greatly impaired. (*Carboneum-sulphuratum*). See "Eye-troubles".

Vision-dim—Dulness and dimness of vision without any ostensible cause. (*Ambra.*). See "Eyes dimness" and "Asthenopia".

Vital-force—*Sil.* affects vital forces bodily and cures many deep-seated diseases. Patient always suffers from vital warmth and is afraid to uncover head or feet in cold weather. (*Sil.*). See "Debility due to various causes".

Vital force exhausted and consequential collapse—When the vital force is nearly exhausted the surface of the body is cold perspiring ; the patient lies motionless as if dying ; voice lost, blueness of fingers, then *Cargo-veg*. is the medicine which is usually used in such serious conditions. (*Carb-v.*). See "Collapse".

Vitamins—(*a*) Vitamin theory is of later origin but vitamins are very important from the point of view of Homoeopathy. As a matter of fact they are group of organic compounds present in very minute quantities in natural foodstuffs required for the normal growth and maintenance of life of animals including man, who as a rule are unable to synthesize these compounds. They are effective in small amounts and do not furnish energy but are essential from transformation of energy and for the regulation of metabolism in the organism. Homoeopathy has appropriate remedies which will not only provide for deficiency but also correct the system enabling it to take the required vitamins from the food. But in actual practice I have found that vitamins are not contra-indicated under homoeopathic treatment. I have found them doing immense benefit to the patients under my treatment. Unless the practitioner is fully conversant with various kinds of vitamins and their properties he should not prescribe them for greater mischief might ensue than good. (*b*) According to Dr. A.Z. Blackwood vitamins are fat soluble and water soluble. The fat soluble vitamins are essential, to the growth and proper nutrition of animals. They are present in butter, the yolk of eggs, cod-liver oil, also in carrots, potatoes and bananas.

The water soluble vitamins are essential for appetite and nutrition. They are present to a greater extent in glandular tissues. Tomatoes are rich in the antineuritic (efficient in neuritis) and anti-scorbute (effective in scurvy). The feeding of oranges, lemons, and tomatoes prevents scurvy. Spinach, turnips and cabbages also possess these qualities.

The antineuratic vitamins are water soluble. They are found in yeast, the outer shall of many cereal foods and orange juice: their absence from the diet are a cause of beriberi while their present is preventive.

Fresh unheated normal milk contains vitamins necessary to health and growth. In some cases it is low in water soluble vitamins and may require of fruit juices specially that of the orange to prevent scurvy in children.

Vitamins-homoeopathic medicines of vitamins group (out of many few are given below) :

Vitamin A—*Calc-phos. 12x, Acid-phos-Q-200, Phos. 200.*

Vitamin B—*Kali-mur. 6x or 12x, Cardiuus-mar-Q, Chelidonium Q 6x, Nat-phos. 3x, Lyco. 200, Hydras-Q.*

Vitamin C—*Kali Phos 6x, Carbo-veg 200; Silicea 200, Graphites 200.*

Vitamin D—*Calc fluor. 12x, Calc-phos. 12, Rhus-tox. 30x.*

Vitamin E—*Sabina Q, Sepia 6.*

Vitamin K—*Geranium Q, Fer-phos-9, Secale-cor. Q.*

Voices hearing—Hearing voices, which are inaudible to others but patient persists that he hears them. This may be due to hallucination. (*Naja-30.*). See "Delution" and "Hallucination".

Voice-hoarse with expectoration of mucus—Acute complaints of the voice. Catarrhal hoarseness. Copious expectoration of mucus from larynx. (*All-c.*). See also "Hoarseness catarrhal with expectoration of mucus".

Voice-loss of—(1) *Lach.* has great effect on respiratory organs and chest. Paralysis of vocal chords, causing loss of voice ; larynx sensitive to least touch, it causes suffocation when the child gets worse in sleep. Pain in the throat usually runs up to ears. (*Lach.*).

(2) Loss of voice from simple catarrh. (*Caust 2* hourly).

(3) Loss of voice when patient exposed to heat. (*Antcrud.*, 3 hourly). See "Croup-loss of voice" and "Paralysis of vocal chord".

Voice-lost suddenly—(1) Sudden loss of voice of singers and public speakers or of a lawyer, who is making his final efforts to sum up a case, speaking for hours, can be cured with *Arum-t.* enabling him to go on with his speech in a clear voice. It is specially suitable if the voice is uncertain and uncontrollable, changing continually in its tone. (*Arum-t.*). Compare *Rhus-tox.* and *Phos.*

(2) Loss of voice at menstrual period. (*Gels.*). See "Clergyman's sore-throat—loss of voice" and "Hoarseness Sudden".

Vomiting periodic and of different types—(1) Sudden vomiting of milk in infants. (*Merc-sol.* 2 hourly). Compare *Aethusa-cynapium.*

(2) Nausea, headache, vomiting of food and bile. (*Petroleum* 1 hourly).

(3) Periodical vomiting spells specially vomiting of sour matter which is so sour that it sets the teeth on edge. (*Iris-v.*). See "Sour-every thing".

(4) The patient vomits as soon as he eats or drinks ; vomiting from an overloaded stomach, from eating indigestible substances, such as fat foods or from the heat of summer ; white coated tongue (*Ant-c.*). See "Over-feeding of children" and "Dyspepsia of adults from brain trouble and constant eating".

(5) Vomiting by even raising the head from pillow. (*Stram.*).

(6) Vomiting due to abuse of tobacco. (*Tabacum.*). See "Tobacco habit" and how to get over it.

(7) Vomiting of drunkards. Burning in stomach. (*Acid-carbolic.*). See "Drunkenness".

(8) Child vomits as soon as it nurses. (*Valeriana*).

(9) *Aethusa* is an excellent remedy for vomiting of children. The child vomits soon after eating or nursing. It is followed by great exhaustion which is the keynote of this remedy. The child falls back exhausted. The vomiting is of green curds of milk. The vomiting starts suddenly without notice in summer. Death is stamped on the face from the very beginning

and if there is any medicine to save the life it is *Aeth-cy*. See "Milk not digested with diarrhoea" and "Summer complaints of children during dentition milk causing diarrhoea".

Vomiting-all things—Vomits all kinds of food and, drink bile and blood. Heart-burn ; cannot bear the sight or smell of food. (*Ars-alb.*). See "Bilious attack" and "Smell of food".

Vomiting-on alternate days—Dr. Clarke cured a case of vomiting on alternate days with *Baptisia* 12. (c).

Vomiting of bile—Vomiting of bile between chill and heat (*Eupar-perf.*).

Vomiting-of curds—Vomiting of large curds (sour) with sour stools, sweaty heads and open foutanelles. (*Calc. ostrearum.*).

Vomiting of all kinds—*Iris-versicolor.* according to Dr. Ribson.

Vomiting of dark blood—(1) When dark give *Ip.*, if not better soon then *Ham.* See "Blood spitting".

(2) Vomiting of blood and blood from rectum. (*Aloe.*). See also "Rectum haemorrhage".

Vomiting-in cholera—*Ip.* and if fails then *Verat-a* ; for vomiting and purging. *Carbo-veg.* for vomiting with collapse symptom. See "Cholera" under its different heads.

Vomiting in dropsy and hysterical vomiting—(a) In dropsical conditions. Abdomen very much distended, his stomach is distended and he must vomit and with distension of his whole body, he drinks and vomits, it is with difficulty he can eat ; he will not digest. Sense of pressure in the epigastrium, in the chest. (*Apoc-can.*). (b) For hysterical vomiting. (*Kreos.*), See "Thirst-water disagrees" and "Hysterical vomiting".

Vomiting-faecal matter—Reversed peristalsis and faecal matter. (*Opium*). It is due to a disease named ilews which is characterized by severe griping pain, vomiting of faecal matter, and costiveness, with retraction and spasm of the abdomen muscles, accompanied by reversed peristalsis and the pumping of bile back into the stomach.

Vomiting-gastric disturbance periodical—(1) Patient has paroxysm of vomiting every 2 or 3 weeks with high fever. Red face ; thirst for ice cold water. He vomits yellow and green and even pure bile. Jaundiced eyes and skin. Constipation. Urine brick-dust. The warmer the weather the severer are the symptoms. Cold hands and damp feet. (*Phos*).

(2) If occasioned by disordered stomach and tongue is coated give *Ip*. See "Fever periodic" and "Gastro-intestinal disturbances".

Vomiting-due to morphine effect of operation—Morphine effect on sensitive persons after operations, awful eructation with retching and vomiting and there is nothing to vomit. Give *Cham*. which will stop these within a few minutes and is practically the only remedy that stops vomiting from morphine. (*Cham*.). See "Morphia-vomiting after operation" and "Chloroform vomiting".

Vomiting persistent—Due to gastric trouble from dietetic error. Efforts to vomiting with empty eructation and accumulation of saliva. Vomiting with clean tongue. (*Ip*.). See "Persistent nausea".

Vomiting-in pregnancy—In pregnancy ; nausea or vomiting at the very thought or smell of cooked food. The patient cannot even pass by the kitchen. *Colchicum* is a good medicine for this but *Sep*. is better in pregnancy (*Sep*.).

(2) Both *Nux-v*. and *Anacard-occidental*e may be useful for the morning sickness of pregnancy, the patient is relieved while eating but the symptoms return soon after. (*Anac*.). See "Morning sickness".

(3) *Natrum-mur*. is for obstinate cases. There is loss of appetite, water brash and pain in pit of stomach. (*Nat-m*.). See "Water-brash".

(4) Dr. Dewey says that *Carbolic-ac*. will cure vomiting of pregnant women, who at the same time have frantic headache and are very irritable. (*Carb-ac*.).

(5) Dr. Hoyne recommends *Cupr. 30* for morning sickness of pregnant lady vomiting many times each day attended by agonising and long continued pain, retching, frequent cramps in legs and limbs and great mental disquiet and restlessness night and day. This medicine relieves symptoms within 24 hours.

(6) *Symphosicarpus* is considered by some as specific if given in 1X potency. It has great nausea and vomiting. (*Sym-R.*). See "Pregnancy-vomiting".

Vomiting-due to rich food—(1) Vomiting of food eaten long before. Dryness of mouth without thirst by rich, greasy food and these rich greasy foods upsetting the stomach. (*Puls.*).

(2) If accompanied by much loud belching of wind and hot face. (*Sep.*). See "Dyspepsia" under its different heads.

Vomiting-starting suddenly in children with serious symptoms—*Aeth.* is one of the best medicines for vomiting of children, with sour stools and extreme prostration. It starts suddenly without notice in hot weather. The milk comes up partly in curds and partly liquid and accompanying the vomiting there is thin, yellow, greenish stool. The child has the appearance as if it were dying, pale hippocratic face. The eyes are sunken and there is sunken condition around the nose. The child sinks into an exhausted sleep. Death is stamped on the face from the very beginning and if there is any medicine to save the life, it is this *Aeth-c.* See "Suddenness of disease in children with redness, swelling and pain and "Diarrhoea of vomiting children in summer starting suddenly."

Vomiting-sour—Every thing from mouth to anus turns sour. Taste in mouth and eructation sour. (*Calc.*). See "Sour every thing ' and "Diarrhoea of children sour smelling."

Vomiting with thirst for large quantities of water—Heaviness in stomach. Nausea, characterised by (*i*) Aggravation by movement. (*ii*) Thirst for large quantities of water. (*iii*) Relief by pressure. (*Bry.*). See "Nausea-heaviness in stomach."

V

Vomiting-with thirst for cold water becoming warm and bleeding tendency—Thirst for large quantities of water. Burning in palms ; vomiting in the morning. Bleeding tendency. Cold water vomiting after it is warm in stomach ; whereas the vomiting of *Ars-a.* is immediately after drinking. (*Phos.*). See "Thirst-cold water."

Vomiting-uncontrollable—Uncontrollable. (*Bell.*). See "Nausea-persistent."

Vomiting with worm symptoms—Vomiting or nausea with clean tongue is found in connection with worm symptoms of *Cina*. (*Cina.*). See "Worms".

Vulva eruptions, inflammation and soreness—

(1) Eruption on : *Cenchris-contortrix.*

(2) Inflammation of : *Copaiva., Itu.*

(3) Soreness of :—*Ovigallinae pellicula.*
See "Oedema (Dropsical swelling)".

W

Wakeful and restless infants—*Coffea*, if this fails then *Opium, Puls.* or *Ipec.* when due to over-loading of stomach. See "Over-feeding of children", "Restlessness" under their different heads and "Sleep-unrefreshing and child wakes at night playing".

Walking-rapidly—Walking rapidly either a habit in *Sepia* patient or it relieves her. (*Sep.*). See "Walking stooped".

Walking-delayed in fat children—Delayed walking in children. Children have no disposition to walk and will not try. Fat and flabby children with enlarged abdomen and sweating during sleep. (*Calc.*). See "Children late in learning to talk and walking".

Walking delayed-thin children not growing—The child cannot walk well and learns to walk late as in *Calc-c* ; he does not grow according to his age. The child is very hungry and even then goes on emaciating. The belly is big as in *Calc. carb.* He has thin limbs with pinched and emaciated face and the face looks cold and creased as in monkey. These children can be saved and made healthy with the help of *Sil.*, provided the generl symptoms of *Sil.* are present (*Sil.*). See "Dental development slow and late in children" and "Hunger-emaciated child".

Walking-stooped—Stooped walk in aged person. Dr. Lippe recommends. *Mezereum*. It may not remove the stoop but may help the patient to over-come this handicap. See "Walking rapidly".

Walking delayed, slow learning and talking—Late learning to talk and walking in children. Children slow in learning in school and who make mistakes and cannot remember things. The patient is sluggish and stupid. Compare *Natrum-*

muriaticum which has late learning to talk and *Calcarea-carb.* which has late learning to walk. These two features are combined with *Agar.* In *Calc.* it is due to defective bones. In *Agaricus* it is mental defect. Any slow development of mind (*Agar*). See "Children late in learning to talk and walking" and "Back-ward, children-who do not develop properly and look idiotic."

Walking-on knees—Children dwarfed and stunted ; legs heavy. Ankles easily turned when walking ; can't walk except on knee. (*Medorrhinum.*).

Wandering joint pains—In *Aur-met.* the pains wander from joints to joint and finally locate in the heart. (*Aur-met.*). Compare *Puls.* See "Pains wandering" and "Flying gout pains."

War-explosion—Any survivor not too close to the centre of the explosion would be helped and comforted by the remedy *Arnica* given in any potency as soon as possible after explosion. (Dr. A.H. Grimmer, M.D.).

Warts-round the anus—A crop of short warts, small in size, like a ring round the orifice. The patient had been vaccinated and had gonorrhoea many years back. He had dyspepsia also. *Thuja 30* with infrequent administration.

Warts-on different parts of body—(1) On face and on eyelids. *Caust.* or *Calc-c* or *Nit-ac.*

(2) On hands. (*Kali-mur.*).

(3) On the palm. (*Nat-m.*).

(4) In crops ; wart like excrescences on back of head or chin. (*Thuja.*). Compare *Antimonium-crudum.*

(5) On the sides of fingers—(*Calc-c., Caust. Sepia.*).

(6) Cauliflower like on upper lip. (*Nit-ac.*). See "Condylomata" and "Corns". (b) Most warts like cauliflower, hard and hagadic having cracks or fissures of skin or in thin pellicles (a thin membrane) often emiting a fetid humour (fluid) and bleeding when touched. (*Nit-ac.*). Dr. Lilienthal.

(2) Isolated warts. Try *Caust, Calc-c.* and *Nat-c.*

(3) Smooth and soft warts, itching and burning (*Ant-c.*)

(4) On tips of fingers and nose. Large warts, jagged (having notches or teeth) bleeding easily. (*Caust.*).

(5) Horny warts on genitals of glands which bleed on washing. (*Nit-ac.*).

(6) On back of hands and fingers. (*Dulc.*).

(7) Red warts on fingers (*Calc-c*).

(8) Fig. warts *i.e.* venereal warts near rectum or genitals. (*Phos-a.*).

(9) Hard warts which split easily. Itch and bleed. (*Thuj*).

(10) According to Dr. Nash *Causticum* is one of the most successful remedies for warts.

Warts-of different types—On skin of different types as a consequence of gonorrhoeal infections or otherwise all symptoms of suppressed gonorrhoea. (*Thuj.*) Paint *Thuja* (*M.T.*) externally for warts around anus. See "Tumour" under different heads.

Warts-prevention of its recurrence—See "Chapter V for details".

Warts-on face and hands—*Calc.*

Warts-on fingers—See "Fingers-warts on".

Warts on hands upon back—See "Hands-warts upon back".

Warts-multiple on back—A bunch of dark warts about 100 in number on the back near lumbar region, skin takes a bluish appearance, eczema on both feet. History of rheumatic fever and frequent colds. Constipative and occasional head-ache. History of breast cancer in family. (Give *Thuja 1M* and *50M* at intervals. *Carcinocin* 200 as intercurrent remedy. *Bacill 200* to *50M* at weekly intervals. As a finishing touch give *Bacill C.M.* to complete the cure. (Dr. Wadia.).

Warts - on palms—On palms. (*Nat-mur.*). Skin burns. (*Anac.*).

W

Washing causing aggravation—Cold washing aggravates except headache which is relieved from cold. (*Act-rac.*). See "Bathing dread".

Washing-hands Always washing one's hand. (*Syphilinum.*).

Wasp-bite For wasp bites, apply *Arnica* mother tincture externally and give *Canth 200* internally. (*Arn-mont.*). See "Insect bites or stings"

Wassermann-reaction In old chronic cases, in which there is one plus or two plus reaction give *Naja*.

Water-brash (gastric burning pain with eructations) (1) With foul taste in the morning. Vomiting of food eaten long before. Bad taste in the mouth. Dryness of mouth caused by rich greasy food. Nothing taste well not even water. (*Puls.*).

(2) During pregnancy. (*Lyco.*).

(3) Water-brash after eating with heart-burn and colic. (*Nux-v.*). See "Dyspepsia with bad taste with rich food."

Watering-from eyes—Watering both from nose and eyes but irritation in the eyes and not in the nose. (*Euphr.*). Compare *Allium-cepa*, if there is irritation in the nose but the eyes have no irritation and simply water. See "Eyes-watering with redness". See also "Acrid fluids" and "Nose watering causing rawness".

Watering-from nose—Watering both from nose and eyes but irritation in the eyes and not in the nose. (*Euphr.*). Compare *Allium-cepa*. if there is irritation in the nose but the eyes have no irritation and simply water. See "Nose watering with irritation in eyes".

Weakness of any kind—Weakness brought on by hot weather, over-exertion, mental, physical or night watching, which leads to sleepiness. (*Selenium.*).

Weakness-anaemia—Emaciation weakness, anaemia, loss of appetite, burning thirst and copious pale urine as a combination calling for the remedy *Acet-ac.* Inherited phthisis patients. (*Acet-ac.*) See also "Delility" and "Emaciation in T.B." and "Anaemea pernicious".

Weakness-anaemic with mental prostration—Anaemic looking patient who is emaciated more on the cheeks and round the neck. The prostration of mind as well as the body is the main feature. In women *Nat-m.* has a hysteric tendency and in men neurasthenic disposition. *Nat-m.* is one of our best remedies for anaemic condition with general weakness and emaciation and the mental condition stated above. (*Nat-m.*). See "Anaemia".

Weakness-of bladder after labour—Paralytic weakness of bladder after a woman has gone through strenuous labour causing retention of urine afterwards is miraculously removed by *Causticum.* See "Labour-retention of urine". and "Bladder weakness after labour".

Weakness-after influenza—Dewey recommends *Phos.* as the great post-influenza tonic. See "Influenza-post-weakness".

Weakness-due to loss of blood and fluids and also due to nursing—In general and other complaints as a result of excessive loss of blood or other fluids (diarrhoea.) Debilitated and broken down from exhausting discharges, *China,* is all the more indicated if the loss of blood has been sudden with faintness. Aversion to work ; unrefreshing sleep : oversensitiveness to touch. Perspiration during sleep ; blackness before eyes and ringing in the ears. Weakness by nursing. (*Chin.*) See "Debility-due to loss of fluids."

Weakness-at midnight with sinking of vital powers—Prostration with hands and feel cold and sinking of vital powers. Restlessness and sinking of strength. Anxiety of mind with thirst. Wants to toss about if still enough to do so. Intense burning and burning pains. *Arsenic symptoms* occur usually at midnight between 12 and 2 and sometimes between 1 and 2 P.M. (*Ars-a.*). See "Prostration with burning pain at midnight with sinking of vital powers".

Weakness-premature old age with impaired function—A man of middle age looks and shows symptoms of old age.

Also for patients weakened by age or over work are anaemic and sleepless. *Ambra.* is a great remedy for the aged with impairment of all functions, weakness, coldness, and numbness usually, of single parts, fingers, arms, etc. Feebleness and forgetfulness. One sided complaints call for it. (*Ambra*), See "Prematurely old with impairment of all functions", "See old age" and "Debility due to excess."

Weakness-in rickety children inspite of nourishment—In children : Thin rickety children. Children who sweat on head easily : emaciated and badly nourished children. Child hungry, wanting food too often but not gaining weight due to bad assimilation. Large head, big belly, thin limbs, emaciated face ; cannot walk, or learning to walk late constipated. Does not grow according to age. Face looks old and creased as in monkey. (*Sil.*). Compare *Calc-c.* See "Assimilation—defective in children" inspite of nourishment and "Rickets".

Weakness in small of back—As if back paralyzed, gives out when walking ; can hardly walk or talk ; hands and feet get numb, asleep ; the whole arm goes to sleep and hands and feet swollen. They all seem to depend upon spinal weakness, spinal trouble. (*Cocculus Ind.*)

Weakness in sprained joints—Weakness and tenderness remaining in the sprained joints and tendons after use of *Arnica* are usually removed by *Rhus-tox.* and subsequently with *Calc.* In isolated cases the pain which persists may require such remedies as *Caust.* or *Staphy.* See "Sprain-in joints" and "Rickets".

Weakness of the tendons and muscles with pain—*Rhus-tox.* follows *Arnica* well in removing the pain and weakness of the tendons and muscles. When weakness persists then use *Calc-carb.* See "Tendons and muscles-their weakness."

Weakness of legs—Weakness of legs. Chronic movements, numbness of legs, must move them constantly. (*Tarent-his.*) (Dr. Boericke).

Weak digestion after typhoid—Weak digestion after typhoid flatulence ; eructations give temporary relief. The simplest food disagree, specially fatty foods. (*Carbo-v.*). See "Digestion-weak after typhoid".

Weak memory—Forgetful of things in his mind but a moment ago foregetful as if in dream. (*Anac.*). See "Memory" under its different heads and "Forgetfulness with absent mindedness loss of memory".

Weak-children waking irritability—Children are weak in body but with well-developed head and intellect. They are irritable usually and when sick wake up from sleep with great irritability, screaming and kicking (*Lyco.*). See "Irritability of child", "Child-frightened" and "Crying of child" under its different heads.

Weather-causing aggravation—(1) Wet stormy weather, electric conditions of atmosphere. (*Rhododendron*).

(2) Change of weather from warm to cold. (*Dulcamara*).

(3) Wet Cold weather. Asthma, loose cough and rattling of mucus. (*Nat-sulph.*).

Weaning-engorgement of breast after weaning—*Puls.* is most useful remedy. Then comes *Calc-c.* Remember *Calc.* follows *Puls. Bryonia* according Dr. Clarke prevents congestion of breast. See "Breast congestion after weaning".

Wedlock-urine trouble after it—Urinary trouble of young nervous women after marriage when urging to urinate becomes trouble-some then *Staphy.* proves most comforting to young wife. See "Micturition-in young wives after marriage".

Weeping-child pretending—Child who makes a pretence of weeping without tears. (*Staphy. 30* or *200*). See "Obstinate" and "Child unmanageable".

Weeping tendency in girls—*Puls.* girls often weeps while stating her symptom. Changeableness is present in her disposition. She is now obstinate, next moment tearful, mild and pleasant under persuation. Consolation and sympathy please her. She weeps on all occasions whether it is an offence without the offender knowing even if sympathy shown to her. (*Puls.*). Compare *Nat-m.* Patient whose weeping alternates with laughing and who is more disturbed and irritated by consolation. See also "Mind-weeping tendency" and "Consolation causing aggravation and weeping".

Weeping tendency causing indifference—Great weeping tendency. Patient weeps while stating her case. Afraid of being alone. She is tearful when she narrates her trouble to any one. Compare *Puls*. But *Puls*. patient is more yielding than *Sepia*. But in *Sepia* she develops a peculiar indifference. She grows indifferent to every thing, *e.g.*, her dress occupation, sense of cleanliness and to her husband and children. She is sad and cries on all occasions without always knowing the reason thereof. (*Sep.*). See also "Hysteria weeping"

Wen-on scalp—A sebaceous cyst occurring in the scalp. Give *Thuja 30* one dose before breakfast, daily and apply externally *Thuja M.T* for weeks together. Give also *Bacillinum 30* one dose once a week to remove its cause. According to Dr. Nash *Graphites* is one of the best remedies for wens found in persons of herpetic dyscrasia a disordered condition of body attributed orginally unsuitable mixing of body fluids. See "Cyst-eyelids".

Wet weather-cold air and full moon causing aggravation—*Calc.* is worse in cold air, in wet weather, cold water and during full moon. (*Calc.*) See "Cold air-extremely sensitive" and "Tendency-to catch cold".

Wetting the bed—(1) (a) Child wets the bed during its first sleep. (*Sep.*). (b) *Bell.*, for a week and *Calcarea* for a week and so on (2) *Nux., Bell., Kali-brom.* If due to worms. *Cina*. See also "Urine-frequent and painful and wetting bed", "Enuresis" in Paediatrics.

Wetting-bladder for children—The action of *Apocynum* is marked on bladder. It is a routine medicine once given to children for wetting the bed. (*Apoc-can.*) See "No. 2 of bladder".

Witlow—(a) *Calcarea fluorica*. Dr. Jahr says that *Sulph, Hepar-s.* have effected such rapid cures in his hands that he scarcely found it necessary to use other remedies. Farrington used *Flour-ac.* with good success in acute throbbing pains and sensation of splinter under nails. According to Dr. Laurie *Silica* should be given when the matter is deeply seated, the swelling very considerable, and attended with excruciating pain. A dose every 4 hours. (b) Dr. Leonard claims that 12x *Calc-sulph.* will abort whitlow. (c) When the pain is unbearable driving patient to despair ; this medicine goes a long way in relieving pain and hastening suppuration. (*Stram.*). (d) Pain does not allow the patient to sleep for several nights. To stay morbid process also. (*Am-c.* 500. 1 or 2 doses sufficient). (e) Apply *Cryptopodium punctuatum* externally to relieve pain and promote suppuration.

Whooping-cough—*Acon.* for fever, *Dros.* and *Cup-met.* for the attacks of cough and convulsions. *Bell.*, *Hyos.* if at night chiefly. (b) R B Bishamber Dass recommends that *Pertussin* which is a nosode should be given at the commencement of treatment. In many cases one dose may prove curative or cut short its duration. As for *Drosera* he thinks that it is almost specific and should be given in 30 potency and to be repeated only after every 4 days. For children who have convulsions with clenching of thumbs and fists he recommends *Cuprum-met. 30*. Dr. Clarke recommends that treatment should begin with *Conquelu-chin 30*, 4 hourly to be alternated with *Ipec.* for spasmodic fit of coughing, *Dros.* for spells of hacking cough with vomiting ; *Cocc.* for frequent passage of urine with vomiting ; *Hydrocy-ac.* for severe spasm threatening convulsion ; *Kali-c.* for puffiness of upper lids ; *Ambra.* for convulsive cough with hoarseness and flow of water from mouth. (b) *Solanum Carolinense Tincture* in drop doses say 10 to 20 or more if needed is said to be specific for such a cough ; spasmodic whooping cough with difficulty in lying down, voice hoarse and larynx sore. (*Mag-p.*). Whooping cough, long and continued paroxysms of coughing unable to get a respiration, restless, face pale yellowish hue. (*Napthal. 1x.*). According to Dr. L. Hartman *Napthaline* is more useful than any other remedy in whooping cough.

Whooping cough-boring fingers and recurring—Violent and recurring. Very restless while asleep. Bores fingers in the nose and grinds teeth while asleep. (*China*.). See "Finger boring-during sleep" and "Boring into the nose".

Whooping cough-breathless and blue—Suffocating cough, child becomes stiff and blue in the face : loses breath, turns purple, bleeding from mouth or nose, vomiting of mucus. There must be nausea and vomiting present. (*Ip.*). See "Cough-child with breathing difficulty".

Whooping cough-choking after midnight with vomiting—Spasmodic dry irritative cough ; chokes, cough very deep and hoarse ; worse after midnight, paroxysm are excited by laughing, playing or violent exercise ; if expectoration is not easy. Vomiting and retching (an unsuccessful attempt at vomiting) ensue. (*Drosera*). See "Cough-dry".

Whooping cough-followed by glands—Inflammation of glands on the right side of neck. Tongue white with bad apitite. *Lach. 6*, T.D.S.

Whooping cough-lessening its frequency and severity—Noisy and agitated breathing, suffocative whooping cough, asthma, *Hydrocyanic acid* exerts an almost magical influence in such cases. (Dr. West).

Whooping cough-preventive—*Pertussin*. According to Clarke, *Dros. 6* night and morning should be given to those who have had no attack. See "Preventives".

Whooping cough-prophylactic—*Dros., Vaccine*.

Whooping cough-child shakes and vomiting—Cough attended with indigestion, vomiting and offensive flatus. The child shakes and shudders and you can see that it dreads the cough, because of tearing pains in the larynx. (*All-c.*). See "Cough child grasping larynx".

Whooping cough-tears flowing—When tears flow from eyes with cough. (*Nat-m.*). See "Tears or watering from eyes with swollen lids".

Widows' remedy-screaming with grief—Sensation of dying ; apathy, indifference ; tearfulness ; cannot concentrate mind when attempting to read or study, dreams full of care and toil ; screams and sudden starting from sleep ; feels as if she could not draw another breath, tearfulness, piercing. screams ; vexation and grief. (*Apis-m.*). See "Grief-ailments due to".

Will-positive and negative—As if he has two wills—one positive and the other negative ; one to commit murder and the other to do otherwise. (*Anac.*). See "Religious mania" and "Delution".

Wind trouble—*Lyco.* is the leading medicine for flatulence of wind trouble mainly in the lower region. Belching relieves. There is almost constant fermenting of gas going on in the abdomen with a loud croaking and rumbling. The distension is most prominent between 4 and 8 P.M. Relieved also by passing of flatus. (*Lyco.*). Compare *Carbo-veg.* and *Chi.* See also "Distension", "Flatus offensive and gurgling" and "Flatulence-lower region".

Wisdom teeth-effects of cutting—Painful effects of cutting of wisdom tooth. (*Cheiranthus.*). See "Teeth aches".

Witty-but indecent—When a person is witty but indecent. (*Stram.*). See "Mania-amorous or religious".

Women-looking as half man—There is a class of women half man, half woman as regards, their appearance and character to those of gross physique with ugly feature, broad pelvis, meagre limbs. In short a remedy which is for a monster. *Thuja 30.* according to Dr. Nobel.

Worms—(1) Constantly digging or boring at the nose. Pitiful weeping while awakes, starts and screams during sleep. Grinding of teeth ; jumps and jerks during sleep. Restless at night. Does not like to be touched or even looked at by strangers. Frequent swallowing as if something is coming up in the throat. Wants things and throws them away, when offered in anger. The *Cina.* child takes time to be at ease. (*Cina.*).

Compare *Cham.* child who is soothed as soon as is taken up and carried. If *Cina* fails then *Santonine* may be tried. *Cina* and *Santonine* will cure most of cases if given alternately 200 or 1000. (b) If child emaciated and vomits give *Ip.* If this fails then give *Puls.*

(2) (*a*) Pale sunken face and eyes surrounded by blue rings, sluggish disposition, fetid breath and passive fever, patient prefers to lie on stomach. (*Stannum.*) (b) *Silicea* passes worms in large numbers. (c) For terrible itching in anus due to worms which are round and pinworms. (*Teucr.*).

(3) For all kinds of worms. An excellent remedy is *Cuprum Oxydatum nigrum.* It should be given in small doses in alternation with *Nux-vom. 30,* 4 or 5 times a day for 4 to 6 weeks. Another most efficient and least harmful for expelling tape worms is *Cucurbita-pepu* in tincture form. It is also useful for vomiting of pregnancy.

(4) Fat, flaby children who have big head, large abdomen and profusely sweat and eat indigestable thing like chalk, earth, slate, pencils etc. (*Calc-Carb.*). See "Anaemia with thread worms" "Nose-child boring fingers in worms" and "Vomiting with worm symptoms".

Worms-its prevention—See "Chapter V for details".

Worry with fear and nervousness—Worries over trifles ; impulsive thoughts of suicide ; constant state of fear and nervousness. (*Butyric-acid.*) See "Melancholia" and "Sadness"

Wounds-bleeding extracted teeth—Even slight wounds bleed a good deal. Phos. patient has a bleeding tendency. Extracted teeth bleed red blood for hours. (*Phos*). See "Teeth-bleeding after extraction".

Wound-incised and clear cut—If it is done with a sharp instrument or even done with a surgeons' scalpel and the wound is unhealthy and there are stinging and burning pains then *Staphy.* is the remedy. See "Incised wound", "Lacerated wound", "Antiseptic-homoeopathic" and "Cuts-sharp with knife".

Wound-dry infected and inflamed with pricks and cuts—*Hypericum* is useful for pricks with needles and severe cuts with swords, *Hypericum oil* and ointment may be applied to wounds, cuts and abrasions. See "Lacerated wound in nerve area".

Wounds on palms and sentient parts—For wounds on palms and other parts with sentient nerves give *Hyper.* See "Shooting pain from wound".

Wound punctured—*Led.* See also "Punctured wound-inflammatory".

Wound forming pus—Every little wound tends to form pus. (*Sil.*). See "Pus formation" and "Glands-glandular or bony ulceration".

Wounds-sloughing—*Hypericum* is used to very good effect for ulceration and sloughing of wounds. See "Sloughing".

Wound on scalp—Give *Calendula* internally as well as applying locally Aqueous *Calendula* dressing. It will prevent the wounds from becoming septic and healing quickly. *Calendula* internally is to be given in potency 3x,3 or 4 doses about an hour apart.

Wound unhealthy no tendency to heal—A wound will sometimes well up, yawn and show no tendency to heal, looking dry, shining on the edges and remain red, inflamed with burning stinging and tearing pains. This type of wound usually needs *Hypericum.* (b) In cases of infected wound *Echinacea M.T.* may be applied. Internally *Galium-aparine* be given for healthy granulation. See "Ulcers delayed healing". (c) Give alternately *Ars-a. 200* and *Hep. 200* at least 3 doses of each for a week or so for healing the wound. (d) For septic wounds which involve the heart and other parts of body, *Pyrogen* has proved very useful. (e) After operation when gangrene sets in, tissues are not strong enough to reproduce healing inflammation, there is sort of blackness and stitches break open. Give *Sulphuric acid* which is a wonderful remedy in such cases. See "Inflammatory complication in the wound", "Gangrene ulcers" and "Septic infections and its prophylactic and also for surgical cases".

Wrinkles in children forehead—The wrinking of forehead is very characteristic of *Lyco.* in lung diseases. For *Lyco.* the characteristic aggravation time of 4 to 8 P. M. is generally found in this condition. *Lyco.* child has wrinkles on forehead whenever the child cries or is disgusted. The child is irritable usually and when sick wakes up from sleep with great irritability, screaming and kicking. (*Lyco.*). See "irritability of child".

Wrist-its affections like boils, pain and paralysis—(1) *Perisca*.

(2) Boils on wrist ; *Sanicula.*

(3) Pain in wrist-*Homarus, Rhododendron, Plectranthus.*

(4) Paralysis of wrists-*Hippomanes.* See "Tennis elbow".

Wrist-rheumatism—*Actea spicala* ; *Voil-od.* according to symptoms.

Writer's and players cramp and contraction of fingers—(1) *Mag-p.* (b) Involuntary contraction of fingers, partial paralysis of fore-arms, swelling of ankles. Writers cramp. *Argentum metallicum.*

(2) Cramps, trembling of hands. Lack of power of muscular control of forearms. (*Gels.*). See "Cramps".

(3) Weakness of fingers with slight cramping. (*Stram.*).

(4) *Zincum-phos.* to be tried when other remedies fail. See "Rheumatism and gout" and "Fingers dropping things and not holding things properly".

Wry neck (stiff neck)—A painful rheumatic affection caused by exposure in a draught of air. *Acon.* or *Bell.* will often suffice. Should they fail give *Bryonia* in repeated doses. After this give *Rhus-t.* and *Arnica* ; only on rare occasions *Puls.* and *Nux-v.* will be required. See "Stiff neck" and "Head drawn back." (c) (1) of "Rheumatism and "Neck-Sprain"!

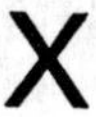

X-Ray-exposure and its bad effects—Give *Fl-ac.* if exposure to radiation is excessive then give *X-ray* 30 or 200. *Rad-b.* 30 or 200 as intercurrent remedies. Compare *Phosphorus* which is best antidote for *Radium-b.* and *Flouric acid* for X-ray.

—: o :—

Y

Yawning without sleep and also after eating—(1) Frequent yawning without sleepiness. (*Acon*.).

(2) Yawning for hours after eating. (*Nux-v.*).

(3) Yawning after sleep. Yawning while eating. (*Ig.*).

(4) Yawning so violent that it threatens to dislocate jaw. (*Rhus-tox.*).

(5) Frequent, with eructations during day. *Sulf.* 3, 2 hrly.

(6) Yawning and sleepiness, stretching after being awake all night. *Chel.*, 3, 2 hrly. "See Jaw carious or cracking with growth, tumour and easy dislocation" and "Sleeplessness due to pain, nervousness and with excessive yawning".

Yellow Saddle across nose with spots on chest, face and abdomen—A yellow saddle across upper part, of the cheek and nose of roundish yellow spots on the face may be cured with *Sepia*. These will be found in a woman along with menstrual trouble. Brown spots on chest, face and abdomen. (*Sep.*). See "Spots brown and yellow saddle on face, on cheeks, face and nose".

—: o :—

CHAPTER II

HOMOEOPATHY IN PAEDIATRICS

Ailments of children and infants have already been sufficiently dealt with under their alphabetical names. It is clearly mentioned there that the disease in question refers to the child and that particular remedy which is suggested is specially meant for a child. The Prescribers therefore should look to that particular diseases under alphabetical group first before looking into this chapter.

For the convenience of the Prescriber I have in this new edition incorporated more than one hundred and fifty 'headings' from the Alphabetical list of general diseases to which the children generally fall prey. This will obviate the necessity of looking into the Alphabetical list of general diseases It will also save the time of Prescriber in finding appropriate medicine for a particular ailment of the child without losing time. For lack of time, the headings of general diseases could not be repeated here.

Abdomen-children—See in the "Alphabetical list of general diseases".

Abdominal enlargement—*Sulf.* 18th attenuation 3 pellets for 4 or 5 weeks to be followed by a similar dose of *Cal-c.*; if accompanied by diarrhoea and general debility, then *Ars-a.* 30, six pellets dissolved in half a tumbler of cooled boiled water and a teaspoonful morning and evening. After this give *Nux-v.* 30 three or 4 pellets dry on tongue and after a week or so give *Sulf.* in a similar manner.

Adenoid growth—See in the "Alphabetical list of general diseases".

Anaemia-in infants—See in the "Alphabetical list of general diseases".

Anger of children—See in the "Alphabetical list of general diseases".

Anus-red rash—Fiery red rash developing about the anus in babies ; fiery old constipation with hard stool. (*Medorrhinum.*)

Appetite of child—See in the "Alphabetical list of general diseases".

Apoplectic condition, body swollen with blackish colour This is caused by long and painful labour. It is not to be confused with Asphyxia; In apoplectic condition the surface of the body seems swollen, the face and the whole body are of violet or rather blackish blue colour ; the muscles do not move. A single dose of *Acon.* 18th attenuation placed on dry tongue changes the unfavourable condition. If no improvement within 10 minutes then use *Tartar emetic* ; but if body is of violet colour then use *Op.*

Apthae or thrush—A disease recognised by small white ulcers on the gums, lips and in the mucous membrane of the mouth. The best remedy for this affection is *Sulphuric acid* six pellets of third attenuation in a half tumbler of cooled boiled water in dessert spoonful every 3 hours. If this fails then *Merc. or Sulf.*, If it also fails then ultimately *Borax. 3x* may be given and also applied with honey locally. See "Ulcers in mouth."

Asphyxia-child not breathing—Generally occurs among feeble children weakened by tedious labour. Breathing and muscular movements wanting. Skin pale. Remove mucus from nostrils. Place 3 pellets of *China 10* on tongue. If no improvement whithin 10 to 15 minutes a similar dose of *Tartarus-emeticus* to be alternated with *China* every 15 minutes. If this fails then give *Lach.* (b) The child with blue asphyxia has no mechanical obstruction but does not breathe. The pulse begins to fail. A dose of *Laur.* will make him breathe and he will then begin to cry. (c) If the child lies limp and cold as if drowned and outward friction does not make him breathe then give him a dose of *Carb-v.* Another effective mean is to hold the childs legs with head down and thump it between the shoulders and also the hip ; then adopt artificial respiration. See "Snuffles stopping nose of infants".

Asphyxia-neonatorum—(Inability of new born to respire.) See "Asphyxia-neonatorum in Alphabetical list of general diseases".

Asthma-children—See in the "Alphabetical list of general diseases".

Asthma-infantile—*Colon-mutable*. "Variable". See "Asthma children".

Assimilation-defective in children—See in the "Alphabetical list of general diseases".

Asphyxia - neonatorum - inability, of new born to respire—See in the "Alphabetical list of general diseases".

Backward children who do not develop properly and look idiotic—See in the "Alphabetical list of general diseases".

Bleeding from navel—See in the "Alphabetical list of general diseases".

Boils—Crops of boils on head growing out of each other's discharges. *Arn. 6* or *Sulf. 30* or *Calc-c. 30, Hep-s 30*; sores behind the ears with thin acid discharge from the ulcer. *Graph. 6*; pimples round the sores. *Cham. 6*. See "Boils" under different heads.

Boils children—See in the "Alphabetical list of general diseases".

Bones rickets—See in the "Alphabetical list of general diseases".

Breast-swelling—If due to improper pressure give *Arnica 30*; otherwise then *Cham. 30.*

Bronchitis—With fever and hoarseness. Give *Acon.*; excessive secretion of mucus suffocating the child with perspiration. *Ip.* See "Bronchitis children" and "Bronchitis infants".

Bronchitis - childern—See in the "Alphabetical list of general diseases".

Bronchitis-infants—See in the "Alphabetical list of general diseases".

Chicken pox—See in the "Alphabetical list of general diseases".

Child-frightened—See in the "Alphabetical list of general diseases".

Child's adenoid—In most cases *Tuber.* alone is sufficient. See "Adenoid growths".

Children-craving for sugar or sweet in excess—Give *Merc. viv: 6x*, or *Nat. Phos. 2x*, 3 times daily and it will dimish such craving.

Children's debilitating diseases—See in the "Alphabetical list of general diseases".

Child-gasping through chord—Child at birth pale, breathless, gasping though the chord still pulsates. (*Antimonium-tart.*).

Children late in learning to talk and walking—See in the "Alphabetical list of general diseases".

Child-not crying when born—Give *Lauròcerasus 6* and it works wonderfully.

Child- unmanageable—See in the "Alphabetical list of general diseases".

Children-vomiting habit—*Iris ver. 6x*, twice daily.

Cholera-infantum—See in the "Alphabetical list of general diseases".

Cholera-infantum sudden and extreme prostration—See in the "Alphabetical list of general diseases".

Cholera infantum worse by milk—See in the "Alphabetical list of general diseases".

Cholera-prophylactic—See in the "Alphabetical list of general diseases".

Cleft-lip—This has to be repaired surgically but to prevent for the deliveries of such a child with such a defect the mother should take *Calc-s. 12*x trituration from 3rd month until the 7th month.

Colic with flatulence and diarrhoea—Can easily be recognised by crying, twisting of the child, drawing of legs and emission of flatulence. *Cham.* is a specific remedy if there is greenish and watery diarrhoea, constant crying, distension of the abdomen and cold feet ; *China* may be given if the colic occurs towards evening with hardness of abdomen, absence of stool or without stool or stool resembling stirred eggs ; *Puls.*, for flatulence ; rumbling, frequent shuddering pale face and no thirst ; *Ip.* for fermented diarrhoea, having a foul smell and the child utterly violent and piercing cries for, frightful colicky children, *Nepeta-cataria* which is a children remedy, is very useful. See "Colic in babies" "Colic of infants" and "Colic of child in dysentery".

Colic in babies—See in the "Alphabetical list of general diseases".

Colic of child in dysentery—See in the "Alphabetical list of general diseases".

Colic infants—See in the "Alphabetical list of general diseases".

Coma in diphtheria, measles, small pox—See in the "Alphabetical list of general diseases".

Constipation also of bottle fed babies—*Bryo. 30 or Nux-v., 30 or Op. 30,* give *1* or *2* pellets, changing the medicine only when no improvement takes place after second dose. For chronic constipation give 3 pellets of *Sulf.* or *Alumina.* If baby has no evacuation then the mother may be administered *Bry.* or *Nux-v.*, or *Ant-c*, or *Op.* according to symptoms. For bottle-fed babies *Podo.* See "Constipation" under its different heads in chapter I of the Book.

Convulsions with fever, diarrhoea and vomiting—Due to fright when the body trembles, the child cries, distension of stool and urine. Give *Op.* : temperature is high and infants body is arched during convulsions. *Verat-v., 3x* : jerking of limbs, twitching of the muscles of the face and eyelids with motion of head from side to side with half closed eyes *Cham.* if the attack comes on without any apparent cause specially every day at the same time or if teething or worms seem to be the cause then give *Ig.* ; if worms are really present then give *Sulf.* and *Cina.* *4* pellets every week alternately ; if due to grips from indigestion then *Nux-v. 6*:when fits are accompanied by nausea, vomiting or diarrhoea *Ip*., when caused by fright, foaming at the mouth and twitching of muscles then *Hyos*. The other medicines *Bell*., *Coff*., *Merc*., *Rheum*, *Stram*, and *Sulf*., as indicated by symptoms. (ii) *Thyrodinum* is also an excellent medicine for convulsions of infants in all cases when there is no temperature. See "Convulsions-during fever of children" and "Convulsions child grinding teeth in chapter I of the Book".

Convulsion during fever of children—See in the "Alphabetical list of general diseases".

Convulsions-child grinding teeth—See in the "Alphabetical list of general diseases".

Convulsions of child with sweat—See in the "Alphabetical list of general diseases".

Coryza with irritating eyes—See in the "Alphabetical list of general diseases".

Convulsions-teething children—See in the "Alphabetical list of general diseases".

Cough child after exposure—See in the "Alphabetical list of general diseases".

Cough child with breathing difficulty—See in the "Alphabetical list of general diseases".

Cough child-grasping larynx—See in the "Alphabetical list of general diseases".

Cough dry of children during sleep—See in the "Alphabeticl list of general diseases".

Cough of children during day only—See in the "Alphabetical list of general diseases".

Croup with loss of voice—Suffocative breathing short and dry Cough with loss of voice *Hep*. should be given followed either by *Hyos*. or *Samb*; *Hep*. in the morning and *Acon*. at night. Dr. Saunder recommends *Calc-p. 12*x and *Kali-s. 12*x alternately every 30 minutes. *Spong*. Then the breathing is rattling. See "Cough" under its different heads.

Crying for a long time without apparent cause—See "Screaming of children"

Crying-propensity—A child develops propensity immediatety after birth and does not cease crying. (*Syphilinum.*).

Croup-loss of voice—See in the "Alphabetical list of general diseases".

Crying baby-not sleeping—Baby not sleeping day and night but cries, frets restless and plays all day, but screaming all night. (*Psorinum.*).

Crying of child-teething trouble—See in the "Alphabetical list of general diseases".

Crying of child before urinating—See in the "Alphabetical list of general diseases".

Crying of child dentition-milk not digested—See in the "Alphabetical list of general diseases".

Cyanosis—Blue discolouration of the infant skin. According Dr. Iyer a drop of the solution of *Sulphur 30* should be given immediately and at an interval of three hours a dose of *Calcarea-carb. 30* be given ; after two months interval a dose of *Digitalis 30* may be followed ; after a fortnight a dose of *Calc.-carb.* 200 may be given.

Deafness with enlarged adenoids—Deafness caused by eustachian catarrh in children with enlarged adenoids. *Agraphis-nutans. 3.* See "No. 12 of Deafness".

Decay of teeth in children—See in the "Alphabetical list of general diseases".

Defected assimilation in children—See in the "Alphabetical list of general diseases".

Deformities—In all deformities of infant a few doses *Sulphur 30* and *Calcarea 30* may be given in alternation at fortnightly intervals. If the deformities of the bone than *Silicea 200* may be given monthly. Dr. Iyer.

Delayed mental development—See in the "Alphabetical list of general diseases".

Delirium muttering in diphtheria, measles, small pox etc.—See in the "Alphabetical list of general diseases".

Dentition-diarrhoea—See in the "Alphabetical list of general diseases"

Dentition-difficulty—See in the "Alphabetical list of general diseases".

Dentition—If there is fever and cold during dentition then give *Ferr-Phos.* 6x for easily coming out of teeth.

Dentition-difficulty pressing gums swollen and teething irregular—See in the "Alphabetical list of general diseases"

Dentition-fever and diarrhoea—See in the "Alphabetical list of general diseases".

Dentition-inability to digest milk and convulsions—See in the "Alphabetical list of general diseases".

Diarrhoea-alternating with constipation—See in the "Alphabetical list of general diseases

Diarrhoea-epidemic in children—Such an epidemic diarrhoea can be prevented by a few doses of *Escherichia-coli.* nosode. Dr. M.G. Blackie.

Diarrhoea of children with changeful colour—See in the "Alphabetical list of general diseases".

Diarrhoea due to various causes—3 globules of *Ip.* 18th attenuation dissolved in half a tumbler of cooled boiled water. Give a dessertful of this solution every 3 hours ; if this fails then give *Rhubarb* if the evacuations and the child's whole body smell sour ; if the child cries a good deal, draws up legs with distension of bowels and frequent emissions of flatulence then give *Cham. ; Ant-c.* if the tongue is coated white or yellow ; *Dulc.* if the diarrhoea arises from cold or from exposure to cold air ; *Bry.* if caused by summer heat : greenish diarrhoea with frequent watery stools high fever, restlessness and sleeplessness *Cuphea* ; *Bell.* if the child sleeps a good deal but the sleep is restless with pale face ; *Sulf.*, *Calc.* or *Nux-m.* in obstinate cases when nothing else will help ; when there is fever with diarrhoea then *Acon.*, when caused by overloading of stomach with nausea and vomiting then *Ip.* ; when due to fright then *Op.* and when with mucous stools with blood, then *Merc-c.* 6. Chronic diarrhoea with vomiting : *Thyroidinum.*

Diarrhoea-during dentition—See in the "Alphabetical list of general diseases".

Diarrhoea-during dentition with green stool and foul order—See in the "Alphabetical list of general diseases".

Diarrhoea-milk disagrees—When milk does not agree and causes diarrhoea accompanied by whitish spots on the lip and sides of tongue then *Nat-c.* is a very good medicine for such diarrhoea. See 'Milk not digested with diarrhoea' and 'Diarrhoea of children causing extreme weakness".

Diarrhoea milk upsets—See in the "Alphabetical list of general diseases".

Diarrhoea of children with changeful colour—See in the "Alphabetical list of general diseases".

Diarrhoea-small pox—See in the "Alphabetical list of general diseases".

Diarrhoea-after vaccination and chronic—See in the "Alphabetical list of general diseases".

Diarrhoea-children offensive—See in the "Alphabetical list of general diseases".

Diarrhoea-frothy of child periodical—See in the "Alphabetical list of general diseases".

Diarrhoea of children sour smelling—See in the "Alphabetical list of general diseases".

Diarrhoea of children (involuntary stool without knowing—See in the "Alphabetical list of general diseases".

Diarrhoea-in children with vomiting milk—See in the "Alphabetical list of general diseases".

Diarrhoea of vomiting in summer starting suddenly—See in the "Alphabetical list of general diseases".

Diarrhoea of children with nausea in summer—See in the "Alphabetical list of general diseases".

Diarrhoea of children after every meal draining the patient and causing weakness—See in the "Alphabetical list of general diseases".

Diphtheria - false membrane—See in the "Alphabetical list of general diseases".

Diphtheria - followed by paralytical condition—See in the "Alphabetical list of general diseases".

Diphtheria - left sided—See in the "Alphabetical list of general diseases".

Diphtheria - preventive—See in the "Alphabetical list of general diseases".

Diphtheria - right sided—See in the "Alphabetical list of general diseases".

Diphtheria-swollen—See in the "Alphabetical list of general diseases".

Diphtheria-when patient progressing—See in the "Alphabetical list of general diseases".

Dreams of dreadful animals and ghosts—See in the "Alphabetical list of general diseases".

Dwarfishness - hands and legs short—See in the "Alphabetical list of general diseases".

Ear discharge offensive in children—See in the "Alphabetical list of general diseases".

Ear deafness- after measles—See in the "Alphabetical list of general diseases".

Earpain - earache of infant—See in the "Alphabetical list of general diseases".

Eating dirty things by children—See in the "Alphabetical list of general diseases".

Ecchymosis caused during delivery—It is an extravasation of blood under the skin as in bruises with swelling caused by instruments during delivery. Bathe head with 10 drops of *Arnica tincture* in half a bucket of water.

Eczema on face—See in the "Alphabetical list of general diseases".

Eczema scalp—See in the "Alphabetical list of general diseases".

Elongation-due to painful labour—Swelling of head due to painful and difficult labour. Wash the child's head with 3 or 4 drops. of *Arn. MT.* in a half tumbler of water and internally give *Rhus-t.*

Emaciation—See in the "Alphabetical list of general diseases".

Emaciation with sweating in head in children—See 'Emaciation' under its different heads in alphabetical list.

Entero-colitis of children—See in the "Alphabetical list of general diseases".

Enuresis-involuntary discharge of urine—Give *Sulf. 200* once weekly and remaining 6 days give *Plantago* and *Equisetum 30* in alternation on the remaining days. See "Wetting the bed".

Epileptic spasms of children—See 'Epilepsy, under its different diseases".

Examination-fussy children—See in the "Alphabetical list of general diseases".

Eyes-sore—(1) If the inflammation is due to exposure of too much light and the eye becomes red. (*Aconite.*).

(2) When there are ulcers along the margins of the eyelid with discharge of yellowish matter. (*Merc.*).

(3) If the eyelids are swollen and discharge pus. (*Argentum Nitricum*).

Face-child creased like monkey and does not grow—See in the "Alphabetical list of general diseases".

Face-creased like monkey—See in the "Alphabetical list of general diseases".

Falling-of rectum—Due to diarrhoea or violent straining when the faeces are hard. The best medicines are *Ig.* or *Nux-v.* to be given at the time when child is passing stool. See "Prolapse of rectum".

Fat patient-tendency of obesity—See in the "Alphabetical list of general diseases".

Fever—Give 3 pellets of *Acon. 18th* attenuation dissolved in cooled boiled water in a half tumbler of water and give a tea spoonful of this solution every 3 hours particularly when the child is hot, restless with quick pulse. See "Fever" and "Dentition" under their different heads.

Fever-child with trembling and startling—See in the "Alphabetical list of general diseases".

Fever-of children with foul smelling stool—See in the "Alphabetical list of general diseases".

Fever-during dentition—See in the "Alphabetical list of general diseases".

Fever-remittent of children drowsy with trembling—See in the "Alphabetical list of general diseases".

Fever-due to vaccination—See in the "Alphabetical list of general diseases".

Feverishness of children—See in the "Alphabetical list of general diseases".

Fidgetiness including constantly moving legs—See in the "Alphabetical list of general diseases".

Flatulence in children—See in the "Alphabetical list of general diseases".

Fracture-green stick of children—See in the "Alphabetical list of general diseases".

Fright-sleep—See in the "Alphabetical list of general diseases".

Gas-in bowels—Poor appetite. Infant unable to digest the fat in normal quantities which causes fat dyspepsia. Infants regurgitate sour milk curds and have a great deal of gas in bowels. Bowels irregular, (*Butyric acid* in potency 30 to 1 M). See "Dyspepsia wind".

Getting blue—*Dig. 3* and if the body is cold then *Ars-a 6*.

Glands in neck—Hardened glands about the neck. (*Silicea*).

Grinding of teeth—See in the "Alphabetical list of general diseases".

Gums-pressing—See in the "Alphabetical list of general diseases".

Habitual vomiting—For habitual vomiting in babies. *Iris*.

Head of child larger—See in the "Alphabetical list of general diseases"

Hernia-congenital of a child—*Calc*., *Carb-b*.

Hernia of navel or groin—Of navel or groin *Nux-v. 6*. and *Sulf. 3* globules alternately every week on the tongue. If not better in 6 weeks, then give *Cocc*. or *Aur*. or *Verat, Lach* or *Sulf-ac*., See "Hernia-infants".

Hernia-infants—See in the "Alphabetical list of general diseases".

Hiccough—*Nux. vomica*. See "Hiccough in "Alphabetical list of general diseases".

Hunger in children-satiety soon—See in the "Alphabetical list of general diseases".

Hunger-emaciated—See in the "Alphabetical list of general diseases".

Hydrocephalus-increase of fluid in skull—See in the "Alphabetical list of general diseases".

Idiocy-physically dwarf—See in the "Alphabetical list of general diseases".

Improperly fed babies—See in the "Alphabetical list of general diseases".

Indigestion of babies due to over-feeding and intolerance of milk—See in the "Alphabetical list of general diseases".

Infantile eczema—Severe eczema face, neck, feet, and hands *Graphites 6*.

Infantile liver—See in the "Alphabetical list of general diseases".

Infants-nose bleed—See in the "Alphabetical list of general diseases".

Infancy-baby dying in infancy and grown up child during early ages—See in the "Alphabetical list of general diseases".

Injury-children tending to form pus—See in the "Alphabetical list of general diseases".

Insomnia—See in the "Alphabetical list of general diseases".

Irritability of child—See in the "Alphabetical list of general diseases".

Involuntary stool in the children :—See in the "Alphabetical list of general diseases".

Jaundice-at birth—(1) Give *Cham.* first for traces of jaundice. If it does not disappear within a week or so then give *Merc-6* and later *China.*

(2) According to Dr. Ghosh *Thyroidine* will bring back the child suffering from jaundice from the jaws of the death. See "Jaundice".

Jaundice-liver hard and painful—See in the "Alphabetical list of general diseases".

Knees—When the knees of child knock against each other when ; walking and he staggers when he tries to walk then give (*Lathyrus.*).

Large-head—*Sulf, Calc., Sil.* and *Merc.* may be tried one after the other separately allowing each medicine to work at least for 3 or 4 weeks. 3 pellets of each medicine may be taken dry on the tongue. Dr. Krichbosem suggests *Mad.* for this defect.

Larynx-in children who grasp larynx—See in the "Alphabetical list of general diseases".

Lice in child's head—See in the "Alphabetical list of general diseases".

Liver-children with hunger—See in the "Alphabetical list of general diseases".

Liver-infantile with spleen—See in the "Alphabetical list of general diseases".

Liver trouble in children with constipation—See in the "Alphabetical list of general diseases".

Marasmus (Emaciation and wasting)—See in the "Alphabetical list of general diseases".

Marasmus—For fatty children give *Calc-c.* and for lean and thin children give *Calc. Phos.* See "Alphabetical list of general diseases".

Marasmus-witn hunger and fever—See in the "Alphabetical list of general diseases".

Marks on the surface on the skin—These may be corrected by *Sulphur 30* followed by a few doses of *Calcarea 30*.

Measles-not coming out properly—See in the "Alphabetical list of general diseases".

Measles-German—See in the "Alphabetical list of general diseases".

Measles-prophylactic—See in the "Alphabetical list of general diseases".

Measles-restlessness—See in the "Alphabetical list of general diseases".

Meconium or first discharge from the bowels—If this first discharge is delayed too long and the child feels uneasy and unrestless, if a few tea spoon full of warm sugar and water will bring this discharge.

Mental development slow and late in children—See in the "Alphabetical list of general diseases".

Milk-causes pain—Child is puny and sickly ; milk causes diarrhoea. Colic, stools green and pain in the stomach (*Mag-carb.*).

Milk-not digested with diarrhoea—See in the "Alphabetical list of general diseases".

Milk crust—It is an eruption of infants having numerous small white pustules with red surface. They first appear on the face and then spread to the cheeks and forehead covering the entire body. They become yellow or dark colour. There is itching and swelling of surrounding parts. The child becomes restless and rubs the affected parts by which the scabs are torn off and the disease is aggravated. If the erruption is red and inflamed then *Aconite* is to be followed by *Rhus-tox.*, *Viola Tricolar* is a principal remedy for such an eczema in child-hood (Dr. Iyer).

Mind confusion on waking—See in the "Alphabetical list of general diseases".

Mouth-ulcers in child's mouth—See in the 'Alphabetical list of general diseases".

Mumps—See in the "Alphabetical list of general diseases".

Mumps changing to testes—See in the "Alphabetical list of general diseases".

Mumps-preventive—See in the "Alphabetical list of general diseases".

Nail-biting—For nail biting in children, *Natrium-mur.* will be very helpful.

Navel—(1) Swollen and painful ; 10 drops of *Calendula M.T.* should be mixed with an ounce of hot water may be applied to the navel or *Calendula* ointment should be rubed gently.

(2) If there is pus in navel then *Silicea 30* should be given.

(3) For swelling with redness and pain give *Beladonna.*

(4) If the pus from the navel is offensive then give. *Ars-alb.* See "Alphabetical list of general diseases".

Navel bleeding—(1) Bleeding from navel of infants (*Abrot*).

(2) Ulceration of navel in new born children. (*Nux-mosch.*). See "Bleeding from Navel".

Neck—When neck is so weak that the child can't hold his head up, and his legs are greatly emaciated then give *Abrot.*

Nephritis-children—See in the "Alphabetical list of general diseases".

Night-terrors—Night terrors in children when no cause can be found and the child cries at night particularly, *Leuticum 200* is almost specific.

Nose-adenoids—See in the "Alphabetical list of general diseases".

Nose-dirty-with fetid discharge—Acrid pus like discharge running down the lips. (*Merc. sol.*)

Nose-children scratching in acute diseases—See in the "Alphabetical list of general diseases".

Nose-child boring fingers in worms—See in the "Alphabetical list of general diseases".

Obesity—See in the "Alphabetical list of general diseases".

Obstinate—See in the "Alphabetical list of general diseases".

Osteogenesis imperfecta (imperfect development of bony tissue ; ossification ; histogenesis)—The child is unable to sit or stand because bones were too weak and had to be strapped ; sweated very profusely around the head and sometime woke up screaming from night terrors. (*Calc-carb.*). in high potency.

Over feeding of children—See in the "Alphabetical list of general diseases".

Paralysis-left arm and leg—See in the "Alphabetical list of general diseases".

Paralysis of lower limbs in infancy—See in the "Alphabetical list of general diseases".

Peralysis of vocal chord—See in the "Alphabetical list of general diseases".

Peevish—See in the "Alphabetical list of general diseases"

Pneumonia of infants—See "Alphabetical list of general diseases".

Pneumonia with constipation or diarrhoea—Rapid breathing, violent thirst and dry cough, *Acon.* ; great difficulty in breathing, sputum of red colour, constipation with great thirst, *Bry.* ; if diarrhoea with thirst then *Ars.* ; dry teasing cough in weak, emaciated boys accompained by irritability on waking, kicking and screaming. *Lyco*. See "Broncho pneumonia".

Pot-bellied children—See in the "Alphabetical list of general diseases".

Prolapse of rectum in child or after child birth—See in the "Alphabetical list of general diseases".

Prostration-child drowsy—See in the "Alphabetical list of general diseases".

Pulling of penis by children—See in the "Alphabetical list of general diseases".

Rapid-growing toddler—To strengthen the child who is growing rapidly give *Ferr-p. 12x* three times a day for a week or two.

Rash-on child's body—See in the "Alphabetical list of general diseases".

Rectum-prolapse with or without diarrhoea—See in the "Alphabetical list of general diseases".

Retention of urine after labour and of infants—See "Alphabetical list of general diseases".

Rickets including curvature or malformation of bone—See in the "Alphabetical list of general diseases".

Ringworm on face and chest—See in the "Alphabetical list of general diseases".

Ring-worm on the scalp—See in the "Alphabetical list of general diseases".

Ring-worm on the scalp of children extending to face, neck, and eye—See in the "Alphabetical list of general diseases".

Screaming of children—See in the "Alphabetical list of general diseases".

Sleep-child gnashing teeth—See in the "Alphabetical list of general diseases".

Sleep-unrefreshing and child awakes at night playing—See in the "Alphabetical list of general diseases".

Slow development with sweating head—See in the "Alphabetical list of general diseases".

Small-pox—See small-pox under different heads in the "Alphabetical list of general diseases".

Snuffle-stuffing nose of infants—See in the "Alphabetical list of general diseases".

Sore throat—Give *Aconite, Belladonna,* and *Merc.* according to Symptoms.

Sore throat tendency—Tendency to sore throat and enlarged glands ; the child being dull and backward. (*Baryta-carb.*)

Spasms-of child during sleep—See in the "Alphabetical list of general diseases".

Spine-deviation—Spine deviation is due to deficient ossification, owing to which the bones do not offer sufficient resistance to the muscles and hence they deviate from the true direction. The following medicines have successfully removed the trouble : *Ammovicum*; *Calc*., *Hep*., *Lyco*., *Merc*., *Phos*., *Plumb*, *Sil*.

Spontneous dislocation of femur thigh bone—The child limps as one limb is shorter than the other. It is most troublesome malady which causes incurable disorganisation in the joints. The best remedies are *Sulf*. and *Calc*. If the child simply limps without complaining of pains in the thighs and symptoms are not fully developed then give *Merc*. and *Bell*. alternately. First give 5 pellets of *Merc*. dry on the tongue and after 3 or 4 doses a similar dose of *Bell*. may be given. This alternate use should he continued at least for a fortnight unless improvement is perceived. If they fail then *Rhus*. 18th attenuation—5 pellets every 4 days may be tried until improvement is noticed. After this, discontinue the use of medicine until the improvement ceases to progress. If *Rhus-t*. does not show any improvement, the *Sulf*. may be given in the way described above.

Stammering—*Merc*. may be given in the beginning to be followed by *Bell*. 4 pellets dry on tongue. A prolonged use of *Hyos*. 3 may also be useful. See "Stammering" in the "Alphabetical list of general diseases".

Startling of child in fever—See in the "Alphabetical list of general diseases".

Stealing habit and tendency—(a) Abnormal children whose moral sense has never been developed and who lie and steal, fit for mental hospital. (*Op*.). (b) Cruel habit in children is cured by *Anac*. See "Stealing" in the "Alphabetical list of general diseases".

Stool involuntry in children and craving to swallow it—See in the "Alphabetical list of general diseases"

Stoppage of nose of new born—See in the "Alphabetical list of general diseases".

Stupor of child with red face—See in the "Alphabetical list of general diseases".

Stupor sudden in eruptive fevers—See in the "Alphabetical list of general diseases".

Styes-on lower lids—See "Alphabetical list of general diseases of Styes" under its different heads.

Sucking of thumb—See in the "Alphabetical list of general diseases".

Sucking-disinclination to take to breast and vomits milk See in the "Alphabetical list of general diseases".

Stuttering (A hesitation in speech due to an inability to enunciate the syllables without repeated efforts)—its treatment should be started immediately. *Belladonna,* followed later by *Merc.* or *Platina or Euphrasia* to be followed later by *Sulpher.*

Suddenness of disease in children with redness, swelling and pain—See in the "Alphabetical list of general diseases".

Summer complaints-of children during dentition and milk causing diarrhoea—See in the "Alphabetical list of general diseases".

Swallowing by child See "Alphabetical list of general diseases".

Swallowing and boring finger in nose by a child See in the "Alphabetical list of general diseases".

Sweat-on head and hands in sleep—See in the "Alphabetical list of general diseases"

Teeth decaying in children—See in the "Alphabetical list of general diseases".

Tear duct in eye obstructed—*Thiosinaminum* can clear this at once.

Teeth gnashing by a child—See in the "Alphabetical list of general diseases"

Teeth-grinding by child—See in the "Alphabetical list of general diseases".

Teething children spasm—See in the "Alphabetical list of general diseases".

Teething-children-distress—See "Alphabetical list of general diseases".

Teething troubles incidental to dentition—See in the "Alphabetical list of general diseases".

Terror of injection—For fear of injection give *Phos. C.M.* before injection.

Terror of child for medical examination—Unreasonable terror in a child for medical examination or with strangers. (*Tuber.*). See "Dread and Fright" in the "Alphabetical list of general diseases"

Thirst absence in fever with cold feet See in the "Alphabetical list of general diseases".

Toxemia intestinal of children—See in the "Alphabetical list of general diseases".

Trouble of migraine—For migraine in children give *Carbolic acid 12*.

Typhoid-of children See "Typhoid under its different heads in the "Alphabetical list of general diseases"

Ulcer corneal with lachrymation and pain in eye brow See in the "Alphabetical list of general diseases"

Under development in children See in the "Alphabetical list of general diseases".

Under-weight child If the child is skinny, underweight, wrinkled and old looking give a dose of *Sulph.*

Undescended testicle In undescended testicles where surgery is recommended, Dr. Wadia has found very good results with *Aur-mur.*, or *Aur. mur. nat.*

Urine-child crying—See in the "Alphabetical list of general diseases"

Urine-milky in children—See in the "Alphabetical list of general diseases".

Urine-retention in infants See in the "Alphabetical list of general diseases".

Vaccination—See in the "Alphabetical list of general diseases".

Vaccination-child unwell since—See in the "Alphabetical list of general diseases".

Vaccination-discomfort from pustules—See in the "Alphabetical list of general diseases".

Vaccination fever See in the "Alphabetical list of general diseases".

Vomiting habitual Vomiting sour bloody, biliary and nausea. Profuse flow of saliva (*Iris-versi.*).

Vomiting of milk in curds with constipation or diarrhoea The mother being dyspeptic the child vomits milk in curds : *Puls.*, when the child is constipated and the vomiting of foul smell : *Nux-v.*, when the child vomits milk as soon as taken and vomit consists of curds then *Aethusia.*, when there is diarrhoea with such vomiting then *Calc-c.*, in chronic cases *Kreos* ; if this fails then *Verat-a.* Compare *Valeriana* when child vomits curdled milk in large lumps after nursing and also compare *Cuphea Visco* which is useful when the child vomits milk on account of hyper accidity of the stomach with frequent, green, watery acid stool which are dysenteric also.

Wakeful and restless child See in the "Alphabetical list of general diseases".

Walking delayed in fat children See in the "Alphabetical list of general diseases".

Walking delayed in thin childern See in the "Alphabetical list of general diseases".

Weakness in rickety children See in the "Alphabetical list of general diseases".

Weak children walking with irritability—See in the "Alphabetical list of general diseases"

Weak-puny child—Rachitic child with big belly, limbs shruken, eyes sunken, large head. The child takes enough nourishment but there is want of assimilation. Growing weaker *Silicea 30*th and upwards. (Dr. Nash)

Weeping child pretending—See in the "Alphabetical list of general diseases".

Weeping without tears child pretending—The child who pretends to weep but without tears then the surest remedy is *Staphy 30* or *200*. See "Weeping tendency indifference" in the Alphabetical list of general diseases".

Weeping—(1) When the child sleeps in the day and weeps at night (*Jalap*)

(2) When the child weeps in the day and sleeps in the night (*Lyco*.)

(3) When the child weeps day and night (*Psorinum*.)

(Dr. Y. Singh)

Wetting the bed due to different causes Children who sleep on belly, of mild disposition, who are inclined to weep, urine offensive ; *Puls*. Children who are obstinate and get angry easily and put their hands or arms above their heads ; *Nux-v*. ; children who have catarrh or cold, whose hands feel easily cold who are prone to cold whenever they go out and who don't like to get up early in the morning *Ferr*. ; children who suffer from boils or swelled neck or whose wounds heal slowly then *Sil* ; children who wet the bed during first sleep, whose urine is acrid and who pass urine while coughing, walking or sneezing : *Caust* ; children whose urine is sticky and who put their arms under or above head and turn over upon belly *Coloc*. ; *Sil*. 30th attenuation 3-pellets dry on the tongue every week until the patient is better. See "Wetting the bed" in the "Alphabetical list of general diseases".

Wetting bladder distended—See in the "Alphabetical list of general diseases"

Whooping cough See it under its different heads in "Alphabetical list of general diseases"

Whooping cough child shakes and vomiting--See in the "Alphabetical list of general diseases".

Worms--(1) See in the "Alphabetical list of general diseases".

(2) For round worms give 10 drops of *Chanopodium* oil mixed with hot water. T.D.S. According to Dr. Yudvir Singh Tape worms are killed and expelled by the following mixture.

(*i*) *Potassium iodide 35* grains.

(*ii*) *Iodine 4* grains.

(*iii*) Distilled water one ounce, give 10 drops of this mixture in a little water T.D.S.

He further suggests that to destroy all sorts of worms give *Lyco. 30*, for two days, then *Verat. A. 12* for four days followed by *Ipecac. 6* for a week. Two doses daily should be given.

Wrinkles-in children forehead See in the "Alphabetical list of general diseases".

——:o:——

CHAPTER III

TREATMENT OF PET ANIMALS

Homoeopathic medicines have been found equally effective in treating pet animals. You may not have veterinary surgeon at hand at times and in his absence the pet may be undergoing great suffering and agony.

Below are given a very few common ordinary troubles from which such pets generally suffer and which can be diagnosed easily on objective symptoms. For serious troubles such as of feet and mouth etc. you may have to take the aid of veterinary surgeon for they can't be diagnosed easily.

Brain affections in Horses—Pupils contracted, teeth clinched, tongue protruding, restlessness, head forced back, stupor frequent changing of position, biting and kicking, furious, rages, desire to escape, with tears. Give *Belladonna 200* in water two teaspoonful every 15 minutes or longer until improvement takes place. (J.S. Mathur)

Cholera of fowls—Dissolve 20 to 30 globules of *Ars. Iod.* in water and give one teaspoonful at interval of 1 to 3 hours according to the severity of symptoms.

Colic in horses and cows—When the animal has over-fed itself and there is flatulent distension of abdomen as if it were to explode, it is also tympanatic, fullness and continuous rumbling, urine suppressed, or scanty. Give *Colchium 200.* At least 3 days at intervals. Compare *Magnesium Phos.* and *Colocynth*, which are useful for wind colic.

According to Dr. Cushing pour a little water in the horse's ear and the pain will disappear promptly.

Cough in horses when ascending or after exertion—Slightest incline causes cough, foam about mouth, breathing with grumbling sound and violent cough. *Nux-vomica 1M.* Compare *Hepar-sulph.* if the horse coughs after exertion as a result of dust in the hay. (Dr. Skinner)

Cows-tendency for abortion and its prevention -*Thyroidinum 30,* just after the heat and a dose later after she is covered will prevent abortion and bring her to full term.

Diarrhoea Cadaverous smelling stools which are watery *Carb-v. 30* and *Ars. 30* alternately every 2 hours. For acute diarrhoea give *Acon. 30* every one hour, if this fails then give *Puls. 30* and *Nux-v. 30* alternately every 2 hours. If still the diarrhoea persists then *Phos. 30* every 3 hours. For chronic diarrhoea *Sulf., Calc-c.* and *Podo.* each of 30 potencies are suggested.

Diarrhoea-in running horses--During acute exercise give *Rheum off.* (Hurndall)

Diarrhoea in racing dogs- Diarrhoea with a state of great prostration. The stools are putrid and during sleep they are involuntary, are accompanied by eructations and flatus smelling sulphurated hydrogen. Give *Arnica-montana.*

Diarrhoea-in fowls *Ars. 30* one dose daily until it stops.

Digestive disorders No appetite, goes near food, smells it but comes back without touching or taking it, constipation, barks or howls, restless or disturbed. No stool. *Nux-v. 30* three times a day. If due to unwholesome meat or diet *Puls. 30* three times a day. If due to eating decayed food or animal matter or other dirty stuff, then *Ars-a. 30* three times a day.

Distemper—It is an infectious disease affecting the dogs up to the age of 2 years. A discharge of thick mucus from the reddish eyes and sore nostrils, loss of appetite, the dog coughs a good deal, lies down most of the time, staggers about, drags hind legs, falls down frequently, is costive and is finally paralysed all. Has diarrhoea and convulsions. *Bell., Cocc., Kali-c* and *Rhus-tox.*

Dogs-belated in intelligence Could not be house-broken, drops urine and faeces on the carpets instead of whinning the door as a house broken dog will soon learn to do, crawls under furniture when any stranger comes. Give *Baryta-carb.* for sometime with interruptions. (Kent)

Ears—Swelling, thick, brown deposit or watery and purulent discharge. Give *Bell. 30* twice daily. Apply *Hydrastis M.T.* on ears twice daily.

Eczema-ear of dogs Eczema round or even in the ears, respond well to *Sulphur* in 12th or 30th potency.

Eyes Inflamed, red, sore, watering, aversion to light and purulent discharge. *Euphrasia-tincture 10* drops in an ounce of boiled water internally and bathe eyes with *Ruta M.T. 20* drops in half tumbler of boiled water.

Fetigue in horses—After hard days, work or in hunting. Give a few doses of *Arnica* internally and rub the tendons with a cloth dipped in *Arnica* lotion.

Fractures—Whatever may be character of the injury whether contusion, sprain, strain, dislocation or fracture if it is due to mechanical violence give *Arnica* internally and apply *M.T. Arnica* dissolved in water as a lotion.

Hair falling—Falling of hair can be stopped by giving. *Arsenic.*

Lameness of horses—*Rhus tox.*

Milk cows—(a) To increase the milk of cows give *Phytolacca 3x* alternating with *Asafoetida.*

(b) Some cows draw up milk when they are milked. Give *Belladonna 4x* one hour before milking. Stop it when the animal becomes normal in giving milk.

Mouth—Simple mouth trouble : If by opening the mouth ulcers are found, gums and tongue seem inflamed then they indicate derangement of digestion Give *Ars-30.* or *Silicea 30* or *Lycopodium 30.* three times a day. The mouth should be washed with *Calendula M.T.* lotion at least 3 times a day.

Mouth-diseases and foot diseases prevention—*Kali-iod.* against mouth and foot diseases in animals.

Panting of dogs—When a dog pants on the least exertion then give *Bryonia* three times a day. **(Anshutz)**

Prophylactic for mouth and foot diseases *Borax*.

Racing dogs When a dog has exhaustion after a hard day's racing. Give *Arnica* every hour internally at least 6 doses and externally rub *Arnica* lotion

Red Mange Infestation of the skin of mammals by mange mites which burrow into the epidermal layer of the skin; characterised by multiple lesions in the skin with vesiculation and papule formation accompanied by intense itching. And baldness of rather large patches entirely denuded of hair being a prominent symptom. Give *Acid fluoricum*, one drop in a powder from every morning for 6 days. Miss a day and likewise resume again until 24 powders of the drug for 24 days are taken in order to ensure complete recovery.

(Edward Thomas)

Respiration with fever Breathlessness. The normal rectum temperature of dogs is 101.4 but can be higher after exercise or excitement. Fever 103 or 105 with cough. restlessness, malaise; no appetite, no normal evacuation. *Aconite 30, Bryonia 30, China 30*. Prepare a solution of each separately with 20 drops of each in one ounce of boiled water and give a table spoonful of each alternately every 2 hours.

Skin diseases—They are very common in dogs and prognosis is unfavourable. Hair falls, skin is red and inflamed, and eruptions. Scratching, rubbing against tree, wall, table or chair or any thing which comes in its way. *Mercurious 200* or *Sulf.* 200 alternately at least 4 doses per day. The potency of Sulf. may be increased to 1 M. if no improvement is noticed. *M.T. Hydrastis* mixed in a cup of water may be applied locally compresses of *Calendula M.T.* may be employed as an alternative method.

Sore Hoofs—Of horses, sheeps and dogs etc. Give *Graphites* internally in water and apply it in vaseline externally.

Udder caking of—Swollen indurated udders, intensely hot, painful and sensitive when not a drop of milk could be drawn. Give a few doses of *Phytolacca*. (Dr. Kent)

Wounds—Lacerated wounds, broken knees. *Hypericum* to be shaken up with water in bottle with spraying arrangement and knees to be constantly sprayed and not to be covered. (Tyler.)

CHAPTER IV

HOMOEOPATHY IN SURGERY

Homoeopathy in surgery largely involves the use of *Arnica; Rhus-tox, Hypericum, Ledum, Staphysagria, Calc-carb., Strontium* and *Ruta.*

These medicines are related to surgery, injuries and after effects of injuries including surgical operations.

The treatment of inflammation and abcesses including internal inflammation has already been given under alphabetical diseases.

For the bruised, black and blue sore appearance of an injured part with intense soreness round about it, there is nothing like *Arnica.* But *Arnica* corresponds specially to the acute *stage* until the soreness and bruised condition disappear from the part injured or from the whole body.

The strains of the muscles and tendons, *Arnica* is unable to remove always, and usually *Rhus-tox* follows *Arnica* well in removing the pain and weakness of the tendons and muscles. But the characteristic symptom of *Rhus-Tox* of removal of pain by motion must be present. Warm application usually helps the *Rhus-tox* cases. Strom and wet weather will increase the pain where *Rhus-tox* is indicated.

When *Rhus-tox* has done its work and has removed the painful condition the weakness may still persist in the muscles which can be then removed by *Calc-carb.*

In these three above mentioned medicines (*Arnica, Rhus-Tox* and *Calc Carb.*) we have a series usually to be used in case of contusion or bruises where skin in any way has been ruptured.

We have quite a different set of remedies for injuries involving laceration and puncture of the skin and underlying tissues. Here we have two prime remedies *Hypericum* and *Ledum* which must be considered when there is a punctured injury to a nerve which later on takes inflammatory condition. Here instead of muscles, bones and blood-vessels being contuised by the injury where the series : *Arnica, Rhus Tox* and *Calc.* is the remedy, the nerves are the injured parts where *Hypericum* or *Ledum* are indicated. When nerve-rich areas as the finger ends or the ends are injured on a nail which has been crushed between hammer above and the bone below and nerve shows signs of inflammation and the pain can be traced up to the nerve, *Hypericum* is the remedy under these conditions.

Hence, all the injuries, *e.g.* punctured, incised, contused and lacerated, as a matter of fact all painful wounds can be cured with medicine without any active surgical intervention.

A wound will sometime swell up, yawn and show no tendency to heal, looking dry, shining on the edges and remain red, inflamed with burning, stinging and tearing pains. This type of wound usually needs *Hypericum.*

The *tetanus* is the commonest complication of all injuries.

Hypericum and *Ledum* are the main remedies for preventing tetanus in Homoeopathy. If after a wound in a nerve-rich area the pain extends up the nerve and where one suspects tetanus complications to appear *Hypericum* is the remedy to be given at once after the injury as well as if any of signs of tetanus are appearing.

It is the remedy for any type of ascending neuritis due to an injury in the nerve.

If there is an old scar which is injured or bruised by coming into contact with something hard and starts burning and stinging with the pain running along the course of the nerve use *Hypericum.*

A painful cicatrix with pain shooting up towards the centre of the body along the course of the nerve always requires *Hypericum.*

Everybody knows that *Arnica* is the only remedy to be used in the injuries ; but the few people know that its sphere of application is very limited. *Arnica* is good only in the first stage of injury *where much bruising has been done, and the pain is intense but diffused and not running along the nerve course as in Hypericum.*

Arnica is an excellent remedy for the first hours for bruised conditions after an injury and shock of an injury. *Arnica* will always remove the shock. Here *Arnica* is the routine remedy. Usually we are against application of *Arnica* locally on the wounded parts, it does no good medicinally, it may be on the contrary that it may cause greater irritations to the injured part.

Ledum is another supreme remedy but it comes in very often as a *preventive medicine of tetanus.*

It is a preventive medicine when an accident happens to the ends to the fingers which are rich in nerves or if a patient steps on a nail or a splinter sticks under the finger nail or into the foot or any other sensitive part give a dose of *Ledum*. This will always prevent the tetanus.

Hence all punctured wounds or rat-bites, dog-bites, cat-bites, etc. are made safe by use of *Ledum* from its subsequent complication of tetanus or any other form of septic condition. *Ledum* will prevent not only the subsequent inflammatory complication but will also prevent the shooting pains that naturally come when nerves are involved in the injury.

There will be no trouble subsequently if *Ledum* can be given at once.

If the pain is dull aching in the part that was injured *Ledum* is still the remedy but *if the pain shoots from the wound up the nerve it is Hypericum.*

Hence, if a person steps on a tack during the day and he feels pain where the tack (short nail) went in and the pain may be violent that he cannot keep still *Ledum*, will most probably prevent further trouble.

But if the trouble continues after *Ledum* and the shooting pain along the nerve starts, the case calls for *Hypericum*. But in all these cases before the typical symptoms of *Hypericum* start *i.e.*, extension of pain along the course of nerve, *Ledum must be used as a preventive.*

Ledum is the *preventive of tetanus* whereas *Hypericum* is the remedy for the tetanus *after the initial symptoms have started.* But, if the wound is not a punctured one but is a lacerated wound involving parts full of small nerves, sentient (having sensation) nerves, give *Hypericum at once and do not start with Ledum.* Do not waste your time with *Arnica* either.

Hence the golden rule is, in a punctured wound give *Ledum* as a preventive and in a lacerated wound in a nerve rich area give *Hypericum* both for prevention as well as for cure of tetanic or inflammatory consequences. Of course, if there is inflammatory cnosequences with formation of pus etc., these must be treated according to the symptom present of such complications

For bruises of bones, cartilages, tendons, insertion of tendons and about joints *Ruta* is better than any other remedy. *Ruta for lingering sore* bruised places on bones, in joints and upon cartilages which have been injured.

Now, let us come to the *injuries to the spine.*

Hypericum usually is the remedy to be used. Injuries of coccyx from a fall are the most trouble-some injuries on the spine at times.

Usually very little symptoms appear at the beginning and hence many times we have not the descriptive pains shooting up the spine or down the extremities and there may be only soreness on pressure on the spot. Here also *Hypericum* is the remedy. Many women sustain injuries of coccyx during labour and the soreness may remain for years thereafter. This little injury may make her quite nervous or even hysterical. This can be cured by *Hypericum.* In inflammatory condition of the lower part of the cord which feels sore after an injury to the spine causing aches etc., these have been cured even after years by remedies like *carbo Animalis, Silicea and Thuja etc.*

Hypericum also relates to injuries of spine higher up. Suppose a person falls down the stair-case and he strikes his back against a step causing great soreness of the spine. *Here neither Rhus Tox nor Arnica will help.*

Hypericum must be given at once to prevent any complications due to inflammatory changes either to the spine or the cord. Of course, later tendencies such as drawings aud rheumatic symptoms might occur and may call for *Rhus Tox* and finally *Calcarea*. *But Hypericum is the immediate remedy.* Painfulness of the back on rising from a seat which is the result of old hurt is often cured by *Rhux Tox* followed if necessary by *Calc.* But *Hypericum* must be given *immediately after the injury of the spine* to take cere of the condition of the fibres and cord and meninges (membrane and especially one of the brain or spinal cord). Meningial injuries of the back are sometimes very troublesome and may linger very long. But the cure of such a condition will be simpler if *Hypericum has been given at the very outset.*

Persons who have been injured in the spine or about the coccyx may linger for years with symptoms that would require many remedies.

.They of course, will require remedies according to the symptoms then present. But for the action of the nerves sheaths and meninges with tearing, burning and stinging pain along the nerves *Hypericum is the remedy.*

Now, there is another type of wound that we want to discuss here. It is the clear-cut incised wound made with a sharp instrument ; even if it is done with the surgeon's scalpal. If the abdominal cavity has been opened and the walls of the abdomen take an unhealthy look and there are stinging burning pain *Staphysagria* is the remedy that will make the granulations healthy. *Staphysagria* is also the remedy where sphincter has been stretched surgically.

As a matter of fact *Staphysagria* is the natural antidote of all stretches. When the urethra has been stretched for removing a stone or by use of bougies and catheter, dilatation of cervix has been done or the anal sphincter for treatment of piles etc. *Staphysagria* will remove the subsequent difficulties.

These stretches after surgical operation may cause great distress with painfulness and symptoms of collapse causing cold sweat etc. *These are also removable by staphysagria.*

Where coldness, congestion of the head and receding tearing pain occur from stretching sphincter or tearing of a sensitive part takes place *Staphysagria* is the remedy *Stretching and tearing are the key words here.*

Collapse symptoms after a surgical operation with great prostration, coldness of body, slow oozing of the blood, cold breath and profuse perspiration will require *Strontium Carb.*

It relieves a shock at once and the patient gets warm and comfortable. Don't think of *Carbo. Veg.* under these circumstances.

Carbo Veg is the physician's remedy for similar symptoms where as *Strontium Carb. is the surgeon's remedy.*

Lastly, as an appendix to this chapter we must say something about antidotes to the *Chloroform* symptoms *Phosphorus is the natural antidote to Chloroform.* It will stop chloroform vomiting. But we have sometime to antidote chloroform for the sake of making other drugs act.

Pains and aches after an operation will not be removed by corresponding medicines unless chloroform is antidoted by *Phosphorus.*

Morphine effects on sensitive person awful eructations retching and vomiting and there is nothing to vomit. Give *Chammomilla* which will stop these within a few minutes and is practically the only remedy that stops the vomiting from morphine.

Ad Ledum.

Convulsions with tetanic rigidity where injured parts are icy cold and where spasms begin in the wounded part, *Ledum* is the remedy.

Ad Hypericum

Convulsions with wounds in such parts as soles, fingers or palms need *Hypericum.* (*Belladonna,* Ledum).

To summarise this chapter we may say that for *Punctured wounds* as preventive give *Ledum.*

For punctured and lacerated wounds of sentient nerve study *Hypericum.*

Where tetanus threatening with coldness of the parts give Ledum.

For *wounds of palms* and other parts with sentient nerves, give *Hypericum.*

For bruises give *Arnica.*

For open laceration and cut with much damaged skin apply *Calendula* and also give *Calendula* internally.

Ad Staphysagria

We have mentioned the *Staphysagria* is the medicine for sharp cuts with knife as well as for stretch of sphincter. To this later category also belongs the urinary trouble of young nervous women after marriage where the painful urging to urinate becomes very troublesome to the young women. *Staphysagria* is the most comforting to the young wife under such circumstances.

Ad Arnica

Arnica is very suitable for sore, bruised condition of the body. Therefore it is an important remedy in injuries, bruises and shock from injury.

Arnica will very often take the soreness out of the *sprained joints. Black and blue appearances* of the sprained parts will go away in a surprisingly short time. Weakness and tenderness remaining in the joints and tendons after the use of *Arnica* are usually removed by *Rhus Tox* and subsequently with *Calc.*

In insolated cases the pain which persists may require such remedies as *Causticum* or *Staphysagria.*

Constant dribbing of urine after labour which is due to the paralytic condition of sphincter, vescae (bladder) on account of contusion is always relieved by *Arnica*.

Causticum : Contracture of muscles and tendons either due to an injury or a burn or any septic process is usually removed by *Causticum* if given high. Paralytic *weakness of the bladder after a women has gone through strenuous labour causing retention of urine afterwards* is miraculously removed by *Causticum*.

: o

CHAPTER V

PAIN KILLERS, PREVENTIVES AND PROPHYLACTICS

A patient suffering from various types of pains, always wants instant relief from it and avoid its recurrence if Physicians so approached is unable to cure it downright as the course of disease whether chronic or acute may take sometime for its eradication.

For facility of Physician and save his time in searching different headings, I have placed them in this chapter for ready reference along with significant symptoms. Such a physician will be rendering a great suffering patient if he is able to relieve such pain.

Pains of different types in different parts of body

Pain—in abdomen (a) Abdomen distended from flatulence ; great pain, bowels loose. Tincture *Dioscorea. 3x* ten drops 3 times a day. (b) Pain in lower side of abdomen, violent stoops over when he stands on feet. (*Sulf. 6*). See under 'A' "Abdomen" under different heads in the list of general diseases.

Pain—in abdomen after eating decayed food—See "Abdomen pains after decayed food," and also "Abdomen colic distress" under 'A' in the list of general diseases.

Pain—in abdomen when cavity opened causing burning pains—Abdominal cavity opened and its wall take an unhealthy look causing burning and stinging pain. *Staphysagria* which is also a remedy where sphincter has been surgically stretched will be effective in this case as well.

Pain—in abdomen causing spasms.—*Mag. Phos* may be given in hot water. It is very helpful as a great spasmodic remedy.

Pain—in abdomen burning causing also pain in the region of third rib—See under 'P' Pain in abdomen burning causing pain in the region of 3rd rib.

Pain—in abdomen due to colic—See "Colic disorders" in the list of general diseases.

Pain—in albunaria (inflammation of kidney)—See "Inflammation of Kidney" under 'I' in the list of general diseases.

Pains—Ague (Malaria) pains in gouts—(a) *Cinchona officinalis.* (b) Pains in bones, limbs and soreness *Eup. perf.* (c) Pains in knees, ankles, wrists and hypogastrium *Pod.* (Dr. W. Boericke). See also "Malaria" in the list of general diseases and also "Ague".

Pain—After pains in delivery—See "After pains" under 'A' in the list of general diseases.

Pain—Amputation neuritis—See "Amputation neuritis" under 'A' in the list of general diseases.

Pain—in angina pectoris, palpitation and pain—See "Angina pectoris, palpitation and pain" under 'A' in the list of general diseases.

Pain—in anus abscess—See "Anus abscess" in the list of general diseases.

Pain—in anus fissure—See "Anus fissure" under 'A' in the list of general diseases.

Pain—in anus—See "Rectum aches" under 'R' in the list of general diseases.

Pain—in appendicitis being septic—See "Appendicitis" also "Septic" in the list of general diseases under 'A'

Pain—in apoplectic condition in which body is swollen with blackish colour—See under chapter II regarding "Homoeopathy in Paediatrics" heading "Apoplectic condition body swollen with blackish colour" under A'

Pain—in appendicitis and to prevent its recurring attacks of pain and necrosis—(a) *Psorinum 200* or C.M. will prevent its such attacks. (b) *Cadmium iodat* will prevent necrosis in appendicitis.

Pain—in arthritis—Acute pain (a) *Ferrum Phos. 3x* three tablets in a tea spoonful of hot water every 2 hours in alternation with *Natrum Sulf 6* three tablets every 3 hours and *Tinature Urtica Urens* T.D.S (3 doses per day). (b) *Arthritis deformans* (chronic rheumatoid particularly of fingers). Fingers stuff and painful, cutting pains in the joint if the hand is closed. *Tr. Caullophyllum 3*x drops every 3 hours. *Phosphat* of *Ammonia 3*x in alternation with *Tr. Thuja 3***x** ten drops every 3 hours.

Pain—Asthma—(1) Pain through lower left chest, expectoration thick, must sit up in bed when coughing. *Natrum Sulf. 6*x, 3 tablets every 2 hours. (2) For paroxys of asthma *Tr. Gelsimium* in alternation with *Tr. Sambucus Ngra* every 15 minutes. (3) In chronic bronchitis, when there is scanty, tenacious and plenty muscus but can not raise it. *Tr. Sanguinaria* every 2 hours. See Asthma attack" and "Bronchitis" under this respective heads in the list of general diseases :

Pain—in backache—(1) Lameness and siffness, pain in thighs and loins when urinating. *Tr. Berb-Vulg 5* drops every 2 hours. (2) The patient may have to set up when turning over. *Nux. V.* three tablets 3 times per day. (3) Backache affecting hips and sacrum worse walking and stooping. *Tr. Aesculus* three drops · T.D.S. (4) *Tr. Tellurium 30*x twice a day cures pain in upper part of column and back. Please see "Backaches" under their different heads under 'B' in the general list of diseases as they are of various natures and types due to different causes and choose the drug which tallies with the symptoms of the patient under your treatment.

Pain—Backache—due to different causes—See "Backache due to different causes" in the list of general diseases.

Pain—Backache—due to old hurt—See "Back-old hurt" in the list of general diseases under 'B'.

Pain—Backache—scarcely able to use or walk—See under 'B' in the list of general diseases.

Pain—Backache—Patient prone to backache—See under 'B' in the list of general diseases.

Pain—Backache—with stiff spine—See under 'B' in the list of general diseases.

Pain—Backache—due to wetting feet, over—lifting—See under 'B' in the list of general diseases.

Pain—Backache—violent due to sudden kink—See "Backache violent" in the list of general diseases.

Pain—Backaching—due to different causes—See "Backaching due to different causes" in the list of general diseases under 'B'.

Pain—Back pain during menstruation—See "Back pain in the back during menstruation" under 'B' in the list of general diseases.

Pain—in Bee stings See under 'B' in the list of general diseases.

Pain—Bilious colic pain—(a) Griping pain, twisting and doubling up relieved by standing. *Tr. Dioscorea Villosa* one dran. in a little water one table spoonful may be given every one hour. (Dr. W. Boericke). (b) Cutting pain relieved by pressure against table or bed. *Tr. Colocymth 3x* five drops in 4 ounces of water every 16 minutes. See "Colic", "Gallstone Colic" "Renal Colic" "Bladder with involuntary Urine" and "Bladder-irritation frequent urination" under their different respective heads.

Pain—in Bladder See "Bladder" in the list of general diseases.

Pain—in Blisters in feet about nails—See under 'B' in the list of general diseases.

Pain—Blisters in mouth extremely painful—See under 'B' in the list of general diseases.

Pain—in Boils—See under 'B' in the list of general diseases

Pain—in Boils in Crops See under 'B' in the list of general diseases.

Pain—Boils painful covered by scab—See "Sore painful covered by a scab" under 'S' in the list of general diseases.

Pain—Boils throbbing, swelling and painful—See under 'B' in the list of general diseases.

Pain—Bonesache—See under 'B' in the list of general diseases.

Pain—Bone pains due to injury or fracture—See under 'B' in the list of general diseases.

Pain—Bones-swelling of fingers and knees—See under 'B' in the list of general diseases.

Pain—Boring with acute pain in the back—This needs *Mag-Phos. 3x* three tablets 2 hourly.

Pain—in Brain concussions—See under 'B' in the list of general diseases.

Pain—in Brain—It may be from a fall or blow to head, patient may be unconcious and vomitting *Tr. Belladonna* five drops in a half glass of water may be given hourly.

Pain—in the breast—(a) If the pain is in both breasts with scanty urine—*Conium*. (b) If the pain is in right breast then give *Sangunaria*. (c) If the pain is in left breast then give *Cimic*.

Pain—Breast in menses with abcess—See "Breast pain with abscess" in the list of general diseases.

Pain—in Bright diseases—(inflammation of kidney with face puffed up—See under 'B' in the list of general diseases.

Pain—in Bruises—See "Bruises" of different nature and types under 'B' in the list of general diseases.

Pain—in Bowels—See "Bowel pains" under 'B' in the list of general diseases.

Pain—Bowels-intussusception—Slipping of one part of the intestine into another—See under 'B' in the list of general diseases.

Pain—in Burns and scalds—See under 'B' in the list of general diseases.

Pain—in Bubo—See under 'B' in the list of general diseases.

Pain—Burning and swelling of eyelids—Weary pain while reading. Rheumatic inflammation of eyelids. Eyes red, hot and painful, opacities of cornea. The following lotion for such eyes is very useful for various troubles of eyes. To be dropped in both the eyes 3 times a day.

(1) *Tr. Euphrasia*—20 drops.

(2) *Tr. Ruta*—20 drops.

(3) *Tr. Zincum*—20 drops.

(4) *Tr. Boric acid*—20 drops.

All mixed together in Damask Rose or distilled water one ounce.

Pain—Calculus in kidney with agonising pain—See this heading under 'C' in the list of general diseases.

Pain—Calculus-stone in liver or gall bladder—See this heading under 'C' in the list of general diseases.

Pain—Carbuncles with pain and discharge—See this heading under 'C' in the list of general diseases. It is requested that all headings of "Carbuncles" should be looked into.

Pain—Carbuncles—hot compresses for it—See this heading under 'C' in the list of general diseases.

Pain—Cartilages-bruised and injured—See this heading under 'C' in the list of general diseases.

Pain—Changing position giving relief—See under 'C' in the list of general diseases.

Pain—in Changeable symptoms—See under 'C' in the list of general diseases.

Pain—in Catheter fever and avoiding its pains—See under 'C' in the list of general diseases.

Pain—in Cicatrix—See "Cicatrix" under 'C' in the list of general diseases.

Pain—in Circumcision—See "Circumcision" under 'C' in the list of general diseases.

Pain—in Chilblains—Pains for it—See 'C' portion of "Chilblains" in the list of general diseases. (Dr. Boericke).

Pain—in Climacteric headache—See "Headache at Climacteric" under 'H' in the list of general diseases. (Note : Since headaches are of different types due to various causes so it is suggested that all "headaches" under 'H' should be studied.)

Pain—in Coccyx due to a fall—(a) *Tr. & Hypericum. 6x* ten drops in a little water 4 times a day. (b) If the coccyx is extremely sensitive to pressure and aches all the times then *Tr. Xanthoxylum 1x* ten drops 4 times a day.

Pain—in Coccyx (the last bone of spine) injured—See under 'C' in the list of general diseases.

Pain—Colic pains in bounds—See under 'C' in the list of general diseases.

Pain—Colic with flatulence diarrhoea—See this heading in Chapter 2. See also several headings of "Colic" in this chapter as well as colics under 'C' in the list of general diseases.

Pain—in colic general with sharp pain and flatulence—See under 'C' in the list of general diseases.

Pain—in colic of infants See under 'C' in the list of general diseases.

Pain—Colic pains at intervals—See under 'C' in the list of general diseases.

Pain—Colic renal (pertaining to kidney) difficult urination with stone in kidney—See this heading under 'C' in the list of general diseases.

Pain—Colic renal with general pain in right kidney—See this heading under 'C' in the list of general diseases.

Pain—Colic renal stone in kidney and its prevention—See under 'C' in the list of general diseases.

Pain—Colitis with pain and mucus—See portion 'B' of "Colitis and its treatment" under 'C' in the list of general diseases.

Pain—in Concussion of brain or spine—See this heading under 'C' in the list of general diseases.

Pain—in Congestion of lungs—See this heading under 'C' in the list of general diseases.

Pain—in Conjunctivitis—See—this heading under 'C' also different troubles of this type under 'C'. Note: For eye lotion see "pain burning and swelling of eyelids" in the list of general diseases.

Pain—Corns inflamed or burning—See under 'C' in the list of general diseases.

Pain—Corns on soles—See under 'C' in the list of general diseases.

Pain—Coronary thrombosis with fever and palpitation See this heading under 'C' in the list of general diseases.

Pain—Crushing of nerve—See this heading under 'C' in the list of general diseases.

Pain—Cystitis inflammation of urinary bladder with burning pain in urethra and frequent urination—See this heading under 'C' in the list of general diseases.

Pain—Cystitis with acute pain—(a) Cutting pain in urethra and bladder while urinating. *Tr. Cantharis* 15 drops in half a cup of water a tea spoonful after every hour. (b) In chronic cystitis with itching in urethra, burning and scalding urine, and passing of bloody and ropy mucus. *Tr Chimphilla umbelatta 20* drops in half glass of water—a tea spoonful every half an hour. (Dr. W. Boericke).

Pain—Cystits—Severe dull pain but at the same time very acute and feeling of fullness of bladder not relieved by urinating. Painful urinating. Sharp and cutting pain in urethra. Mucus in urine. *Tr. Equestrium* 6th potency in hot water. A tea spoonful of this hot water every half an hour. Compare *Epigea Repens* and *Terebinth*.

Pain—in Dentition—See 'Dentition difficulty' in the list of general diseases.

Pain—in Dislocation—See 'Dislocation' in the list of general diseases.

Pain—Dull at the injured part—If the pain is dull in the part that has been injured then *Ledum* is still the remedy. But if the pain shoots to nerve, then *Hyper.*

Pain—'Dysmenorrhoea'—Irregular with leucorrhoea with pain (difficult or painful menstruation). See this heading under 'D' in the list of general diseases. *Note*: It is important that all headings of "Dysmenorrhoea" due to different causes should be studied.

Pain—in Dysuria (painful urination)—See under 'D' in the list of general diseases.

Pain—in Ear—See "Earache" "Ear boils on it", "Ear inflammation spreading during cold" and other different headings under "Ear" in the list of general diseases and "Otitis" (inflammation of ear) under 'O'.

Pain—Ear pains of various types—See under 'E' in the list of general diseases.

Pain—Excoriation—(Abrasion of position of skin) due to walking—*Agnus castus*.

Pain—Eye strain with headache—See under 'E' in the list of general diseases.

Pain—Reading causing pain—See under 'E' in the list of general diseases.

Pain—Eye troubles—and troubles after operation—See under 'E' "Eye troubles and troubles after operation" in the list of general diseases.

Pain—Eyes watering with redness and pain—See under 'E' in the list of general diseases.

Pain—Fatigue corporeal or mental—Causing pains, headache or confusion. See under 'F' in the list of general diseases.

Pain—Felous (whitlow) and its aborting—*Calc. Sulf.* 12x will abort whitlow and boils and their resulting pains.

Pain—Fever colicky with sweat—See under 'F' in the list of general diseases.

Pain—Fever glandular due to swollen and enlarged tonsils See under 'F' in the list of general diseases.

Pain—Fever puerperal—See under 'F' in the list of general diseases.

Pain—Finger ends or toe ends or nails injured causing pains—See under 'F' in the list of general diseases.

Pain—Fissure—See under 'F' No. 2 of fissure in the list of general diseases.

Pain—Flying pains—See under 'F' this heading in the list of general diseases.

Pain—Flying gout pains—See this heading under 'F' in the list of general diseases.

Pain—Fracture—compound getting suppurated—See this heading under 'F' in the list of general diseases.

Pain—Fracture—no union, swelling pain, sepsis and compound fracture—See this heading under 'F' in the list of general diseases.

Pain—Gall bladder colic which forming stone—*Tr. Hydrastis* ten drops in a table spoonful of hot water every half an hour. See "Gall stone, colic and prevention of formation of stone" under 'G' in the list of general diseases.

N.B.—Since there are different types of gall stone colics so the entire list of gall stone colics should be studied.

Pain—Gall stone shifting causing pain—See this heading under 'G' in the list of general diseases.

Pain—Gastro-enteritis (Intestinal inflammation acute or chronic) in the stomach—See this heading under 'G' in the list of general diseases. Please look into other "Gastric troubles" in the same list.

Pain—Gastric ulcer and arresting its formation—See this heading under 'G' in the list of general diseases.

Pain—Glands of ear swollen—See this heading under in the list of general diseases. See other troubles of "Ear" under 'E' in the same list.

Pain—Glaucoma and its checking—See this heading under 'G' in the list of general diseases.

Pain—Glossitis (inflammation of tongue)—See this heading under 'G' in the list of general diseases.

Pain—Gonorrhoea(Chronic and painful)—See this heading under 'G' in the list of general diseases.

Pain—Gonorrhoea painful with inflammation—See this heading under list of general diseases under 'G'.

Pain—Gout acute pain—See this heading under 'G' in the list of general diseases.

Pain—Gout in different parts including arthritis deformans—See this heading under 'G' in the list of general diseases.

Pain—Gout pains flying—See this heading under 'G' in the list of general diseases.

Pain—Gout in long bones—See this heading under 'G' in the list of general diseases.

Pain—Gout of toe and heels—See this heading under 'G' in the list of general diseases.

Pain—Granulations after operation of abdomen—See this heading under 'G' in the list of general diseases.

Pain—in Groin—(a) Pain in the right groin. The patient feels light headache and staggers when trying to walk. *Iris factissima*. (b) Old abscess in left groin with pain. *Silica 30* T.D.S.

Pain—in Gums—Apply Gum Paint as mentioned under 'G' in the list of general diseases.

Pain—in Gum boil throbbing pain—See "Gum-boil throbbing" in the list of general diseases under 'G'.

Pain—in Hands—When hands swell and are painful *Apis Mel. 3x* fifteen drops in a half glass of water out of which a tea spoonful may be given every hour.

Pain—in Headache congestive—(a) Pain in fore-head and temples increasing gradually at noon of malarial origin. Worse on left side, falling asleep. Inability to remain standing *Chininum sulf.* 3rd trituration. (b) Congestion of brain and headache following great loss of blood *Ferrum Pyrophosph* 12. (Dr. Boericke).

Pain—in Headache migraine—Dull heavy pressing pain starting in the occiput and extending to front region, worse in in the morning, chiefly on left side. For pain in the eyeballs. Caused by overstrain. For dilution *Onosmodium 3x* dilution fifteen drops in half glass of water, a tea spoonful may be given hourly. See "Headache migraine" under 'H' in the list of general disease.

Pain—Headache sick—The pain is the fore-head chiefly over the eyes, eyeballs painful, vomiting, bitter matter with Jaundice. Tr. *Chionanthus 2x*. Five drops every hour during the headache. (Dr. E.J. Jones)

N.B. : There are different types of headaches due to various causes. The Prescriber is requested to go through the book comprising headaches and to choose the right medicine according to mental and physical symptoms and in keeping with the miasmatic principle of the patient before him. Above I have generally but briefly mentioned in this Chapter which do not find place in the book.

Pain—Heart palpitation and pain—See this heading under H' in the list of general diseases.

Pain—Heaviness of the head, throbbing carotids and burning in the ears—(a) Tr. *Verat Viride 1x* five drops in a little water may be given hourly. (b) Sensation of burning in the forehead and eyeballs. Patient desires to be on a high pillow. Tr. *Gelsemium 3x* thirty drops of it be mixed in 4 ounces of water out of which a tea spoonful be given hourly. (c) Morning headache. It begins on waking. *Codenium 2*x. Three tablets every half an hour until relief. (d) Headache nervous caused by over exertion, worse on left side. Constant desire to expectorate. Tr. *Epiphegus Orabanche 30*. Five drops of tincture in a little water be given every 15 minutes

Pain—Heels and Heels painful—See both these heading under 'H' in the list of general diseases.

Pain—in Hips and small of back—Tr. *Staphysagria 3*x. Five drops of tincture in a little water be given every 2 hours. (a) If the pain is in left hip then give Tr. *Stramonium 3*x ten drops in a little water every hour. (b) If the pain happens to be in the right hip then give Tr. *Lilium Tigrinum 3*x ten drops every hour in a little water.

Pain—in Hepatitis-liver enlarged—See this heading under 'H' in the list of general diseases.

Pain—in Hernia—See "Hernia pain" under 'H' in the list of general diseases.

Pain—in Herpes Zoster—See this heading under 'H' in the list of general diseases.

Pain—in Hydrocephalus-increase of fluid in the skull—See No. 3 of this Heading under 'H' in the list of general diseases.

Pain—Hypersensitiveness of pain—See "Hypersensitiveness" under 'H' in the list of general diseases.

Pain—in Hypochondrium (The upper lateral region of abdomen below the lower ribs) the hepatic region—See this heading under 'H' in the list of general diseases.

Pain—Ill effects of stretches—See under 'I' this heading in the list of general diseases.

Pain—Injury to finger causing inflammation in arm-pit—See this heading under 'I' in the list of general diseases.

Pain—in Injuries at different parts of body—See "Injury" under 'I' in the list of general diseases.

Pain—in the Incised wound made with a sharp instrument—*Staphysagria*.

Pain—in Intense itching—See "Itching intense" under 'I' in the list of general diseases.

Pain—in Jar (shaking causing upleasant vibration and shock)—See under 'I' in the list of general diseases.

Pain—Jaundice liver hard and painful—See this heading under 'G' in the list of general diseases.

Pain—Jaw carious or cracking with growth of tumour and easy dislocation—See this heading under 'G' in the list of general diseases.

Pain—in Jaw swelling—See this heading under 'J' in the list of general diseases.

Pain—in Joints small like fingers, toes, ankles and wrists Severe drawing, erratic pain and stiffness in small joints. Cutting pains on closing hands. Tr. *Caulophylum* 3rd attenuation. (Dr. W. Boericke)

Pain—in Kidney-cessation of its function—See this heading under 'K' in the list of general diseases.

Pain—Labour pain causing blindness—See this heading under 'L' in the list of general diseases.

Pains—Labour pains-distinction between true pains and false pains—See this heading under 'L' in the list of general diseases.

Pain—Spasmodic in child birth—See this heading under 'L' in the list of general diseases.

Pain—Labour pains ineffectual—See this heading under 'L' in the list of general diseases.

Pain—Labour pains irregular—See this heading under 'L' in list of general diseases.

Pain—Lightning character—Pain is coming and going and is usually of cutting and piercing variety. Relieved by warmth and pressure. Such pains can be found along the nerves of muscles in the stomach or abdomen or in the pelvic region *i e.* uterus—*Mag Phos*. See Neuralgia pain in nerve lightning like under 'N' in the list of general diseases.

Pain—Leucorrhea old with pain in hips—See this heading under 'L' in the list of general diseases.

Pain—in Lumbago—See "Pain—Backache" in this chapter and also under 'L' in the list of general diseases.

Pain—in Mastoid abscess—See under 'M' this heading in the list of general diseases.

Pain—in Menopause rheumatism—See this heading under 'M' in the list of general diseases.

Pain—in Meninges-membrane of spinal cord injuries—See this heading under 'M' in the list of general diseases.

Pain—Menorrhagia—excessive menstruation—See this heading under 'M' in the list of general diseases.

Pain—in Menstruation colic—(a) For such a pain give *Chamomilla* 20 drops in half a cup of water-one tea spoonful every hour. (b) In such a colic when belching of gas does not lessen the pain give, *Phosphate of Magnesia* 10 drops in hot water—a teaspoonful every 15 minutes. See—"Menstruation with colic and diarrhoea" and "Vomiting" under 'M' in the list of general diseases.

Pain—in Muco—entritis (inflammation of mucous coat of intestine)—Severe pain drawing the patient frantic with a painful, muddy and thick discharge. *Kali bich. 3x* two grains every 2 hours

Pain—in Myelitis (inflammation of spinal cord)—See this heading under 'M' in the list of general diseases.

Pain—in Nail of finger hurt—See this under heading 'N' in the list of general diseases.

Pain—in Nails blue, falling, pains and soft nails—See this heading under 'N' in the list of general diseases.

Pain—in Nail-fingers and abnormal out-growth of finger and toe nails—See this heading under 'N' in the list of general diseases.

Pain—in Navel—See this heading "Navel" under Chapter 2 under 'N'.

Pain—in Nail—mis-shapen, due to tight shoes—See this heading under 'N' in the list of general diseases.

Pain—in the Neck—In the right side of neck and down the right arm. *Picrate of iron 3x* three tablets every 3 hours. See "Neck" under its different headings in the list of general diseases under 'N'.

Pain—in Nephritis (inflammation of Kidney with acute pain)—According to Dr. Jones Tr. *Gelsemium* is an ideal remedy for this pain. It reduces the albumin in the urine and has permanent soothing influence in the nerves of entire urinary tract in a most satisfactory manner.

Pain—in Nerve injury—See this heading under 'N' in the list of general diseases.

Pain—in Nerve sheath (the connective tissue covering vessels, muscles, nerve tendons, etc.) Spine—See this heading under 'N' in the list of general diseases.

Pain—in Nerve of face due to exposure—See Neuralgia of face pain in nerve due to exposure. See this heading under 'N' in the list of general diseases.

Pain—in Nerve of face being crampy relieved by pressure See 'Neuralgia' of face pain crampy, pressure relieves, under 'N' in the list of general diseases.

Pain—in Nerve—all left sided—See Neuralgia—of left side (pain in nerve). See this heading under 'N' in the list of general diseases.

Pain—Neuralgia pain in nerves lightning like—See "Neuralgia pains in nerves lightning like" this heading under 'N' in the list of general diseases.

Pain—Neuralgia pains in anywhere in the body relief by pressure—See this heading under 'N' in the list of general diseases.

Pain—Neuralgic pains with numbness—See this heading under 'N' in the list of general diseases.

Pain—Neuralgic pains right sided—See "Neuralgia of right sided" in the list of general diseases under 'N'.

Pain—Neuralgia nerve pain with trembling of limbs—See this heading in the list of general diseases.

Pain—Neuralgia (Severe paroxysmal pain along the course of nerve) of eye—See "Neuralgia eye" heading in the list of general diseases.

Pain—Neutritis (inflammation of nerve) in retrobulbon (behind the eye ball) area—See "Neutritis (inflammation of nerve behind the eye-ball)" under 'TV' in the list of general diseases.

Pain—Neutritis in stump (inflammation of nerve)—See this heading under 'N' in the list of general diseases.

Pain—in Nose-diseased bone of nose red tipped and pain See this heading under 'N' in the list of general diseases.

Pain—Numbness of head with pain—See this heading under 'N' in the list of general diseases.

Pain—Operation causing pain and aches—(a) Pain and aches after operation will not be relieved unless Chloroform is antidoted by *Phosphorus*. (b) Awful eructations retching and vomiting due to Morphine effect after operation will stop if *Chamomilla* is given.

Pain—in Orchitis (inflammation of testicles)—See under 'O' this heading in the list of general diseases.

Pain—in Orchitis (inflammation of testicles) due to mumps pain transferred to testicles—See under 'O' in the list of general diseases.

Pain—in Otalgia (ear-ache)—(a) Dr. E.G. Jones recommends to take a table spoonful of hot water, not too hot, sprinkle some powder of black pepper into hot water, then pour some or all of it into the ear in which there is pain. It will stop pain when other remedies have failed. (b) For mastoid (Beast shaped), as the mastoid process of the (temporal bone) disease give Tr. *Capsicum* 6x, ten drops every half an hour. See "Mastoid" under its different heads in the list of general diseases.

Pain—in Otitis (inflammation of ear)—See this heading under 'O' in the list of general diseases.

Pain—in Ovary of right side—See this under 'O' in the list of general diseases.

Pain—in Ovary with sweating—See this under 'O' in the list of general diseases.

Pain—Ovarian Colic (right sided)—See this under 'O' in the list of general diseases.

Pain—due to overlifting, mis-step and strains—See this heading in the list of general diseases under 'O'.

Pain—in Oxaluria and infantile colic. (Calcium, Oxalats and Phosphates in urine)—See this heading under 'O' in the list of general diseases.

Pain—in Palpitation from noise and heart failure of the aged—See this heading under 'P' in the list of general diseases.

Pain—in Pancreatic troubles—See this heading under 'P' in the list of general diseases.

Pain—Piles throbbing in both types—See this heading under 'P' in the list of general diseases.

Pain—in Pelvis—See under 'P' in the list of general diseases.

Pain—Piles with pain and ulcerated pimples—See this under 'P' in the list of general diseases.

Pain—in Pluerisy (inflammation of the pleura)—Give Tr. *Asclepias Tuberosa* fifteen drops every hour. See "Pleurisy dry and wet" under 'P' in the list of general diseases.

Pain—Post operative gas pain—*China.*

Pain—in Proctalgia (Pain in anus)—Smarting pain in rectum after stool with burning sensation. *Nitric Acid 3x* fifteen drops in half a glass of water every 2 hours. See "Anus" and "Rectum" under their respective heads in the general list of diseases.

Pain—Prostration—with burning pain at mid-night—See this heading in the list of general diseases.

Pain—in the Punctured wound—*Ledum* will prevent not only the subsequent inflammatory complications in the wound but also prevent the shooting pains that naturally come when nerves are involved in the injury. Apply *Ledum M.T. Lotion* externally. See also "Wound punctured" in the list of general diseases under 'W'.

Pain—in Quinsy-acute inflammation of the tonsil with pain—See under 'Q' in the list of general diseases.

Pain—Relief in pain by shaking the part or hanging it down—(a) If the pains are better by shaking the part then give *Fl-Ac* (b) If the pains and sufferings are better by letting the limb hang, *Conium m* See "Leg hanging down unbearable" under 'L' in the list of general diseases.

Pain—in Rat bites with shooting pain—(a) See under 'R' in the list of general diseases. (b) For external application of such bites including scorpion bites apply M.T. of *Ledum pal.*

Pain—in Rash causing a good deal of itching—See under 'R' in the list of general diseases.

Pain—in Renal colic—For pain in such a colic give *Dioscorea* sixty drops in 2 ounces of hot water every 15 minutes until relief. See also "Renal Colic-severe pain caused by efforts to pass stones locked up in ureter" under 'R' in the list of general diseases.

Pain—Rectum-aches—See in the list of general diseases under 'R'.

Pain—Renal (pertaining to Kidney) Colic severe pain caused by efforts to pass a stone locked up in urater and suppression of urine—See this heading under 'R' in the list of general diseases.

Pain—in Retina detachment, haemorrhage and its re-absorption and apoplexy of retina—See this heading under 'R' in the list of general diseases.

Pain—in Retina Hyperasthesia (exaggerated sensibility of nerve filaments)—See this heading under 'R' in list of general diseases.

Pain—in Rheumatism—(a) The pains that rendered the patient wild with numbness of affected parts. *Cham. 3x* ten drops every hour. (b) Lameness, stiffness, with getting up in the morning after rest. *Rhus-tox 2x.* ten drops every hour.

(c) In case of rheumatism when the painful parts are puffed up and swollen *Apoc Cann.* twenty drops in water—a tea spoonful every hour. See "Rheumatism general" in different parts of body under 'R' in the general list of diseases.

Pain—in Rheumatism aggravated in damp wheather—See this heading under 'R' in the list of general diseases.

Pain—in Rheumatism which are spreading over other parts of body—See "Rheumatism" pains spreading in the list of general diseases under 'R'.

Pain—in Rheumatism with swelling—See "Rheumatism pain and swelling" under 'R' in the list of general diseases.

Pain—in Rheumatism with cold extremities—See under 'R' in the list of general diseases.

Pain—in Rheumatic dysmenorrhea—See this heading under 'R' in the list of general diseases.

Pain--in Rheumatic fever—See this heading under 'R' in the list of general diseases.

Pain—in Rheumatic heart—See this heading under 'R' in the list of general diseases.

Pain—Rheumatic—the patient being over sensitive to pain and of peevish temper—See this under 'R' in the list of general diseases.

Pain—in Rheumatism in different parts of body and its line of treatment—See under 'R' in the list of general diseases.

Pain—in Rheumatism in joints aggravated in bad weather See under 'R' in the list of general diseases.

Pain—in Rheumatism of any type without taking the totality of symptoms—See this heading under 'R' in the list of general diseases.

Pain—in Rheumatism in upper limbs and also in lower limbs—See this under 'R' in the list of general diseases.

Pain—in Rheumatic pains spreading at neck and extremities—See this under 'R' in the list of general diseases.

Pain—in Rheumatism with swelling in all joints—See this heading under 'R' in the list of general diseases.

Pain—Rheumatic inflammation—See this under 'R' in the list of general diseases.

Pain—in Right arm--Shooting pain in right arm and shoulder with stiffness to raise arm. Such pains leave the heart and appear in arm. *Phyt*. See portion VII of "Angina pectoris, palpitation and pain".

Pain—in Sciatica—See under 'S' in the list of general diseases.

Pain—in Small Joints—Pains in fingers, toes, ankles and wrists of rheumatic nature. They increase on movements swelling of joints from slight fatigue. Pain in Knees. Wrist swollen red, worse any motion. Lame feeling in arms. *Actea Spicata*. (Dr. W. Boericke, M.D.)

Pain—Preventing patient to sleep due to nervousness and yawning—(a) The patient oversensitive to pain and also of peerish temper. *Cham.* will often put the patient to sleep if along with this sleeplessness over-sensitiveness to pain and peevishtemper are present and for children desire to be carried are present—(*Cham.*). (b) For excessive yawning-*Ig.*

Pain—in Shock of operation collapse and resulting in various troubles—See this heading under 'S' in the list of general diseases.

Pain—Shooting from wound—See this heading under 'S' in the list of general diseases.

Pain—Shooting in eye-brows, head, jaw and ears—See this heading under 'S' in the list of general diseases.

Pain—in Sore throat with pain in mouth and fever—See this heading under 'S' in the list of general diseases. Please look into different kinds of "Sore throat" and "Tonsillitis" in the same list.

Pain—in Sore throat with raw mouth and swollen glands See under 'S' in the list of general diseases.

Pain—in Sore throat with redness and throbbing pain—See under 'S' in the list of general diseases.

Pain—in Sprained joints with black—blue appearances—See "Sprained joints sore and ankles" under 'S' in the list of general diseases.

Pain—in Spondilitis (inflammation of one or more vartibrae with complete stiffness of back and lower part of neck)—Inflammation of vartebrae with pain. *Lachnanthus 200* one dose to be taken in the morning and 1 dose in the evening. From next day *Mag Phos 30x, Calc. Flour 30x, Kali Mur 30x,* four tablets of each should be taken alternately and this process to be continued for some time until relief.

P ain—in Stiff neck—Rheumatic pains in stiff neck, and back, for *Cimicifuga 18x* ten drops once an hour See under 'N' "Neck Stiff" in the list of general diseases.

Pain—Striking against a stair—case or such like thing when a person falls from a high place—A person falls from height or strikes against a wall etc. causing great soreness and pain in spine then *Hypericum* is to be given frequently.

Pain—in stomach relief by eating—(a) Such a pain is sometimes relieved by giving *Anac.* (b) For pain in stomach give *Bell. 200* in water every five minutes. (c) If the patient feels pain on empty stomach *Anac.* 30 four times daily. (d) If the pains occur after eating *Abies N* 30 four times a day.

Pain—Stone in Kidney causing such pain—See under 'K' "Kidney stone in" in the list of general diseases.

Pain—Stretches and catheter insertion causing great distress with pain—When the urethra has been stretched for removing a stone or by use of bougies and catheter, dilation of cervix has been done or anal sphincter for treatment of piles etc. *Staphysagria* will remove the subsequent difficulties. The stretches after surgical operation may cause great distress with painfulness and symptoms of collapse causing cold sweat etc. These are also removable by *Staphy.* (b) A dose of *Aconite* given shortly before passing a catheter will prevent pain if there is any difficulty (Dr. Clarke). See "Catheter fever and avoiding its pain in the list of general diseases under 'C'.

Pain—Stomach pain after eating—Severe pain in stomach always comes after eating, distressing constriction just above the pit of stomach. Total loss of appetite in the morning but great desire for food at noon and night. *Abies N.* (Dr. W. Boericke).

Pain—in Sun-burn—When exposed parts to Sun's rays become painful, bathe them with succus (a vegetable juice, of *Calendula*). It may be mixed with little water.

Pain—in Sun headache—Sun headache due to exposure to Sunheat. The patient is distressed with a headache every time he is exposed to Sun's heat for sometime—*Lach.* See "Headache due to exposure to Sun" under 'H' in the list of general diseases.

Pain—in Sun stroke (apoplexy) with headache, laboured respiration and its prevention—(a) Pale face, fixed eyes, white tongue along with laboured respiration. The temperature is high and often times there is unconsciousness. Severe headache jaws clenched—Involuntary eructations (belching). *Glonine* every five minutes—later larger intervals. (b) For Sun stroke *Nat. m.* is an excellent medicine. (c) Much flushing of heat ; tremor of limbs, surging of blood to head and face ; throbbing throughout whole body—*Amyl. n.* (d) Face flushed, blood shot eyes. Throbbing headache with high fevers—*Bell.* (e) For prevention of Sun stroke *Gelesimum* is an excellent medicine. See "Apoplexy" in the list of general diseases.

Pain—in Sun stroke with pain and mental sluggishness—(1) Growing pain in the back of head extending to spine. Mental sluggishness. Throbbing in the back of neck. Bowels constipated—*Nat Sulf.* (2) Breathing difficult or obstructed and face bloated—*Opium.* (3) For Collapse—*Camphor.* (4) For Nausea and Vomiting—*Silicea* and *Theridion.*

Pain—Swelling of abdomen with pain extending to lower limbs—See this heading under 'S' in the list of general diseases.

Pain—in Swelling of joints spreading over large surface—Rheumatic pains spread over large surface of neck, loins and extremities better by motion, limbs stiff. Pain along ulnar nerve. Tenderness about knee joint, loss of power in fore-arms and fingers, crawling sensation in the tips of fingers—*Rhus Tox.* See "Swelling with inflamed glands" under 'S' in the list of general diseases.

Pain—in Glands with swelling—See under 'S' in the list of general diseases.

Pain—with Swelling in localised inflammation—See "Swlling localised" under 'S' in the list of general diseases.

Pain—Swelling with pus formation with pain—See Swelling with pus formation under 'S' in the list of general diseases.

Pain—in Synovitis (inflammation of Synovial membrane) inflammation of knee joints—See under 'S' in the list of general diseases.

Pain—Syphilis pain in bone—See under 'S' in the list of general diseases.

Pain—Syphilitic iritis eyes with ulcers, discharge, inflammation with stiching pains—See this heading under 'S' in the list of general diseases.

Pain—Cutting pain in Tachycardia (Abnormal rapidity of cardiac action)—See under 'T' in the list of general diseases.

Pain—Tearing and stretches after operation—See under 'T' in the list of general diseases.

Pain—in terrible disease of cancer—See under 'T' in the list of general diseases and also read about the further cancer at the following parts of body :

(a) Cancer Gastric—Acidum Carb. and *Ornithogalum*.

(b) Cancer Pancreas—*Calc. arsen.*

(c) Cancer Liver—*Cholesterinurm.*

(d) Concer of Carcinoma—*Arsen brom.* (Dr. Blackwood).

Pain—in Teethaches of various types and also due to false teeth—See under 'T' this heading in the list of general diseases.

Pain—in Teeth bleeding after extraction and nervousness See under 'T' in the list of general diseases.

Pain—Colicky in teething children distress—See under 'T' in the list of general diseases.

Pain—in Teething troubles incidental to dentetion being very painful and difficult—See under 'T' in the list of general diseases.

Pain—in Tendons and muscles due to their weakness with pain—See under 'T' in the list of general diseases.

Pain—in Tenesmus of rectum and bladder with pain in dysentery—See this heading under 'T' in the list of general diseases.

Pain—in Testicles and its different troubles—See under 'T' in the list of general diseases.

Pain—in Throat inflammation spreading and glands swollen—See under 'T' in the list of general diseases.

Pain—in sore throat, sore with pain and fever—See under 'T' in the list of general diseases.

Pain—in Thrombosis (a blood clot in the heart) including hemiplegia and cardiac asthma—See this heading under 'T' in the list of general diseases.

Pain—in Tibia—(a) See this under 'T' in the list of general diseases.

(b) Pain of aching type in lame feeling in the sharp anterior margin of tibia. *Lach.*

Pain—in Tongue cancer and hard nodules—(1) Ulcer of tongue with indurated edges. Power of speech lost but intelligence in tact *Kali. cyanatum.*

(2) Stony hard nodules. *Calcarea-fluorica.*

(a) small aggregation of cells (*i.e.* nodes) *Aurum-Met.*

Pain—Tongue maped and painfully cracked—See under 'T' in the list of general diseases.

Pain—in Tongue papilla (Conic eminence) bleeding and cracked—See under 'T' in the list of general diseases.

Pain—in Tonsils—red with throbbing pain—See this heading under 'T' in the list of general diseases.

Pain—in Tonsillitis with swelling left sided causing paralysis of vocal chord—See this heading under 'T' in the list of general diseases.

Pain—in Tonsillitis with swelling right sided causing suppuration—See this under 'T' in the list of general diseases.

Pain—in Tonsillitis—Sore throat with throbbing pain— See this under 'T' in the list of general diseases.

Pain—in Toothache during pregnancy—See under 'T' in the list of general diseases.

Pain—Traumatic (pertaining to wounds) neuritis amputation and fever—See under 'T' in the list of general diseases.

Pain—in Tumours in brain—the pain being stitching, lightning and lancinating—See "Tumour in brain" under 'T' in the list of general diseases.

Pain—in Tumour in ovary with neuralgia—See this under 'T' in the list of general diseases.

Pain—Ulcers of different types painful—See this heading under 'U' in the list of general diseases.

Pain—in Ulcers corneal with lachrymation and pain in eye brow—See this under 'U' in the list of general diseases.

Pain—in ulcer of stomach being gastric ulcer with burning pain—See "Ulcer of stomach" under 'U' in the list of general diseases.

Pain—in Ulcers—Syphilitic and offensive with a shooting pain outwards from the ulcer—See "Ulcers Syphilitic and offensive" under 'U' in the list of general diseases.

Pain—in Urethra for stretching it for removing stone—See heading "Urethra stretching for stone" under 'U' in the list of general diseases.

Pain—Urine—involuntary escape when walking or coughing or just after urinating with pain—See—"Urine involuntary escape when walking or coughing" in the list of general diseases.

Pain—Urine—pus in Kidneys with pain—See "Urine-pus in" under 'U' in the list of general diseases.

Pain—in Urine with painful micturition—See "Dysuria" under 'D' in the list of general diseases.

Pain—Urine prostatic hypertrophy with dancing agony—See heading "Urine with prostatic hypertrophy" in the list of general diseases under 'U' in the list of general diseases.

Pain—in Uterine colic—See this under 'U' in the list of general diseases.

Pain—Uterine pains darting to sided—See this under 'U' in the list of general diseases.

Pain—Uvula—different complaints with pain—See this under 'U' in the list of general diseases.

Pain—in Varicose with ulceratia left leg hanging down unbearable and scarcely able to move about due to pain—See this under 'V' in the list of general diseases.

Pain—Varicose leg with pain—See this heading under 'V' in the list of general diseases.

Pain—Voice loss of with pain in throat—See "Voice loss of" under 'V' in the list of general diseases.

Pain—Vomiting faecal matter with severe griping pain—See "Vomiting—faecal matter" under 'V' in the list of general diseases. As a matter of fact this trouble is due to a disease named 'ileus' which is characterised by severe griping pain, vomiting of faecal matter.

Pain—in Pustules of vaccination causing pain and discomfort without neutralising the effects of vaccination—See under 'V' the heading "Vaccination discomfort from Pustules" in the list of general diseases.

Pain—Wandering joint pains—See this heading under 'W' in the list of general diseases.

Pain—Weakness at midnight with sinking of vital power with burning pain—See under 'W' in the list of general diseases.

Pain—Weakness in sprained joints with persisting pain—See this under 'W' in the list of general diseases.

Pain—in Weakness of the tendons and muscles with pain See in the list under 'W'.

Pain—in Whitlow with throbbing and excruciating pain—See "Whitlow" under 'W' in the list of general diseases.

Pain—in Whooping cough—See under "W" in the list of general diseases.

Pain—Whooping cough with tearing pains in the larynx, child shakes and vomiting—See "Whooping Cough—Child shakes and Vomiting" under 'W' in the list of general diseases.

Pain—in Wisdom teeth—effects of cutting—See under 'W' in the list of general diseases.

Pain—in Wound incised and clear-cut with burning and stinging pain—See wound incised and clear-cut with no tendency to heal under 'C' in the list of general diseases.

Pain—in Wrist its affections like boils, pain and paralysis—See under 'W' in the list of general diseases.

Pain—in Wry neck with painful rheumatic affections—See "Wry neck, stiff neck" under 'W' in the list of general diseases.

Pain—in Zona or herpes zoster—See "Herpes Zoster" under 'H' in the list of general diseases.

PREVENTIVES

Preventive—Abdomen operation—To prevent sepsis after its operation—Give *Rhus Tox 6x* every 2 hours before abdominal surgery as this medicine has power to prevent sepsis.

Preventive—Appendicitis and its recurring attacks and necrosis—(a) See "Appendicitis also septic" under 'A' in the list of general diseases.

(b) As for necrosis give *Psorinum* 200 or C.M. and *Cadmium Iodat* which will prevent necrosis.

Preventive—of Pain in Arthritis, gout and rheumatism—Gultheria Oil in 10 to 20 drops if given never fails to arrest such pains.

Preventive—Arthritis causing deformations—*Actaea spicata* 3x and *Caulophyllum* 3x if put directly under the tongue three times a day wili prevent deformaties and stiffness in fingers before any deformaties and stiffness sets in.

Preventive of Bronchitis—See under 'B' Bronchitis and prevention of its attack in different weather. Also see "Bronchitis of different types due to different causes" in the list of general diseases.

Preventive—of Bites and its shooting pains—See under 'B' "Bites—prevention of its complications" in the list of general diseases.

Preventive—of Bites by rabid animals causing its injurious effects in cases like rabies and snake poisoning—*Anagallis Arvensis* will prevent ill-effects of bites by rabid animals.

Preventive—Caries of teeth and pyorrhoea—(a) *Calcarea renalis* is preventive of these troubles.

(b) For local application use for *Plantago Major* in lower potencies in toothache in hollow teeth. According to Dr. W. Boericke local application is useful in otorrhoea, pruritus and incised wounds.

Preventive—of Chicken pox—*Antimoniam Tart* and *Rhus Tox* are preventive against chicken pox (Dr. Mackenzie).

Preventive--Chill causing cold and other ailments—(a) *Fucus Vesiculosis 2x* is useful in preventing the cold in the head or illness due to chills. (According to Dr. A. Margittal).

(b) According to Dr. Y. Singh if there is yawning and bruised feeling all over the body due to sensation of cold in the body then 2 or 3 drops of mother tincture of *Spirit of Camphor* should be taken in sugar every one or two hours which will cut-short the attack of cold.

(c) If 4 or 5 drops of *Spirit of Camphor* are taken with sugar it will protect one from catching cold.

Prevention—of cold—(a) *Ammon. Carb.* will often abort a recent cold while *Cistus Canandensis* aborts a cold which centres in posterior nose.

(b) *Nux V* 3 may prevent a cold if given early before running of nose.

Preventive—Calculus—preventive of formation of stone and dissolving of stone—See under 'C' in the list of general diseases. Various forms of this disease. Please also see under 'G' "Gall Stone colic" under its various heads as well as under 'K' "Kidney" under its various heads in the list of general diseases.

Preventive—Cat bites and prevention of their subsequent complications—See under 'C' in the list of general diseases.

Preventive—of cataract— See 'cataract' in the list of general diseases under C'.

Preventive—Cerebral meningitis—*Cicuta Virosa*.

Preventive—Dengue fever—*Eupat Pur*.

Preventive—Diphtheria—*Diph. 200, Mercurious Cynatum 30* to be given in small quantity of water.

Preventive—Diseases of different types—(1) Against mumps—*Pilocarpinum, Parotidinum*.

(2) Against Poliomyelitis—*Lathyrus Sativa*.

(3) Against small pox—*Varolinum Vaccinum*.

(4) Against measles—*Malandrinums Morbitinum*.

(5) Against influenza—Influenzinum, *Arsenic a*, 3 night and morning.

(6) Against Diphtherea—*Diphtherinum*.

(i) Dr. Jahr says that a dose of *Sulf* followed by a dose of *Nux V* acts like a magic.

(ii) As for puerperal mania (following child birth) there is aimless wandering from home, delusion of impending misfortune, melancholy with stupor and manias, sullen, indifference, frenzy excitment, shrieks, curses—*Verat*.

(7) Against whooping cough—*Pertussion*.

Preventive—Dysentery amoebic and its recurrence—See under 'D' Dysentery—amoebic and its prevention of recurrence in the list of general diseases. Please also see under 'D' "Dysentery of different types."

Preventive—Epilepsy and its attacks—(a) Attacks due to mortification or vexation may be prevented by timely giving of *Ignatia*. (Dr. Hahnemann).

(b) According to Dr. Nash along with *Ignatia* Tincture *Amyl Nitrate* 30 a few drops may be sprinkled on a handkerchief for inhaling for prevention. See "Epilepsy" under 'E' under its different heads.

Preventive—Excoriation (abrasion due to walking)—*Agnus Castus*.

Preventive—Eyes Cataract—See "Cataract prevention" under 'C' and "Eyes Cataract prevention" under their respective heads. But don't forget to look "Eye troubles and troubles after operation" in the list of general diseases.

Preventive—Felons (Whitlow) and boils—*Calc. Sulph.12x* will abort whitlow and also boils. See "Whitlow" under 'W' and "Boils—pus aborted" under 'B' in the list of general diseases as well as "Boils" of different kinds.

Preventive—Fever intermittent—*Ars. a. Chininum sulf.* and *Natrum Mur.* if given in the order given above, then it will remove the tendency to intermittent fever restoring patient to health and taking away the susceptibility to cold and periodicity. (Dr. Kent). See under 'F' "Fever—pernicious intermittent" and under 'I' "Intermittent fever prophylactic" in the list of general diseases.

Preventive—Gall stone colic—See under 'G' in the list of general diseases of different types of gall stone colics.

Preventive—Gall stone colic and prevention of formation of stones—*China 6x*, six pills twice a day till 10 doses are taken, then 6 pills of the above medicine every other day till 10 doses are taken, then after this 6 pills of the same medicine every third day till 10 doses are taken and so on till at length the dose is taken once a month. Dr. Thayer has never failed to cure in a single instance permanently with a gall stone. Please see under 'C' "Colics" of different natures and types.

Preventive—Gout and preventing its attack—See under 'G' "Gout preventing" in the list of general diseases. Also don't forget to look into different types of "Gout" under the same head in the same list.

Preventive—Grayness of hair—See under 'G' "Grayness of hair and its prevention" in the list of general diseases. Also under 'H' "Hair Gray" and also different ailments of "Hair".

Preventive—Headache sick—(a) Before an attack of sick headache when the patient feels its coming on, then put two tea spoonfuls of powdered charcoal, (Not Carbo. Veg.) in a half glass of water and drink it. This will frequently prevent the attack of sick headache.

(b) One or two tea spoonfuls of *Cascara Cordial* taken in the morning will avert the appearance of such a headache many times (Dr. E. Jones).

Preventive—Harnia—*Coculus* is said to prevent it when there is weakness in abdomen though this symptom is probably of nervous character. (Dr. Cowperthwaite) See "Hernia" in its different aspects under 'H' in the list of general diseases.

Prevention—(a) **Hydrocephalic (water in brain) children and preventing birth of such children and** (b) **Birth of syphilitic children**—(a) If mother gives birth to such children then she may be given alternately *Sulf. 6* and *Calcarea Phos 6* during the time of pregnancy. (Dr. Ruddock).

(b) For birth of syphilitic children and to prevent them from this disease give *Aurum Mur, nat 3x* to syphilitic mother during course of her pregnancy (D. Clarke).

Prevention—of Inflammation—See under 'P' in the list of general diseases

Prevention—of Ill-effects of carbon mono-oxide—See under 'I' "ill-effects of high attitude and No. IV" in the list of general diseases.

Preventive—of Influenza—See under 'I' "Influenza preventive" and "Influenza prophylactic" in the list of general diseases.

Preventive—Injury causing putrefaction—See "Injury preventing from putrefaction" in the list of general diseases under 'I'.

Preventive—Mastoid and obviate it from surgery—See under 'M' "Mastoid and its prevention from surgery" in the list of general diseases.

Preventive—Malformed children and preventing their birth—"Malformed children such as suffering from club foot, twisted hands, curvature of spine, and cleft palate on lip etc. may be prevented being born with such defects if pregnant mother is being given *Phosphorus* throughout the course of her pregnancy, see under 'C' curvature of bones including curvature of hip joint and vertebra" in the list of general diseases.

Preventive—of Melancholia—*Kali phos. 3x* should be given to prevent the development to a victim of melancholia (Dr. Meta Gumpertz).

Preventive—of Measles—According to Dr. H. Clarke when measles break out in a house let all those not affected take *Acon. 3* and *Puls. 3* each twice a day or *Morbilinum 12* twice daily.

Preventive—of Mumps—See under 'M' "Mumps preventive" and "Mumps prophylactic" in the list of general diseases.

Preventive—Perspiration profuse—See "Perspiration profuse and its prevention" under 'P' in the list of general diseases.

Preventive—Piles—*Tuberculinum* 1000 acts well as an intercurrent medicine to avoid the tendency to piles.

Preventive—Piles and their recurrence—Continuous oozing of mucus staining the linen. Disagreeable to the patient. *Antimonium Crudum*.

Preventive—of Poliomyelitis (inflammation of gray matter in the spinal cord)—See under 'P' in the list of general diseases.

Preventive—of Pulmonary (pertaining to or affecting the lungs or any anatomic component of the lungs Tuberculosis—*Arsenic Iod.*

Preventive—of Quinsy—*Baryta Carb. 30 or Hepar Sulf 30* according to symptoms.

Preventive—Rat bites causing inflammation—See "Rat bites" under 'R' in the list of general diseases.

Preventive—of Rachitis (Rickets)—*Calc. Phos.* is an excellent medicine to prevent rickets. If it fails then try *Silicea.*

Preventive—Respiration laboured due to Sun stroke, with fever and headache—Pale face, fixed eyes, white tongue, laboured respiration. The temperature is high and often times there is unconsciousness. Severe headache, jaws clenched. Involuntary eructations. *Glonine* every five minutes later longer at intervals.

(1) For Sun stroke *Nat. M.* is an excellent medicine.

(2) Much flushing of heat, tremour of limbs, surging of blood to head and face, throbbing headache, throbbing throughout whole body. (*Amyl-n*).

(3) Face flushed blood shot eyes. Throbbing headache with high fever. (*Bell.*).

(4) For prevention of Sun stroke *Gelsinium* is an excellent medicine.

Preventive—of Rubella (German measles)—(i) *Puls. 6* night and morning for 10 to 14 days after contact with other cases. (ii) Rubella which is a nosode of German measles is also curative.

Preventive—Small pox causing disfigurement—See "Small pox preventive and for disfigurement" in the list of general diseases under head 'S'.

Preventive—Small pox causing eruptions and pitting on face—See "Small pox with eruptions on face and to prevent pitting" in the list of general diseases under head 'S'.

Preventive—Still birth child (The birth of dead child)—*Arnicafuga 3x* one dose per day for 2 or 3 months may be given to mother before birth. See also "Pregnancy its affections" under 'P' in the list of general diseases.

Preventive—of Sore throat—Children subject to recurrent sore throat may be given a course of *Baryta Carb.* 6x for two weeks.

Preventive—of Stricture and passing sound in urethra—See under head 'S' "Stricture inability to pass sound and removal of this inability" in the list of general diseases.

Prevention—of Suppuration—*Sulphuric acid prevents* excessive suppuration.

Preventive—Syphilitic birth of a child—If trituration of *Aurum Muriaticum Nat-Mur.* 3x is given to syphilitic mother during the course of her pregnancy with certain short gaps then it prevents the syphilis in her child (Dr. Clarke).

Preventive—of Tartar and its removal from teeth—*Calcarea renalis* prevents formation of tartar from birth while *Fragania* removes it if tartar already formed.

Preventive—Teething trouble of a child—*Calc. Phos.* prevents teething troubles of a children passing through this stage (Dr. Boericke).

Prevention—of Tonsillitis—*Baryta Carb.* not only prevents tonsillitis but also prevents otitis media (inflammation of middle ear) that so frequently results from it. (Dr. Blackwood).

Preventive—of Tonsils from surgery—See under head 'T' "Tonsils to be prevented from surgery" in the list of general diseases.

Preventive—of Tetanus—*Ledum* and *Hypericum* are the chief remedies for its prevention. *Hypericum* is the remedy for the tetanus after the initial symptoms have started.

Preventive—of Typhoid Fever—*Typhoid* vaccine in higher potency is prevention of such a fever.

Preventive—of Ulceration in lungs not healing—See "Ulceration in lungs not healing" under 'U' in the list of general diseases.

Preventive—of warts and their recurrence—*Thuja* or *Acid nit.* or *Flouric acid* should be used according to symptoms.

Preventive—of Whooping cough—See "Whooping cough preventive" in the list of general diseases.

Prevention of Worms—*Calc. C.*

PROPHYLACTICS

Prophylactic—for Abortion—(i) For abortion of second month—*Kali Carb. 1M.*

(ii) For abortion for second and third month—*Apis.*

(iii) For abortion for seventh month—*Sepia.* Dr. Hale says that *Viburnum Opulus* will prevent miscarriage if given before membranes are injured and when pains are threatening. See "Abortion" under 'A' under its different heads in the list of general diseases.

Prophylactic—Cholera—See "Cholera prophylactic" under 'C' in the list of general diseases.

Prophylactic—Diphtheria—*Apis* 30, *Dipht* 30.

Prophylactic—Epilepsy—According to Dr. Das Gupta M.B *Kali Brom.* is recognised as the best prophylactic by most authors, next comes *Glon.*

Prophylactic—Erysipelas-*Graphites* 30.

Prophylactic—Influenza—*Ars.* See also "Influenza prophylactic" and "Influenza preventive" under head 'I' in the list of general diseases.

Prophylactic—Jaundice—*China.* See 'Jaundice' under 'J' in its different phases in the list of general diseases.

Prophylactic—Labour difficult—See "Labour prophylactics for difficult labour" under 'L' in the list of general diseases.

Prophylactic—of Measles—Dr. Hartmann is said to have good results by giving *Puls.* and *Acon.* one dose of 6th or 12th, every other day during the whole course of epidemic. An occasional dose of *Sulph.* as an intercurrent remedy. Dr. Gaudy thinks *Ars. a.* to be a good prophylactic. See also "Measles-prophylactic" under 'M' in the list of general diseases.

Prophylactic—Mump—See "Mumps preventive" and "Mumps prophylactic" under letter 'M' in the list of general diseases.

Prophylactic—Plague—See "Plague also its prophylactic" under head 'P' in the list of general diseases.

Prophylactic—Small pox—*Variolinum* is the best preventive and curative medicine. Drs. Jahr and Kippax give *Variolinum* 30 twice daily on alternate days and think it will be sufficient, and occasional dose of *Sulf.* 30 should be taken inter-currently for *Variolinum* is said to act very well after *Sulf.* See also "Small pox preventive and disfigurement" under 'S' in the list of general diseases.

Prophylactic—for snake poison—*Euphorbia—prostata* is employed as a prophylactic to snake poison (Dr. Blackwood). See also "Snake poisoning prophylactic" under 'S' in the list of general diseases.

Prophylactic—Styes recurring—See under 'S' in the list of general diseases.

Prophylactic—Whooping cough—See "Whooping cough prophylactic" under head 'W' in the list of general diseases.

Prophylactic for other diseases :—(1) Catheter fever—Camph

(2) Cholera—Ars., Cupr-ac ; Veratrum album.

(3) Diphtheria—Apis 30 ; Diph. 30.

(4) Hydrophobia (rabies)—Bell., Canth., Hyos., Stram.

(5) Intermittent fever—Ars. ; Chin-s.

(6) Measles—Acon ; Ars ; Puls.

(7) Mumps—Tritole-rep.

(8) Pus infection—Arn.

(9) Quinsy (Acute inflammation of tonsil and peritosillar tissue usually tending to suppuration) : Bar-c. 30.

(10) Variola (small pox)—Ant-t ; Hydr ; Kali-cy.

(11) Whooping cough—Dros ; Vaccin. (Dr. Boericke, M.D.).

(12) Antidote to snake poison and is thus a prophylactic—Glondrina. (Boericke)

(b) **The other medicines having prophylactic powers are :**

(i) *Aconite* prevents abortion from excitment or fright. (Coperthwaite)

(ii) *Arnica* prevents suppuration and septic conditions. (H.C. Allen)

(iii) *Baptisia* against Typhus or typhoid. (A.H. Grimmer).

(iv) According to Hahnemann *Belladonna* is the surest preventive of hydrophobia.

(v) *Berberis* prevents the recurrence of boils. (Dewey)

(vi) *Calcarea sulphurica* will abort felons and boils. (Dr. Leonard)

(vii) *Calendula tincture* 1x diluted with an equal part of water is used to check bleeding and to prevent a wound from going septic. (P.H. Sharp)

(viii) *Caulophyllum* is a powerful agent for the prevention of premature labour and miscarriage provided the premonitions are pains of spasmodic character. (Tyler)

(ix) *Fluoric acid* will prevent the manifestation or disease (oedema of prepuce in sycotic subjects), and will prevent formation of warts. (Kent)

(x) *Frgaria* prevents the attacks of gout. (Boericke)

(xi) *Helonias Dioica* prevents abortions which occur after result of slightest over-exertion of irritating emotions. (Blackwood)

(xii) Attacks of even chronic epilepsy, which only occur after mortification or similar vexation (and not from any other cause) may always be prevented by timely administration of *Ignatia*. (Hahnemann)

(xiii) *Nux-vomica 3* may prevent a cold if given early before the commencement of running of nose. (Carter)

(xiv) *Pilocarpine*, should be used once daily as a preventive against mumps. (Clarke)

(xv) *Saponaria* will often 'break-up' a cold. (Boericke)

(xvi) *Silicea* is a remedy to prevent boils. (Dewey)

(xvii) If *Tuberculinum* be given in 10 m., 500 m., and C.M. potencies, two doses of each potency at long intervals, all children and young people who have inherited tuberculosis may be inmuned from this inheritance and their resilience will be restored. (J. T. Kent)

(xviii) *Lathyrus sativa* (already mentioned under head 'Preventives') has given the most certain protection in thousands of cases through many epidemics. (A.H.Grinner)

Note :—According to Dr. A. H. Grinner these prophylactics never cause any susceptibility or hyper-sensitivity, shock of secondary infection. He suggests that 10 M. is a protective potency and the reaction is good at least for that epidemic period.

Atrophies of different parts of body .

It was not my idea to include "Atrophies", in this Chapter but I have found that this disease is the most nasty trouble and is rather difficult to be treated but Homoeopathy gives some rays of successful treatment. So I have taken liberty to describe a few cases in the following :

(1) **Atrophy from above downwards**—*Lyc* ; *Nat. m.*

(2) **Atrophy from below upwards**—Abrot.

(3) **Atrophy of legs**—*Abrot. Am. m.*

(4) **Atrophy of neck, flabby, loose skin**—*Nat. m., Sanic.*

(5) **Atrophy, rapid**—Thuyai Tub.

(6) **Atrophy, progressive, muscular**—Phos, Plumb.

(7) **Atrophy, rapid, with cold sweat and debility**—Ars. Ver. a.

(8) **Atrophy with shrivelled up look**—Arg. N., Kreos, Sul. (Dr. Boericke)

Clinical Relationships of Medicines

APPENDIX I

Clinical Relationships of Medicines

List of remedies suggested in the Quick Bed Side Prescriber. Those in column I should be in varying strengths preferably in different forms. Two potencies at least of those mentioned in Col. 1 should be at least of 30th and 200th potencies to be kept ready. Intercurrent remedies should be used wherever suggested and should at least be of 200 or 1 M. potency. The nosodes should not be less than of 1 M. Potency.

Principal Remedy with abbreviations	Complementary Remedies	Remedy is followed well by	Incompatible Remedies	Remedy Antidotes	Remedy is Antidoted by
Abies Nigra (Abies-n.)	—	—	—	—	—
Abrotanum (Abrot.)	—	—	—	Bam. (Sometimes)	—
Absinthium (Absin.)	—	—	—	—	—
Acalypha Indica (Acal-Ind.)	—	—	—	—	—

Principal Remedy with abbreviation	Complementary Remedies	Remedy is followed well by	Incompatible Remedies	Remedy Antidotes	Remedy is Antidoted by
Acetic acid (Acet-ac.)	China in haemorrhages		Disagrees when given after Bor., Caus., Nux, Rn. B., Sars.	Aco., Anaesthetics, Ar.t., Asr., Cof., Eub., Hep., Ign., Opi., Ph., (colic), sausage poisoning, Sep., Stm., Tab.	Potencies by Aco. and Tab. for depressing agonising feeling, Mag. c. Large doses, by Calc. (water) Mag. (fluid). For gastric, pulmonary, and febrile symptoms Na. m. and afterwards Sep.
Aconitine (Acon.)					
Note : Heavy feeling as of lead ; pains in supra orbital nerve ; ice cold symptoms creep up ; hydrophobia symptoms.					
Aconitum (Aconi)					
Aconitum napellus (Acon. n.)	Arn. (bruises, injury to eye), Cof. (fever,	Arn., Ars., Bel., Bry., Cac., Cth., Coc-i., Hep.		Arn., Asp.(some times), Ast. f., Bel., Bry., Cac.	Ac.x Alcoh., Bel Ber., Cham. Cit Cof., Nux, Par

Principal Remedy with abbreviation	Complementary Remedies	Remedy is followed well by	Incompatible Remedies	Remedy Antidotes	Remedy is Antidoted by
	sleeplessness, intolerance of pain). Sul.	Ips., K. br, Merc., Pul., Rhs., Sep., Sil., Spo., Sul., (also for abuse of Aco.), Sul.		Cth. Cham. Chel., Cinm., Cit., Coff., Cro., Dol. Glon., Gph., Klm. (Kre.) Lyc., Mrl., Mez., Morphia (secondary effects of). Nux. Pet., Sep., Sol., Spo Sty. (?) Sul., Ther. (sensitiveness to noise), Ver. Vb. o. (epididymitis).	Sul., Ver., Wine
Actaea Racemosa also known Cimicifuga (Actea or Ciml).	—	—	—	Tansy poisoning.	Aco. (the Sleeplessness). Bap. (ameliorates the headache and nausea) ; Lcs.

Principal Remedy with abbreviation	Complementary Remedies	Remedy is followed well by	Incompatible Remedies	Remedy Antidotes	Remedy is Antidoted by
Actaea Spicata (Actea sp.)	—	—	—		
Adonis Vernalis (Adon-v.)	—	—	—		
Adrenalin (Adren.)	—	—	—	—	—
Aesculus hippo-castanum (Aes.)	—	—	—	—	Nux. (pile symptoms)
Aethusa-cynapium (Aeth-c).	Calc.	—	—	Opium,	Vegetable acids.
Agaricin		—	—	—	
Agaricus muscarius, (Agar-m.)		Bel., Calc., Cup., Mer., Opi., Pul., Rhs., Sil., Trn. (typhoid with "rolling of the head").	—	—	Brandy Calc. (ameliorates Icy-coldness) Cam., Charcoal, Cof., Fat or Oil ameliorates stomach Pul., Rhs., (nightly backahce). Wine

Principal Remedy with abbreviation	Complementary Remedies	Remedy is followed well by	Incompatible Remedies	Remedy Antidotes	Remedy is Antidoted by
Agnus Castus (Agn.)		Ars., Bry., Ign., Lyc., Pul., Sel. Sul.			Cam., Na. m. (headache), strong solutions of table salt.
Agraphis Nutans (Agraph-n)				—	
Ailanthus. g.	*Note* : Nervous sensitive persons ; bilious temperament, stout and robust.				
Alfalfa (Alf.)	—		—		
Atetris farinosa (Alt-f.)	—	—	—	—	—
Allium cepa (All-c.)	Fho,, Pul., Sars., Thu.	Calc. and Sil. in polypus.	All., Alo., Cep., Scil.	Clp.,	Arn, (toothache), Cham, (abdominal pains), Cf. t. (onion breath), Nux (coryza recurring in August), Thu, (offensive breath and diarrhoea after eating onions), Ver, (colic with despondency).

Principal Remedy with abbreviation	Complementary Remedies	Remedy is followed well by	Incompatible Remedies	Remedy Antidotes	Remedy is Antidoted by
Allium Sativum (all-s).	Ars.		Alo., Cep., Scil.		Lyc.
Alnus.	—	—	—	—	—
Aloe.	*Note* : Old people, phlegmatic and indolent persons ; Aloe has many symptoms like Sulf and is equally important in chronic diseases with abdominal plethora.		All., Cep.	Paeo	Aln. (vomiting blood), Cam. ameliorates for a while, Lyc. and Nux ameliorates the earache, Mustard. Sul.
Alumen (Alumn.)				Lead poisoning, calomel and other mercurials, Alo. (vomiting blood)	Cham. (cramps in abdomen), Ipc. (nausea and vomiting), Nux, Sul.
Alumina (Alum.)	Bry, Fer.	*Note* : Constipation of children stool green, acidity, puberty, chlorosis with longing for indigestible substances.		Bry., Cham., Lach., Lead.	Bry., Cam., Cham., Ipc., Pul.
Ambra grisea. (Ambra).	Lyc., Pul., Sep., Sul.			Nux, Stp. (esp the voluptuous itching of scrotum).	Cam., Cof Nux, Pul., Stp.
Aluminum-met. (Alumi-m).					

Principal Remedy with abbreviation	Complementary Remedies	Remedy is followed well by	Incompatible Remedies	Remedy Antidotes	Remedy is Antidoted by
Ammonium bromatum (Am-br.)	—	—			—
Ammonium carbonicum (Am-c.)	— —	Bell., Calc., Lyc., Pho., Pul., Rhs., Sep., Sul.	Lach.	Bro., Cen., Char-coal fumes, Plo. Rhs., and stings of insects.	Vegetable acids Arn., Cam., Fixed Oils, Hep., Lah.
Ammonium formald Am-formal)	*Note* : Prevents decomposition of urine in bladder, kidneys and ureters turbid urine rendered clear and non-irritating, phosphatic deposits dissolved and growth of pyogenic bacteria arrested.				
Ammonium muriaticum (Am-m).	—	Ant. c, Cof., Hot-bath, Merc., Nux, Pho., Pul., Rhs.		—	Bitter almonds, Cam., Cof., Hep., Nux.
Ammonium ph.		—	—	—	—
Amylenum nitrite (Aml-n.)	—	—	—	Chlf. (failure of respiration) Sty. (convulsion).	Cac. (cardiac con-striction.)
Anacardium Occid (Anac.)	*Note* : Gastric and nervous disorders during pregnancy ; nervous and hysterical females.				Iodine (locally) Rhs.
Anacardium or.	Lyc., Plat., Pul			Rhs. if there are gastric symptoms, or symptoms go-ing from r. to 1	Clem, Cof., Ctn. Jg., C., Rn., b, Rhs.

Principal Remedy with abbreviation	Complementary Remedies	Remedy is Followed Well by	Incompatible Remedies	Remedy Antidotes	Remedy is Antidoted by
Anagallis arv. (Anag).		—	—	—	—
Anantherum (Anan.)			Wines and spirits		Aromatic liquors.
Anthracinum (Anthrac).		An. m. n, (periosteal swelling of lower jaw), Sil., (cellulitis)			Aps., Ars., Cam., Cbl., x., Cb. v., Kre., Lach., Pul., Rhs., Sil., Sl. x.
Anthrokokali (Anthrok).	—	—	—	—	—
Antimonium a. (Ant-a.)					
Antimonium cudum (Ant-c.)	Scil.	Calc., Lach., Merc., Pul., Sep., Sul.		Pb., Pl. n., Sep., Stings of insects.	Calc., Hep., Merc.
Antimonium tart (Ant-t.)		Ba. c., Cam., Cin., Ipc., Pul., Sep., Sul., Ter.		Ba.c., Bry. (dyspepsia), Cam., Caus. (dyspepsia), Ctn., Iod, (relieves the vertigo of Mil.), Sep., Vac., Var.	Asa., Chi., Coc. i., Con. (pustules on genitals), Ipc., Lau. Merc., Opi. Opium in large doses is the best antidote.

Principal Remedy with abbreviation	Complementary Remedies	Remedy is Followed Well by	Incompatible Remedies	Remedy Antidotes	Remedy is Antidoted by
					in poisoning., Pul., Rhs., Sep.
Antipyrinum (Atp.)			Cof. in excess.		Bel.
Apis mellifica (Apis)	Na. m. (the "chronic" of Apis).	Ars (hydrothorax), Gph, (tetter on earlobe). Iod. (swollen knee), K. bi. (scrofulous ophthalmia), Lyc. (staphyloma), Pho. (diphtheria), Pul., Stm. (mania), Sul. (hydrothorax, pleurisy, hydrocephalus.)	Pho., Rhs , (in eruptive diseases)	Athra., Asp., Cth (the cystitis). Chi. Dig. Iod., Na. P. (urticaria), Vac , Vsp.	Cth., Ipc., Lach., Lc, x., Led., Na. m., Massive doses, poisonings and stings are antidoted by Na. m. (the crude salt, solutions, and potencies); Sweet-oil (which contains salt), Onions; Ammonia Urtica; powdered Ipec. applied locally.
Apocynum Cannabinum (Apoc.)	—	—	—	—	—
Aranea diadema (Aran.)	—	—	—	Chi., Merc, Quinine	Smoking tobacco.

Principal Remedy with abbreviation	Complementary Remedies	Remedy is Followed Well by	Incompatible Remedies	Remedy Antidotes	Remedy is Antidoted by
Argentum metallicum (Arg-m.)		Calc., Pul., Sep.			Merc., Pul., (an occasional dose of Pul. favours action of Ag. n. in ophthalmia).
Argentum nitricum (Arg-n.)		Calc. Hfb, K. ca., Lyc. (flatus), Merc., Pul., Sep., Sil.	Cof. (it increases the nervous headache), Vsp.	Amm., K.i. (fulness and indigestion after each dose), Op. effects of tobacco	Ars., Iod., Merc., Milk. Na. m (chemical and dynamic). Antidotes to Ag. n and Nt. x. are Calc. Pul., Sep., next in importance Lyc. Pho., Rhs., Sil., Sul.
Arnica (Arn.)	Aco., Ipc., Ver.	Aco. Ars (action aided by Ars, in dysentery and varicose veins), Bel. Bry., Cac. Cal., Cham., Chi., Con., Hep, Iod, Ipc, Nux.	Injurious in bites of dogs or rabid or angry animals Wine aggravates unpleasant effect of Arn.	Amc., Am. C., Caln. Cep (toothache), Chi., Ch. s., Cic. v., Fer., Ham., Ign., Ipc., Phst., Sga.	*If potencies*: Aco., Ars., Cam., Chi., Cic. v., Fer., Ign., Ipc., Sga. *If massive doses*; Cam., Ip. c. Coffee.

Principal Remedy with abbreviations	Complementary Remedies	Remedy is Followed Well by	Incompatible Remedies	Remedy Antidotes	Remedy is Antidoted by
		Pho., Pul., Rhs , Sul., Su. x.			(headache).
Arsenicum album (Ars.)	All., Cb. v., Na. s., Pho., Thu.	Aps., Aran., Bel., Cac., Cham., Chel., Chi., Cic., Fer., Fl.x, Hep., Iod., Ipc , K. bi., Lyc., Merc., Nux ; Rhs. follows well in skin affections, esp. in cases treated allopathically with large doses of arsenic ; Sul, Ver.	—	Athra., Ag. n., Arn., Cb. a., Cb. v., Chi., Ch.s., Elp., Fer., Gph., Hep., Hyp. (weakness or sickness on moving), Iod., Ipc., K. bi , Lach., Leo., Mag. c , Mag. m., Mlr. No. II., Merc., Na m. (bad effects of sea-bathing), Nux., Pho , Pb., Smb n., Sty, Tab., Thri, Ver.	*Chemical antidotes* : Animal Charcoal, Hydrated peroxide of iron, Lime-water, Magnesia. *Dynamic antidotes :* Opium ; it may be administered by Clyster if not retained on stomach ; Brandy and stimulants if there is depression and collapse ; Sweet spirit of nitre in large quantities of water if urine is suppressed. *If poisonous doses*.

Note : Lead poisoning and evil effects of alcohal. Complaints of drunkards.

Principal Remedy with abbreviations	Complementary Remedies	Remedy is Followed Well by	Incompatible Remedies	Remedy Antidotes	Remedy is Antidoted by
					Milk, Albumen, Demulcent drinks followed by emetics of Mustard, Sulphate of Zinc or Sulphate of Copper (Tartar emetic is too irritating.) Castor oil is the best purgative. *If potencies* : Gph., Hep., Iod., Ipc., Lach., Merc., Nx. m, Nux., Smb. n., Sul., Tab., Ver.
Arsenicum brom. (Ars-b.)	—	—	—	—	Veratum A.
Arsenicum iodatum (Ars-i.)	Pho.			Relieves the diarrhoea of Mil.	Bry. ameliorates pain and pyrosis

Principal Remedy with abbreviation	Complementary Remedies	Remedy is Followed Well by	Incompatible Remedies	Remedy Antidotes	Remedy is Antidoted by
Arsenicum Sulphuratun Flavun (Ars-s-f.)	—	—	—	—	—
Artemisia Vulgaris (Art-v.)	Art. v. acts better when given with wine than with water.	Caus.	—	—	—
Arum triphyllum (Arum-t.)		Eub.	Cld.		Ac. x., Bel., Butter-Milk, Lc. x., Ful.,
Asafoetida *Note* : Phlegmatic temperament, scrofulous, bloated clumsy children ; venous, haemorrhodial constitution ; nervous people ; syphilitics who have taken much mercury.		Chi., Merc., Pul,		Alcohol, Ant. t., Caus., Ln. u.(?) Merc., Pul.	Cam., Caus., Chi., Merc., Pul., Val.
Asarum-can. (Asa-c.)	...	Bis., Caus., Pul., Sil.		Cit.	Ac. x., Cam., vegetable acids and vinegar.
Asparagus (Aspar.)	---		-- --	Cof.	Aco. (prostration, feeble pulse, pain in shoulder), Aps,

Principal Remedy with abbreviation	Complementary Remedies	Remedy is Followed Well by	Incompatible Remedies	Remedy Antidotes	Remedy is Antidoted by
Astacus fluriatilis. (Astac.)	—	—	—	—	Aco.
Asterias rubens. (Astan.)			Cof., Nux (Ipc. ameliorates after Nux aggravates		Pb., Zin.
Aurum chloride (Aur-c.)	—	—	—	—	—
Aurum metallicum Aur-met.)			Aco., Bel, Calc., Chi., Lyc., Merc., Nt. x., Pul., Rhs., Sep., Sul.	Chronic effects of alcohol, K/i., Merc., Spi.	Bel., Cam. Chi., Cac.i., Cof., Cup., Merc., Pul., So. n., Spi.
Note : Girls at puberty ; old people, weak vision, sanguine temperament scrofulous, syphilitic and mercurial patients.					
Aurum muriaticum (Aur-m.)	—	—	—	—	Bel., Cnb., Merc.
Aurum muriaticum natronatum (Aur-m-n.)	—	—	Alcohol, Cof.		
Avena sativa. (Aena-s.)					Mor.

Principal Remedy with abbreviations	Complementary Remedies	Remedy is Followed Well by	Incompatible Remedies	Remedy Antidotes	Remedy is Antidoted by
Bacillinum. (Bacill.)	Calc-p goes with medicine very well, so do Hdr. Lach and C. carb.	—	—	—	—
Bacillinum testum (Bac-test)	—	—	—	—	—
Badiaga (Bad.)	Iod., Merc., Sul.	Lach.	—	—	—
Baptisia tinctoria (Bap-t.)		Ham., Nt. x., Ter.			Phyt., Sang.
Baryta carbonica (Bar-c.)	Dul.	Ant. t., (Calc), Con., Pho., Pul., Rhs., Sep., Sil., Sul.	Calc.		Ant. t., Bel., Cam. Dul., Merc., Zin.
Note : Old fat people, scrofulous children dwarfed in body and mind ; general emaciation.					
Baryta muriatica (Bar-m.)	—	—	—	—	Absinthe (the vomiting).
Belladonna (Bell.)	Calc.	Aco., Ars., Cac. Calc., Cb. v., Cham., Chi., Con., Dul., Hep., Hyo..	Dul., Vinegar. aggravated bo Ac. acid	Aco., Atp., As. mt. (Sometimes), Ar. t. Atr., Aur., Au. m., Ba. c.,	If effects of large doses, Vegetable acids, infusion of galls, or green tea.

Principal Remedy with abbreviations	Complementary Remedies	Remedy is Followed Well by	Incompatible Remedies	Remedy Antidotes	Remedy is Antidoted by
		Lach., Merc., Mos., Mu. x, Nux., Pul., Rhs., Sga., Sep., Sil., Stm., Sul , Val., Ver.		Ber,, Ced., Chi., Clch., Cop., Cro., Cup., Fer., Grt., Hep., Hyo., Iod , Jab., K. m., Klm., Lach., Mag. p. Mrl., Merc., Mor., Nt., o. (?) Nux., Opl., Osm. (laryngeal catarrh), Pal (headache). Phyt., Plat., Pb., Rhs., Rum., Sars., Sga., Sol., Stm., Val., Oil of turpentine ; Sausage poisoning.	Cof. Hpo. If effects of small doses, Aco., Cam., Cof., Hep., Hyo., Opi., Pul., Sbd. (saliv-ation), Vinum

Note : Bell suits plethoric, lymphatic constitutions, who are jovial and entertaining when well, but irritable and violent when sick. Women, children, blue eyes, light hair, fine complexion, deilcate skin.

Principal Remedy with abbreviations	Complementary Remedies	Remedy is Followed Well by	Incompatible Remedies	Remedy Antidotes	Remedy is Antidoted by
Bellis perennis (Bell-p.)	Van.				
Benzoicum acid (Benz-a).			Wine, which aggravates pains in kidneys, drawing in knees, & c.		

Note : Rheumatic or gouty diathesis, especially in syphilitic or gonorrhoeal patients.

Principal Remedy with abbreviations	Complementary Remedies	Remedy is Followed Well by	Incompatible Remedies	Remedy Antidotes	Remedy is Antidoted by
Berberis vulgaris (Berb.)	An occasional doses of Lyc. helped action of Ber.			Aco	Bel., Cham.
Blatta orientala (Blatta).	—	—	—	—	—
Boracicum acidum (Bor-ac.)	—	—	—	—	—
Borax (Bor.)	—	Calc., Nux.	Ac. x, Vinegar., Wine	Cham.	Cham., Cof.
Bothrops lanceolatus (Both.)	—	—	—	—	—
Bovista		Alm., Calc., Rhs., Sep.	Cof.	Effects of tar applied locally.	Cam.

Note : Palpitation in old maids, children, stammering in children.

Principal Remedy with abbreviation	Complementary Remedies	Remedy is Followed Well by	Incompatible Remedies	Remedy Antidotes	Remedy is Antidoted by
Bromium (Brom.)	—	Ag. n., K. ca.	—	—	Am, c., Cam., Clch., (?), Mag. c., Opi.
Bryonia (Bry.)	Alum, Rhs. Alumina is the "chronic" of Bry. ; and Kali c. and Nat. m. hold a similar but less pronounced relation to it.	Alum., Ars., Bel., Cac., Cb. v, Drs., Hyos., Kali. c., Mu. x., Nux. Pho., Pul., Rhs., Sbd., Sep., Sil., Sul.,	Calc.	Alum., Amc., Ang. (sometimes) relieved pain and pyrosis of As. i., Chi., Chim., Clem. (sometimes), Dph., Frg., Jg. c. (angina pectoris), Lc. x. (sometimes partly), Mlr, No. I, II and III., Mns., Merc., Mez., Mu.x. (small doses), Cst.; Rn. b., Rho., Rhs., Sil., Scro. (chest symptoms), Sga.	Aco., Alum., Ant.t. (sometimes), Cam., Cham., Chel., Clem., Cof. Teste found by accident, Fe. m. the best antidote in his experience ; Ign., Mu.x., Nux, Pul., Rhs., Sga.

Note : Complaints from warm wheather following cold cold days, exposure to heat and fire.

Principal Remedy with abbreviations	Complementary Remedies	Remedy is Followed Well by	Incompatible Remedies	Remedy Antidotes	Remedy is Antidoted by
Bufo.	Salamandra in epilepsy and brain-softening.	—	—	—	Lach., Sga.
Cactus grandiflorus (Cact.)	—	—	—	Aml. (cardiac constriction).	Aco., Cam., Chi., E. pf,
Cadmium sulphuratum (Cad.)	—	Alet. (nausea of pregnancy), Bel. (rolling of head with open eyes in cholera infantum), Cb. v., Lo. i. (in yellow fever), Nt. x.	—	—	—
Caladium (Calad.)	Nt. x.	Aco., Caus., Pul., Sep.	Ar. t, ; the Araceae.	Cap., Merc.	Cap., Cb. v. (rash) Hyo. (night cough) Ign. (stitches in pit of stomach and fever), Merc. (preputial symptoms), Zng. (asthma).

Principal Remedy with abbreviation	Complementary Remedies	Remedy is Followed Well by	Incompatible Remedies	Remedy Antidotes	Remedy is Antidoted by
Calcarea arsenica (Calc-ars.)		Con., Glo., Opi., Pul.			Cv. b. palpitation, Glo. (headache), Pul. (headache, tearing pains in face).
Calcarea bromata (Calc-bro.)	—	—	—	—	—
Calcarea carbonica (Calc-c.)	Bel., Rhs.	Aga., Bel., Bis., Drs., Gph., Ipc., Lyc., Na. c., Nt. x., Nux, Pho., Plat., Pul., Rhs., Sars., Sep., Sil., Ther	Ba. c., Bry. ; Kali b. (before Calc.) Nt. x, (after) ; Sul (after).	Relieves icy coldness of Aga. ; Ant. c., Bis., Chi., Ch. s., Cop., Dig. Mez. (headache), Nt. s. d., Nt. x. Ox. x (?) Pho.	Bry, Cam., Chi., Hep., Iod., Ip., Nt. s.d., Nt. x., Nux., Sep., Sul.
Note : Leuco-phlegmatic Temperament ; for, plump children, with open fontanelies and sutures, ex essive obesity of young people.					
Calcarea fluorica (Calc-f.)	—	—	—	—	—
Calcarea iodata (Calc-i.)	—	—	—	—	—

Principal Remedy with abbreviations	Complementary Remedies	Remedy is Followed Well by	Incompatible Remedies	Remedy Antidotes	Remedy is Antidoted by
Calcarea phosphorica (Calc-p.)	Hep., Rut., Sul., Zin.	Rhs., Sul.		Pul. (air passages).	
Calcarea renalis (Calc-r.)	—	—	—	—	—
Calcarea sulphurica (Calc-s.)	—	—	—	K m.	—
Calendula (Calend.)	Hep.	Arn., Ars., Bry., Hep., Nt. x, Pho., Rhs.	Cam.	—	—
Camphora (Camph.)	Cth.	Ant.t., Ars., Bel., Coc. i., Nux, Rhs., Ver.	Caln., after Cof, (sometimes), aggravates sufferings from Kalinatrum agg. effects of Sac., 1	Am. c., Canth Cb. v., Cup., Lau., Led., Lyc., Mag. m., Men., Mep. (temporarily). Mos, (unconsciousness and coldness), Mu. x. (small doses), Na. c., Na. m., Scil. so called	Cth. Dul. Nt.s. d , Opi., Pho.

Principal Remedy with abbreviations	Complementary Remedies	Remedy is Followed Well by	Incompatible Remedies	Remedy Antidotes	Remedy is Antidoted by
				worm medicines, tobacco, bitter almonds, and other fruits containing prussic acid ; also the secondary affections remaining after poisoning with Acids, salts, metals, poisonous mushrooms, & c.	
Camphora acid (Camp-a.)	—	—	—	—	—
Cannabis indica (Cann-i.)	—	—	—	—	—
Cantharis (Canth.)	Cam.	Rel., K. bi., Merc., Sul., Pul., Sep., Sul.	Cof.	Alcohol, Cam., Vinegar	Aco., Aps, antidotes the cystitis of Cth ; Cam. the strangury and retention

Principal Remedy with abbreviations	Complementary Remedies	Remedy is Followed Well by	Incompatible Remedies	Remedy Antidotes	Remedy is Antidoted by
					of urine, K. n. the renal symptoms ; Lau.' Pul., Rhe., Symt.
Capsicum (Caps.)		Bel., Lyc., Pul. Sil.		Effects of Alcohol, Bis., Cof., Cf. t,, Merc-high (?) Opi., Quinine.	Cam., Chi., Cin., Cld., Su. x., vapour of burning sulphur.
Note : Phlegmatic, awkward, easily offended, indolent, melancholic, lack of reaction, dread of open air, lazy, fat, unclean, light hair, blue eyes.					
Carbo animalis (Carb-a.)	Ca. p.	Ars., Bel , Bry., (Cb. v. ?), Nt. x., Pho., Pul., Sep., Sil., Sul., Ver.	Cb. a, (?)	Effects of Quinine, Ziz.	Ars., Cam,, Cof., Lach., Nux., Vinegar, Vinum.
Note : Useful in elderly people, with venous plethora, blue cheeks and lips : young scrofulous subjects.					
Carbo vegetabilis (Carb-v.)	Chi., Drs., K. ca. (stitches	Aco., Ars., Chi, Drs. K. ca., Lyc.	Cb. a. (?)	Athra, Cld. (rash) Ca. ar., (palpitation),	Ars., Caus., Cof. Fer., Nt. s. d.

Principal Remedy with abbreviations	Complementary Remedies	Remedy is Followed Well by	Incompatible Remedies	Remedy Antidotes	Remedy is Antidoted by
	in heart, & c.). Pho.	Nux, Ph. x., Pul., Sep., Sul.		Chi., Ch.s., Lach., Merc., Nt. s. d., effects of putrid meats or fish, rancid fats, sal or salt meats, relieved effects, of Sla.	
Carbolicum acid (Carb-ac.)	—	—		Athra.	Chalk, Saccharated Lime. In burns milk gives immediate relief, also copious draughts of milk in poisoning cases.
Carboneum sulphuratum. (Carb-s.)	—	—	—	—	—
Canduus benedictus Carduus marianus (Card-m.)	—	—	—	—	—

Principal Remedy with abbreviations	Complementary Remedies	Remedy is Followed Well by	Incompatible Remedies	Remedy Antidotes	Remedy is Antidoted by
Carlsbad (Carsl.)	—	—	—	—	—
Caulophyllum (Caul.)	—	—	Cof.	—	—
Causticum (Caust.)	Col., Pts., Mr. c. assists the action of Caus. and *vice versa* (in small-pox).	Ant. t., Calc., Gui., K.i., Lyc., Nux, Pul., Rhs., Rut., Sep., Sil., Stn., Sul.	Acids, Coc. i., Cof., Pho.	Asa., Chi., Co., Ephr., Grt., Lyc , Nt. s. d., Pb. (lead poisoning), type poisoning, abuse of Merc., and Sul., in scabies. Relieves paralysis of wrist of Hpm.	Ant. t. (sometimes), Asa., Cof., Col., Dul., Gui. (rheumatic contractions). K.n. (renal symptoms) Nt. s.d., Nux
Ceanothus americanus (Ceon.)	—	Ber., Con., My. c., Qer.	—	—	Na. m.
Cedron (Cedr.)	—	—	—	Lach.	Bel., Lach.

Principal Remedy with abbreviations	Complementary Remedies	Remedy is Followed Well by	Incompatible Remedies	Remedy Antidotes	Remedy is Antidoted by
Chamomilla (Cham.)	Bel. in diseases of children (Cham, acts more on nerves of abdomen, Bel. more on cranial nerves), Mgn. c, Pul.	Aco., Arn., Bef., Bry., Cac., Calc., Coc. i., For., Merc., Nux, Pul., Rhs., Sep., Sil., Sul.	Nux., Zin.	Coffee and the narcotics, esp. Opium (useful in nerve storm when morphia is discontinued) the nightly toothache of Thu.	Aco., Alm., Bor., Cam. Coc.i., Cof., Col., Con., Ign., Nux, Pul., Val.

Note: Children, light brown hair nervous, excitable temperament. Adult and aged persons with arthritic or rheumatic diathesis.

Principal Remedy with abbreviations	Complementary Remedies	Remedy is Followed Well by	Incompatible Remedies	Remedy Antidotes	Remedy is Antidoted by
Chaparro amar. (Chaprro.)					
Chelidonium majus (Chel.)		Aco., Ars., Bry., Ipc., Led., Lyc., Nux, Sep., Spi. Sul.		Ang. (sometimes) Bry.	Acids, Aco, Cam., Cham., Cof., Coffee. Wine.

Note : Spare subject disposed to abdominal plethora, cutaneous diseases, catarrhs or neuralgia, Blondes.

Principal Remedy with abbreviations	Complementary Remedies	Remedy is Followed Well by	Incompatible Remedies	Remedy Antidotes	Remedy is Antidoted by
Chimaphila umbel. (Chim.)					

Principal Remedy with abbreviations	Complementary Remedies	Remedy is Followed Well by	Incompatible Remedies	Remedy Antidotes	Remedy is Antidoted by
China officin (Chin.)	Fer.	Ac., x. Arn., Ars, Asa., Bel., Calc., Ca. p., Cb.v., Fer Lach., Merc., Pho. Ph. x., Pul., Sul., Ver.	After Dig., Kre (when following Chi), after Sel.	Ant. t., Arn., Ars., Asa., Aur., Cac., Calc., Cap, Cham., Cin., Cof., Cu. a., Fer., Gel., Gph., Ham., Hel., Hyo., Iod., Ipc., Merc., Mns., Pal. (diar-rhoea), Ped. (sometimes) Sul. is useful in bad effects of tea-drinking and after abuse of chamomile tea (uterine	Aps., Aran., Arn,. Ars., Asa., Bel., Bry., Calc., Cb. v., Caus., Cin., E. pf., Fer., Ipc., Lac., Led., Lyc., Men., Merc., Na. c., Na. M., Nux, Pul., Rhs., Sep., Sul., Ver.

Principal Remedy with abbreviations	Complementary Remedies	Remedy is Followed Well by	Incompatible Remedies	Remedy Antidotes	Remedy is Antidoted by
				haemorrhages) Ver., Vis.	
Note : Swarthy persons ; debilitated, broken down from exhausting discharges ; pleurisy, dropsy.					
Chininum arsenicosum (China-a.)	—	—	—	—	—
Chininum sulphuricum (Chion-s.)	—	—	—	Ars., Iod.	Aran., Arn., Ars., Calc., Cb. v., Fer., Hep., Lach. and esp. Na. M., which antidotes overdosing with Quinine, Pul.
Chionanthus vir. (Chion.)	—	—	—	—	—
Chloralum (Chlol.)	—	—	—	—	Ammon., Atr., Dig (heart), Electricity, Mos.
Cholesterinum. (Cholest.)	—	—	—	—	—

Principal Remedy with abbreviations	Complementary Remedies	Remedy is Followed Well by	Incompatible Remedies	Remedy Antidotes	Remedy is Antidoted by
Chrysarobinum (Chrysar.)	—	—	—	—	—
Cicuta virosa. (Cic.)	—	Bel., Hep., Opi., Pul., Rhs., Sep.		Cup., Opium.	Arn., Cof., Cu. a., Opi., Tobacco for massive doses.
Cimex. (Cimex.)	—	—	—	—	—
Note :—Climacteric years ; nervousness from anxiety and exertion ; rheumatic persons, etc.					
Cimicifuga (Cimic.)	—	—	—	—	—
Cina (Cina)	—	Calc , Chi., Ign., Nux., Plat., Pul., Rhs., Sil. Stn.		Cap., Chi , Merc. val.	Cam., Cap., Chi., Pip.n.
Cineraria maritima (Cinerar-mar.)	—	—	—	—	—
Cinnabaris (Cinnb.)	—	—	—	Au m.	Hep., Nt. x., Opi , Sul ,
Cistus can (Cist.)	Bel., Cb. v., Magnesium, Pho.		Coffee		Cam., Rhs. Sep.

Principal Remedy with abbreviations	Complementary Remedies	Remedy is Followed Well by	Incompatible Remedies	Remedy Antidotes	Remedy is Antidoted by
Clematis erecta (Clem.)		Calc., Rhs., Sep , Sil., Sul.		Bry., Merc., Rho , Rs v. (sometimes) Tab. (sometimes).	Anac. Bry. (toothache, urinary symptoms), Cam., Cham., Ctn., Rn. b., Rhs.
Note :—Torpid cachetic conditions ; light hair					
Coca (Coca)					Gel.
Cocculus (Cocc.)		Ars., Bel., Hep., Ign. Lyc., Nux., Opi , Pul., Rhs., Sul.	Caus., Cof.	Alcohol, Ant. t., Aur., Cham., Cup., Ign., Nux, Pet., Pb., Spi., the fever of Thu., Yuc.	Cam., Cham., Cup. Ign., Nux, Stp.
Coccus cacti (Coc-c.)	—	—	—	—	—
Codeinum (Cod.)	—	—	—	—	—
Coffea cruda (Coff.)	Aco.	Aco., Aur., Bel., Lyc., Nux, Opi., Sul.	Ast. r. ; inimical to Ag. n. (nervous	Amb., Am. m. Aha. Ang., Aur., Bel.,	Ac. x, Aco., Asp. Cham., Ign., Merc. Nux, Sul., and esp.

Principal Remedy with abbreviations	Complementary Remedies	Remedy is Followed Well by	Incompatible Remedies	Remedy Antidotes	Remedy is Antidoted by
			headache); Cth. Caus , Cis , Coc. i., Ign., aggravates symptoms of Lc. x Mil. (is equal to congestion to head) Stramonium	Bor., Cb. v , Caus., Cham., Cic., Col., Con., Cyc., Gam., Gel., Glo., Hy x., Ign., Iod , K. ca , Lach., Lau. Lyc., Man., Mos., Nux. Par., Ph. x. Pho., Pul., Rhs., Sty., Tab., Val.	Tab.
Colchicum (Colah.)		Cb. v. (ascites) Merc., Nux, Pul., Rhs , Sep.	Ac. x. disagrees whei given after Clch.	Cai., Castor, Plai , Thu.	Bel., Cam , Coc. i., Led. Nux., Pul. (heart), Spi., honey and sugar. In poisoning give Amm. in sugar water.

Note :—Gout in persons of vigorous constitutions.

Principal Remedy with abbreviations	Complementary Remedies	Remedy is Followed Well by	Incompatible Remedies	Remedy Antidotes	Remedy is Antidoted by
Collinsonia can. (Coll.)					Nux.
Colocynthis (Coloc.)	Merc. (dysentery with much tenesmus).	Bel., Bry., Caus., Cham., Merc., Nux., Pul., Spi., Sep.		Caus., Cham., Gam., Magnes, Pod., Rhe.	Cam., Cam., Cham., Cof., Opi., Stp. Large doses are counteracted by Cam-infusion of galls, tepid milk Opi.
Conium mac. (Con.)	—	Arn., Ars., Bel., Calc., Cic., Drs., Lyc., Nux. Pho., Pul., Rhs., Stm., Sul.	Conium sometime disagrees with patients who have been taking Psorinum	Ant. t. (Sometime) cham., Cu. a, Cup. Merc. Nit s.d., Nt-acid Rumex., Sbd. Sul.	Cof., Dul., Nt. acid., Nitri Spirtus Dulcis. (wine)
Copaiva (Cop.)	—	—	—	—	Bel., Calc., Merc., Sul., Mr.c. in the male, and Mr. sol. in the female, according to

Principal Remedy with abbreviations	Complementary Remedies	Remedy is Followed Well by	Incompatible Remedies	Remedy Antidotes	Remedy is Antidoted by
					Teste, neutralise the action of Cop. almost in stantaneously.
Coqueluchin (Coquel.)					
Note :—Taken from the virus of whooping cough for the treatment of whooping cough & other spasmodic cough.					
Cotyledon (Cotyled.)					
Crataegus (Crataeg.)		Dig., Naja, strophantus.			Acon., Bel, Opi.
Crocus-sativa (Croc-s.)	—	Nux, Pul., Sul.	—	—	—
Crotalus horridus. (Crot-h.)	—	—	—	It relived eye symptoms of Mep.	Lach. Its effects are modified by Alcohol, Ammon. Com., Cof., Opi., and radiant heat.

Principal Remedy with abbreviations	Complementary Remedies	Remedy is Followed Well by	Incompatible Remedies	Remedy Antidotes	Remedy is Antidoted by
Croton tiglium (Crot-t.)	—	Rhs.	—	Rhs.	Anac., Ant. t., Clem., Rhs., Rn. b.
Cucurbita pepo. (Cucur-b.)	—	—	—	—	—
Cuprum aceticum (Cupr-acet.)	Calc.., Gel. (over worked brain), Cicut. and Solanaceae (Mental symptoms) Zin. (hydrocephalus and convulsions from suppressed exanthems).	—	—	—	Bel., Chi., Cicut., Dul., Hep., Ipc., Merc., Nux. In poisoning cases, by sugar or white of egg given freely.
Cuprum arsenitum (Cupr-ars.)	—	—	—	—	See under Arsen
Cuprum metallicum (Cupr-met.)	Calc.	Ars., Bel., Calc., Caus., Cic.. Hyo.,		Coc. i., Dul.	*Dynamic* : Aur., Bel., Cham., Chi.,

Principal Remedy with abbreviation	Complementary Remedies	Remedy is Followed Well by	Incompatible Remedies	Remedy Antidotes	Remedy is Antidoted by
		K. •n., Pul., Stm., Ver.			Con., Cic., Dul., Hep , Ipc., Merc., Nux, Pul., Ver., Aggravations are Ameliorated by smelling Cam. Hep., or potash soap may be used after *poisoning* from food prepared in copper vessels. Suger, or white of egg mixed with milk, and given freely.
Cuprum oxyd. (Curpur-oxy.)	—	—	—	—	—
Cyclamen (Cycl.)		Pho., Pul, Rhs., Sep., Sul.			Cam., Cof., Pul.
Cypripedium (Cypr.)	—	—	—	Rhs. poisoning	—

Principal Remedy with abbreviations	Complementary Remedies	Remedy is Followed Well by	Incompatible Remedies	Remedy Antidotes	Remedy is Antidoted by
Daphne indica (Daph.)				Chr. x. Merc.	Bry. Dig., Rhs., Sep., Sil., Zn.
Damiana	*Note* : Sexual neurasthenia ; impotency incontinence of old people, chronic prostate discharge. Aids the establishment of normal menstrual discharge in young girls.				
Digitalis (Dig.)	—	Bel., Bry., Cham., Chi., Lyc., Nux, Opi., Pho., Pul., Sep., Sul., Ver.	Chi. (increases the anxiety), Nt. s.d.	Chi. h.(heart), Dph., Gel., My. c. (jaundice), Wine.	Vegetable acids, Aps, Calc., Camphor, (Clch.), Ether, infusion of galls, Nt. x., Nux, Opi., Serpentaria, Vinegar.
Dioscorea (Dios.)	—	—	—	—	—
Diphtherinum (Dipth.)	—	—	—	—	—
Dolichos (Dol.)	—	—	—	—	Aco., and "in cases of dentition with fever, Aco.

Principal Remedy with abbreviations	Complementary Remedies	Remedy is Followed Well by	Incompatible Remedies	Remedy Antidotes	Remedy is Antidoted by
					should be given before Dol. to prevent convulsions" (Hering).
Drosera (Dros.)	Nux.	Calc., Cin., Pul. Sul., Ver.	—	—	Cam.
Duboisinum (Dub.)	—	—	—	—	Cof., Lemon-juice.
Dulcamara (Dulc.)	Baryta Carb.	Bel., Calc., Lyc., Rhs., Sep.	Bel., Lach.	Ba. c., Cam., Con., Cup., Merc.	Cam., Cup., Ipc., Kalicarb., Merc.

Note : Phlegmatic, torpid scrofulous persons who are restless and irritable susceptible to changes of weathar and taking cold easily.

Principal Remedy with abbreviations	Complementary Remedies	Remedy is Followed Well by	Incompatible Remedies	Remedy Antidotes	Remedy is Antidoted by
Echinacea (Ech.)	Locally as cleaning and antiseptic wash.	Bathrops, lach. Ars., Baptisia, Rhus, Hepar.,	—	—	—
Elaps corallinus (Elaps.)	—	—	—	—	Alcohol, Ars., Radiated heat,

Principal Remedy with abbreviation	Complementary Remedies	Remedy is Followed Well by	Incompatible Remedies	Remedy Antidotes	Remedy is Antidoted by
Elaterium (Elat.)	—	—	—	—	—
Equisetum (Equis.)	—	—	—	—	—
Eserinum (Eser.)	—	—	—	Sty. poisoning	—
Eucalyptus (Eucal.)	—	—	—	—	—
Euonyminum (Euonym.)	—	—	—	—	—
Eupatorium pur. (up-pur.)	—	—	—	—	—
Euphrasia (Euphr.)	—	Aco., Clc., Con., Nux, Pho., Pul., Rhs., Sil, Sul.	—	—	Cam., Caus., Pul.
Epihysterinum (Epihyst.)	—	—	—	—	Gph. (effect on eye lids.)

Principal Remedy with abbreviations	Complementary Remedies	Remedy is Followed Well by	Incompatible Remedies	Remedy Antidotes	Remedy is Antidoted by
Ferrum aceticum (Ferr-a.)					
Note :—Alkaline urine in acute diseases. Pain in right deltoid ; asthma ; philtisis ; Constant Cough. Vomiting of food after eating ; haemoplysis.					
Ferrum-metallicum (Ferr-met.)	Alm., Chi., Ham.	Aco., Arn., Bel., Chi., Con. Lyc., Merc., Pho., Pul., Sul., Ver.	Ac. x., Beer. Thea.	Alcoholic drinks, Ars., Chi Hy. x, Iod., Merc., Tea.	Arn., Ars., Beer., Bel., Chi., Hep., Ipc., Pul.
Note :—Persons who, though weak and nervous, have a very red face Delicate, chlorotic women, sanguine, choleric people.					
Ferrum arsenicum (Ferr-ars.)	—	—	—	—	—
Ferrum phosphoricum (Ferr-p.)	—	—	Par.	According to Cooper, Fe. p. antidoted "violent	—

Principal Remedy with abbreviations	Complementary Remedies	Remedy is Followed Well by	Incompatible Remedies	Remedy Antidotes	Remedy is Antidoted by
				dysuria, night and day." caused by Sto. b.	
Ferrum picricum (Ferr pic.)	—	—	—	—	—
Ficus religosia (Ficus-r.)	—	—	—	—	—
Fluoricum acid (Fl-ac.)	Sil.	Gph., Nt. x.	—	Sil.	—
Fragaria (Frag.)	—	Apis., Calc.	—	—	Bry.
Fraxinus americanus (Frac-am.)	—	—	—	—	—
Fucus vesiculosus (Fucus-ves.)	—	—	—	—	—
Galium-aperine (Gal-ap.)	—	—	—	—	—

Principal Remedy with abbreviations	Complementary Remedies	Remedy is Followed Well by	Incompatible Remedies	Remedy Antidotes	Remedy is Antidoted by
Gelsemium (Gels.)	—	Bap., Cac., Ipc.	Gel. antagonises Atr., Opi.	Coca, Mag. p., Nx. m, Sol, Tab. (sometimes).	Atr., Chi., Cof. Dig., Na. m., Nx. m. In cases of poisoning, artificial respiration and faradisation of respiratory muscles. Foy tound Nitro glycerine a perfect antidote in one case. Jephson antidoted his case with strychnine.
Gentiana lutea (Gent-l.)	—	—	—	—	—
Geranium (Ger.)	—	—	—	—	—
Glycerinum (Glycerin.)	—	Gels., Calc.	—	—	—
Ginseng (Gins.)	—	—	—	—	—

Principal Remedy with abbreviations	Complementary Remedies	Remedy is Followed Well by	Incompatible Remedies	Remedy Antidotes	Remedy is Antidoted by
Glonoinum (Glon.)	—	—	—	Ca. ar. (headache), Pal. (headache), Sol.	Aco., Cam., Cof., Nux.
Gnaphalium (Gnaph.)	—	—	—	—	—
Gossypium (Goss.)	—	—	—	—	Vh. p.
Golondrina (Golond.)	—	Euphorbias, Cedron.	—	—	—
Graphites (Graph.)	Ars., Caus., Fer., Hep., Lyc.	Eub.. Ntr. s., Sil.	—	Ars effect on eyelid of Eupionum, Iod., Lyc., Rhs. Ther., (more chronic effects of)	Aco., Ars., China., Nux. Wine.

Principal Remedy with abbreviations	Complementary Remedies	Remedy is Followed Well by	Incompatible Remedies	Remedy Antidotes	Remedy is Antidoted by
Gratiola. (Gra.)	—	—	—	Iod. —	Caus., Bel , Eub., Nux.
Guaiacum (Guaic.)		Calc , Merc.		Caus., Merc., Natrum hypo-chlor, Rhs.	Nux.
Guarea (Gunp.)	—	—	—		
Gun-powder (Gump.)	—	—	—	—	—

Note : Septic suppuration ; protractive against wound infection, herpes facialis ; crops of boils, carbuncles.

Principal Remedy with abbreviations	Complementary Remedies	Remedy is Followed Well by	Incompatible Remedies	Remedy Antidotes	Remedy is Antidoted by
Hamamelis (Ham.)	Fer. in haemorrhages.	—	—	—	Arn., Cam., Chi., Pul. (toothache).
Hecla Lava (Hecla.)	—	—	—	—	—
Helix tosta (Helix-t.)	—	—	—	—	—
Helleborus niger (Hell.)	—	Bel., Bry., Chi, Ly., Nux., Pho.,		—	— Cam., Chi.

Principal Remedy with abbreviations	Complementary Remedies	Remedy is Followed Well by	Incompatible Remedies	Remedy Antidotes	Remedy is Antidoted by
		Pul., Sul., Zin.			
Note : During dentition brain symptoms, weakly serofulous children.					
Heloderma (Helo.)					
Helonias (Helon.)				The prolapse of Lil and the mental depression of K. br.	
Hepar-sulphuris (Hep.)	Caln. in injuries	Aco., Arn, Bel., Bry, Iod., Lach., Merc., Nt. x, Nux., Pul., Rhs., Sep., Sil., Spo., Sul., Zin.	Spo. does not follow well, according to C.C. Smith ; but see under Follows Well	Am. c., Ant. c., Ars., Bel., Calc., Ch. s., Cnb., Cit., Cod-liver oil. It may be used after poisoning from food prepared in copper vessels. It removes the weakening effets of Ether. Cu. a., Cup.,	Ac. x., Bel., Cham., Sil.

Principal Remedy with abbreviations	Complementary Remedies	Remedy is Followed Well by	Incompatible Remedies	Remedy Antidotes	Remedy is Antidoted by
				Fer., Iod., Iof,, K. i., Lach., Metals, and especially Mercurial preparations. Nt. x., Osm. (pain in larynx), Pb., Sil.	
Hippozaeninum (Hippoz.)	—	—	—	—	—
Hydrastinum muriatica (Hydr-mur.)	—	—	—	—	—
Hydrastis (Hydr.)	—	—	—	Chlorate of potash, Merc. Ss. x. (constipation)	Sul. (head symptoms and aciatic pains).
Hydrocotyle (Hydrc.)	—	—	—	—	—

Principal Remedy with abbreviations	Complementary Remedies	Remedy is Followed Well by	Incompatible Remedies	Remedy Antidotes	Remedy is Antidoted by
Hydrocyanicum acid (Hydr-ac.)	—	—	—	—	Cam., Chlm., Cof., Fer., Ips., Nux, Opi., Ver.
Hydrophobinum (Hydpob.)	—	Na. m.	—	—	Agn., Bel., Ced., Fgs., Hyo., Lach., Stm.
Hydrobromic acid (Hydrobr-a)	—	—	—	—	—
Hyoscyamus (Hyos.)	—	Bel., Pho., Pul., Stm., Ver.		Bel., Cld., (night cough) Eth., Merc., Plumb., Rum., Stm., Sty. (drowsiness).	Ac., x., Bel., Chi., Citric ac., Stm., Vinegar.
Note : Sanguine temperament ; nervous ; irritable, excitable, hysterical subjects, drunkards, old men, children.					
Hypericum (Hyper.)	—	—	—	Effects of mesmerism (Sul.)	Ars. (weakness or sickness on moving) Cham. (pains in face).
Ictodes foe. (Pothos foetidus) (Poth.)	—	—	—	—	—

Principal Remedy with abbreviations	Complementary Remedies	Remedy is Followed Well by	Incompatible Remedies	Remedy Antidotes	Remedy is Antidoted by
Ignatia (Ign.)	Na. m.	Ars., Bel., Calc., Chi., Lyc., Nux., Pul., Rhs., Sep., Sil., Sul.	Cof., Nux (sometimes), Tab.	Arn., Brandy Cld. (sometimes), Chamomile tea, Cham., Coc. i., Cof., Mgt., Mgt. n., Mgt.s., Phyt., Pul., Sel., Tab., Zin.	Ac. x., Arn., Cam., Cham., Coc. i., Cof., Nux., Pul., (chief antidote).
Note :—Suitable to nervous, hysterical females of mild, but easily excited nature.					
Indol. (Ind.)					
Iodium (Ind.)	Bad., Lyc.	Aco., Ag. n., Calc., K. bi., Lyc., Mr. sol., Pho., Pul.		An. oc. (locally), Ars., Merc. (glands).	Starch or wheat-flour mixed with water (to large doses). *Antidotes to small doses* ; Ant. t., Aps. Ars., Bel., Cam., Ch. s. Cof. Fer., Gph.,

Principal Remedy with abbreviations	Complementary Remedies	Remedy is Followed Well by	Incompatible Remedies	Remedy Antidotes	Remedy is Antidoted by
					Grt., Hep , Opi., Pho., Spo., Sul., Thu.

Note :—Suitable particularly to persons with dark eyes and hair ; overgrown boys with weak chests; serofulous diathesis ; old people.

Principal Remedy with abbreviations	Complementary Remedies	Remedy is Followed Well by	Incompatible Remedies	Remedy Antidotes	Remedy is Antidoted by
Ipecacuanha (Ip.)	Arn., Cup.	Ant. t., Arn. Ars. (cholera infantum, debility, colds, croup, chills), Bel , Bry., Calc., Cd. s., (yellow fever), Cham., Chi., Cup., Ign., Nux, Pho., Pul., Rhe., Sep., Sul., Tab., Ver.		Ago., Alum , Ant. t., Aps. (Ipc. low antidotes medium doses and poisoning of Aps., also powdered Ipc. applied locally); Arn , Ars., Calc., Chi., Chl. Chlf. Copper fumes, Cu. a. Cup; Dul., Fer., Hy.	Arn., Ars., Chi. Nux, Tab.

Principal Remedy with abbreviations	Complementary Remedies	Remedy is Followed Well by	Incompatible Remedies	Remedy Antidotes	Remedy is Antidoted by
				x., it relieved the cough of K. n., Lau., Ln.u. Lo. i., Med. (dry cough), esp. useful for secondary effects of Mor., (Teste says it is the surest antidote to Mu. acid.), Opi., Stil. (nausea from the fumes), Su. acid. Tab., (primary effects; vomiting).	
Ipomea (Ipom.)					

Note : Kidney disorders with pain in back. Much abdominal flatulence. Pain in left lumbar region on stooping ; aching in small of back and extremities. Aching in top of right shoulder ; renal colic.

Principal Remedy with abbreviations	Complementary Remedies	Remedy is Followed Well by	Incompatible Remedies	Remedy Antidotes	Remedy is Antidoted by
Iris tenax (Iris-t.)	—	—	—	—	—
Iris versicolor (Iris-v.)				Merc , Nux. Ol j. (sometimes). Phyt.	Nux.
Jaborandi (Jab.)	—	—	—	— Bel.	—
Jacaranda caroba (Jac-c.)	—	—	—	Ana.	—
Juglans cin (Jay-c.)					
Juglans regia (Jug-r.)	—	—	—	—	Rhs.
Kali bichromicum (Kali-b.)	—	Ant. t. (in catarrhal affections diseases) Pul.	—	Arsenical vapour, effect of beer, Merc., Mr. i. f. ; also it is the best general antidote to the effect of	The same antidotes as for poisoning by acids ; Chalk, Eggs, Hydrated peroxide oi iron. Magnesia Milk, Almond or Olive Oil, soap, Bicarbonates of

Principal Remedy with abbreviations	Complementary Remedies	Remedy is Followed Well by	Incompatible Remedies	Remedy Antidotes	Remedy is Antidoted by
				metallic poisoning among brass worker.	Soda. and Potash any one of which should be administered almost immediately after the dose.
Note :—Fat, light haired persons; fat, Chubby children.					
					Among the *dynamic antidotes* are Ars., Lach (croup. diphtheria etc.) Puls. (wandering pains.)
Kali bromatum (Kali-br.)	—	—	—	Lead poisoning	Vegetable acids, Cam., Hlon. (mental depression), Oils, Nux, Zin.
Kali carbonicum (Kali-c.)	K. ca. is complementary to: Cb.v., Na. m., Nt. ac.	Ars., Chs. v., Fl. x., Lyc. Nt. ac., Pho.. Pul., Sep. Sul.		Dul., Gambogia Nitri spiritus dulcis	Camphor, Cof. Nt. Spiritus dulcis

Principal Remedy with abbreviation	Complementary Remedies	Remedy is Followed Well by	Incompatible Remedies	Remedy Antidotes	Remedy is Antidoted by
	Pho., Sep, Complementary to K. ca. are Cb. v., Nux.				
Note :—After loss of fluids on vitality; specially anaemic persons.					
Kali chloricum (Kali-chl.)	—	—	—	Merc.	Hdr.
Kali cyanatum (Kaly-cy.)	—	—	—	—	Nitrate of cobalt
Kali Hydriodicum (Kali-hy)	—	Iod., Mercur., sulf.	—	—	Hepar.
Kali muriaticum (Kali-m.)	—	—	—	Merc.	Bel., Ca. s., Hdr., Pul.
Kali nitricum (Kali-n.)	—	Bel., Calc., Nux in dysentery, Pul., Rhs., Sep., Sul.	Smelling Cam intensified the sufferings.	Cth. (sometimes) the renal symptoms of Caus., Nt. s.d.	Ipc. ameliorates the cough, smelling Ntr. spiritus dulcis.
Kali phosphoricum (Kali-p.)		—	—	—	—

Principal Remedy with abbreviations	Complementary Remedies	Remedy is Followed Well by	Incompatible Remedies	Remedy Antidotes	Remedy is Antidoted by
Kali Sulphuricum (Kali-s.)	—	Ac. x., Ars Calc., Hep., Pul., Rhs., Sep., Sil., Sul.	—	Rhs. poisoning	—
Kalmia (Kalm)	Benz-ac.	Spigelia, Puls.	—	—	—
Kreosotum (Kreos.)	—	Ars. (in malignant diseases), Bel., Calc., K. ca., Lyc., Nt. x., Nux., Rhs., Sep., Sul.	After Cb. v., also after China.	Athra, Guac., Pb.	Aco. (vascular erethism). According to Teste Fer. is the best antidote. esp. for overaction of Kre. in lively, sanguine, and vigorous children. Nux. (violent pulsation in every part of body).

Note :—Young people tall for their age; dark complexion, slight, lean. Complexion livid, disposition sad, irritable, often indicated for old women.

Principal Remedy with abbreviations	Complementary Remedies	Remedy is Followed Well by	Incompatible Remedies	Remedy Antidotes	Remedy is Antidoted by
Lac caninum (Lac-c.)	—	—	—	—	—
Lachesis (Lach.)	Hep., Lyc., (the chief complement). Iod and K.i., which are complementary to Lyc., are probably Complementary to Nt. ac.	Aco., Alm., Ars., Bel., Bro., Cac, Cb. v., Caus , Chi. Cic., Con., Eub., Hep., Hyo., L. bi. Lc. c., Lyc., Merc., Mr. i.f, Na. m., Nt., ac. Nux, Pho., Pul., Rhs., Sil., Sul., Trn.	Aggravated by and incompatible with Ac. x; Am. c , Dul., Nt. x. inimical to Pso. Sep.	Athra., Aps., Ars., Buf., Ch. s., Crt. h., K. bi. (croup, diphtheria & c.) Mag. p. (cough), Rhs., Rum.	Alcohol inwardly, radiate heat outwardly, Salt (for effects of bite). *Antidotes to dilutions:* Alum, Ars., Bel., Calc., Cb. V. according to Tests the chief antidote is Ced.; Cham Coc. i. Cof. Hep., Led., Merc., Nt. ac. Nux, Pho. ac., Sep. (the visible tenesmus of rectum) Tarentula (Hering)

Note :—Useful in women during climacteric period.

Principal Remedy with abbreviations	Complementary Remedies	Remedy is Followed Well by	Incompatible Remedies	Remedy Antidotes	Remedy is Antidoted by
Lachnanthes (Lachn.)	—	—	—	—	—
Lacticum acid (Lac-ac.)	—	—	Coffee aggravates symptoms.	Art. t. Pod.	Bry. (ameliorates sharp pains upper third r. side, but soreness remained).
Lactuca-virosa (Lac-v.)	—	—	—	—	Vegetable acids and Coffee. In a proving of Lactucarium, Acetic Ether and Hock were more effectual the Coffee.
Lapis albus (Lap-a.)	—	—	—	—	—
Lathyrus (Lath.)	—	—	—	—	—
Laurocerasus (Laur.)	—	Bel. Ch. v., Pho., Pul., Ver.		Ant. t. Cth., Nx. m.	Cam., Cof., Ipc., Nx. m., Opi.

Principal Remedy with abbreviations	Complementary Remedies	Remedy is Followed Well by	Incompatible Remedies	Remedy Antidotes	Remedy is Antidoted by
Ledum (Led.)	—	Aco., Bel., Bry., Chel., Nux., Pul., Rhs., Sul.	Chi ("Cinchona bark given for the debility produced by Ledum is very injurious.", —Hahnemann).	Effects of alcohol, Aps. Chi., Vsp.	Cam., Rhs. (the best antidote, according to Teste).
Lemna minor (Lem-m.)	—	—	—	—	—
Leueticum (syphilinum (Luet.)		merc. ; Nit-ac Aur., Kal-hyd.		—	—
Liatris spic. (Liat.)	—	—	—	—	—
Lilium tigrinum (Lit-t.)	—	—	—	—	Hion. (anteversion) Nux. colic), Plat., Pul.—
Lithium carbonicium (lith.)	—	—	—	—	

Principal Remedy with abbreviations	Complementary Remedies	Remedy is Followed Well by	Incompatible Remedies	Remedy Antidotes	Remedy is Antidoted by
Lycopodium (Lyco.)	Chel., Iod., Ign., Ipc. (in capillary bronchitis aggravates right side, sputa yellow and thick.) Kali Iodide, Lach., Pul.	Ana., Bel., Bry., Clch., Drs., Gph., Hyo., Kali Carb, La-chases. Ledum Nux, Pho., Pul. Sep., Sil., Stm., Ther., Ver.	Cof; after sul. except in cycle of Sul., Calc. Lyc., Sul. etc.	All. Alo. (relieves earache) Chi., (yellow face, liver and spleen swollen, flatulence, tension under short ribs aggravates right side, pres-sure in stomach and Constipation), Chlorine (effects of the fumes when they cause inpotence), Merc., Mr. i.f., Tab. (some times).	Aco, Cam. caust., Cham., Cof., Gph Nux, Pul.

Note :—Often useful in old women, persons of keen intellect, but muscular development, lean and predisposed to Lung and hepatic effections.

Principal Remedy with abbreviations	Complementary Remedies	Remedy is Followed Well by	Incompatible Remedies	Remedy Antidotes	Remedy is Antidoted by
Lyssin (Hydrophobinum) (Lyss.),	—	—	—	—	—
Macrotinum (Macro.)	—	—	—	Ost.	—
Magnesia carbonica. (Mag-c.)	Cham.	Caus, pho., Pul., Sep., Sul.	—	—	Ars., Cham. (neuralgia), Col., Mr. sol., Nux., Pul., Rhe. (abdominal troubles.) Bel., Gel., Lach. (cough).
Magnesia phosphorica (Mag-p.)	—	—	—	—	
Magnitis polus Austrealis. (Mag-Aust.)	—	—	—	Mgt. s.	Mgt. s. Ign., Zin.
Malandrinum (Maland.)	—	—	—	Vac., Var.	—
Mancinella (Manc.)	—	—	—	—	—

Principal Remedy with abbreviations	Complementary Remedies	Remedy is Followed Well by	Incompatible Remedies	Remedy Antidotes	Remedy is Antidoted by
Medorrhinum (Med.)	—	—	—	—	—
Melilotus (Meli.)	—	—	—	—	—
Menyanthes (Meny.)	—	Cap., Lach., Lyc., Pul., Rhs.	—	Effects of China and Quinine.	Cam.
Mephitis (Meph.)	—	—	—	—	Cam., but cnly temporarily. Crotal ameliorates eye symptoms.
Mercurius (Merc.)	Bad.	Ars., Asa., Bel. Calc , Cb. v, Chr., Gui., Hep., Iod., Lyc., Mu. x., Nt. x., Pho., Pul , Rhs., Sep., Sul., Thu.	It is aggravated by Ac. x., Sil. (Merc. and Sil. should never be given immediately before or after each other.)	Ailments from arsenic or copper vapours, stings of insects, bad effects of sugar. Ant. c., Ant. t , Arg., Asa., Aur., Ba. carb., Bel., Cld. (sometimes) Can. s. (small doses), Chi., Cof.,	Aran., Ars., Asa. (bone affections—Asa. is distinguished by extreme sensitiveness of diseased parts, extreme soreness of bones round eye), Aur. suicidal manal

Principal Remedy with abbreviations	Complementary Remedies	Remedy is Followed Well by	Incompatible Remedies	Remedy Antidotes	Remedy is Antidoted by
				Cop, (in the female) Cu. a , Cup., Dul., Ja. g., Mag. c., Man., Mez., Mr. c., Nt. ac., Opi., Osm. (laryngeal catarrh). Plant. (tooth-ache), Rhs., Sars., Sul., Vi. t.	caries of bones, esp. of patella and nose). Bel., Bry., Cld., Cap., (abuse of Merc.), Cb. v., Caus. (sometimes) Chi. (chronic ptyalism), Cin., Clem., Con., Cup., Dph., Dul. (ptylism aggravate by every damp change). Elc., Fer., Gui., Hep. (mental symptoms-anxiety, distress, sucidial and even homicidal mood—bone pains, (sore mouth, ulcers and gastric symptoms), Hdr., Hyo., Iod. (glands), Iris,

Principal Remedy with abbreviation	Complementary Remedies	Remedy is Followed Well by	Incompatible Remedies	Remedy Antidotes	Remedy is Antidoted by
					Ja. g., K. bi., K. chl., K. i. (syphilis and mercurialism combined, bones, periosteum, glands ozoena, thin watery discharge upper lip sore and raw, repeated catarrhs after Merc., every little exposure to damp or wet air-coryza, eyes hot, watery, swollen, neuralgic pains in one or both cheek, nose stuffed and swollen and at the same time profuse watery, scalding coryza, sore throat

Principal Remedy with abbreviations	Complementary Remedies	Remedy is Followed Well by	Incompatible Remedies	Remedy Antidotes	Remedy is Antidoted by
					aggravated every fresh exposure) Kali Mur. (scorbutus) fetor, Lyc., Mag. M. (metorrhagia), Mez., (nervous system, neuralgia in eyes, face, any where), Mu. x., Nux, (tremors), Opi., Pod., (vapours) Puls., Spi., Stp. (depressed system, wasted, sallow, darkings round eyes, spongy gums, ulcers on tongue, Stil., Sul., Ter., Thu., "all symptoms agreeing Merc., high" (Guernsey).

Principal Remedy with abbreviations	Complementary Remedies	Remedy is Followed Well by	Incompatible Remedies	Remedy Antidotes	Remedy is Antidoted by
Mercurius biniod (Merc-bin.)	—	—	—	—	Hep.
Mercurius corrosivus (Merc-c.)				Chr. ox. (sometimes), Trb. (diarrhoea).	(*Poisonous doses*) While of egg. *Dynamic antidotes*: Lo. i. (Teste), Mr. sol., Sep., Sil., (Hering). Also antidotes to the Mercuries generally (*see* Merc.)
Mercurius cyanatus (Merc-cy.)	—	—	—	—	
Mercurius dulcis (Merc-d.)	—	—	—	—	Hep.
Mercurius Vivus or Sol. (Merc-s)	Badiaga	Mer. Phos, Syph.	—	—	—
Mezereum. (Mez.)	—	Calc., Caus., Ign., Lyc., Merc. Nux, Pho., Pul.	—	Alcohol, Merc., Nt. x., Pho., Phyt.	Acids, Aco., Bry., Calc. (headache) Cam., K. i., Merc., Nux.
Note : Phlegmatic temperament.					
Millefolium (Mill.)	—	—	Coffee (congestion to the head).	Ar. m.	—

Principal Remedy with abbreviations	Complementary Remedies	Remedy is Followed Well by	Incompatible Remedies	Remedy Antidotes	Remedy is Antidoted by
Morbillinum. (Morbil.)					
Morphinum (Morph.)			Vinegar (it increases the painful symptoms, vertigo & c.)	Elc. (Mo. a., see Electricitas).	Aco. and Ipc., esp. useful for secondary effects, Art., Avn., Bel., Strong Coffee (poisoning), Oxg., Oxygen inhalations. Keaney (*H.P.* xv. 195) cured with one dose of Sul. c.m. (Swan)a man who had taken 2 grs. of morphine daily for 15 years.
Moschus (Mosch.)	—	—	—	Chl. h, Ther. (headaches).	Cam. (unconsciousness and coldness), Cof.
Murex . (Murx.)	—	—	—	—	—
Muriaticum acid (Mur-ac.)		Calc , K. ca., Nux, Pul , Sep., Sil., Sul.		Bry., Merc., Opi (it "cures the muscular	Carbonates of alkalies and earths (poisoning cases),

Principal Remedy with abbreviations	Complementary Remedies	Remedy is Followed Well by	Incompatible Remedies	Remedy Antidotes	Remedy is Antidoted by
				weakness following the excessive use of Opium"—Hering). Sel.	small doses : Bry., Cam. (Teste says the surest antidote is Ipc.)
Mullein Oil (Mullein-oil.)	—	—	—	—	Dig. (jundice).
Myrica (Myric.)	—	—	—	—	—
Myristica seb. (Mst-s.)	—	—	—	—	—
Naja tripudians. (Naja).	—	—	—	—	Ammonia, stimulants (effects of bite), Tab. (potencies.)
Napthalinum. (Nepthal).	—	—	—	—	—
Nasturtrum. (water-reress). (Nasturt.)	—	—	—	—	—

Note :—Useful in scorbutic affections and constipation, related structures of urinary apparatus ; sedative in neurasthenia and hysteria, cirrhosis of liver and dropsy.

Principal Remedy with abbreviations	Complementary Remedies	Remedy is Followed Well by	Incompatible Remedies	Remedy Antidotes	Remedy is Antidoted by
Natrum carbonicum (Nat-c.)	Sep, (Kali-salts)	Calc., Nt. ac., Nux, Pul., Sed., Sul.		As., mt. Chi., Nt. s.d.	Cam., Nt. s.d.
Natrum hypo-sulph (Nat-hyposulph)	Sep.	—	—	—	Gui, Pul. (rheumatic and myalgic symptoms ; also; probably; the antidotes to Na. m.)
Natrum cholenicum (Nat-chol.)	—	—	—	—	—

Note : Constipation, chronic gastric, intestinal catarrh ; cirrhotic liver ; diabetes ; nape of neck pains ; tendency to sleep after eating ; much flatus ; ascitns.

Principal Remedy with abbreviations	Complementary Remedies	Remedy is Followed Well by	Incompatible Remedies	Remedy Antidotes	Remedy is Antidoted by
Natrum Muriatium (Nat-m.)	Aps., Cap., Ign., Sep., Na. m. is the *Chronic* of : Aps., Cap., Ign. (its vegeta-	Bry., Calc., Hep. K. ca., Pul., Rhs., Sep., Sul. Thu.	It increases the action of Pod.	Ac. x (for gestric pulmonary, and febrile symptoms), Agn. (headache) Aps. (bee-stings) Ag n	Ars. (bad effects of sea-bathing), Cam.; Smelling Nt. s.d. ; Nux will ameliorates headache if persistent, or prostration if prolon-

Principal Remedy with abbreviations	Complementary Remedies	Remedy is Followed Well by	Incompatible Remedies	Remedy Antidotes	Remedy is Antidoted by
	ble analogue).			(abuse of as in cautery) Cean., Cin., Nt. s. d., Quinine (when diseases continue intermittent, and patients suffer from headache, constipation, disturbed sleep) Na. m. should not be given *during* the paroxysm of fever.	ged after Na. m.; Pho. (esp. abuse of salt in food), Sep.
Natrum Phosphoricum (Nat-p.)	—	—	—	—	Aps. (urticaria Sep. (esp. eruption and swelling about joints).
Natrum sulphuricum (Nat-s.)	— Ars., Thu.	—	—	—	—
Niccolum sulphuricum. (Nicc-s.)	—	—	—	—	—

Principal Remedy with abbreviations	Complementary Remedies	Remedy is Followed Well by	Incompatible Remedies	Remedy Antidotes	Remedy is Antidoted by
Nitroso-muriatic acid (Nit-m-ac.)	—	—	—	—	—
Nux moschata (Nux-m.)	—	Ant. t., Lyc., Pul., Rhs., Stm.	—	Alcohol, bad yeasty beer, Ars. Gel., Lau., Lead colic, Rho., Turpentine.	Cam., Gel., Lau., Nux, Opi. Val., Zin.
Note :—Suits mostly women and children and the aged.					
Nux vomica (Nux-v)	(Calc.), K. ca., Sep., Sul.	Act. s., Ars. Bel., Bry., Cac., Calc Cb.v., Clch., Coc.i., Hyo., Lyc., Pho., Pul., Rhs., Sep., Sul.	Ac. x disagrees when given after Nux. Nux disagrees when followed by Ac., acids Ast. r., Ign., (sometimes), Zin.	Narcotic, drastic and vegitable remedies. Bad effects of anomalies in foods *e.g.*, Ginger, Nutmeg., Papper, and so called "hot" medicines, Aesc. (pile symptoms). Ail., Alcohal, Alo. (relieves earache.), Aln (nausea and	Aco., Amb., Ars., Bel., Cam., Cham., Coc. i., Cof., Eub., Ign., Iris. Opi., Pal., Plat., Pul., Stm., Thu., Wine.

Principal Remedy with abbreviations	Complementary Remedies	Remedy is Followed Well by	Incompatible Remedies	Remedy Antidotes	Remedy is Antidoted by
				vomiting), Amb. Am. m., Ars., As. h., Bis., Bry., Calc., Cb. a., Caus., Cep. (coryza recurring in August)., Cham., Chi., Coc. i., Cof., Cich., Coll., Cu. a., Cup., Ether, Glo., Gph., Grt., Gui., Hy. x., Ind, Ipc., Iris, K. br., Kre. (sometimes) Lach., Lil., Lyc., Mag. c., Mag. cil., Mag. m., Mlr. (effects of No. 1.), Merc., Mez. (neuralgia), Nux will relieve headache if persistent or prostation or if	

Principal Remedy with abbreviations	Complementary Remedies	Remedy is Followed Well by	Incompatible Remedies	Remedy Antidotes	Remedy is Antidoted by
				prolonged after Na. m., Ol., a. Opl. Ost. (lumbago), Pet., Pho., Plumb., Pod., Pul., Rhe., Sin. n., Stm., Tab., (sometimes). Tel. (epigastric oppression) Thu. (urination).	

Note :—Suitable for thin, irritable, choleric persons with dark hair, who make great mental exertion or lead a tendentary life. Debauchers, who are irritable and thin.

Principal Remedy with abbreviations	Complementary Remedies	Remedy is Followed Well by	Incompatible Remedies	Remedy Antidotes	Remedy is Antidoted by
Nyctanthes (Nyct.)	—	—	—	—	—
Ocimum canum (Oci)	—	Dio.	—	—	—
Oenanthe croc. (Oena.)	—	—	—	—	—

Principal Remedy with abbreviations	Complementary Remedies	Remedy is Followed Well by	Incompatible Remedies	Remedy Antidotes	Remedy is Antidoted by
Oleander (Olnd.)	—	—	Con., Lyc., Na. m, Pul., Rhs., Sep., Spi.	—	Cam. (acute effects), Sul. (chronic effects).
Oleum-jacoris aselle (Ol-j.)	—	—	Sep.	—	—
Opium (Op.)	—	—	Aco., Ant. t., Bel., Bry., Hyo., Nux, Nx. m.	Amg. (convulsions), Ant. t. (Opium in large doses is the best antidote to Ant. t.) Atr., Bel., Bro., Cam., Cic., Cnb Col. (large doses). Cro., Dig., Eub., Gam., Hur., Hur.c., Hy. acid., Iod, Lach.,	Strong Coffee, Kali pm. solution (about 1. gr. to the pint of water the patient is made to swallow half a-pint every five minutes, and then caused to vomit; later a somewhat stronger solution may be given and retained) ; Oxygen

Principal Remedy with abbreviations	Complementary Remedies	Remedy is Followed Well by	Incompatible Remedies	Remedy Antidotes	Remedy is Antidoted by
				Lau,, Merc., Nt. s. d., Nx. m., Nux, Ol. a., Pb., Phyt. (large doses.) Stm., Sty.	inhalations; (patient must be kept walking about ; if allowed to sleep, it may be impossible to wake him again); Ag.n., Bel., Cam., Cham. (nervous irritability), Ipc., Nux, Sars., Sul. (marasmus), Vanil., Vinum.

Note:—Especially suitable for children and old person. Frequently suited to persons addicted to liquors.

Principal Remedy with abbreviations	Complementary Remedies	Remedy is Followed Well by	Incompatible Remedies	Remedy Antidotes	Remedy is Antidoted by
Orchitinum (Orchit.)	—	—	—	—	—
Osmium (Osm.)	—	—	—	—	Bel. and Merc. (laryngeal catarrh) Hep. and Spo. (pain in larynx), Sulphurated Hy-

Principal Remedy with abbreviations	Complementary Remedies	Remedy is Followed Well by	Incompatible Remedies	Remedy Antidotes	Remedy is Antidoted by
		—			drogen, Ph. x., Sil. (swollen gums). Carbonates of Lime and Magnesia.
Oxalicum ac. (Ox-ac.)	—	—	—	—	Alo., Rat. —
Paeonia. (Paen.)	—	—	—	—	—
Paraffinum (Parf.)	—	—	—	—	—
Pareira (Pareir.)	—	—	—	—	—
Parotidinum (Parot.)	—	—	—	—	—
Passiflora (Passi-fl.)	—	—	—	— Sty.	—
Pertussin (Pertuss.)	—	—	—	—	—

Note :—Contains the virus of whooping cough for the treatment of whooping cough & other spasmodic cough.

Principal Remedy with abbreviations	Complementary	Remedy is Followed Well by	Incompatible Remedies	Remedy Antidotes	Remedy is Antidoted by
Petroleum (Petr.)	Before Sep.	Bry., Calc., Lyc., Nt. x., Nux, Pul., Sep., Sil., Sul.		Lead poisoning (one of the best remedies), Nt. ac.	Aco., Coc., i., Nux, Pho.
Petroselinum (Petros.)	—	—	—	—	Rhe. (Diarrhoea).
Phellandrium (Phel.)					
Phosphoricum acid	—	Ars., Bel., Ca. p., Caus., Chi., Fer., Fe. p., K. phos., Lyc., Na., p., Nux, Pul., Sep., Sul., Ver.	—	—	Cam., Cof., Stp.

Note : Bad effects from growing too rapidly ; as if beaten in back and limbs.

Principal Remedy with abbreviations	Complementary	Remedy is Followed Well by	Incompatible Remedies	Remedy Antidotes	Remedy is Antidoted by
Phosphorus (Phos.)	Ars. Cep. (all three have alliaceous	Ars., Bel., Bry., Calc., Cb. v., Chi., K. ca., Lyc.,	Aps., Caus.	Cam., Iod., Na. m. (excessive	Ars., Calc., Cam., Chlf. Cof., K. pm. well diluted

Principal Remedy with abbreviations	Complementary Remedies	Remedy is Followed Well by	Incompatible Remedies	Remedy Antidotes	Remedy is Antidoted by
	odours), Cb. v., Ipc.	Nux, Pul., Sep., Sil., Sul.		use of salt), Pet., Rs. v., Rum., it relieved the effects of Sla., Tab. (sometimes), Ter.	and given freely (Dr. Antal), Mez., Nux, Sep., Ter., Wine,

Note :—Tall, slender, (slim) women disposed to stoop. Nervous, weak; grow too rapidly.

Principal Remedy with abbreviations	Complementary Remedies	Remedy is Followed Well by	Incompatible Remedies	Remedy Antidotes	Remedy is Antidoted by
Physostigma (Phys.)	—	—	—	Atr.	Injection of Atr., antagonises its effects, Arn., Coffee; Emetics are of the first importance. Lil. cured astigmatism of Phst., Sinapisms.
Phytolacca (Phyt.)	—	—	—	Bap.	Bel., Coffee (vomiting), Ign., Iris., Merc., Mez., Milk, Nt. s. d., Opi. (large doses) Salt, Sul. (eyes).

Principal Remedy with abbreviations	Complementary Remedies	Remedy is Followed Well by	Incompatible Remedies	Remedy Antidotes	Remedy is Antidoted by
Picricum acid (Pic-a.)	—	—	—	—	—
Pilocarpinum-mur, (Piloc.)	—	—	—	—	Atr., Am. c. (sal volatile), Braddy.
Note :—Rapidly progressive phithises with free haemorrhages; profuse sweating.					
Pituitrin (Pituitrin.)	—	—	—	—	—
Note :—Used for its action on the uterus either to aid in child birth or to check bleeding after child-birth.					
Plantago (Plan.)	—	—	—	Aps., Rhs., Tab.	Merc. (toothache
Platinum (Plat-met)	Pal (both affect r. ovary, but Pal. has amelioration from pressure).	Ana., Arg., Bel., Lyc., Pul., Rhs., Sep., Ver.		Lead, Sil (?), Nux.	Bel., Nt. s.d., Pul., (Tests, who classes Plat. with Thu., Bro., and Castor, says Colch. is the best antidote to all four).
Note :—Especially suited to women with dark hair, rigid fibre.					
Plumbum-metallicum (Plb-met.)	—	Ars., Bel., Lyc., Merc., Pho., Pul., Sil., Sul.		Ast. r., bad effects of long abuse of vinegar.	Ac. x. (colic), Alcohol is a preventive, Alm., Aln., Ant. c.,

Principal Remedy with abbreviations	Complementary Remedies	Remedy is Followed Well by	Incompatible Remedies	Remedy Antidotes	Remedy is Antidoted by
					Bel., Caus, (lead poisoning), Coc. i., Hep., Kre., Na. n. (?) Nx. m. (lead colic), Nux, Opi., Pet., Plat., Ppz., Sulphuric acid diluted is one of the best antidotes to the chronic effects of lead, Zin (Taste, who classes Pb. with Merc. and Ars. says. Aeth. is the best antidote in his experience he names also Elc., Hyo.; Ple., Strm.).
Plumbum iodatum (Plumb-iod.)	—	—	—	—	—
Podophyllum (Podo.)	(Sul.)	—	Salt, which increases its action.	Merc., it relieved the diarrhoea of Lo. s., but not the	Col., Lc. x., Lpt.; Nux.

Principal Remedy With abbreviations	Complementary Remedies	Remedy is Followed Well by	Incompatible Remedies	Remedy Antidotes	Remedy is Antidoted by
				acute abdominal pains, Src.	

Note :—Bilious temperament specially after mercurialization.

Principal Remedy With abbreviations	Complementary Remedies	Remedy is Followed Well by	Incompatible Remedies	Remedy Antidotes	Remedy is Antidoted by
Pothos-foetidus. (Poth.)					

Note :—Asthmatic complaints worse from inhaling dust. Hysteria, inflation and tension in abdomen.

Principal Remedy With abbreviations	Complementary Remedies	Remedy is Followed Well by	Incompatible Remedies	Remedy Antidotes	Remedy is Antidoted by
Prunus-spinosa (Pru-s.)	—	—	—	—	—
Psorinum (Psor.)	After Arn. (blow on ovary), Bac. (Bac. is the *acute* of Pso.), after Lc. x. (vomiting of pregnancy), (Sul., after Pso. in mammary cancer.	Alm., Bor., Cb. v., Chi., Hep., Sul.	Con (sometimes) Lach., Sep.		Coffee.

Note :—Scrofulous; nervous, restless, easily startled. Psoric constitutions, specially when other remedies fail to permanently improve. Lack of reaction after severe diseases. Pale, sickly, delicate children,

Principal Remedy With abbreviations	Complementary Remedies	Remedy is Followed Well by	Incompatible Remedies	Remedy Antidotes	Remedy is Antidoted by
Pulsatilla (Puls.)	Ag. n. (if Ag. n. flags give Pul.,	Ana., Ant. t. Ars., Asa., Bel., Bry., Calc., Eub.,		Amb., Ant. t., Athra., Arg., Ar. t., Asa.,	Acids, Ant. t., Cen., Cham (Cham. and Pul. antidote each

Principal Remedy with abbreviations	Complementary Remedies	Remedy is Followed Well by	Incompatible Remedies	Remedy Antidotes	Remedy is Antidoted by
	Ag. n. follows Pul. in ophthalmia), Cham. Cep., Lyc., Sel., Stn. (Stn. has menses too early and too profuse), Sux.	Gph., Ign., K. bi., Lyc., Nt. x., Nux, Pho., Rhs, Sep., Sul.		Aur., Bel., Bry., Ca. ar. (sometimes) Cth., Cham., Chi., Ch. s., Cof., Clch., Cyc., Ephr., Fer. (in chlorotic girls who have been damaged by Iron Pul. has an excellent effect), Gel., Ham. (toothache) Ign. (chief antidote) K. bi. (wandering pains), K. m., Lil., Lyc., vapours of Murcury and Copper, Mag. c., Na. hch. (rheumatic and myalgic symptoms), Pip. m. (partially) Plat., Rn. b, Rn.	other and follow each other well. If either one has over acted the other will probably neutralise the ill-effect and carry on the good) ; Cof., Ign., Nux, Stn. (Teste adds Sul., and says when the improper use of Pul. has affected the air passages Ca. p. has proved the best antidote).

Principal Remedy with abbreviations	Complementary Remedies	Remedy is Followed Well by	Incompatible Remedies	Remedy Antidotes	Remedy is Antidoted by
				s., Rhe., Sbd., Sbl. (sometimes), Sbi., Sel., Spi., Stn., Stm., Sul., Su. x., Tab. (sometimes), Thu., Toadstool poisoning, Val., Vi. t., Whisky, Ziz. (migraine).	

Note :—Sandy hair, blue eyes, plane face, inclined to grief and submissiveness; easily moved to tears or laughter. Often indicated with women and children.

Principal Remedy with abbreviations	Complementary Remedies	Remedy is Followed Well by	Incompatible Remedies	Remedy Antidotes	Remedy is Antidoted by
Pyrogenium (Pyrog.)	—	—	—	—	—
Radium (Rad.)	—	—	—	—	—

Note :—Effective in rheumatism and gout; severe aching pains all over; chronic rheumatic arthritis.

Principal Remedy with abbreviations	Complementary Remedies	Remedy is Followed Well by	Incompatible Remedies	Remedy Antidotes	Remedy is Antidoted by
Ranunculus bulbosus (Ran-b.)		Bry., Ign, K. ca., Nux, Rhs., Sep.	Ac. x. disagrees when given after Rn. b. Rn. b.,	Rs. v. (Rheumatic pains agravates on taking cold).	Anac. Bry., Cam., Clem., Ctn., Pul., Rhs.

Principal Remedy with abbreviations	Complementary Remedies	Remedy is Followed Well by	Incompatible Remedies	Remedy Antidotes	Remedy is Antidoted by
			disagrees when followed by Ac. x., Alcohol, Nt. s. d., Stp., Sul., Vinegar, Wine.		
Raphanus (Raph.)	—	—	—	—	Copious draughts of cold water. (Milk and water. aggravate the pains in abdomen).
Ratanhia (Rat.)	—	—	—	Paeo.	—
Rheum (Rheum)	After Mag. c. when milk disagrees and child has sour odour.	Bel., Pul., Rhs., Sul.		Cth., Mag. c. ("Rhe. may be given after abuse of Magnesia, with or without hubbub of stool are Phel.	Cam., Cham., Col., Merc., Nux, Pul.

Principal Remedy with abbreviations	Complementary Remedies	Remedy is Followed Well by	Incompatible Remedies	Remedy Antidotes	Remedy is Antidoted by
Rhus radicans (Rhus-r.) Rhus toxicodindron (Rhus-t.)	Bry., Calc.	Arn., Ars., Bel., Bry., Cac., Calc., Ca. p., Cham., Con., Drs., Gph., Hyo, Lach., Merc., Mu. x., Nux, Pho., Pul., Sep., Sul.	Aps. Before or after, esp. in skin affections.	Aga., Ail., An. oc., Ant. t. Athra., (Ars.), Bry., Cai., Chi., Cis., Dph., Jg. r., Mir. (effects of No III.), Pip. m. (partially), Pop. c., Rn. b., Rho., Sap., Sep., Sin. n, Sul., Vi. t.	Ana. (if there are gastric symptoms or symptoms going from r. to l.), Am. c., Bel., Bry., Cam, Clem., Cof., Ctn., Cup. (poisoning), Gph., Gnd., Gui. (poisoning) K. sc., Lach., Leb. (Teste), Merc., Plnt., Rn. b., Sang., Sep., Sul, Vbn.
Rhus venenata (Rhus-v.)	Rhs.	—	—	—	Bry., Clem. (itching on hands and genitals, anus, lips, mouth and nose) Nt. x. (sprained pain in right hip). Pho., Ranun. (rheumatic pains aggravates on taking cold). Blue clay

Principal Remedy with abbreviations	Complementary Remedies	Remedy is Followed Well by	Incompatible Remedies	Remedy Antidotes	Remedy is Antidoted by
					applied externally ameliorates itching and burning entirely (Hering). Coffee had no effect on the symptoms.
Ricinus-communis (Ricin-com.)	—	—	—	—	—
Robina (Roba.)	—	—	—	—	—
Ruta (Ruta)	Ca. p. in joint affections.	Calc., Caus., Lyc., Ph. x., Pul., Sep., Sul., Su., x.,		Merc.	Cam.
Sabadilla (Sabab.)	Sep.	Ars., Bel., Merc., Nux, Pul.		Bel. (salivation).	Cam., Con., Pul.
Note :—Children ; old people, light hair. Muscles lax.					
Sabal serrulata (Sabal.)	—	—	—	—	Sil. (Sbl. grows on the sandy shore).

Principal Remedy with abbreviations	Complementary Remedies	Remedy is Followed Well by	Incompatible Remedies	Remedy Antidotes	Remedy is Antidoted by
					Pul. (delayed menses, Pul. also grows on sandy soils).
Sabina (Sabin.)	Thu.	Ars., Bel., Pul., Rhs., Spo., Sul.	—	—	Cam., Pul.

Note :—Chronic ailments of women ; arthritic pains, tendency to miscarriage.

Principal Remedy with abbreviations	Complementary Remedies	Remedy is Followed Well by	Incompatible Remedies	Remedy Antidotes	Remedy is Antidoted by
Saccharum lactis (Sacchar-lac.)	—	—	—	—	—
Sacharum off. (Sachar-of.)	—	—	—	—	Ac. x.
Salicylicum acidum (Salc-ac.)	—	—	—	—	—
Sambucus nigra (Samb)		Ars., Bel., Con.,		Ars. (ameliorates ailments:	Ars., Cam.

Principal Remedy with abbreviations	Complementary Remedies	Remedy is Followed Well by	Incompatible Remedies	Remedy Antidotes	Remedy is Antidoted by
		Nux, Pho., Rhs, Sep.		from abuse of Ars).	

Note :—People formerly fat and robust become emaciated. After violent emotions, grief, anxiety or excess in sexual indulgence.

Principal Remedy with abbreviations	Complementary Remedies	Remedy is Followed Well by	Incompatible Remedies	Remedy Antidotes	Remedy is Antidoted by
Sanguinaria (Sang.)	—	—	—	Bap., Iof. (skin), Opium, Rhs.	—
Sanicula (Sanic.)					
Santonimum (Sant.)	—	—	—	—	—
Sarracenia (Sarr.)	—	—	—	Var.	Pod.
Sarsaparilla (Sars.)	Cep., Merc., Sep.	Bel., Cep., Hep., Merc., Pho., Rhs., Sep., Sul.	Ac., x., (it disagrees when given after Sars.)	Merc., Opi.	Bel., Merc., Sep.

Note :—Vinegar appears at first to increase the effects of Sars.

Principal Remedy with abbreviations	Complementary Remedies	Remedy is Followed Well by	Incompatible Remedies	Remedy Antidotes	Remedy is Antidoted by
Scilla maritima (Scil.)	—	Ars., Ign., Nux, Rhs. Sil.	All., Cep.	—	Cam.
Scrophularia (Scrophul.)	—	Dig. (in enlarged glands—R.T.C.).	—	—	Bry, (chest Symptoms).
Scutellaria (Scut.)	—	—	—	—	—
Secale cornutum (Sec.)	—	—	Aco., Ars. Bel., Chi., Merc., Pul.	—	Cam., Opi.

Note :—Similar to Ars. but heat and cold not oppositely. Irritable plethoric subjects, women of very lax muscular fibre; feeble, cachetic, thin, scrawny. Old decrepit persons. Nervous temperament.

Principal Remedy with abbreviations	Complementary Remedies	Remedy is Followed Well by	Incompatible Remedies	Remedy Antidotes	Remedy is Antidoted by
Selenium (Sel.)	—	Calc., Merc., Nux, Sep.	Chi., Wine.	—	Ign., (Mu. x. in a case of mine—J.H.C.) Pul.
Senega (Seneg.)	—	Calc , Lyc., Pho., Sul.	—	Bry., Buf.	Arn., Bel., Bry., Cam.

Principal Remedy with abbreviations	Complementary Remedies	Remedy is Followed Well by	Incompatible Remedies	Remedy Antidotes	Remedy is Antidoted by
Senna (Senn)				Stm. (cerebral symptoms)	
Sepia (Sep.)	Na. c., Na. m. (the cuttlefish is a *salt water* animal), and other *Natrum* salts, Nux, Sbd., Sul.	Bel., Calc., Cb. v., Con., Eub., Gph., Lyc., Nt. x., Nux, Pho., Pul., Rhs., Sars , Sil., Sul.	Bry., Lach. (but in one case is which *Lach*. in very high potency had caused intensely distressing rectal tenesmus with alternate inversion of the anus, *Sep*., high proved to be the antidote).	Ac. x. (gastric pulmonary and febrile symptoms). At. t., Calc., Chi., Cis., Cit., Dph., Lach., (sometimes), Merc., Mr. c. (dynamic), Na. m., Na. p. (esp. eruption and swelling about joints). Nt. s. d., Sil., Tab. (sometimes).	Vegetable acids, Aco., Ant. c. Ant. t., smelling Nt. s. d., Rhs., Sul.

Note : Especially suited to persons with dark hair for women and particular's during pregnancy in child-bed and while nursing.

Principal Remedy with abbreviations	Complementary Remedies	Remedy is Followed Well by	Incompatible Remedies	Remedy Antidotes	Remedy is Antidoted by
Silica or silicea (Sil.)	Fl. x., Pul. (Sil. is the "chronic" of Pul.), Snc., Thu.	Ars., Asa., Bel., Calc., Clem., Fl. x., Gph., Hep., Lach., Lyc., Nux, Pho., Pul., Rhs., Sep. (If improvement ceases under Sil., a dose or two of Sul. will set up reaction and Sil. will then complete the cure.)	Merc.	Artha., Dph, Hep.., Mr. c., Osm. (swollen gums), Sbl., Sul., Vac.	Cam., Fl. x.,

Note : Specially suitable for children with large heads, open sutures ; much sweat about the head ; large abdomen. Weak persons, imperfectly nourished from imperfect assimilation stonecutters : chest affections and total loss of strength.

Principal Remedy with abbreviations	Complementary Remedies	Remedy is Followed Well by	Incompatible Remedies	Remedy Antidotes	Remedy is Antidoted by
Silica maritima (Sil-m.)	—	—	—	—	—
Spigelia (Spig.)		Aco., Arn., Ars., Bel., Calc., Cimic., Dig., Iris, K. ca., Nux, Pul., Rhs., Sep., Sul., Zin.		Aur., Clch. (heart). Merc., Tab. (sometimes.)	Aur. (restlessness in limbs) ; Cam., Coc. i., Pul.
Spirit glandium quercus (S-quercus.)	—	—	—	—	

Note : Chronic spleen affections ; spleen dropsy, takes away craving for alcoholics. Dropsy & liver affections ; useful in gout, old malarial cases with flatulence.

Principal Remedy with abbreviations	Complementary Remedies	Remedy is Followed Well by	Incompatible Remedies	Remedy Antidotes	Remedy is Antidoted by
Spongia tost (Spong.)	—	Bro., Bry., Cb. v., Com., Hep., K. br., Nux, Pho., Pul.		Iod., Osm. (pain in larynx.)	Aco., Cam.

Principal Remedy with abbreviations	Complementary Remedies	Remedy is Followed Well by	Incompatible Remedies	Remedy Antidotes	Remedy is Antidoted by
Squill *see* Scilla-mar (Squil.)	—	—	—	—	—
Stannum-metallicum (Stann-met.)	Pul.	Bac., Calc., Hfb., Nux, Pho., Pul., Rhs., Sel., Sul.	—	—	Pul.
Stannum iod. (Stann.)	—	—	—	—	—
Staphisagria (Staphy.)	Caus., Col.	Calc., Caus., Col., Ign., Lyc., Nux, Pul., Rhs., Sul.,	Rn. b., before and after	Amb., Coc. i., Col., Merc., Ph. x., Tax. sometimes), Thu., Trb. (toothache), Ver. (most cases—Teste)	Cam.
Sticta pulmonaria (Stic-pul.)	—	—	—	—	
Streptoccin (Streptoccin)	—	—	—	—	—
Note : Anti-febrile action, septic symptoms in infectious diseases. Rapid in its action, specially in its effect on temperature.					
Stramonium (Stram.)		Aco., Bel, Bry. Cub., Hyo., Nux.	Cof.	Dor., Hyo., Merc., Nux. Pb.	Lemon-juice, Senn for cerebral symp-

Principal Remedy with abbreviations	Complementary Remedies	Remedy is Followed Well by	Incompatible Remedies	Remedy Antidotes	Remedy is Antidoted by
					toms, Tobacco injections, Bel , Cam. (particularly—Teste) Nux, Opi, Pul., Cam.
Strontium carb. (Stront-c.)	---	Bel., Caus., K. ca., Pul., Rhs., Sep., Sul.	---	—	
Strophantus (Stroph.)	—	—	— —	—	—
Strychninum (Stry.)	—	—	—	Bz.n., large doses ef Can. s., Gel., (poisoning-Jephson).	Aco., Cam., Chlf., and Tobacco have been advised. Aml. (convulsions), Ars. Black draught (Senna and Epsom Salts) relieved the constipation better than any other aperient Cof. (poisoning), Hyo , (drowsiness respiratory affection), See also

Principal Remedy with abbreviations	Complementary Remedies	Remedy is Followed Well by	Incompatible Remedies	Remedy Antidotes	Remedy is Antidoted by
					under Nux, Opi (large doses), Pas., (suggested by Hale). Osterwald found inhalation of Oxygen an effective antidote in, animals. Ve. v., Sul. 30 in globules dry on the tongue brought about a rapid and almost complete relief of all the rectal symptoms of Robinson's male prover.
Sulphur (Sulf. or Sulph.)	Aco., Nux, Pul. (Sul. is the "chronic" of these three. If a patient is sleepless.	Aco., Alm., Ars., Bel., Bry., Calc., Cb. v., Drs., Eub., Gph., Gui., Merc., Nt. x., Nux,	Sulphur springs are incompatible with Au. m. Hahnemann said Sul. should not	Aco., Aln., Alo., Calc., Chi., Cub., Cof., Con., Cop., Guac. (sometimes) Hdr. (Sometimes), Iod., Ln. c. (headache), Merc., Nt.	Aco., Cam., Cham., Chi., Merc., Pul., Rhs., Sep., Sil., Thu.

Principal Remedy with abbreviations	Complementary Remedies	Remedy is Followed Well by	Incompatible Remedies	Remedy Antidotes	Remedy is Antidoted by
	Sul. may be given at night ; If the patient sleeps well it is best given in the morning, as it may disturb sleep if given at night ; Nux may be given at night and Sul. in the morning when their complementary action is desired). Alo. (Sul.	Pho., Pul., Sars., Sep.	be given after Calc.	x. Oln. (chronic effect), Opi. (marasmus), Phyt. (eyes), Pul. Rhs., Sep., Sul. 30 in globules dry on the tongue brought about a rapid and almost complete relief of all the rectal symptoms of Robinson's male prover of Sty., Thu., Vac., ailments from abuse of metal generally.	

Principal Remedy with abbreviations	Complementary Remedies	Remedy is Followed Well by	Incompatible Remedies	Remedy Antidotes	Remedy is Antidoted by
	is generally the remedy when Alo. has been abused as a purgative). Sul. follows and complements Ant. t. and Ipc. in lung affections, specially left, and at electasis. Ars., Bad., Pso. complements Sul., Pso. loves heat, Sul. hates it. Sul.				

Principal Remedy with abbreviations	Complementary Remedies	Remedy is Followed Well by	Incompatible Rémedies	Remedy Antidotes	Remedy is Antidoted by
	complements Rhs. in paralysis. An interpolated dose of Sul. helps Sil.				

Note :—Sulf. is specially suited for lean stoop should derid persons. If frequently serves to rouse the reactive power of the system, when carefully selected remedies have fails to produce a favourable effect specially in acute cases.

Principal Remedy with abbreviations	Complementary Remedies	Remedy is Followed Well by	Incompatible Rémedies	Remedy Antidotes	Remedy is Antidoted by
Sulphur iodatum (Sul-i.)					
Sulphuricum acidum (Sul-ac.)	Pul.	Arn., Calc., Con., Lyc., Plat., Sep., Sul.		Cap., Lead poisoning. "Sulphuric acid, diluted, taken as a lemonade. one of the best	Ipc., Pul.

Principal Remedy with abbreviations	Complementary Remedies	Remedy is Followed Well by	Incompatible Remedies	Remedy Antidotes	Remedy is Antidoted by
				tidotes to the chronic effects of lead."	
Note :—Frequently indicated for old people, particularly women. Light-haired people. Flushes of heat In elimacteric years.					
Sumbul (Sumb.)	—	—	—	—	—
Symphoricapus rac. (Sympe-r.)	—	—	—	—	—
Symphytum (Symph.)	—	—	—	Cantharis (Green's *Herbat*).	—
Syphilinum (Syph.)	—	—	—	—	—
Syzygium-Jambolanum (Syz.)	—	—	—	—	—
Tabacum (Tab.)	—	**Cb.** v. Hfb.	Ign.	Ac. x., Ars., Cic., Cof., Ipc., Naj. (potencies), Sko., Stm.	Ac. x., Ars. (effects of chewing tobacco), Cam., Clem. (toothache),

Principal Remedy with abbreviations	Complementary Remedies	Remedy is Followed Well by	Incompatible Remedies	Remedy Antidotes	Remedy is Antidoted by
					Cof, Gel. (occipital headache and (vertigo) ; Ign., Ipc., (primary effects : vomiting), Klm, Lyc. (impotence), Nux (bad taste in mouth in morning amblyopia), Pho. (palpitation, tobacco heart, amblyopia, sexual weakness). Plnt. has sometimes caused aversion to tobacco. Pul. (hiccough), Sep. (neuralgia in face and dyspepsia, chronic nervousness), Sour Apples, Spi. (heat affections). Tab. 200, or 1,000 for the craving when

Principal Remedy with abbreviations	Complementary Remedies	Remedy is Followed Well by	Incompatible Remedies	Remedy Antidotes	Remedy is Antidoted by
					discontinuing its use, Ver., Vinegar, Wine (spasms), cold sweat from excessive smoking).
Tannic acid (Tan-ac.)	—	—	—	—	—

Note :—Nasal haemorrhage; elongated uvula; gargle; constipation. Corrects fetor of perspiration. Haematuria; obstinate constipation.

Principal Remedy with abbreviations	Complementary Remedies	Remedy is Followed Well by	Incompatible Remedies	Remedy Antidotes	Remedy is Antidoted by
Tarentula-hispania. (Tarent-h.)	—	—	—	Lach. (Hering).	*Partial antidotes* : Bov., Cb. v., Chel., Cup., Gel., Mg., c., Mos., Pul.
Tarentula cub. (Tarent-c.)	—	—	—	—	
Tartaricum acid (Tart-ac.)	—	—	—	—	—
Tellurium Tell.)	—	—	—	—	Nux (epigastric oppression).

Principal Remedy with abbreviations	Complementary Remedies	Remedy is Followed Well by	Incompatible Remedies	Remedy Antidotes	Remedy is Antidoted by
Tela-aranearum (Tela-aran.)	—	—	—	—	—
Note :—Cardiac sleeplessness, excitment and nervous agitation in febrile states; dry asthma, harrassing cough; obstinate intermittents.					
Terebinthina (Ter.)	—	Mr. c.	—	Merc., Pho.	Pho.
Teucrium marum (Teacr.)	—	—	—	—	Cam.
Theridion (Ther.)	—	—	—	—	Aco, (sensitiveness to noises), Mos. (nausea), Gph. (more chronic effects).
Thlaspi bursa paslori (Thlasp-b-p.)	—	—	—	—	—
Thuja (Thuj.)	Ars., Med., Na. s. in sycosis, Sbi., Sil.	Merc., Sul. (these follow best—H.N.G.); also Asa., Calc., Ign., K. ca., Lyc., Pul.,		Cop. (offensive breath and diarrhoea after eating onions). Iod., Merc, Nux, Sul., Tea., Vac., Var. (Ailments from ab-	Cam. Cham. (nightly toothache), Coc. i. (fever); Teste found Clch. the best antidote in his experience;

Principal Remedy with abbreviations	Complementary Remedies	Remedy is Followed Well by	Incompatible Remedies	Remedy Antidotes	Remedy is Antidoted by
		Sbi., Sil., Sul., Vace.		use of metals generally.)	Merc., Nux (sometimes), Pul., Stp., Sul.
Thyroidinum (Thyr.)	—	—	—	—	Ars.
Tongo (Tongo.)	—	—	—	—	Vinegar.
Trifolium repens (Trif-r.)					
Trillium-cernum (Tril-c.)	Ca. p. (menstrual and haemorrhagic affections).	—	—	—	—

Note :—Eye Symptoms-everything looks bluish; haemorrhages; menorrhagia; epistaxis; haematuria; haematosis; bleeding piles.

Principal Remedy with abbreviations	Complementary Remedies	Remedy is Followed Well by	Incompatible Remedies	Remedy Antidotes	Remedy is Antidoted by
Trimethylaminum (Trimethyl.)	—	—	—	—	—
Triticum repens (Tritic.)	—	—	—	—	—
Tuberculinum (Tuber.)	—	—	—	—	—

Principal Remedy with abbreviations	Complementary Remedies	Remedy is Followed Well by	Incompatible Remedies	Remedy Antidotes	Remedy is Antidoted by
Turnera aph. or Damiana (Tur. or Damiana)	—	—	—	—	
Tussilago petasites (Tus-p.)	—	—	—	—	—
Uranium nitricum (Uran-n.)					
Urea (Urea)	—	—	—	—	—
Urtica urens (Urt-u.)				Apis (bee-stings.)	Dock leaves (Rumux obtus.) rubbed on the stung part lessen the pain; also nettle's own juice, and the juice from the common snail.
Ustilago maydis (Ust.)	—	—	—	—	
Uva-ursi (Uva.)	—	—.	—	—	

Principal Remedy with abbreviations	Complementary Remedies	Remedy is Followed Well by	Incompatible Remedies	Remedy Antidotes	Remedy is Antidoted by
Vaccininum (Vac.)	—	—	—	Var.	Aps., Ant, t. Mld., Sil., Thu.
Valeriana (Valer.)	—	Pho., Pul.	—	Asa., Merc., Nx. m. abuse of Chamomile tea.	Bel., Cam., Cin., Cof., Merc., Pul.
Vanadium (Vanad.)	Bis.	—	—	—	—
Variolinum (Variol.)	—	—	—	—	Ant. t. Mld., Src., Thu., Vac.
Veratrum album (Verat.)	Arn.	Aco., Arn. Ars., Bel., Cb. v., Cham., Chi., Cup., Drs., Ipc.. Pul., Rhs., Sep., Sul.		Ars., Cai., Cep. (colic with despondency), Chi., Cup. (colic), Hdm. (some of its effects), Hy. ac., Opi., Tab., Vb. o. (diarrhoea).	Aco. (anxious, distracted state with coldness of body, or burning in brain Hahn.), Ars., Cam. (pressive pain in head with coldness of body and unconsciousness after-Hahn.)- Chi. (other chro-

Principal Remedy with abbreviations	Complementary Remedies	Remedy is Followed Well by	Incompatible Remedies	Remedy Antidotes	Remedy is Antidoted by
					nic affections from abuse of Ver.—*e.g.* daily forenoon fever—Hahn.) Cof., Stp. (most cases—Teste). Poisonous doses : Strong Coffee.
Note : Lean, choleric or melancholic persons, anaemia, children.					
Veratrum viride (Verat-v.)		—	—	Sty.	Hot Coffee.
Verbascum (Verb.)		Bel., Chi., Lyc., Pul., Rhs., Sep., Stm.	—	—	Cam.
Vesicaria (Vesic.)	—	—	—	—	—
Veronica officinalis (Veronica-off.)		—	—	—	—
Viburnum opulus (Vib-o.)			—	—	Aco. (epididymitis). Ver. (diarrhoea).

Principal Remedy with abbreviations	Complementary Remedies	Remedy is Followed Well by	Incompatible Remedies	Remedy Antidotes	Remedy is Antidoted by
Vinca minor (Vinc-m.)	—	—		—	—
Viola odorata (Viol-o.)	—	Bel., Cin., Crl., Nux., Pul.	—	Used externally, stings and snake-bites.	Cam.
Viscum album (Vis.)	—	—	—	—	Cam., Chi.
Wiesbaden (Wiesbaden)	—	—	—	—	—
Xanthoxylum (Xan.)	—	—	—	—	—
X-Ray (x-ray.)	—	—	—	—	—

Note :—Vial Containing alcohol exposed to x-ray. Anaemia Sexual glands are particularly, affected. Sterility. Brings to the surface suppressed symptoms, specially sycotic and those due to mixed infection.

Principal Remedy with abbreviations	Complementary Remedies	Remedy is Followed Well by	Incompatible Remedies	Remedy Antidotes	Remedy is Antidoted by
Yohimbinum (Yoh.)	—			—	—

Principal Remedy with abbreviations	Complementary Remedies	Remedy is Followed Well by	Incompatible Remedies	Remedy Antidotes	Remedy is Antidoted by
Zincum metallicum (Zinc-m.)	Ca. p. in hydrocephalus.	Hep., Ign., Pul., Sep., Sul. (best-H.N.G.).	Cham., Nux, Wine.	Ba. c.	Cam., Hep., Ign. (Lobel.—Teste).
Zincum sulphuricum (Zinc-s.).	—	—	—	—	—

—:o:—

Appendix II

CONSTITUTIONAL REMEDIES

In medicine, constitution means the total individuality of the persons, including his inherited qualities and the cumulative effects of his reactions to all the environmental factors which influenced his physical and emotional development.

The following are the names of a few constitutional remedies. The list is only illustrative and not exhaustive. The Prescriber will study others from any reliable Materia Medica.

A. Acetic acid ; Aconite ; Agaricus ; Agnus castus ; Ammonia carb ; Arsenic ; Aurum met ; Arnica.

B. Bacillinum ; Baryta carb ; Belladonna.

C. Calcarea carb ; Camphor ; Cannabis sativa ; Capsicum ; Carbo veg ; Causticum ; Cinnabaris ; China.

H. Hyoscyamus.

I. Ignatia.

K. Kali carb ; Kreosotum.

L. Lycopodium.

M. Medorrhinum.

N. Nitric acid ; Nux vomica.

P Phosphorus ; Phosphoric acid ; Platinum ; Psorinum ; Pulsatilla.

S Secale cor ; Sepia ; Senega ; Silicea ; Stramonium ; Sulphur ; Syphilinum.

T. Tuberculinum ; Thuja.

V. Veratrum Alb.

Z. Zincum.

Appendix III

DR. GIBSON'S HOT AND COLD REMEDIES

Remedies predominantly aggravated by cold :—

A. **Abrot**., Acet-ac., Agar., Agn., Alumen, Alum., Al-ph., Alum-sil., Am-c., Apoc., Ars., Ars-s-fl., Asar., Aur., Aur-ars., Aur-sulp.,

B. Bad., **Bar-c**., Bar-m., Benz-ac., Bor-ax., Brom.

C. **Cadm**., Calc-ars., Calc-c., Calc-fl., Calc-ph., Calc-sil., Camph., Canth., **Caps**. Carb-an., Carb-veg., Carbn-s., Card-m., Cauloph., **Caust**., Cham., Chel., **China**., Chin-a., Cimic., Cistus., Cocc., Coff., Colch., Con., Cyl.

D. **Dulc**.

E. Euphras.

F. **Ferr**., Ferr-ars., Form.

G. **Graph**., Gauc.

H. Hell., Helon., Hep., Hyos., Hyper.

I. Ign.

K. Kali-ars., Kali-bich., **Kali-carb**., Kali-Chlor., Kali-phos., Kali-sil., Kalm., Kreos.

L. Lac-defl.

M. **Magn-carb**., Mag-Phos., Mang., Mosch., Mur-ac.

N. Natr-ars., Natr-carb., Nitric-ac., Nux-m., Nux-vom.

O. Oxal-ac.

P. Petrol., Phos., Phos-ac., Plb., Pod., Psor., **Pyrogen**.

R. **Ran-B**., Rheum., Rhodo., **Rhus**., **Rumex**., **Ruta**.

S. Sabad., Sars., Sepia., **Sil**., **Spig**., Stann., Staph., Stram., Stront., Sul-ac.

T. Therid.

V. Valer., Viol-t.

Z. Zinc.

Remedies predominantly aggravated by heat :

A. Aes-h., Aloe., Ambra., **Apis**., **Arg-nit**.; Asaf., Aur-iod., Aur-m.

B. Bar-iod., Bry.

C. Calad., Calc-iod., Calc-sul., Cocc-cacti, Comoc., Crocus.

D. Dros.

F. Fer-iod., Fluor-ac.

G. Grat.,

H. Ham.

I. Iod.

K. Kali-iod., Kali-sul.

L. Lach., Led., Lit-t., Lyc.

N. Nat-mur., **Nat-s**., Niccol.

O. Op.

P. Picric-ac., **Plat**., Ptelea., **Puls**.

S. **Sabina**., **Secale**., Spong., Sul., Sul-iod.

T. Thuj., Tuberc. (Rabe).

U. Ustil.

V. Vespa, Viburn.

Remedies sensitive to both extreme of temperature :—

Merc., Ip., Nat-carb., Cinnabar.

Ant-cr. aggravated both by heat and cold : aggravated by over-heating and radiated heat though many symptoms ameliorated by heat.

(Merc. in chronic troubles aggravated by cold ; in acute aggravated by heat.)

Appendix IV

BIBLIOGRAPHY

(1) Therapeutic notes given by Dr. B.C. Guha, M.D., L.R.C.P's (Edin.).

(2) Notes in the short form of a Materia Medica on a number of medicines both of ordinary daily use and some rare and peculiar medicines and (b) Notes on Homoeopathic philosophy given by Dr. B.C. Guha, M.D., L.R.C.P's (Edin.).

(3) Lectures on Homoeopathic Materia Medica by W. Boericke, M.D.

(4) Dr. J. T. Kent's Repertory of the Homoeopathic Materia Medica.

(5) Leaders in Homoeopathic Therapeutics by E.B. Nash, M.D.

(6) Practical Homoeopathic Therapeutics by W.A. Dewey, M.D.

(7) Key notes and characteristics with comparisions of some of the leading remedies of the Materia Medica by H. C. Allen, M.D.

(8) The Prescriber—a Dictionary of the New Therapeutics by J.H. Clarke, M.D.

(9) Homoeopathic Domestic Physician by C. Herring, M.D.

(10) An epitome of the Homoeopathic Domestic Medicine by Dr. J. Laurie, M.D.

(11) A Hand-Book of the diseases of Children and their Homoeopathic Treatment by Dr. Charles E. Fisher, M.D.

(12) "Select your Remedy" by Rai Bahadur Bishamber Das.

(13) The Homoeopathic Treatment of the Diseases of females and infants at the breast by Dr. G.H.G. Jahr, translated from the French by Charles J. Hempel, M.D.

(14) Therapeutic hints by Dr. Dhirendra Chandra Das Gupta, M.B., Author of Characteristic Materia Medica.

(15) Guide to Health by Father Muller.

(16) Primers by Novel Puddephatt.

(17) Homoeopathic Guide for family use by Dr. Laurie.

(18) Pocket Manual of Homoeopathic Materia Medica by W. Boericke, M.D.

(19) Balkiston's illustrated pocket Medical Dictionary

(20) A Clinical Repertory to the dictionary of Materia Medica by Clarke.

(21) The Homoeopathic Prescriber by Professor Dr. K.C. Bhanja of Bombay formerly professor of Materia Medica, H.M. College, Calcutta.

(22) Clinical Relationship of Drugs with their Modalities compiled by Dr. B.K. Sarkar, Chairman of the Homoeopathic Pharmacopeia Committee, Government of India.

(23) Homoeopathy cures Asthma By Dr. S. R. Wadia, M.B.B.S M.F. Hom. (London), P. Gr. Hom. (U.S.A), President, Maharashtra Homoeopathic Board, Bombay.

(24) Homoeopathy in skin Diseases by Dr. S.R. Wadia, M.B.B.S., M.F. Hom. (Lon.), P. Gr. Hom. (U.S.A.)

(25) Duration of Action and Antidotes of the Principal Homoeopathic Remedies with their complementary and Inimical Relations by F.H. Lutze, M.D.

(26) Clinical Tips compiled by Dr. V. Sundara Vardhan, Homoeopathic Physician, Madras-1.

(27) Hints from Masters Compiled by Shri· P. Rajgopala Rao., B.A.

(28) Diabetes Mellitus, its diagnosis and treatment by Dr. K.N. Mathur, M.F. (Hom.) London.

(29) Influenzas by Dr. Douglas M. Borland, M. B., Ch., B. Glas, F.F. Hom.

(30) Enlarged tonsils cured by medicines by Dr. J.C. Burnett, M.D.

(31) Domestic Homoeopathic Practice by Pandit Kishanlal Kichlu, B. Sc., L.T. (Retd. U.P.E.S.)

(32) Therapeutic By-ways by Dr. E.P. Anshutz.

(33) Homoeopathic Vyavaharik Chikitsa by Dr. G. N. Chauhan, M.A., S.R. Mahavir Homoeo Clinic, Jaipur.

(34) Haryana Homoeo Journal.

REVIEWS

Dr. Shinghal is among the Grand Old Men of Homoeopathy, he having served and practised this science for over half a century-longer than the existence of many of us on this earth. So one can well imagine what wealth of experience must have gone into the compilation of this handy volume.........

Another big merit of the book is that the entries are arranged alphabetically, with copious cross references, which make for quick consultation. This treatment has enabled the author to explain several medical terms and guiding principles of administration of medicine, dose, potency etc. and in simple, direct language. He has also given wise guidance and warnings where ever called for.

However, what will endeavour the book most to the amateur homoeopath is the fact that it suggests just one or rwo medicines to begin the treatment of a particular disease or its phase. This eliminates the confusing details that most bulky books on therapeutics contain. Dr. Shinghal seems to know the amateur's difficulties too well and has therefore produced their best guide so far.

—**Haryana Homoeo Journal.**

"......Shri J. N. Shinghal, an amateur homoeopath, appears to have published his compilation in 1959, and since then the book with a few additions has managed to run into the third edition, most probably due to the enterprising distribution network of M/s. Harjeet & Co."

".. As the author himself had planned, the book follows the arrangement of Clarke's Prescriber and will be useful to many Indian readers because the author has also incorporated some useful data here and there culted from medical text books, to which the lay practitioners generally do not take recourse to".

"......The clinical relationship of medicines, added as an Appendix is another useful feature of the book"

—The Homoeopathic Sandesh.

"With growing faith in the remedial and curative powers of its fold is now religion. Be it a poor, hurried patient, an amateur practitioner or a trained professional, this system of medicine has held an attraction of its own due in no small measure to its simple, economical therapeutics and this in spite of some spectacular results produced by other ancient and modern systems. It is this fascination that has stimulated Dr. J.N. Shinghal to bring out a gem of an epitome of Homoeopathic medicine. Indeed this revised and enlarged editon, the third one, is a remarkable improvement upon its predecessors with new chapter on use of medicines in surgery and on pet animal diseases. But what really marks it out as a must for all concerned is its rare wealth of information on medicines (disease-wise), tried and proved by Indian and foreign wizards of Homoeopathy. And yet this condensation does not suffer from the lack of traditional method of repertorisation."

—The Hindustan Times

" .....In its new format, Dr. Shinghal's well known work is even more welcome than its first edition which was widely acclaimed when it appeared five years ago. In the cases of reference it stays unbeatable."

"...Unlike most books on therapeutics it is compact and successfully keeps confusion at bay with its scope encompassing human beings as well as animals (especially pets) and chapters on pediatrics as well as on surgery, the book is bound to be a long time favourite of the profession".

—The Homoeo Journal.

—: o :—